CLINICAL MANUAL OF
HEALTH ASSESSMENT

Clinical manual of
Health
assessment

JUNE M. THOMPSON, R.N., M.S.

The Ohio State University School of Nursing, Columbus, Ohio

ARDEN C. BOWERS, R.N., M.S.

The Ohio State University School of Nursing, Columbus, Ohio

Illustrated by
ANN L. SCHRECK

Columbus, Ohio

with 487 illustrations

The C. V. Mosby Company

ST. LOUIS · TORONTO · LONDON   1980

Printed in the United States of America

The C. V. Mosby Company
11830 Westline Industrial Drive, St. Louis, Missouri 63141

Library of Congress Cataloging in Publication Data

Thompson, June M   1946-
    Clinical manual of health assessment.

    Bibliography: p.
    1. Physical diagnosis. 2. Nursing. I. Bowers,
Arden C., joint author. II. Title. [DNLM: 1. Health.
WA900.1 T473c]
RT48.T48   616.07'54   79-28832
ISBN 0-8016-4935-8

TS/VH/VH 9 8 7 6 5 4 3   01/A/048

With love to
Terry, Donald, Bruce,
Spencer, and Martin

Preface

This manual is designed to be used in a clinical or laboratory setting as a procedural guideline for students who are learning health assessment. Each chapter outlines the knowledge necessary to proceed with a given portion of assessment, explicit skills for the student to perform, and expected findings that result from individual assessment efforts. Because of the procedural nature of the content, the knowledge base related to assessment is not offered. The student should refer to the suggested textbooks to prepare for successful use of this manual. Further learning is facilitated if a preceptor or clinical instructor is available as a resource to ensure proper interpretation and application of the written material.

Each chapter includes integrated information concerning the adult, the child, and the elderly client. Clinical and behavioral differences and similarities are presented in separate sections of each chapter for the reader's convenience. Some of the information is repeated in the separate, age-related sections so that the student can extract a specific portion for immediate clinical reference. Although this approach is somewhat redundant, it allows each section to stand alone.

The manual is divided into three major areas: the health data base chapter, fourteen clinical chapters that present specific systems or body regions for study, and the integration chapter, which offers a detailed outline of the entire health assessment process. Each chapter can be used as a single unit of study. The fourteen clinical chapters follow a consistent format, comprising the following thirteen sections:

1. *Cognitive objectives:* an outline of defined learning needs.
2. *Clinical objectives:* an outline of clinical entities that must be assessed.
3. *History in addition to data base:* an in-depth system or a regional history which investigates common problems, complaints, and client risk potential.
4. *Clinical guidelines:* a procedural outline including (a) examiner behaviors and clinical entities to be assessed, (b) expected normal findings, and (c) common deviations from normal findings. Throughout the manual this section is supported with illustrations.
5. *Clinical strategies:* notes and helpful hints for the beginning student regarding examination techniques and client behaviors.
6. *Sample recording:* an example of a written description of normal findings.
7. *History and clinical strategies associated with the pediatric client:* a discussion of approaches to the child and additional history data.
8. *Clinical variations associated with the pediatric client:* a detailed outline of the examination procedure for the child, anticipated normal findings, and commonly identified deviations.
9. *History and clinical strategies associated with the geriatric client:* a discussion of approaches to the older adult and additional history data.
10. *Clinical variations associated with the geriatric client:* a detailed outline of the examination procedure for the older adult, anticipated normal findings, and commonly identified deviations.
11. *Vocabulary:* a list of terms associated with the system or region of study. There is space available for the student to write definitions or interpretations of each term.
12. *Cognitive self-assessment:* a quiz section to demonstrate understanding of the related textbook and manual material and to monitor progress. The answers are provided at the end of the book.
13. *Suggested readings:* because of the procedural nature of this text, additional reading is necessary. The suggested reading list complements the information in each chapter of this manual.

The assessment procedures are elaborate and detailed throughout the manual. The beginning student examiner must be exposed to an inclusive pattern of behavior for collecting subjective and objective data related to a client.

We have found that the clinical guidelines are extremely useful in the laboratory setting. We suggest to our students that they read aloud and discuss procedures while following along with a fellow student. They are asked to describe the procedure, their rationale for their behaviors, and the characteristics of the findings as they progress. They frequently complete a practice session by writing out their actual findings for one another to critique.

We wish to express sincere thanks to the individuals who assisted in the development of these materials and who participated as models for the photographs. We are especially grateful to Joanne Littell, who typed the manuscript, and to Ann Schreck, the photographer and illustrator.

June M. Thompson
Arden C. Bowers

Contents

Introduction, 1

1 Total health data base, 2

2 General and mental status assessment, 31

3 Assessment of the integumentary system, 44

4 Assessment of the head and neck, 67

5 Assessment of the nose, paranasal sinuses, mouth, and oropharynx, 87

6 Assessment of the ears and auditory system, 115

7 Assessment of the eyes and visual system, 134

8 Assessment of the thorax and lungs, 169

9 Assessment of the cardiovascular system, 199

10 Assessment of the breasts, 240

11 Assessment of the gastrointestinal system, the abdomen, and the rectal/anal region, 259

12 Assessment of the male genitourinary system, 294

13 Assessment of the female genitourinary system, 315

14 Assessment of the musculoskeletal system, 346

15 Assessment of the neurological system, 412

16 Physical examination integration format, 460

Answers, 474

CLINICAL MANUAL OF
HEALTH ASSESSMENT

Introduction

Assessment of an individual begins with careful, deliberate, and concrete observations of the whole person. Textbooks traditionally divide the remainder of the examination process into parts composed of body systems or regions. This division is convenient for the learner who functions cognitively and clinically in logically sequenced segments, gradually coordinating the segments to form a total process of assessment.

This manual proceeds in a logical fashion. The whole person is assessed (from a personal viewpoint) through the use of the data base chapter. Simultaneously, the examiner must be aware of the information provided in the chapter on general and mental status assessment. The examiner begins collecting objective data as soon as the client is encountered and throughout the history-taking session. Dress, mannerisms, general body movement and behavior are observed and noted as contributions to the final summary. Thereafter the student can proceed through the remaining clinical chapters, segment by segment, gradually using and synthesizing knowledge until all the parts are fitted together. The final chapter offers a detailed outline for fitting examiner behavior and clinical findings into a coordinated procedure and total summary.

We certainly acknowledge that human beings are more than the sum of their parts. They are dynamic entities interacting with the environment to attain or maintain a state of maximum well-being. As the student begins to pool information about a person, the development of a problem list, a client profile, and a risk profile should take place. The therapeutic application of the information in that final summary requires further professional knowledge beyond the scope and intent of this book. Recognizing client strengths, setting priorities with the client for seeking solutions to problems, and taking into account all the environmental variables that alter the client's state of well-being involve additional professional preparation.

This manual is designed to provide the student with an orderly, thorough method of collecting and categorizing accurate and well-defined data in preparation for subsequent professional care.

CHAPTER 1

Total health data base

Cognitive objectives

At the end of this unit the learner will demonstrate knowledge of the effective techniques and components of the health history by the ability to do the following:

1. Define the terms in the vocabulary section.
2. Discuss the rationale and options for examiner behaviors when gathering and analyzing health data for
   a. the well adult
   b. the well child
   c. the well elderly adult
   d. the ill (or symptomatic) client
3. Define the ten components of the adult data base.
4. List the sections and provide at least one example of relevant information gathered in each section of the social history.
5. List and define the eleven components of the analysis of a symptom.
6. Recognize the characteristics of the pediatric data base that are collected in addition to or as substitution for the adult data base.
7. Recognize the characteristics of the geriatric data base that are collected in addition to or as substitution for the adult data base.

Clinical objectives

At the end of this unit the learner will be able to do the following:

1. Demonstrate the application of effective nurse behaviors for establishing a nurse/client relationship during the data base collection session.
2. Conduct a systematic and accurate assessment of an individual's health status (adult, pediatric, geriatric) using a predesignated format.
3. Organize health assessment data to establish a preliminary problem list that accurately reflects the client's priorities, concerns, and physiological state.

4. Systematically record a full data base and subsequent problem list using a predesignated format.
5. Create a client profile that summarizes the lifestyle and the client's assessment of the ability to provide self-care.

Data base overview

The purpose of this chapter is to provide complete information about the subjective data that may be collected about the client. The reader might initially view this as overwhelming and repetitive in places; however, the subjective data available about overall health are vast and in many areas do overlap. The examiner must initially be exposed to this total information and then learn to use the data as a reference to individualize the information collected from each client. Not every client will need to be asked every question.

The examiner's goal is to develop a holistic subjective data profile about the client's health. This is an intellectual process and will depend on (1) the examiner's knowledge base, (2) the questions the examiner chooses to ask, (3) the method by which questions are asked, (4) the examiner's ability to interpret the responses, (5) the examiner's ability to synthesize and assign priority to all data collected, and (6) the philosophy and policies of the health agency (a full data base must be valued, read, and used).

The following format provides a method for collecting data about the client's physiological, psychological, and sociocultural health. It also includes questions about the client's past health and the health of the family. When integrated, the information becomes the client's *health data base*. The practitioner must analyze and organize the data base to formulate the following:

1. A subjective data problem list (including physiological symptoms and psychological, social, or environmental factors that concern the client and/or the examiner). This will later be com-

bined with the physical assessment problem list to develop a total problem list in the final write-up.

2. A risk profile (risk factors related to certain body systems are listed in subsequent chapters).
3. A client profile (a summary, from the *client's* viewpoint, of his life-style and ability to cope with self-care).

These data will serve as a constant resource for comparison as the client changes and provides new information in future assessments.

The collection of the data base may occur during one or more contact periods. The examiner must initially assess the reason for the client's visits and the severity of the concern. The examiner may decide to use an abbreviated history form during the client's initial visit (symptom analysis is discussed under *clinical strategies*) and to reschedule another appointment period to collect the total data base. Each client cared for deserves to have a total data base collected at some early point during his association with the agency or clinic. Each year following that time the data base must be updated.

Following is an outline of the components included in the total health data base:

Data base outline

1. Biographical data
2. Reason for visit
3. Present health status
4. Current health statistics
   a. Immunizations
   b. Allergies
   c. Last examinations
5. Past health status
   a. Childhood illnesses
   b. Serious or chronic illnesses
   c. Serious accidents or injuries
   d. Hospitalizations, operations
   e. Emotional health
   f. Obstetrical health
6. Family history
7. Review of physiological systems/regions
   a. General
   b. Nutritional
   c. Integumentary
   d. Head
   e. Eyes
   f. Ears
   g. Nose, nasopharynx, and paranasal sinuses
   h. Mouth and throat
   i. Neck
   j. Breast
   k. Cardiovascular
   l. Respiratory
   m. Hematolymphatic
   n. Gastrointestinal
   o. Urinary
   p. Genital
   q. Musculoskeletal
   r. Central nervous system
   s. Endocrine
   t. Allergic and immunological
8. Psychological history
   a. General status
   b. Interpersonal relationships
   c. Activities of daily living
   d. General coping skills
   e. Occupations
   f. Stressors/changes
   g. Stressors/coping skills
   h. Response to illness
   i. Psychiatric counseling history
   j. Anxiety
   k. Depression
   l. Personality changes
   m. Medications or specific techniques for stress
   n. Habits
   o. Financial status
9. Health maintenance efforts
   a. General statement
   b. Exercise
   c. Dietary regulations
   d. Mental health
   e. Cultural or religious practices
   f. Frequency of physical, dental, and vision health assessment
10. Environmental health
    a. General assessment
    b. Employment
    c. Home
    d. Neighborhood
    e. Community

Expanded data base outline
BIOGRAPHICAL DATA

1. Name
2. Age
3. Race
4. Culture
5. Address
6. Marital status
7. Children and family in home
8. Occupation
9. Means of transportation to health care facility, if pertinent
10. Description of home; size and type of community

REASON FOR VISIT

One statement that describes the reason for the client's visit, or the chief complaint. State in the client's own words.

PRESENT HEALTH STATUS

1. General health status of the client in the past 1 year, 5 years, now
2. Summary of client's current major health concerns
3. If illness is present, include (symptom analysis) history (pp. 10 and 11)
   a. When was client last well
   b. Date of problem onset
   c. Character of complaint
   d. Nature of problem onset
   e. Course of problem
   f. Client's hunch of precipitating factors
   g. Location of problem
   h. Relation to other body symptoms, body positions, and activity
   i. Patterns of problem
   j. Efforts of client to treat
   k. Coping ability
4. Current medications
   a. Type (prescription, over-the-counter drugs, vitamins, etc.)
   b. Prescribed by whom
   c. Amount per day
   d. Problems

CURRENT HEALTH STATISTICS

1. Immunization status (note dates or year of last immunization)
   a. Tetanus, diphtheria
   b. Mumps
   c. Rubella
   d. Polio
   e. Tuberculosis tine test
   f. Influenza
2. Allergies (describe agent and reactions)
   a. Drugs
   b. Foods
   c. Contact substances
   d. Environmental factors
3. Last examinations (note physician/clinic, findings, advice, and/or instructions)
   a. Physical
   b. Dental
   c. Vision
   d. Hearing
   e. ECG
   f. Chest radiograph
   g. Pap smear (females)

PAST HEALTH STATUS

Although each of the following is asked separately, the examiner must summarize and record the data *chronologically*.

1. Childhood illnesses: rubeola, rubella, mumps, pertussis, scarlet fever, chickenpox, strep throat
2. Serious or chronic illnesses: scarlet fever, diabetes, kidney problems, hypertension, sickle cell anemia, seizure disorders, blood infections
3. Serious accidents or injuries: head injuries, fractures, burns, other trauma
4. Hospitalizations: elaborate, reason for, location, primary care providers, duration
5. Operations: what, where, when, why, by whom
6. Emotional health: past problems, help sought, support persons
7. Obstetrical history
   a. Complete pregnancies: number, pregnancy course, postpartum course, and condition, weight, and sex of each child
   b. Incomplete pregnancies: duration, termination, circumstances (including abortions and stillbirths)
   c. Summary of complications

FAMILY HISTORY

Family members include the client's blood relatives, spouse, and children. Specifically the interviewer should inquire about the client's maternal and paternal grandparents, parents, aunts, uncles, spouse, and children, as well as about the general health, stress factors, and illnesses of other family members. Questions should include a survey of the following:

Cancer	Retardation
Diabetes	Alcoholism
Heart disease	Endocrine diseases
Hypertension	Sickle cell anemia
Epilepsy (or seizure disorder)	Kidney disease
Emotional stresses	Unusual limitations
Mental illness	Other chronic problems

The most concise method to record these data is by a family tree. Fig. 1-1 is an example.

REVIEW OF PHYSIOLOGICAL SYSTEMS

The purpose of this component of the data base is to collect information about the body regions or systems and their function.

1. General—reflect from client's previous description of current health status.
   a. Fatigue patterns
   b. Exercise and exercise tolerance
   c. Weakness episodes
   d. Fever, sweats
   e. Frequent colds, infections, or illnesses

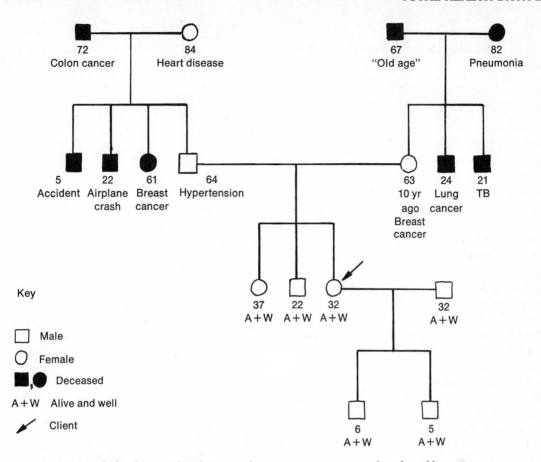

Fig. 1-1. Sample family tree (identifying grandparents, parents, aunts and uncles, siblings, spouse, and children).

f. Ability to carry out activities of daily living
2. Nutritional
   a. Client's average, maximum, and minimum weights during past month, 1 year, 5 years
   b. History of weight gains or losses (time element; specific efforts to change weight)
   c. Twenty-four–hour diet recall (helpful to mail client chart to fill in prior to visit) (Fig. 1-2)
   d. Current appetite
   e. Who buys, prepares food?
   f. Who does client normally eat with?
   g. Is client able to afford preferred food?
   h. Does client wear dentures? Is chewing a problem?
   i. Client's self evaluation of nutritional status
3. Integumentary
   a. Skin
      (1) Skin disease or skin problems or lesions (wounds, sores, ulcers)
      (2) Skin growths, tumors, masses
      (3) Excessive dryness, sweating, odors
      (4) Pigmentation changes or discolorations
      (5) Pruritus (itching)
      (6) Texture changes
      (7) Temperature changes
   b. Hair
      (1) Changes in amount, texture, character
      (2) Alopecia (loss of hair)
      (3) Use of dyes
   c. Nails
      (1) Changes in appearance, texture
4. Head
   a. Headache (characteristics, including frequency, type, location, duration, care for)
   b. Past significant trauma
   c. Dizziness
   d. Syncope
5. Eyes
   a. Discharge (characteristics)
   b. History of infections, frequency, treatment
   c. Pruritus (itching)
   d. Lacrimation, excessive tearing
   e. Pain in eyeball
   f. Spots (floaters)
   g. Swelling around eyes
   h. Cataracts, glaucoma

	Food eaten	Amount	Calories
Breakfast			
Lunch			
Dinner			
Snacks			
Total			

Fig. 1-2. Twenty-four–hour diet record.

    i. Unusual sensations or twitching
    j. Vision changes (generalized or vision field)
    k. Use of corrective or prosthetic devices
    l. Diplopia (double vision)
   m. Blurring
    n. Photophobia
    o. Difficulty reading
    p. Interference with activities of daily living
6. Ears
    a. Pain (characteristics)
    b. Cerumen (wax)
    c. Infection
    d. Hearing changes (describe)
    e. Use of prosthetic devices
    f. Increased sensitivity to environmental noise
    g. Vertigo
    h. Ringing and cracking
    i. Care habits
    j. Interference with activities of daily living
7. Nose, nasopharynx, and paranasal sinuses
    a. Discharge (characteristics)
    b. Epistaxis
    c. Allergies
    d. Pain over sinuses
    e. Postnasal drip
    f. Sneezing
    g. General olfactory ability
8. Mouth and throat
    a. Sore throats (characteristics)
    b. Lesions of tongue or mouth (abscesses, sores, ulcers)
    c. Bleeding gums
    d. Hoarseness
    e. Voice changes
    f. Use of prosthetic devices (dentures, bridges)
    g. Altered taste
    h. Chewing difficulty

    i. Swallowing difficulty
    j. Pattern of dental hygiene
9. Neck
    a. Node enlargement
    b. Swellings, masses
    c. Tenderness
    d. Limitation of movement
    e. Stiffness
10. Breast
    a. Pain or tenderness
    b. Swelling
    c. Nipple discharge
    d. Changes in nipples
    e. Lumps, dimples
    f. Unusual characteristics
    g. Breast examination: pattern, frequency
11. Cardiovascular
    a. Cardiovascular
      (1) Palpitations
      (2) Heart murmur
      (3) Varicose veins
      (4) History of heart disease
      (5) Hypertension
      (6) Chest pain (character and frequency)
      (7) Shortness of breath
      (8) Orthopnea
      (9) Paroxysmal nocturnal dyspnea
    b. Peripheral vascular
      (1) Coldness, numbness
      (2) Discoloration
      (3) Peripheral edema
      (4) Intermittent claudication
12. Respiratory
    a. History of asthma
    b. Other breathing problems (when, precipitating factors)
    c. Sputum production

d. Hemoptysis
e. Chronic cough (characteristics)
f. Shortness of breath (precipitating factors)
g. Night sweats
h. Wheezing or noise with breathing

13. Hematolymphatic
    a. Lymph node swelling
    b. Excessive bleeding or easy bruising
    c. Petechiae, ecchymoses
    d. Anemia
    e. Blood transfusions
    f. Excessive fatigue
    g. Radiation exposure

14. Gastrointestinal
    a. Food idiosyncrasies
    b. Change in taste
    c. Dysphagia (inability or difficulty in swallowing)
    d. Indigestion or pain (associated with eating?)
    e. Pyrosis (burning sensation in esophagus and stomach with sour eructation)
    f. Ulcer history
    g. Nausea/vomiting (time, degree, precipitating and/or associated factors)
    h. Hematemesis
    i. Jaundice
    j. Ascites
    k. Bowel habits (diarrhea/constipation)
    l. Stool characteristics
    m. Change in bowel habits
    n. Hemorrhoids (pain, bleeding, amount)
    o. Dyschezia (constipation due to habitual neglect to respond to stimulus to defecate)
    p. Use of digestive or evacuation aids (what, how often)

15. Urinary
    a. Characteristics of urine
    b. History of renal stones
    c. Hesitancy
    d. Urinary frequency (in 24-hour period)
    e. Change in stream of urination
    f. Nocturia (excessive urination at night)
    g. History of urinary tract infection, dysuria (painful urination, urgency, flank pain)
    h. Suprapubic pain
    i. Dribbling or incontinence
    j. Stress incontinence
    k. Polyuria (excessive excretion or urine)
    l. Oliguria (decrease in urinary output)
    m. Pyuria

16. Genital
    a. General
       (1) Lesions
       (2) Discharges
       (3) Odors
       (4) Pain, burning, pruritus (itching)
       (5) Venereal disease history
       (6) Satisfaction with sexual activity
       (7) Birth control methods practiced
       (8) Sterility
    b. Males
       (1) Prostate problems
       (2) Penis and scrotum self-examination practices
    c. Females
       (1) Menstrual history (age of onset, last menstrual period [LMP], duration, amount of flow, problems)
       (2) Amenorrhea (absence of menses)
       (3) Menorrhagia (excessive menstruation)
       (4) Dysmenorrhea (painful menses); treatment method
       (5) Metrorrhagia (uterine bleeding at times other than during menses)
       (6) Dyspareunia (pain with intercourse)

17. Musculoskeletal
    a. Muscles
       (1) Twitching
       (2) Cramping
       (3) Pain
       (4) Weakness
    b. Extremities
       (1) Deformity
       (2) Gait or coordination difficulties
       (3) Interference with activities of daily living
       (4) Walking (amount per day)
    c. Bones and joints
       (1) Joint swelling
       (2) Joint pain
       (3) Redness
       (4) Stiffness (time of day related)
       (5) Joint deformity
       (6) Noise with joint movement
       (7) Limitations of movement
       (8) Interference with activities of daily living
    d. Back
       (1) History of back injury (characteristics of problems, corrective measures)
       (2) Interference with activities of daily living

18. Central nervous system
    a. History of central nervous system disease
    b. Fainting episodes
    c. Seizure
       (1) Characteristics
       (2) Medications
    d. Cognitive changes
       (1) Inability to remember (recent vs. distant)
       (2) Disorientation

   (3) Phobias
   (4) Hallucinations
   (5) Interference with activities of daily living
  e. Motor-gait
   (1) Coordinated movement
   (2) Ataxia, balance problems
   (3) Paralysis (partial vs. complete)
   (4) Tic, tremor, spasm
   (5) Interference with activities of daily living
  f. Sensory
   (1) Paresthesia (patterns)
   (2) Tingling sensations
   (3) Other changes
19. Endocrine
  a. Diagnosis of disease states (thyroid, diabetes)
  b. Changes in skin pigmentation or texture
  c. Changes in or abnormal hair distribution
  d. Sudden or unexplained changes in height and weight
  e. Intolerance to heat or cold
  f. Exophthalmos
  g. Goiter
  h. Hormone therapy
  i. Polydipsia (↑ thirst)
  j. Polyphagia (↑ food intake)
  k. Polyuria (↑ urination)
  l. Anorexia (↓ appetite)
  m. Weakness
20. Allergic and immunological (Optional; use if client indicates allergic history. Note precipitating factors in each case.)
  a. Dermatitis (inflammation or irritation of skin)
  b. Eczema
  c. Pruritus (itching)
  d. Urticaria (hives)
  e. Sneezing
  f. Vasomotor rhinitis (inflammation and swelling of mucous membrane of nose; nasal discharge)
  g. Conjunctivitis (inflammation of conjunctiva)
  h. Interference with activities of daily living
  i. Environmental and seasonal correlation
  j. Treatment techniques
21. Does client have any other physiological problems or disease states not specifically discussed. If so, explore in detail (e.g., fatigue, insomnia, nervousness).

PSYCHOSOCIAL HISTORY

1. General statement of client's feelings about self
2. Feelings of satisfaction or frustration in interpersonal relationships
  a. Home; occupants
  b. Client's position in home relationships
  c. Most significant relationship (in and out of home)
  d. Community activities
  e. Work or school relationships
  f. Family cohesiveness patterns
3. Activities of daily living
  a. General description of work, leisure, and rest distribution
  b. Significant hobbies or methods of relaxation
  c. Family demands
  d. Community activities and involvement
  e. During period of day/week is client able to accomplish all that is desired?
4. General statement about client's ability to cope with activities of daily living
5. Occupational history
  a. Jobs held in past
  b. Current employer
  c. Educational preparation
  d. Satisfaction with present and past employment
  e. Time spent at work vs. time spent at play
6. Recent changes or stresses in client's life-style (e.g., divorce, moving, new job, family illness, new baby, financial stresses)
7. Patterns in which client copes with situations of stress
8. Response to illness
  a. Does the client cope satisfactorily during own or others' illness?
  b. Do the client's family and friends respond satisfactorily during periods of illness?
9. History of psychiatric care or counseling
10. Feelings of anxiety or nervousness (characteristics and coping mechanisms)
11. Feelings of depression (symptoms such as insomnia, crying, fearfulness, marked irritability or anger)
12. Changes in personality, behavior, or mood
13. Use of medications or other techniques during times of anxiety, stress, or depression
14. Habits
  a. Alcohol
   (1) Kinds (beer, wine, mixed drinks)
   (2) Frequency per week
   (3) Pattern over past 5 years, 1 year
   (4) Drinking companions
   (5) Alcohol consumption increased when anxious or stressed?
  b. Smoking
   (1) Kind (pipe, cigarette, cigar)
   (2) Amount per week/day
   (3) Pattern over past 5 years, 1 year
   (4) Smoking with others

(5) Smoking increased when anxious or stressed?

(6) Desire to quit smoking? (method, attempts)

c. Coffee and tea

(1) Amount per day

(2) Pattern over past 5 years, 1 year

(3) Consumption increased when anxious or stressed?

(4) Physiological effects

d. Other

(1) Overeating or sporadic eating (e.g., always in refrigerator, soft drink abuse, cookie jar syndrome)

(2) Nail biting

(3) Street drug usage

(4) Nervous noneating

15. Financial status

a. Sources

b. Adequacy

c. Recent changes in resources and expenditures

HEALTH MAINTENANCE EFFORTS

1. General statement of client's own physical fitness
2. Exercise (amount, type, frequency)
3. Dietary regulations; special efforts (describe in detail)
4. Mental health; special efforts such as group therapy, meditation, yoga (describe in detail)
5. Cultural or religious practices
6. Frequency of physical, dental, and vision health assessment

ENVIRONMENTAL HEALTH

1. General statement of client's assessment of environmental safety and comfort
2. Hazards of employment (inhalants, noise, heavy lifting, psychological stress, machinery)
3. Hazards in the home (concern about fire, stairs to climb, inadequate heat, open gas heaters, inadequate toilet facilities, concern about pest control, inadequate space)
4. Hazards in neighborhood (noise, water, and air pollution, inadequate police protection, heavy traffic on surrounding streets, isolation from neighbors, overcrowding)
5. Community hazards (unavailability of stores, market, laundry facilities, drugstore; no access to bus line)

Clinical strategies

1. Complete data base collection and symptom analysis take practice and constant validation with an experienced practitioner. Complete your problem list *before* checking with your clinical resource advisor. Use *all* the steps; each is important.
2. Write up as many histories for review by an experienced practitioner as possible. It takes practice to write successfully.
3. The examiner needs ample time to formulate an accurate and complete data base. Negotiate for time and space with your employer. Next, contract for an extended time period with your client. Collecting a full data base from an individual may take an hour or more.
4. Frequently the client may come to see the examiner because of an episodic care problem. It may not be appropriate for the examiner to collect a complete data base, so a systematic and routine manner of collecting episodic care data must be developed. Following is a list of data that should be collected about every episodic care problem:

a. Chief complaint

b. Analysis of the symptom or complaint (see pp. 10 and 11 for details)

c. Interrelationship of current problem to other body systems (would include a review of associated body systems; vague symptoms such as weakness or fatigue must be thoroughly explored by reviewing all body systems)

d. Relation of current problem to past health and health maintenance

5. Following are several "nuggets" of interviewing that facilitate data collection:

a. Pose questions without suggesting answers: "Tell me about your pain," not "Does your pain travel down your arm?"

b. Begin questioning with the most *recent* episode (if client has experienced a number of "attacks" over a period of time), then move on to preceding episodes. The client is most likely to remember specific details of the most recent episode.

c. Begin questioning with the most *urgent* problem (if client presents a number of complaints that are worrying him): "What brought you to the clinic today?"

d. Chronology is the anchor of the history: request calendar dates and clock times.

e. Use simple language (e.g., instead of saying *void*, use *urinate* or *pass your water*).

f. Pose one question at a time.

g. Keep the client politely on track: "Before we go on to that, I would like to hear more about. . . ."

h. Clarify the client's responses: what do these

really mean to the client? do they mean the same to you?

    (1) Quasimedical terms

        (a) tumor

        (b) nervous breakdown

        (c) sick-to-the-stomach

        (d) pneumonia

        (e) sciatica

        (f) dizziness

        (g) heart attack

        (h) diarrhea

    (2) Quantities (unclear)

        (a) a lot

        (b) often

        (c) once in a while

  i. If you accept a diagnosis from a client, record it in quotations. Follow up with a summary of the symptoms that prompted diagnosis (e.g., *hemorrhoids*—involves five or six droplets of bright red blood on tissue; associated with once-a-week constipation; pain localized at anus with each daily bowel movement; palpable tags at anal area).

  j. At the end of the interview, summarize (aloud) what the client has said.

6. Following are several "hazards" of interviewing that will hinder data collection.

  a. The need to hurry. Clients will sense this, and thus incomplete data may be collected.

  b. Nonverbal cues. If the examiner is uninterested, the client may sense this and provide incomplete data.

  c. Environment. The examiner and client need a quiet, private environment with adequate chairs and writing space. If the facility or environment is busy, noisy, nonprivate, or confusing, incomplete data may be collected.

  d. "Nonhuman" techniques. This includes the "just the facts" approach. The examiner rapidly moves from one question to the next without taking time to build a relationship with the client.

  e. "Aha!" This technique is more a hazard for the experienced practitioner. The temptation is to leap to a "diagnosis" without collecting ample information; incorrect assessment can be based on incomplete data.

  f. "Oh, my!" This response allows the examiner to indicate disapproval, which could stifle examiner-client communication. For example, the client admits that he has not taken his hypertension medication for 4 months because he "felt so good." The examiner responds with "oh, my."

  g. "Halo effect." This hazard might prohibit the examiner from collecting all relevant data about a client. For example, the client is a 42-year-old new widow, and the examiner neglects to ask if the client is sexually active.

  h. Use of *normal, negative, healthy,* or *well.* Each of these terms has a different meaning to individual examiners with different levels of expertise. The beginning practitioner is encouraged to use descriptive terminology to define significant findings, or significant negatives to describe "normal" states.

  i. Limited knowledge is perhaps the biggest hazard of all. The beginning examiner must be disciplined enough to use the suggested data collection tools and to continue to study and learn.

7. Write an outline of the data collection format on small cards to use as a reference while taking histories. The beginning examiner cannot memorize all the data categories.

8. Use a clipboard or a small notebook for taking notes during the interview. The examiner will need a portable, hard surface to write on. This will permit seating comfort with maintenance of eye contact.

9. During progression of data base collection skills, monitor efficiency in terms of collecting, organizing, and recording a data base. Cost effectiveness is an issue in most employment settings.

10. *Note:* The client often does not present a tidy package of symptoms for analysis at the onset of the interview. Symptoms will be uncovered as the examiner pursues information in the review of systems. The examiner *must* stop and analyze these problems as thoroughly as those presented initially.

Analysis of a symptom

In addition to the health data base, the examiner must be prepared to collect in-depth information about a symptom. The following format is a data collection tool that can be used for physiological, psychological, or sociological symptoms.

CHIEF COMPLAINT

A one-sentence or brief statement using the client's words to describe the reason for the visit. (Details about the complaint follow in the *symptom analysis* or *history of present illness* section.)

ANALYSIS APPROACH

Reconstruction from the client's words of the body or mental processes underlying the symptom.

1. Last time client was entirely well
   a. Patient may confuse onset of symptom with the first time he was *concerned* about it.
   b. Major symptom may have been preceded by other less alarming ones (e.g., fatigue) that the client will not recall unless questioned.
2. Date of current problem onset
   a. Name specific date and time if possible.
   b. Inquiry about the setting at the time of onset may help establish chronology (time of day, month).
   c. How was client feeling prior to symptom onset?
3. Character (describe the qualities of the problem)
   a. Move back to quoting the client: What is the pain like? "like being stabbed"; "squeezed in a vice."
   b. Severity (does it interfere with activities of daily living?)
4. Nature of problem onset
   Was the onset slow? Abrupt? Noticeable to others? Use quotes if possible.
5. Client's hunch of precipitating factors
   In determining aggravating or alleviating factors, word questions to avoid influencing answers. For example, angina: "What effect does walking have?" vertigo: "What happens if you move your head?"
6. Course of problem (did client continue with normal activity during episode?)
   a. Consistent
   b. Intermittent
   c. Duration
7. Location of problem
   a. Pinpoint
   b. Generalized, vague
   c. Radiation patterns
8. Effect on other systems and activities
   a. Symptoms, signs
   b. Body functions or positions
   c. Activities (body movement, exercise)
   d. Eating
9. Patterns
   The client may exhibit a symptom that has been occurring intermittently over a period of time. Most previous questions have elicited data about the quantity and quality of *one* episode. This section concerns multiple episodes, identifies pat-

terns, and provides an overview of chronology.
   a. *Timing.* Relate incidences to number of times per hour, day, week, month; inquire about client's well-being during the intervals.
   b. *Duration* and quality variations. May indicate a stepping up or increase in intensity over a period of time. ("Has it been getting any better? Worse? Staying the same?")
   c. If there have been exacerbations or remission, try to associate with other symptoms, activities, or precipitating factors.
10. Efforts to treat
    a. Home remedies (what and when)
    b. Body positions (e.g., bed rest)
    c. Over-the-counter medications
    d. Prescription medications and physician visits (give details)
11. In-depth exploration of client's life-style and coping ability as related to the symptom
    a. Pose questions to discover an association between daily activities and the symptom.
       (1) What mandatory activities make the symptom worse? For example, if stair climbing causes chest pain, does the client have to use stairs at home or at work?
       (2) What activities are altered or curtailed because of the symptom? For example, if the client complains of nocturnal urination, how much sleep is lost? Is fatigue a problem? Possible to sleep during the day?
       (3) Do altered activities pose a threat to the client? If client complains of diminished vision or glare, is driving hazardous? Is reading part of job?
    b. Pose questions that indicate an association between client's ability to deal with current life-style and the symptom. For example, if a mother complains of marked fatigue, does this interfere with child-rearing activities or management of the home?
    c. A general question such as, "What does this problem *mean* to you?" might help to summarize the previous questions. It also permits the client to voice an emotional response to changes or problems. It may help the examiner to grasp more fully the impact or severity of the symptom.

Sample adult data base write-up

Once the data base is collected, it must be organized, synthesized, and documented. Following is a sample data base write-up. Refer to the pediatric and geriatric sections of this chapter to make the appropriate changes.

Biographical data

Cynthia M. Stoner; 32 years old; white; female; married; two sons, ages 6 and 7; 3792 Hedge Creek Lane, Maysville, Ohio; lives in single-family dwelling owned by family; described as three-bedroom "comfortable" home in midst of rural community.

Reason for visit

Time for Pap smear; "lower abdominal discomfort off and on"; desire to lose weight.

Present health status

Health during past 5 years has been good; during past year has noted 15-pound weight gain and periods of not feeling "up to par"; complains of being "tired" much of the time; no fatigue pattern identified; currently most significant concern is lower abdominal discomfort.

Initial problem onset 8 months ago; since then increased episodes and severity; increased discomfort prior to menses, with increased flatus and full bladder; discomfort described as nonradiating, sharp, and stabbing; pinpoint location in LLQ; client perceives problem associated with uterus or left ovary; coping methods: client aware of discomfort but problem not interfering with activities of daily living.

Currently taking no medications.

Current health statistics

Immunizations
Polio: 1972
Diphtheria, tetanus: 1978
Tuberculosis tine test: 1978
Influenza, mumps, rubella: none
Allergies
Seasonal and environmental: pollen, dust, grass; no treatment
Last examination
Physical, Pap smear, chest x-ray examination: Sept., 1979
Dental: June, 1979
Vision: Oct., 1978
Hearing: high school
ECG: 1972

Past health status

1946 to 1956 Childhood diseases: measles, mumps, chickenpox
1958 Tonsillectomy: Marion, Ohio, Dr. Harris
1961 Appendectomy: Marion, Ohio, Dr. Spencer
1962 Hospitalized for hepatitis
1964 Fracture of left tibia from riding accident; uncomplicated
1970 Surgery: benign left breast cyst removed, Delaware, Ohio, Dr. Southwood
1972 Pregnancy: delivered healthy 7-lb, 2-oz boy; vaginal delivery, uncomplicated

1973 Pregnancy: delivered healthy 7-lb, 9-oz boy; vaginal delivery; complications—high blood pressure, fluid retention, hospitalized 3 weeks prior to induced delivery; recovered to healthy state within 2 weeks following delivery
1973 Tubal ligation, Delaware, Ohio, Dr. Southwood

Family history

See Fig. 1-1.

Review of physiological systems

1. General: Client considers herself in "good health" but has periods of fatigue with physical and emotional stress. Feels rested following sleep periods. Client states she would feel better if she could lose 20 lb and exercise more regularly.
2. Nutritional
   Current weight: 142 lb; height: 5 feet, 4 in
   Weight past year: 138 to 140 lb
   Weight past 5 years: 120 to 138 lb

Twenty-four–hour dietary recall

Food eaten	Amount	Calories
Breakfast		
Toast with peanut butter and butter	1 slice	214
Coffee with cream	8 oz	30
Orange juice	4 oz	100
		344
Lunch		
Hamburger sandwich	1	250
Salad with ranch dressing	6 oz	105
Coffee with cream	8 oz	30
		385
Dinner		
Swiss steak	3 oz	300
Baked potato	1	230
Green beans	4 oz	27
Bread	2 slices	228
Water		
		785
Snacks		
Iced cupcake	1	200
Carbonated beverage	8 oz	105
		305
TOTAL		1819

Client considers the accompanying dietary recall to be typical. She states, "I know better than to eat all that junk." Dietary efforts have been sporadic; major methods involved skipping meals (breakfast and lunch) and protein (meat and salad) diets; no efforts in past 8 months.

Client considers current appetite "too good." She enjoys eating and eats more when nervous or worried. Client does grocery shopping. States she buys food that her children and husband like. Money or transportation not a problem.

Review of physiological systems—cont'd

3. Integumentary
    a. Skin: denies skin problems or diseases. Some pruritus during winter; clears with lotion.
    b. Hair: denies any problems with hair; uses color rinse monthly to maintain lightened color; no scalp irritation reported from the rinse.
    c. Nails: states she has always had brittle nails.
4. Head: periodic headaches in occipital area and back of neck usually follow tension period and are relieved by aspirin and rest (no more than four aspirin tablets/week consumed).
5. Eyes: denies infections or discharge from eyes; seasonal periorbital swelling associated with pollen allergy. Denies visual changes, diplopia, blurring, photophobia, pain in eyeball, or excessive tearing. Client wears glasses for reading (past 3 years).
6. Ears: complains of chronic hearing problem (multiple ear infections as child); states hearing difficulty does not interfere with activities of daily living; "just certain sounds are not clear." Denies pain, infections, or vertigo; frequent complaints of ringing and cracking in ears. Cares for ears with cotton-tipped swabs.
7. Nose, nasopharynx, and paranasal sinuses: denies epistaxis, sinus problems, postnasal drip, or olfactory deficit; seasonal sneezing and discharge associated with allergies.
8. Mouth and throat: denies sore throats, lesions, gum irritation, chewing or swallowing difficulties, hoarseness, or voice changes. Brushes teeth two times a day and uses dental floss.
9. Neck: denies tenderness or range of motion difficulties.
10. Breast: Breast tenderness prior to menses; breasts "feel lumpy"; "small amount of yellow" bilateral nipple discharge present since birth of second child. Examines own breasts each month following menstrual period. Breast biopsy with cyst removed in 1970. Client considers breasts to be "cystic, lumpy."
11. Cardiovascular: denies chest pain, shortness of breath, or palpitations. No known history of heart murmurs, heart disease, or hypertension. Feet always feel cold. Denies discoloration or peripheral edema.
12. Respiratory: denies any breathing difficulties, chronic cough, or shortness of breath.
13. Hematolymphatic: describes periods of fatigue related to stress or excessive work. Denies lymphatic swelling, excessive bleeding, or bruising. Never tested for anemia.
14. Gastrointestinal: denies eating or digestion problems. Periodic pyrosis usually follows rapid food ingestion or during stressful period. Denies hematemesis, jaundice, or ascites. Bowel movement once each day. Stools are soft and brown. Denies difficulty with diarrhea or constipation. No known hemorrhoids.
15. Urinary: describes urine as yellow and clear. Voiding frequency 4 or 5 times in 24 hours. Denies voiding difficulties, dysuria, urgency, or flank pain. Infrequent nocturia. Denies polyuria or oliguria. Complains of frequent episodes of stress incontinence since birth of second child. Condition becoming no worse but does present problem during laughing, running, or lifting heavy objects.
16. Genital: LMP, 6-14-79. Periods normally 28 to 30 days apart; regular intervals; heavy flow with clotting and cramps in first 24 hr. Cramps controlled by aspirin. LLQ pain increases just prior to menses. Denies genital lesions, discharges, or VD history. Sexually active, satisfied with sexual activity.
17. Musculoskeletal and extremities: denies muscular weakness, twitching, or pain; gait difficulties or extremity deformities; joint swelling, pain, stiffness, or noise; history of back injury problems.
18. Central nervous system: denies changes in cognitive function, coordination, or sensory defects.
19. Endocrine: denies endocrine disease, history of skin changes, polydipsia, polyuria, polyphagia, anorexia, or weakness.
20. Allergic: describes allergy problems as seasonal (August to October). Treatment consists of symptomatic relief by a "cortisone shot" and an unidentified prescription. During allergic season client reports sneezing, vasomotor rhinitis, conjunctivitis; no interference with activities of daily living.

Psychosocial history

Client states she feels good about herself most of the time. She experiences episodes of depression and fatigue and expresses a feeling that she should "do more" with her life.

Client expresses feelings of satisfaction with family members and friends. She considers her husband her best friend but also speaks of two other very close female friends. She counts on her friends to help her "talk through" stress periods. Considers family very close; communication channels are open.

Client's energies revolve around maintaining home, raising two small sons, and working part-time (12 hr/wk) at a local flower shop. Denies membership in clubs or church. Spends weekends just relaxing with family. Feels stress and at times "angry" when husband's business keeps him away on weekends. Client stated that much of her time is spent meeting the needs of others. States she would like more time for herself.

As soon as children are older, client hopes to return to college to complete degree in horticulture (5 terms to go). Client loves work at flower shop and would like to either take a college course or two or work a few more hours at the flower shop. Husband supports career goals but for now believes client's job is at home with the children (seemed to be a stress point).

Husband just accepted job promotion. Now travels approximately 12 days out of the month. This seems to cause direct stress and creates child care problems during client's working hours.

Client denies previous psychiatric counseling or feelings of anxiety or nervousness that she could not cope with. Methods of coping most frequently are (1) easy and sometimes inappropriate expression of anger, (2) increased sleeping, and (3) eating. To relax, client enjoys reading, playing with children, and going out with husband.

Continued.

Sample adult data base write-up—cont'd

Psychosocial history—cont'd

Client denies use of drugs or medications.
Alcohol: three or four glasses of wine a week
Smoking: none
Coffee: four or five cups a day. No increase over the past 5 years. Increased consumption with stress (6 to 8 cups a day).
Overeating: increased with stress; eats most when alone and after children go to bed.
Financial status: client feels they could do more as a family if there were more money but states there are no serious financial problems.

Health maintenance efforts

No specific health maintenance efforts. Health care patterns inconsistent, as previously stated.

Environmental health

Client believes her home and neighborhood environment are safe and without hazards. Client is exposed to fertilizer fumes at flower shop, but ventilation is adequate.

Subjective problem list

1. Periods of fatigue
2. LLQ pain: cyclical with menses? does not interfere with activities of daily living; increased severity and frequency past 8 months
3. Stress incontinence past 5 years, not increased in severity
4. Seasonal allergies: symptomatically treated; do not interfere with activities of daily living
5. Feet cold "most of time"
6. Long-standing hearing difficulty since childhood; does not interfere with activities of daily living

7. Overweight for height and build; 22-lb weight gain in past 5 years; 4 lb in past year
8. Poor dietary habits
9. Needs Pap smear
10. Feels trapped at times by home and child-raising responsibilities; husband travels approximately 12 days a month

Final problem list is developed, and priorities are established following physical assessment.

Risk profile

1. Family cancer history
   Maternal: mother, breast cancer; uncle, lung cancer
   Paternal: aunt, breast cancer; grandfather, colon cancer
   Client: cystic breasts; already has had one cyst removed (1970); client performs breast examination regularly
2. Weight: Steady weight gain since 1972; attempts at regular dieting and exercise programs have failed
3. Irregular health maintenance program: health care visits, diet, exercise
4. At times, client does not feel self-fulfilled; believes she is always meeting needs of others and neglecting self

Client profile

Client views herself as a healthy and resourceful 32-year-old female. Physiologically she is bothered by (1) LLQ discomfort, (2) overweight state, and (3) periodic fatigue.

Psychologically and sociologically, stresses viewed by client are (1) husband traveling too often, (2) feeling burdened periodically by family and household responsibilities, (3) a desire to return to college or become more actively involved in outside activities, and (4) fear of breast cancer. In summary, client views coping skills as adequate to meet present stresses.

Pediatric total health data base

Data base collection for the pediatric client is basically similar to that for the adult. Exceptions include prenatal, growth and development, behavioral, and school status histories. The following format parallels the adult history but includes the significant pediatric data.

INFORMANT

Who is giving the history (relation to client)?

BIOGRAPHICAL DATA

1. Name
2. Age
3. Race
4. Culture
5. Address and telephone
6. Children and family in home

7. Means of transportation to health care facility, if pertinent
8. Description of home; size and type of community

REASON FOR VISIT

One statement that describes the reason for the client's visit, preferably in the client's own words.

PRESENT HEALTH STATUS

1. Describe general health status of the client past 1 year, 5 years, now
2. Summary of client's major health concerns
3. If illness present, record symptom analysis (pp. 10 and 11).
   a. When was client last well
   b. Date of problem onset
   c. Character of complaint
   d. Nature of problem onset

e. Course of problem
f. Client's hunch of precipitating factors
g. Location of problem
h. Relation to
   (1) Other body symptoms
   (2) Body positions
   (3) Activity
   (4) Eating
i. Patterns of problem
j. Efforts of client to treat
k. Coping ability
4. Current medications: type (prescription, over-the-counter drugs, vitamins, etc.), prescribed by whom, amount per day, problems
5. *Current* development of the child
   The examiner must develop a profile of the child's current developmental status. It is expected that the examiner will have a working knowledge of the appropriate developmental progression for the child's age. Developmental screening questions should reflect the following areas:
   a. Children from 1 month through preschool age
      (1) *Motor development,* including rolling over, sitting, standing, walking, skipping, climbing, etc.
      (2) *Prehension,* including playing with hands, using pincer grip, using cup and spoon to feed self, stacking blocks, drawing with crayon, buttoning, drawing multiple-part persons, etc.
      (3) *Vision and hearing,* including ability to follow movement with eyes to midline and past midline, turn head to follow sound, smile at mirror image, recognize name when spoken to, etc.
      (4) *Cognitive development,* including ability to bring hands to mouth, suck thumb, recognize that actions can cause personal pleasure, search for object that has fallen, play peek-a-boo, drop object from chair to watch where it falls, remember solutions to simple problems, understand different points of view to conflicting problems, etc.
      (5) *Vocalization,* including ability to coo, smile, produce different tones, gurgle, and generate multiple verbal tones, single words, multiple words, and sentences.
   b. School-age children
      (1) *Gross motor development,* including assessment of running, jumping, climbing, general and eye-hand coordination, awkwardness, ability to ride a bicycle, etc.
      (2) *Fine motor development,* including assessment of ability to tie shoe, use scissors, draw

with detail, print name and numbers, etc.
      (3) *Vocalization,* including assessment of child's verbal communication ability, vocabulary, ability to read and tell time, etc.
6. Common behaviors
   General statement about child's behavior pattern.

Wants too little or too much attention	Bangs head
	Rocks
Accident prone	Encopresis (bowel incontinence)
Unsure of self	
Bites nails	Enuresis (wets bed)
Sucks thumb	Has temper tantrums
Stutters	Has breath-holding spells
Fearful	Smokes
Lies	Takes drugs, sniffs glue
Masturbates	Sets fires
Eats paint or dirt (pica)	

CURRENT HEALTH STATISTICS

1. Immunization status (note dates administered)
   DPT no 1 (2 mo)
   DPT no. 2 (4 mo)
   DPT no. 3 (6 mo)
   DPT booster no. 1 (18 mo)
   DPT booster no. 2 (4 to 6 yr)
   Last DPT, DT, or T
   Trivalent Sabin no. 1 (2 mo)
   Trivalent Sabin no. 2 (4 mo)
   Trivalent Sabin no. 3 (18 mo)
   Trivalent Sabin no. 4 (4 to 6 yr)
   Tuberculin test no. 1 (15 mo) then yearly thereafter (note results of tests)
   Measles (15 mo)
   Mumps (15 mo)
   Rubella (15 mo)
2. Allergies
   a. Drugs
   b. Foods
   c. Contact substances
   d. Environmental factors
3. Last examinations (note physician/clinic, findings, advice, and/or instructions)
   a. Physical
   b. Dental
   c. Vision
   d. Hearing
   e. Developmental assessment such as Denver Developmental Screening Test
4. Is there a public or visiting health nurse working with client?

PAST HEALTH STATUS

1. Perinatal history
   a. General health of mother during pregnancy
   b. Complications of pregnancy: bleeding, falls,

swelling of hands and feet, high blood pressure, unusual weight gain

  c. Medications taken during pregnancy

  d. Radiographs taken

  e. Emotional state of mother during pregnancy: crying or depression states

  f. Was pregnancy planned?

  g. Father's attitude

  h. Pregnancy history (para, gravida, abortions, miscarriages)

2. Labor and delivery
  a. Date and place of birth
  b. Complications
  c. Anesthesia used for delivery
  d. Number of weeks of gestation
  e. Type of delivery—breech, vertex, cesarean section
  f. Weight
  g. Length
  h. Did baby cry immediately?
  i. Was there cyanosis, jaundice, or respiratory problems?
  j. Did baby go to the regular nursery?
  k. Was any special equipment used for the baby?
  l. Was baby discharged with mother?

3. Newborn
  a. Initial problems with feeding, formula, colic, diarrhea
  b. Choking spells
  c. Blue spells
  d. Excessive crying

4. Growth and development
   Unlike the developmental data collected under *current health status,* this section includes a survey of significant developmental milestones.
  a. General statement as to how this child compares with siblings
  b. Does parent feel that the child's growth and development have been normal?
  c. Note age: rolled over, sat up, walked, first tooth, first words, toilet trained

5. State age and complications of each: chickenpox, rubella, measles, mumps, whooping cough, hay fever

6. State age and complications of each serious or chronic illness: meningitis or encephalitis, pneumonia or chronic lung problems, rheumatic fever, asthma, hay fever, scarlet fever, diabetes, kidney problems, hypertension, sickle cell anemia, seizure disorders, blood infections, etc.

7. State age and extent of each serious accident or injury: head injuries, fractures, burns, traumas, poisonings, etc.

8. Hospitalizations: list reason, location, primary care providers, duration, and how child reacted to hospitalization

9. Operations: what, where, when, why, by whom

10. Emotional health: past behavior problems, help sought, support persons, how child reacted to stress

FAMILY HISTORY

Family members include the client's blood relatives. Specifically the interviewer should inquire about the client's maternal and paternal grandparents, parents, aunts, uncles, and siblings. The interviewer should inquire about the general health, stress factors, and illnesses of family members. Questions should include a survey of the following:

Cancer	Hypertension
Diabetes	Sickle cell anemia
Heart problems	Blindness
Mental retardation	Endocrine diseases
Learning problems	Kidney diseases
Cystic fibrosis	Birth defects
Asthma	Infant deaths
Other allergies	Other chronic problems
Seizure disorders	

REVIEW OF PHYSIOLOGICAL SYSTEMS

1. General
  a. Frequent colds, infections, or illnesses
  b. Frequent fevers, sweats
  c. Fatigue patterns
  d. Energetic or overactive patterns

2. Nutritional
  a. Recent weight gain or loss (describe)
  b. Appetite
  c. 24-hour diet recall, including types, amount of food eaten (formula, breast milk, meat, fruits, vegetables, cereals, juices, eggs, sweets, milk, snacks), and frequency (i.e., how many times a day or week)
  d. Child feeding self?
  e. Where does child eat?
  f. Who does child eat with?
  g. Parents' perception of child's nutritional status (note problems)
  h. Vitamins?
  i. Junk food consumption (amount and kinds)

3. Integumentary
  a. Skin
    (1) Chronic rashes
    (2) Easy bruising or petechiae
    (3) Easy bleeding
    (4) Acne (treatment pattern)
    (5) Excessive sweating
    (6) Skin diseases, problems, or lesions

      (7) Itching
      (8) Pigmentation changes, discolorations, mottling
      (9) Excessive dryness
      (10) Skin growths or tumors
  b. Hair
      (1) Changes in amount, texture, characteristics
      (2) Infections, lice
      (3) Alopecia
  c. Nails
      (1) Changes in appearance
      (2) Cyanosis
      (3) Texture

4. Head
  a. Headache (frequency, type, location, duration, care for)
  b. Past significant trauma
  c. Dizziness
  d. Syncope

5. Eyes
  a. Crossed eyes
  b. Strabismus
  c. Discharge
  d. Complaint of vision changes
  e. Reading difficulty
  f. Sitting close to television
  g. History of infections
  h. Pruritus
  i. Excessive tearing
  j. Pain in eyeball
  k. Swelling around eyes
  l. Cataracts
  m. Unusual sensations or twitching
  n. Excessive blinking
  o. Eye injury history
  p. Currently wear glasses
  q. Diplopia
  r. Blurring
  s. Gives history of inability to see distant images

6. Ears
  a. Multiple infections or earaches
  b. Myringotomy tubes in ears
  c. Discharge
  d. Cerumen
  e. Care habits
  f. Cracking or ringing
  g. Parent perceives problem in child's hearing

7. Nose, nasopharynx, and paranasal sinuses
  a. Discharge (character of)
  b. Epistaxis
  c. Allergies
  d. General olfactory ability
  e. Pain over sinuses
  f. Postnasal drip
  g. Sneezing
  h. Nasal stuffiness

8. Mouth and throat
  a. Sore throats (frequency)
  b. Tonsils present
  c. Mouth sores
  d. Toothaches, caries
  e. Voice changes
  f. Hoarseness
  g. Mouth breathing
  h. Chewing difficulties
  i. Swallowing difficulties
  j. Teeth brushing pattern

9. Neck
  a. Swollen glands
  b. Tenderness
  c. Limitations of movement
  d. Stiffness

10. Breast: applicable only with teenagers; refer to adult data base

11. Cardiovascular
  a. History of murmur
  b. History of heart problem
  c. Palpitations
  d. Hypertension
  e. Postural hypotension
  f. Cyanosis (what precipitates)
  g. Dyspnea on exertion
  h. Limitation of activities
  i. Frequent complaints of extremity coldness

12. Respiratory
  a. Breathing trouble
  b. Chronic cough
  c. Wheezing (precipitating factors)
  d. Croup history
  e. Noisy breathing
  f. Shortness of breath

13. Hematolymphatic
  a. Lymph node swelling (note frequency and location)
  b. Excessive bleeding or easy bruising
  c. Anemia
  d. Blood dyscrasias
  e. Lead exposures; deleading in past

14. Gastrointestinal
  a. Ulcer history
  b. Previously diagnosed problem
  c. Vomiting
  d. Diarrhea
  e. Constipation or stool-holding problems
  f. Rectal bleeding
  g. Stool color change

h. Abdominal pains
i. Pinworms by history
j. Perianal pruritus
k. Use of evacuation aids
l. Toilet trained? If not, is it planned? Any problems?

15. Urinary
   a. Urinary tract infections during past year
   b. Previously diagnosed problems
   c. Characteristics of urine (cloudy, dark)
   d. Suprapubic pains
   e. Steadiness and force of urination stream
   f. Dysuria
   g. Nocturia
   h. Bed wetting (associated with emotional upsets? family history of bed wetting?)
   i. Urinary frequency
   j. Dribbling or incontinence
   k. Polyuria/oliguria
   l. Bubble bath used?

16. Genital
   a. Birth defects
   b. Discharges
   c. Odors
   d. Rashes, irritation
   e. Pruritus
   f. How is sexuality education handled in the home?
   g. Areas of concerns
   h. If client is female and menstruating, refer to adult data base for appropriate questioning

17. Musculoskeletal
   a. Muscles
      (1) Twitching
      (2) Cramping
      (3) Pain
      (4) Weakness
      (5) Pain with use
   b. Extremities
      (1) General complaints of pain, weakness, deformity
      (2) Night pains in legs
      (3) Gait ability—strength and coordination
   c. Bones and joints
      (1) Joint swelling
      (2) Joint pain
      (3) Redness, stiffness
      (4) Joint deformity
      (5) Fracture or dislocation history
   d. Back
      (1) History of back injury
      (2) Curvature of spine
      (3) Characteristics of problems and corrective measures

18. Central nervous system
   a. General
      (1) Unusual episodic behaviors
      (2) History of central nervous system diseases
      (3) Birth injury
   b. Seizure: febrile vs. afebrile
   c. Speech
      (1) Stuttering
      (2) Speech misarticulations
      (3) Language delay
   d. Cognitive changes
      (1) Hallucinations
      (2) Passing out episodes
      (3) Staring spells
      (4) Learning difficulties
   e. Motor-gait
      (1) Coordination
      (2) Developmental clumsiness
      (3) Balance problems
      (4) Tic
      (5) Tremor, spasms
   f. Sensory
      (1) Pain patterns
      (2) Tingling sensations

19. Endocrine
   a. Diagnosis of disease states (e.g., thyroid, diabetes)
   b. Changes in skin texture (e.g., ↑ or ↓ dryness or perspiration)
   c. Pigmentation
   d. Abnormal hair distribution
   e. Sudden or unexplained changes in height and weight
   f. Intolerance to heat or cold
   g. Exophthalmos
   h. Goiter
   i. Polydipsia (↑ thirst)
   j. Polyphagia (↑ food intake)
   k. Polyuria (↑ urination)
   l. Anorexia (↓ appetite)
   m. Weakness
   n. Precocious puberty

20. Allergic and immunological
   a. Dermatitis (inflammation or irritation of the skin)
   b. Eczema
   c. Pruritus (itching)
   d. Urticaria (hives)
   e. Sneezing
   f. Vasomotor rhinitis (inflammation and swelling of mucous membrane of nose; nasal discharge)
   g. Conjunctivitis (inflammation of conjunctiva)

h. Interference with activities of daily living
i. Environmental and seasonal causes
j. Treatment techniques

PSYCHOSOCIAL HISTORY

1. General status
   a. General statement of child's feeling about self
   b. Parents' observations of child's feelings of self
2. Caretakers and family
   a. Who lives in the child's home
   b. Primary care provider for child
   c. Child's position in home environment
   d. Relationships among members
3. Friends
   a. How does child get along with friends, classmates, siblings?
   b. Plays with older, younger, same age children?
   c. Does child make friends easily?
4. Activities of daily living
   a. General
      (1) General description of typical day
      (2) Sleep patterns and naps: sound sleeper or fretful; number of hours per 24 hours; nightmares; other nighttime activity (e.g., wakes up at night); how does parent respond?
      (3) Kinds of play: amount of active and quiet play per 24 hours; television time per 24 hours
      (4) Significant hobbies or methods of relaxation (for older child)
   b. Family
      (1) Does family do things as unit?
      (2) What are methods of discipline within family?
      (3) Is discipline effective?
      (4) Who disciplines child?
      (5) How does child react to discipline?
      (6) Parents or providers: type of employment; type of child care provided if both parents work
      (7) Does mother have emotional support for her care of child as well as time away from child?
   c. School
      (1) Present grade in school or level of nursery care
      (2) School performance
      (3) Behavior problems
      (4) Grades skipped
      (5) Learning problems; in special class?
      (6) Attitude about school
      (7) Rate of absenteeism

5. Ability to cope with stress
   a. General statement: activities of daily living, family, school
   b. How does child adapt to new situations?
   c. Have there been any recent changes or stresses in child's life-style (home, school)?
   d. Behavior patterns child uses to cope with stress
   e. Changes in personality, behavior, or mood
   f. History of psychiatric care or counseling

HEALTH MAINTENANCE EFFORTS

1. General statement about physical fitness (parent attitudes and child opinion)
2. Dietary regulations to maintain health
3. Frequency of physical, dental, and vision health assessment
4. Statement reflecting parents' attitude about the importance of health maintenance education, including:
   a. Self-care techniques
   b. Poison control safety
   c. First aid
   d. Toy safety
   e. Environmental safety

ENVIRONMENTAL HEALTH

1. General statement of parents' assessment of environmental safety and comfort
2. Hazards in the home, to include survey of the following:
   a. Toys appropriate for age
   b. Special protection from poisons, household products, or medications
   c. Stairway protection (e.g., use of gates for toddlers or handrails for older children)
   d. Yard equipment for play and safety
   e. Type of bed (protection device to prevent falling)
   f. Pest control problems
   g. Unsafe building (e.g., no heat, poor toilet facilities, open gas heaters)
3. Hazards in neighborhood
   a. Unsafe play area
   b. Heavily traveled streets
   c. No sidewalks
   d. Water or air pollution
   e. Noise factor
   f. Isolation or overcrowding from neighbors

Clinical strategies

1. Depending on the age of the child, it might be helpful to set a time that the examiner may collect information from the parent without the child's pres-

ence. It would be quite disappointing to collect an inadequate or incomplete profile because of the child's impatience.

2. A second option facilitating complete data base collection is to divide the content to be collected into several visits. Once the total information is collected, it should be documented as a single entry.

3. It is undesirable to try to collect a complete data base when the child is ill. The examiner, child, and parent are all likely to become frustrated. The most likely solution is to schedule a well visit specifically for data collection.

4. If the child is old enough to participate in the interview, be sure to include his information.

5. For older children and adolescents the child and parent may conflict on details of the problem or concern. The examiner should collect separate stories from each source, record each story, and at the end analyze all the data. During the examination the examiner should ask the client if the parent's presence is desirable or not.

6. It is also appropriate to excuse the parent from the room while recording the history from the child or teenager. Our experience has been that most children or teenagers are direct with their information when not stressed by the presence of their parent. This is particularly true when discussing sexual, social, or psychological screening questions.

7. It has long been debated at what age to terminate using the pediatric data base tool and to begin using the adult data base tool. Although there is no easy solution to this question, the ages 12 to 14 seem to be a fairly common breakoff point. Other examiners desire to make minor adjustments to the pediatric tool and to continue using it through adolescence. The choice is yours.

8. For additional strategies refer to *clinical strategies* in the adult data base.

Total health data base for geriatric client

Geriatric clients are not "different" from adults. There is no specific age when concerns related to the aging process warrant additional screening questions to complete an accurate data base.

The following questions and concerns are directed toward elderly adults. Many of the questions concern problems of disability, chronic illness, or normal changes that take place with aging. There are many older people who do not have chronic illnesses, disabilities, or marked aging changes that affect their daily lives. The practitioner can use the following format when it seems to be appropriate.

BIOGRAPHICAL DATA

1. Name
2. Age
3. Race
4. Culture
5. Address
6. Marital status
7. Children and family in home
8. Occupation/retirement status
9. Means of transportation to health care facility, if pertinent
10. Description of home and size and type of community

REASON FOR VISIT OR
CHIEF COMPLAINT

Some elderly clients present a multitude of problems. Some complaints are long-standing (e.g., stiff joints, hypertension, dry skin, chronic constipation), and others are more acute. Other problems are not easily identified and, with skilled questioning, emerge as the assessment progresses (e.g., depression, weight loss, weakness, difficulty caring for self at home).

Other clients tend to minimize pain or other symptoms. Older individuals may not manifest fever associated with infection to the extent that younger clients do. Some elderly individuals complain less of pain (e.g., cholecystitis, angina) or seem to experience less pain. New symptoms may be attributed to "getting old" and therefore are not reported as significant.

It takes time and patience to identify the *priorities* of the client's concerns (which may be different from the examiner's priorities). It often takes time and patience to establish the actual reason for the visit.

The final statement describing the reason(s) should be brief, stated in the client's own words, and limited to the *client's* immediate concerns. The final problem list, risk profile, and client profile can absorb (identify) the multiplicity of concerns that are not directly related to the chief complaint.

PRESENT HEALTH STATUS

1. Describe general health status of the client in past year, 5 years, now
2. Summary of client's current major health concerns
3. If illness present, record symptom analysis (pp. 10 and 11)
   a. When was client last well
   b. Date of problem onset
   c. Character of complaint
   d. Nature of problem onset
   e. Course of problem

f. Client's hunch of precipitating factors

g. Location of problem

h. Relation to

   (1) Other body symptoms

   (2) Body positions

   (3) Activity

i. Patterns of problem

j. Efforts of client to treat

k. Coping ability

4. Current medications (include prescriptions, over-the-counter drugs, vitamins, home remedies)

   a. Name of drug

   b. Prescribed when and by whom

   c. Amount prescribed per day

   d. Amount taken per day

   e. Problems with compliancy: complicated or inconvenient dosage schedule, large number and variety of drugs prescribed, visual difficulty (unable to read label), unpleasant side effects, unable to afford drugs, difficulty swallowing or administering, unable to get to pharmacy, client fearful of addiction, client feels drug ineffective, client overdosing to relieve symptoms. If the client is taking a large number of prescribed drugs (often prescribed by different physicians), request that all medications be brought in for review. Clients are often unaware of the names or the purposes of all their drugs.

CURRENT HEALTH STATISTICS

1. Immunization status (note dates or year of last immunization)

   a. Tetanus, diphtheria

   b. Mumps

   c. Rubella

   d. Polio

   e. Tuberculosis tine test

   f. Influenza

2. Allergies (describe agent and reactions)

   a. Drugs

   b. Foods

   c. Contact substances

   d. Environmental factors

3. Last examination (note physician/clinic, findings, advice, and/or instructions)

   a. Physical

   b. Dental

   c. Vision

   d. Hearing

   e. ECG

   f. Chest radiograph

   g. Pap smear (females)

   h. Proctoscopic

   i. Tonometry

PAST HEALTH STATUS

1. Childhood illnesses: rubeola, rubella, mumps, pertussis, scarlet fever, chickenpox, strep throat

2. Serious or chronic illnesses: Parkinson disease, diabetes, hypertension, arthritis, bone diseases, cardiovascular disease, stroke, respiratory disease, kidney or urinary problems, nervous or seizure disorders, blood diseases or infections, gastrointestinal dysfunction, gynecological disorders, cancer, thyroid problems, diseases of eyes or ears

If client offers a diagnosis that is not confirmed by health records, record it in quotes.

3. Serious accidents or injuries: head injuries, fractures, burns, other trauma

4. Hospitalizations: elaborate, listing reason, location, primary care providers, duration

5. Operations: what, where, when, why, by whom

6. Emotional health: past problems, help sought, support persons

7. Obstetrical history

   a. Complete pregnancies: number, pregnancy course, postpartum course, condition, weight, and sex of each

   b. Incomplete pregnancies: duration, termination, circumstances, including abortions and stillbirths

   c. Summary of complications

An elderly individual's past health history may be quite lengthy, complicated, and time-consuming to amass and organize. If the individual has no difficulty with vision or writing skills, it is helpful to have this portion completed at home in advance of the assessment.

FAMILY HISTORY

Family members include the client's blood relatives, spouse, and children. Specifically the interviewer should inquire about the client's maternal and paternal grandparents, parents, aunts, uncles, spouse, and children, as well as the general health, stress factors, and illnesses of family members. Questions should include a survey of the following:

Cancer	Retardation
Diabetes	Alcoholism
Heart disease	Endocrine diseases
Hypertension	Sickle cell anemia
Epilepsy (or seizure disorder)	Kidney disease
Emotional stresses	Unusual limitations
Mental illness	Other chronic problems

The most concise method to record these data is by a family tree. An elaborate family history may be less meaningful with the geriatric client, in terms of serving as a predictor of potential medical problems, since many familial diseases are contracted at an earlier age.

Cancer and diabetes are exceptions. However, the family tree serves as a reference for knowing what past experiences (perhaps fears) the client has had with diseases, disabilities, and causes of death.

REVIEW OF PHYSIOLOGICAL SYSTEMS

1. General—reflect from client's previous description of current health status.
   a. Fatigue patterns
   b. Exercise and exercise tolerance
   c. Weakness episodes
   d. Fevers, sweats
   e. Frequent colds, infections, or illnesses
   f. Activities of daily living assessment (optional package; to be used if the client has multiple complaints or disabilities, such as visual loss, limited energy, motor skill deficits, mental difficulties, arthritic changes). When the multiplicity of diseases, symptoms, and side effects strikes an individual, the general health status is sometimes best assessed in terms of the *impact of disability* on one's daily life. This tool is particularly helpful if the client is living alone or with an elderly companion or spouse.

Activities of daily living (ADL) assessment

A. Self-care
   1. Dressing, undressing, clothing
      a. Keeping clothes in good repair (mending)
      b. Access to clothes
      c. Getting into and out of underwear (bra, girdle, underpants, pantyhose, stockings, garter belt)
      d. Putting on and removing pants
      e. Getting arms in sleeves
      f. Managing zippers, buttons, snaps (especially in back), ties
      g. Putting on socks, shoes, tying laces
      h. Applying prostheses (e.g., glasses, hearing aids)
   2. Grooming and hygiene
      a. Washing, drying, brushing hair
      b. Brushing teeth
      c. Cleaning and putting in dentures
      d. Shaving
      e. Nail care (feet and hands)
      f. Applying makeup
      g. Preparing bath water and testing temperature
      h. Getting into and out of tub, shower
      i. Reaching and cleaning all body parts
   3. Elimination
      a. Position altered for urination or sitting on toilet
      b. Ability to wipe self
      c. Lowering onto and rising from toilet
B. Mobility
   1. Difficulty climbing or descending stairs (is bedroom/bathroom on upper level? how many stairs/flights to apartment or house?)
   2. Sitting up, rising from bed
   3. Lowering to or rising from chair
   4. Walking (short and long distances); describe necessity for walking

5. Opening doors
6. Reaching items in cupboards
7. Necessity for lifting (and any difficulty)
C. Communication
   1. Dialing telephone
   2. Reading numbers
   3. Hearing over telephone
   4. Answering door
   5. Immediate access to neighbors, help
D. Eating (see nutritional section for details about appetite, weight, food consumption)
   1. Access to market
   2. Preparing food (opening cans, packages, using stove, reaching dishes, pots, utensils)
   3. Handling knife, fork, spoon (cutting meat)
   4. Getting food to mouth
   5. Chewing, swallowing
E. Housekeeping, laundry, house upkeep
   1. Making bed
   2. Sweeping, mopping floors
   3. Dusting
   4. Cleaning dishes
   5. Cleaning tub, bathroom
   6. Picking up clutter (to client's satisfaction)
   7. Taking out trash, garbage
   8. Use of basement (stairs, cleaning)
   9. Laundry facilities (in home or near residence, washtub, clothesline)
   10. Yard care (garden, bushes, grass)
   11. Other home maintenance concerns (e.g., access to fuse box, storm windows, furnace filters, painting)
F. Medications
   1. Large number of prescriptions
   2. Difficulty remembering
   3. Able to see labels/directions
   4. Medications kept in one area
G. Access to community
   1. Busline
   2. Walking
   3. Driving (self or service from others)
   4. Church, dry cleaning, drugstore, bank, health care facility, dentist, other community agencies
H. Other
   1. Caring for spouse/relative/companion
   2. Financial management (able to write checks, make payments, cash checks)
   3. Care of pet(s)

2. Nutritional
   a. Client's average, maximum, and minimum weights during past month, year, 5 years
   b. History of weight gain or loss (time element); specific efforts to change weight—if dieting, describe efforts and type of diet used
   c. If client on a special diet, describe
   d. Current appetite patterns—food type preferences (e.g., sweets, fruits, convenience foods), amounts consumed at one time, hunger more marked at certain times of day or night, any loss or gain in appetite recently or over past year
   e. Food consumption patterns (e.g., three meals

a day, smaller meals five or six times a day, eating at night); does client have a similar eating pattern from day to day? does client eat with others or alone? A 24-hour recall may not be indicative of client's real eating pattern, which may vary greatly from day to day.

f. Specific foods and amounts consumed; A 24-hour recall, if appropriate, or foods consumed over a week's or a month's time

g. Fluid intake (24-hour estimate)

h. Who buys, prepares food?

i. If someone else prepares and buys food, is it to the client's liking? Ability to maintain special diet?

j. If client buys own food, ask about access to market, walking (clarify distance), bus, driving, taxi, frequency of trips to market

k. If client prepares food in own home, is preparation a problem (e.g., fatigue, eating alone, decreased vision, refrigerator, stove, water in rural area)?

l. Problem with chewing (dentures fit or loose, teeth loose or painful, edentulous)

m. Problem with swallowing, choking

n. Is client able to afford the food desired and needed?

o. Client's summary of own nutritional status

3. Integumentary

a. Skin
   (1) Skin disease or skin problems or lesions (wounds, sores, ulcers)
   (2) Growths, tumors, masses
   (3) Excessive dryness, sweating, odors
   (4) Pigmentation changes or discolorations
   (5) Pruritus (itching), scratching
   (6) Texture changes
   (7) Temperature changes
   (8) Increased or excessive bruises, excoriations (especially in skinfolds), redness, or trauma marks
   (9) Healing pattern of bruises, cuts, etc. (time element)
   (10) Decreased sensation to pain, heat
   (11) Increased sensation to pain, heat, cold, itching
   (12) History of chronic sun exposure

b. Hair
   (1) Thinning, falling out, dulling
   (2) Texture changes
   (3) Brittleness, breaking
   (4) Use of dyes, permanents

c. Nails
   (1) Brittleness, peeling, breaking
   (2) Changes in appearance, texture
   (3) Toenails: thickening, difficulty cutting

4. Head
   a. Headache (do full symptom analysis)
   b. Past significant trauma
   c. Dizziness (associated with body position or change—sitting up, standing, or head/neck movement)
   d. Syncope

5. Eyes
   a. History of glaucoma
   b. Cataracts, infections (frequency, treatment)
   c. Discharge characteristics
   d. Itching
   e. Lacrimation, excessive tearing
   f. Loss (or decrease) of tears
   g. Pain in eyeball
   h. Swelling around eyes
   i. Spots, floaters
   j. Unusual visual effects (e.g., light flashes, halos or rainbows around lights)
   k. General vision changes
   l. Loss of lateral vision (narrowing fields, tunnel vision)
   m. Double vision
   n. Sensitivity to glare
   o. Difficulty with night vision
   p. Difficulty distinguishing colors (e.g., traffic lights)
   q. Photophobia
   r. Blurring
   s. Difficulty reading
   t. Use of corrective or prosthetic devices (bifocals)
   u. Unusual sensations, twitching
   v. If bifocals, any problems with adjusting to far vision (e.g., stepping up on a curb)
   w. Do vision changes interfere with activities of daily living?

6. Ears
   a. Pain (pattern, position related?)
   b. Cerumen (wax)
   c. Infection
   d. Vertigo
   e. Ringing and cracking
   f. Care habits
   g. Hearing changes
   h. Use of prosthetic devices
   i. Increased sensitivity to environmental noise
   j. Interference with activities of daily living
   k. Does conversation (of others) sound garbled or distorted?
   l. If hearing aid is used, does client feel it is effective? Who prescribed it? How long ago? Does client wear it all the time?

7. Nose, nasopharynx, paranasal sinuses
   a. Discharge (characteristics)
   b. Epistaxis
   c. Allergies
   d. Pain over sinuses
   e. Postnasal drip
   f. Sneezing
   g. Dry nasal passages/crusting
   h. Painful nose breathing
   i. Mouth breathing
   j. General olfactory ability
8. Mouth and throat
   a. Sore throats
   b. Sore mouth
   c. Dry mouth
   d. Lesions (sores, ulcers, bumps on tongue, mouth, gums)
   e. Bleeding gums
   f. Burning mouth, palate, tongue
   g. Toothache
   h. Loose teeth
   i. Missing teeth
   j. Altered taste
   k. Chewing difficulty
   l. Swallowing difficulty
   m. Prosthetic devices (dentures, bridges)
   n. If client has dentures:
      (1) Wearing habits (e.g., for meals only, for appearance only, always, seldom, or never wears)
      (2) Wearing problems (e.g., rubbing or tenderness, looseness, clicking noises, talking difficulty, whistling dentures)
      (3) Cleaning habits and problems
   o. Sores at corner of mouth (associated with edentulous patients or ill-fitting dentures)
   p. Bad breath
   q. Bad taste in mouth
   r. Hoarseness
   s. Voice changes
   t. Pattern of dental hygiene
9. Neck
   a. Node enlargement
   b. Swellings, masses
   c. Tenderness
   d. Limitation of movement
   e. Stiffness
10. Breast
    a. Pain or tenderness
    b. Swelling
    c. Nipple discharge
    d. Changes in nipples
    e. Lumps, dimples
    f. Unusual characteristics
    g. Irritated skin under pendulous breasts, rubbing bra
    h. Breast examination pattern, frequency
11. Cardiovascular
    a. Cardiovascular—chest pain may be reduced, even absent, in elderly. Dyspnea on exertion may be a primary symptom.
       (1) Chest pain (full symptom analysis)
       (2) Dyspnea on exertion (specify *amount* of exertion, e.g., three stairs vs. one flight with 2-minute rest at landing; walking one block vs. walking from bed to bath)
       (3) Palpitations
       (4) Unusual breathing patterns (e.g., Cheyne-Stokes)
       (5) Orthopnea
       (6) Paroxysmal nocturnal dyspnea
       (7) Episodes of confusion
    b. Peripheral vascular
       (1) Coldness
       (2) Loss of sensation to pain, touch
       (3) Exaggerated response to cold (pain)
       (4) Pain associated with exercise
       (5) Color changes (especially feet and ankles: bluish-red or ruddy, mottling, pallor, associated with position)
       (6) Swelling (specify time of day; do full symptom analysis)
       (7) Varicosities
       (8) Does client wear constrictive clothing (e.g., girdles, garters, or stockings rolled at knees?)
    c. Heart and hypertension medications: toxicity symptoms
       The examiner need not pose questions about all these symptoms but should be alert to symptom groupings or patterns of drug reactions. Many clients take digitalis preparations, diuretics, and/or antihypertensive medications. Following are the major side effects and chief symptoms associated with toxicity.

Digitalis	Diuretics	Anti-hypertensives
Anorexia	Fatigue	Lethargy
Nausea, vomiting, diarrhea	Weakness	Mood disturbances
Headache	Muscle cramps	Sedation
Drowziness	Gastrointestinal distress	Postural syncope
Vision changes, (yellow, brown, green vision, halos around lights)	Confusion	Dizziness
		Nausea
		Diarrhea
Arrhythmias (all varieties)		Fluid retention
Confusion		Drug rash

12. Respiratory
    a. History of wheezing, bronchitis, other breathing problems
    b. Painful breathing (on deep or regular inspiration)
    c. Smoking (detailed questions covered in *Habits*)
    d. Chronic cough (full symptom analysis—specify time of day or night that cough is bothersome)
    e. Sputum production (amount, color, time element)
    f. Hemoptysis
    g. Night sweats
    h. Exertional capacity (report present status and any recent change)
        (1) Shortness of breath (SOB) with heavy, sustained work (e.g., lifting, digging, snow shoveling)
        (2) SOB with sudden high-speed exercise (e.g., jogging, brisk walk, bicycling)
        (3) SOB with exertion at slower pace (e.g., slow walk around the block, light housekeeping)
        (4) SOB with slight exertion (e.g., rising from chair, walking from one room to another)
    i. Has client been less active or immobilized recently or in past year, for reasons other than respiratory (e.g., foot problems, fractured hip, arthritic pain)?
13. Hematolymphatic
    a. Lymph node swelling
    b. Excessive bleeding or
    c. Easy bruising
    d. Anemia
    e. Blood transfusions
    f. Excessive fatigue
    g. Radiation exposure
14. Gastrointestinal
    a. Abdominal pain (heartburn, indigestion, pain in lower abdomen; specify if pain associated with eating, before or after; do full symptom analysis)
    b. Excessive belching (sour taste, associated with pain?)
    c. Anorexia
    d. Nausea, vomiting
    e. Food idiosyncrasies (long-standing or recent)
    f. Bloating
    g. Flatulence
    h. Grumbling bowel
    i. Diarrhea
    j. Swollen abdomen
    k. Jaundice
    l. Hemorrhoids (pain, bleeding, amount)
    m. Bowel habits (frequency, defecation difficulty, straining)
    n. Change in bowel habits
    o. Describe stool (color, size, consistency)
    p. Constipation (describe client's concern in detail, including use of digestive or evacuation aids)
15. Urinary
    a. Characteristics of urine; note changes (color, odor, clarity)
    b. Voiding pattern (in 24-hour period), note number of times client is up at night; note any recent change in pattern
    c. Characteristics of urine
    d. Urination pattern/problems (retention, incomplete emptying, straining to void, change in force of stream—does man have to stand closer to toilet? hesitancy, dribbling, incontinence with stress, sneezing, coughing)
    e. Painful urination
    f. Urgency, frequency
    g. Oliguria (decrease in output)
    h. Polyuria (increase in output)
    i. Pyuria
    j. Hematuria
    k. Flank, groin, low back, or suprapubic pain
16. Genital
    a. General
        (1) Lesions
        (2) Discharges
        (3) Odors
        (4) Pain, burning, pruritus (itching)
        (5) Venereal disease history
        (6) Sexually active? If so, satisfaction with sexual activity
    b. Males
        (1) History of prostate trouble
        (2) Scrotal lumps, masses, surface changes
        (3) If uncircumcised, difficulty retracting foreskin
        (4) Scrotum self-examination practices
        (5) Does client have full erection, can he maintain erection to his satisfaction, complete ejaculation?
        (6) Pain preceding, during, or following erection
    c. Females
        (1) Menopause history (onset, course, LMP, associated problems, residual problems, any bleeding since LMP)
        (2) Any severe problems with menstrual history

(3) Soreness or tenderness of vagina

(4) Pressure sensation within vagina

(5) Dyspareunia (pain with intercourse)

17. Musculoskeletal—history of injuries, fractures, dislocations, whiplash

   a. Muscles

      (1) Twitching

      (2) Cramping

      (3) Weakness or pain with use (location of weakness; activity such as stair climbing altered by weakness)

      (4) Manual dexterity problems

      (5) Other interferences with activities of daily living

   b. Extremities

      (1) Deformity or coordination difficulties

      (2) Problems with shoes (fit, rubbing)

      (3) Restless legs

      (4) Transient paresthesia—need to move legs at night

   c. Gait

      (1) Any alterations noted by client (e.g., weakness, balance, difficulty with steps, fear of falling)

      (2) Walking aids (cane, walker, special shoes; does client feel that aids are effective; any difficulty maneuvering aid?)

   d. Bones and joints

      (1) Joint swelling, pain, redness, deformity

      (2) Stiffness (pronounced at certain times of day, associated with or following activity or inactivity)

      (3) Limited movement (specify location, which joint)

      (4) Crepitation (creaking noise on movement)

      (5) Interference with activities of daily living

   e. Back

      (1) Pain (full symptom analysis)

      (2) Stiffness

      (3) Corrective measures (use of bed board, special mattress, prosthetic devices)

      (4) Interference with activities of daily living

      (5) Client's assessment of effectiveness of prosthetic devices; any difficulty applying?

18. Central nervous system—history of any disease

   a. Seizure (characteristics, medications for)

   b. Speech

      (1) Unusual speech patterns

      (2) Aphasia

      (3) Dysarthria (stammering)

   c. Cognitive changes

      (1) Inability to remember (recent vs. remote)

      (2) Disorientation

(3) Phobias

(4) Hallucinations

(5) Passing out episodes

(6) Interference with activities of daily living

   d. Motor-gait

      (1) Coordinated movement

      (2) Ataxia, balance problems

      (3) Paralysis (partial vs. complete)

      (4) Tic

      (5) Tremor, spasm

      (6) Interference with activities of daily living

   e. Sensory

      (1) Tingling sensations

      (2) Areas of paresthesia (patterns)

      (3) Other changes

19. Endocrine

   a. Diagnosis of disease states (e.g., thyroid, diabetes)

   b. Changes in skin pigmentation or texture

   c. Changes in or abnormal hair distribution

   d. Sudden or unexplained changes in height and weight

   e. Intolerance to heat or cold

   f. Exophthalmos

   g. Goiter

   h. Hormone therapy

   i. Polydipsia ($\uparrow$ thirst)

   j. Polyphagia ($\uparrow$ food intake)

   k. Polyuria ($\uparrow$ urination)

   l. Anorexia ($\downarrow$ appetite)

   m. Weakness

20. Allergic and immunological (Optional; use if client indicates allergic history. Note precipitating factors in each case.)

   a. Dermatitis (inflammation or irritation of skin)

   b. Eczema

   c. Pruritus (itching)

   d. Urticaria (hives)

   e. Sneezing

   f. Vasomotor rhinitis (inflammation and swelling or mucous membrane of nose; nasal discharge)

   g. Conjunctivitis (inflammation of conjunctiva)

   h. Interference with activities of daily living

   i. Environmental and seasonal causes

   j. Treatment techniques

21. Does client have any other physiological problems or disease states not specifically discussed? If so, explore in detail.

PSYCHOSOCIAL HISTORY

1. General statement of client's feelings about self

2. Relatives and friends, in home, or nearby (sexual needs, affection, support). If individual lives alone: (a) to what extent is being alone tolerated;

(b) does client have sufficient and satisfactory access to family and friends; (c) does client have a pet? If client lives with family: (a) are relationships satisfactory (with spouse, children, grandchildren); (b) does client participate in activities (meals, recreation) with family; (c) does client participate in family decisions; is there conflict?

3. Environment: is it adequately warm, sufficiently and conveniently spacious, sufficiently private, comfortable, safe, affordable?

4. Time/energy: too much or too little time to carry out daily life; does client have sufficient energy to meet needs?

5. Activities of daily living (see *general health status* for details)
   a. General description of work, leisure, and rest distribution
   b. Significant hobbies or methods of relaxation
   c. Family demands
   d. Community activities and involvement (e.g., church, club)
   e. Transportation
      (1) Automobile: estimate amount of driving; does client consider himself safe (last driving test); financial problems with gas, upkeep, insurance
      (2) Bus: easy access; availability to necessary and desired destinations; problems getting onto bus, tolerating wait
      (3) Taxi: estimate amount used (financial burden)
      (4) Driving services from others: availability, convenience
      (5) Walking: problems with distance, carrying packages, using curbs, stairs, bad weather, fear of traffic
   f. Occupational/volunteer history
      (1) Major jobs held in past
      (2) Current employment
      (3) Volunteer and community activities
      (4) Satisfaction with present activities
   g. Work/retirement concerns
      (1) Reduced/fixed income
      (2) Moving or selling home
      (3) Role change/time adjustment
      (4) Problems in relationship with spouse because of retirement

6. General statement about client's ability to cope with activities of daily living

7. Recent changes or stresses in life-style: illness of self or family, death of spouse, close friends, or family; retirement, moving, financial changes

8. Patterns in which client copes with stress: use of resources, worry pattern

9. Is there any history of psychiatric care or counseling?

10. Feelings of anxiety or nervousness; describe characteristics and coping mechanisms

11. Feelings of depression (consider symptoms such as insomnia, crying, fearfulness, marked irritability, or anger; review medication intake)

12. Changes in personality, behavior, or mood

13. Specific feelings of satisfaction/or frustration: aging changes, setting goals and meeting them, work activities, use of leisure time, mental capacity, intellectual capacity, aspirations

14. Use of drugs or other techniques during times of anxiety or stress

15. Response to illness
    a. Does the client cope satisfactorily during times of own or others' illness?
    b. Do the client's family and friends respond satisfactorily during periods of illness?

16. Physical well-being, particular fears and concerns about death

17. Habits
    a. Alcohol
       (1) Kinds (beer, wine, mixed drinks)
       (2) Frequency per week
       (3) Pattern over past 5 years, 1 year
       (4) Drinking companions?
       (5) Drinks when anxious?
    b. Smoking
       (1) Kind (pipe, cigarette, cigar)
       (2) Amount per week/day
       (3) Pattern over past 5 years, 1 year
       (4) Smokes with whom?
       (5) Smokes when anxious?
       (6) Desire to quit smoking? (method of attempts)
    c. Coffee and tea
       (1) Amount per day
       (2) Pattern over past 5 years, 1 year
       (3) Drinks more coffee when anxious?
       (4) Physiological effects
    d. Sleep
       (1) Has sleep pattern altered recently or in past year?
       (2) Sleep needs being met (fatigue)?
       (3) Concerns about interruptions at night (e.g., pain, SOB, nocturia, light sleeping, insomnia—specify difficulty falling asleep, staying asleep, awakening too early in morning)
       (4) Excessive napping during day
       (5) Inability to stay awake
       (6) Describe *all* client efforts to regulate sleep (e.g., drugs, prescriptions, alcohol, warm milk, reading)

   e. Other
     (1) Overeating, sporadic eating
     (2) Nail biting
     (3) Withdrawal (e.g., sleeping)
18. Financial status
   a. Sources
   b. Adequacy
   c. Recent changes in resources/expenditures

HEALTH MAINTENANCE EFFORTS

1. General statement of client's own physical fitness
2. Exercise: amount, type, frequency
3. Dietary regulations: special efforts (describe in detail)
4. Mental health: special efforts, such as group therapy, meditation, yoga
5. Cultural or religious practices
6. How often does the client seek:
   (a) Physical health assessment
   (b) Dental health assessment
   (c) Vision health assessment

ENVIRONMENTAL HEALTH

1. General statement of client's assessment of environmental safety and comfort; is client's community safe?
2. Hazards of employment: inhalants, noise, heavy lifting, psychological stress, machinery
3. Hazards in the home: concern about fire, stairs to climb, inadequate heat, open gas heaters, inadequate toilet facilities, concern about pest control, inadequate space
4. Hazards in neighborhood: noise, water pollution, air pollution, inadequate police protection, heavy traffic on surrounding streets, isolation from neighbors, overcrowding
5. Community hazards: unavailability of grocery stores, laundry facilities, drugstore; no access to bus line
6. Safety assessment (Optional; to be used if client is disabled or has difficulty with activities of daily living. This section suggests some major hazards.)
   a. Gait and balance problems
     (1) Slippery or irregular surfaces (floors, icy sidewalks, rug edges, small rugs, risers on stairs not fastened down)
     (2) Obstructions or clutter (on stairs, extension cords)
     (3) Steep, dark stairs (cellar)
     (4) Bathtub slippery (oil in bath water)
     (5) Shoes without support, laces untied
     (6) Climbing: use of ladders to paint, make home repairs, replace light bulb, etc.

     (7) Clothing too long
     (8) Walking in heavy traffic areas
   b. Decreased vision
     (1) Insufficient illumination in home (dark hallways, stairways, no night light)
     (2) Glare from polished floors, excess lighting
     (3) Missing the bottom step
     (4) Bifocals (client has difficulty with far vision, descending stairs, curb)
     (5) Medication errors
   c. Decreased sensation to pain and heat
     (1) Hot bath water
     (2) Heating pads, hot water bottles
   d. Other
     (1) Fire hazards: loose sleeves over stove burner, electric cords frayed, open heaters, stove burners left on, smoking (especially in bed)
     (2) Driving and traffic accidents: slow reaction time, decreased vision, difficulty turning head with upper torso (arthritis), walking too slow for traffic signals

Clinical strategies

1. Many older people don't seem to "fit" into traditional clinics. If there is a tight appointment schedule, the examiner and client have time for little other than assessing immediate, acute problems.
   a. Older clients often have a long story to tell (especially medical history).
   b. Their reaction time may be slower. It takes longer for them to reflect and respond to questions.
   c. Many of them have had unpleasant experiences being hurried or pressured (in department stores, heavy traffic, etc.). They may enter the health care facility with a reluctance to take up your time.
   d. It takes *time* to develop trust with clients so that they will be willing to share their concerns.
2. If clinic (or employer) policies cannot be altered to meet geriatric client needs, some alternatives might be helpful.
   a. Gather and organize all available history data from other sources before interviewing the client.
   b. Ask the client to complete the medical history at home (if no vision or writing problems exist).
   c. Spread out the data base collection over several appointments.
   d. Supplement clinic visits with a home visit.
   e. Set aside 1 day a week or month for prolonged appointments to collect initial data base from new clients.

f. Insist that time be made available! Otherwise, the client's needs are not being fully assessed.
3. Visual and hearing losses can distort information exchange. The examiner may believe the client is confused; the client may merely have difficulty hearing the examiner. Limitations of hearing and sight must be assessed early in the interview.

4. Do not shout. This rarely helps in communicating with those who have diminished hearing. It often further distorts conversation.
5. Directly face the client for a full view of your face. Speak slowly and distinctly.
6. Refer to *clinical strategies* in the adult data base section for further suggestions.

Vocabulary

1. Chief complaint

2. Client (patient) profile

3. Closed question

4. Data base

5. Exacerbation

6. Health assessment

7. History

8. Incidence (of a symptom)

9. Incomplete data base

10. Open-ended question

11. Precipitating factor

12. Predisposing factor

13. Remission

14. Sign

15. Significant negative

16. Symptom

17. Symptom analysis

SUGGESTED READINGS
General

Bates, Barbara: A guide to physical examination, ed. 2, Philadelphia, 1979, J. B. Lippincott Co., pp 8-30.

Diekelmann, Nancy: Primary health care of the well adult, New York, 1977, McGraw-Hill Book Co., pp. 213-235.

Engle, George L., and Morgan, William L.: Interviewing the patient, London, England, 1973, W. B. Saunders Co., Ltd.

Mahoney, Elizabeth A., Verdisco, Laurie, and Shortridge, Lillie: How to collect and record a health history, Philadelphia, 1976, J. B. Lippincott Co.

Malasanos, Lois, Barkauskas, Violet, Moss, Muriel, and Stoltenberg-Allen, Kathryn: Health assessment, St. Louis, 1977, The C. V. Mosby Co., pp. 11-41, 56-61.

Patient assessment: taking a patient history, Programmed instruction, Am. J. Nurs. **74**(2): 293-324, 1974.

Prior, John A., and Silberstein, Jack S.: Physical diagnosis: the history and examination of the patient, ed. 5, St. Louis, 1977, The C. V. Mosby Co., pp. 5-35.

Pediatric

Bates, Barbara: A guide to physical examination, ed. 2, Philadelphia, 1979, J. B. Lippincott Co., pp. 15-18.

Brown, Marie Scott, and Murphy, Mary Alexander: Ambulatory pediatrics for nurses, New York, 1975, McGraw-Hill Book Co., pp. 1-34.

DeAngelis, Catherine: Basic pediatrics for the primary health care provider, Boston, 1975, Little, Brown & Co., pp. 1-14.

Erickson, Marcene: Assessment and management of developmental changes in children, St. Louis, 1976, The C. V. Mosby Co.

Malasanos, Lois, Barkauskas, Violet, Moss, Muriel, and Stoltenberg-Allen, Kathryn: Health assessment, St. Louis, 1977, The C. V. Mosby Co., pp. 419-421.

Pillitteri, Adele: Nursing care of the growing family: a child health text, Boston, 1977, Little, Brown & Co., pp. 121-141, 163-169, 187-193, 213-224, 241-249.

Geriatric

Brown, Mollie: Readings in gerontology, ed. 2, St. Louis, 1978, The C. V. Mosby Co.

Burnside, Irene M.: Nursing and the aged, New York, 1976, McGraw-Hill Book Co., pp. 81-91, 398-419, 488-503.

Combs, Karen L.: Preventative care in the elderly, Am. J. Nurs. **78**(8):1339-1341, Aug., 1978.

Diekelmann, Nancy: Pre-retirement counseling, Am. J. Nurs. **78**(8):1337-1338, Aug., 1978.

Dresen, Shiela E.: Autonomy: a continuing developmental task, Am. J. Nurs. **78**(8):1334-1346, Aug., 1978.

Gotz, Bridget E.: Drugs and the elderly, Am. J. Nurs. **78**(8):1347-1351, Aug., 1978.

Hogstel, Mildred: How do the elderly view their world? Am. J. Nurs. **78**(8):1335-1336, Aug., 1978.

Kalish, Richard: Late adulthood: perspectives on human development, Monterey, Calif., 1975, Brooks/Cole Publishing Co., pp. 22-46.

Katz, Sidney, Ford, Amasa B., Moskowitz, Roland, Jackson, Beverly A., and Jaffe, Marjorie: Studies of illness in the aged. The index of ADL: a standardized measure of biological and psychosocial function, J.A.M.A. **185**:94-99, Sept., 1963.

Storz, Rita R.: The role of a professional nurse in a health maintenance program, Nurs. Clin. North Am. **7**(2):207-223, June, 1972.

CHAPTER 2

General and mental status assessment

When a practitioner first encounters a client (perhaps from across the room), a steady stream of data can be observed. Some of it may not operate at a conscious level. The examiner may quickly decide that the client looks "ill," "depressed," "alert," or "pleasant." Many of those observations cannot be classified under body systems, but they are vitally important and must be reported in concrete terms. The word *ill* does not convey a clear message to the reader. The following description does:

Skin is ashen, cool to touch, and moist. The client is slumped in a chair, and body and extremities appear limp. Client does not establish eye contact and responds to all questions in a monotone "yes" or "no."

Observation skills are enhanced through practice and a concentrated awareness of incoming perceptions. Every element of the examiner's behavior should be deliberate and focused on the client. A simple handshake indicates the client's ability to extend the arm, to firmly grip the hand, to respond with a smile or facial expression acknowledging an introduction, and to establish and maintain eye contact. It also permits the examiner to feel the coolness, warmth, dryness, or moisture of the palm.

The purpose of this chapter is to clarify and organize specific, observable behaviors that are valid indications of the client's general state as well as emotional and mental well-being. Note that it is impossible to include all possible behaviors which a client might exhibit. This chapter contains descriptions representative of some more commonly found behaviors.

Cognitive objectives

At the end of this unit the learner will demonstrate knowledge of assessment of the client's general and mental status by the ability to do the following:
1. Identify meanings associated with the holistic concept.
2. Identify major components of the general assessment.

3. Identify some common behaviors associated with mild to moderate anxiety.
4. Identify some common behaviors associated with moderate to severe anxiety.
5. Identify some common behaviors associated with depression.
6. Identify methods by which an examiner can validate the suspicion that a client is disoriented.
7. Identify characteristics of behaviors associated with hallucinations.
8. Identify some disorders that can disrupt thought content.
9. Identify selected pediatric and geriatric variations of behaviors associated with general and mental status.
10. Define the terms in the vocabulary section.

Clinical objectives

At the end of this unit the learner will perform a systematic assessment of the general and mental status of the client, demonstrating the ability to do the following:
1. Describe specific behaviors related to observation of:
   a. Client's initial response to examiner
   b. Body appearance
   c. Posture
   d. Body movements
   e. Gait
   f. Facial expression
   g. Vocal tones
   h. Speech patterns: pace, clarity, word and sentence delivery, accent or foreign language
   i. Apparel
   j. Grooming/hygiene
   k. Client odors
   l. General mannerisms
2. Describe specific behaviors indicating the client's cognitive functions:
   a. Orientation to person, place, time
   b. Attention span and concentration ability

c. Memory—recent and remote
d. Ability to make judgments
e. Abstract reasoning ⎫
f. Underlying intelligence ⎪
  (1) Client's access to basic ⎬ Optional history
     information ⎪ questions
  (2) Vocabulary ⎪
  (3) Similarities ⎪
g. Ability to read and write ⎭

3. Describe specific behaviors indicating the client's emotional status.
4. Describe specific behaviors indicating the client's ability to sustain a clear thinking process: coherency, thought content, clarity of perceptions.
5. Summarize results of the assessment with a written description of findings.

History related to mental status assessment additional to data base

Most of the information needed for the assessment of the "normal" client's mental status can be obtained through the use of the general questions in the *psychosocial history* in Chapter 1. Basically, these questions ask the client: How do you feel about yourself? Are you living in a relatively low-stress environment? and Are your coping abilities adequate to meet the stressors that you encounter in your daily living?

The answers to these questions can become more apparent by observing the client's general behavior (described subsequently). If the client's self-assessment and the examiner's assessment are congruent and if the results indicate that the client is coping adequately to meet personal needs, it is not necessary to pursue further questioning. However, if there is an incongruity between what the client states and the behavior displayed, if behavior disturbances are noted, or if activities of daily living are interrupted, the following detailed questions are helpful.

1. Anxiety or depressive states
   a. Do you have difficulty falling asleep, staying asleep, or being wakeful early in the morning?
   b. Describe your general mood in the morning.
   c. Have you noticed any marked changes in appetite or eating habits?
   d. Have you recently lost or gained weight?
   e. Do you have periods of despondency or nervousness to the extent that you feel unable to cope? If so, how do you treat yourself? Is it effective?
   f. Do you ever have crying spells?
   g. Have there been any marked changes in your sexual habits or desires?
   h. Have you noticed any change in the amount of energy you have to accomplish daily functions?
   i. Do you have any difficulty making decisions?
   j. Have you noticed any increase in irritability? Restlessness? Listlessness?
   k. Do you ever feel as though you do not care about anything?
   l. Do you spend much of your time alone? (Estimate number of waking hours per day, per week.)
   m. Who are your significant friends, that is, individuals you trust and who are available when you need them?
   n. If you had a crisis in the middle of the night, is there a resource you could seek; someone whom you know would be available?
   o. Have you ever thought of hurting yourself or ending your life? (If so, describe past methods and any specific plans for future attempts.)
   p. History of psychiatric counseling and use of medications have already been inquired about in the original data base, but they need to be carefully reviewed again.

2. Orientation
   a. Person: Can you give me your full name, address, and telephone number? Do you recall what my name is? Can you give me the full name of your closest relative?
   b. Place: Do you recall the name of this health agency? What part of town do you live in? What is the name of this town? This county?
   c. Time: Do you recall what day it is? The month? What year is it?

3. Attention span/concentration
   This can best be tested by giving the client a series of directions to follow—a sequence of behaviors. For example, "I would like you to reach into your purse, pull out your billfold, find an identification card, and show it to me. Then I would like you to empty your change purse on the table and put all the dimes and nickels in one stack and the quarters and pennies in another stack." Assuming there is no hearing, vision, or motor dysfunction, the client can be observed (and timed) going through the sequence of behaviors. If immobilized, the client can repeat a short story that you have related or describe a personal story. The examiner should be alert for (a) a total shift in direction of subject matter or sequence of behavior midway through the process, or (b) conversation or sequenced behavior dwindling into silence or inactivity before being completed.

4. Memory
   a. Recent: What did you have for breakfast this

morning? What time did you arrive at the agency today? What time was your appointment? Ask client to repeat a series of three to six numbers.

b. Remote: Can best be tested by having the client describe past medical history, high school graduation, first job, when married, etc. (provided the examiner is able to verify the information).

5. Ability to make judgments (offering solutions to hypothetical situations)
   a. What would you do if you saw a man picking someone's pocket right in front of you?
   b. What would you do if the newspaper deliverer came to the door to collect and you discovered you had no available change?

6. Abstract reasoning
   Ask the client to describe what the following proverbs mean:
   a. A bird in the hand is worth two in the bush.
   b. Not to decide is to decide.
   c. Every cloud has a silver lining.

7. Emotional status alterations (previous questions related to anxiety and depression are relevant in this area)
   a. Inquire again about stressors (e.g., money, intimate relationship, death or illness in family or friends, employment problems).
   b. How are you feeling right now?
   c. Do you consider your present feelings to be a problem in your daily life? If so, do you feel the problem is temporary or curable?
   d. Describe a typical day at home (and/or at school, work), and tell which times or experiences are easiest for you and which are difficult.
   e. Do you think you need help with your problem?

8. If underlying intelligence appears to be minimal, the following questions or tests will be helpful.
   a. Client's access to basic information. In what direction does the sun set? How many months are in a year? What month follows July? In what state is Philadelphia?
   b. Client's vocabulary level. Ask the client to define a list of words. The list should begin with simple words and progress to more diffi-

cult ones, for example, chair, trouble, tender, posture, maximum.

   c. Ability to see similarities. Ask the client to describe how the following words are alike: a carrot and a potato, a dog and a cat, a lantern and a candle, a rose and perfume, an automobile and a train, etc.
   d. Ability to read and write. Ask the client to write his name and address on a sheet of paper. Ask the client to read newsprint (also a test for near vision). *Note:* The inability to read and write is not always a measure of intelligence; however, this is useful information for a practitioner when devising a care plan.

9. Coherence and relevance dysfunction
   This is best tested by listening to the client talk. A detailed account of an event will usually not be completed if the client is incoherent.

10. Thought content disruptions
    a. Do you have certain thoughts or feelings that consistently return or disrupt your thinking? Are you able to control them?
    b. Do you ever lose control of your thoughts?
    c. Is your thinking the same as, as good as, or better than it was 5 years ago?
    d. Do you ever have trouble making decisions about everyday events?
    e. Do you have any dreadful or uncontrollable fears that keep returning?
    f. Do you ever have the feeling that something dreadful is going to happen?
    g. Do you feel that you have enemies? Is anyone trying to harm you, discredit you, or control you?
    h. Are you being watched or followed?
    i. Do you ever feel guilty about your behavior or your feelings?
    j. Do you ever have the feeling that you are losing touch with what is happening around you?

11. Perception distortion
    Do you ever hear voices or strange noises? Do you ever see visions, lights, or people that others cannot see? Do you ever experience strange odors or tastes? Have you ever experienced strange sensations (warm, cold, or pressure) on your skin?

Clinical guidelines

The student will:	To identify:	
	Normal	**Deviations from normal**
1. Observe the whole client and the client's interaction with the environment for: **a.** Client's initial response to examiner 1. Examiner introduces self, clarifies client's name, offers hand in greeting, and sits down to be at eye level with client	Client responds with smile or facial expression acknowledging examiner's presence Establishes eye contact Offers own name Extends hand in greeting	Client does not attain or maintain eye contact; does not acknowledge presence of examiner with facial expression, body gesture, or extension of hand Client may jump up, interrupt, or talk through examiner May be tearful or grimacing with pain
2. Examiner explains own role to client and begins interview with broad, open question	Client attentive, nodding head, maintaining eye contact, leaning toward examiner	Client looking away, eyes closed, eyes wandering around room Body pulled back in chair or leaning forward, tense posture
2. Make more specific observations regarding: **a.** Body appearance	(Height and weight measured with scale and results compared with standards) Body appears symmetrical in terms of size and placement of parts Body fat is sparse or moderate and evenly distributed Body parts present and in proportion Arm span equals height; distance between crown and pubis nearly equal to distance between pubis and soles of feet Skin color evenly distributed; skin smooth Muscles well or moderately developed or defined Hair evenly distributed over scalp, present in brows, lashes; moderate to light distribution over extremities, torso	Excessively tall or short Unilateral wasting or hypertrophy Asymmetrical body alignment Wasted, cachectic appearance; obesity, odd fat cushion distribution (e.g., confined to abdomen, hips, or buttocks) Arms or legs exceptionally short Extremities missing Arm span exceeds body height Prognathism Sallow, pale, flushed Patchy discoloration Marked wrinkling (localized or general) Muscle wasting (localized or general) Hirsutism Absence of scalp or body hair or excessive thinning
b. Posture	Shoulders back and relaxed; arms resting at sides or on chair; feet resting on floor; body relaxed in chair or on examining table	Asymmetrical posture (e.g., guarding or contractures) Tense posture, client at edge of chair, curled up in bed; back/neck rigid (client must move torso to view side) Slumped in chair
c. Body movements	Deliberate, smooth, and coordinated Client sits motionless for brief periods, alternating with body position shifts and gestures Client able to sit up in bed, swing legs to side; able to rise to standing position from sitting position with smooth even movements	Jerky, fidgety, constant movement; tremors (localized or general) Movements very slow or very fast; client fails to move certain parts (e.g., may be splinting or guarding a painful area) Hemiplegia or paraplegia Total absence or paucity of movement of arms, torso, or legs Movement uncoordinated (e.g., client slips when trying to rise; falls into chair rather than easing into it)
d. Gait	Steps even and smooth Heel-strike, midstance, push-off, and swing phases easily executed	Client watches feet while moving Stumbles, shuffles, staggers, limps (midstance phase shortened with painful leg or foot) Steps uneven

The student will:	To identify:	
	Normal	**Deviations from normal**
e. Facial expression	Eye contact maintained good part of time	One leg not functioning, lurching or propulsive, spastic or scissors gait No eye contact Staring fixedly (*Note:* A fixed gaze may indicate an effort to lip-read.)
	Smile alternating with serious or thoughtful expressions appropriate to conversation	Face immobile, expressionless Constant smile Grimacing (pain associated) Face puffy, flushed, pale; excessive perspiration on forehead, upper lip Dark circles under eyes (may be normal)
	Facial features symmetrical	Asymmetrical features Tearful expression Brow constantly furrowed Eyes darting around or constantly wandering about room Tics, tremors, lip biting or licking Squinting (inability to see)
f. Vocal tones	Moderate in pitch and volume; voice clear, firm, and audible; plentiful and varied inflections of tone in conversation	Very high pitched, loud, weak, inaudible Hoarseness Monotone
g. Speech 1. Pace	Moderate; may slow down with difficult or serious topic; may accelerate with excitement	Constantly rapid or very slow
2. Clarity	Words easily understood Enunciation of vowels and consonants clear	Slurred, garbled Client misses particular consonants at beginning of words or mispronounces vowels
3. Word and sentence pattern	Style of verbal response may be brief or loquacious; client pauses to think	Paucity of words (e.g., confined to yes/no responses) Constant flow of words and sentences Stammering Injection of numerous pauses (e.g., uhs, umms)
4. Accent or foreign language	Varies according to origin	Accent very heavy (determine whether client able to use English language sufficiently to convey and receive messages)
h. Apparel	Clothing fits body	Clothing too tight, too small, too large (*Note:* May indicate recent weight loss or gain.)
	Clean, pressed and "appropriate" for occasion (*Note:* Appropriate must be *broadly* defined; dress varies with age, life-style, financial resources, culture, climate.)	Dirty, rumpled Distinctly bizarre dress or combination of colors
i. Grooming/hygiene	Hair brushed, shiny Men: shaved or trimmed facial hair Nails clean (*Note:* Some employment leaves nails chronically dirty.) Women: moderate or no makeup Shoes fitted and clean (*Note:* Cleanliness is subjective and may or may not be an indication of normalcy.)	Hair disheveled, dull, broken ends Unshaved Dirty, ragged nails Bizarre makeup Shoes ill fitted, dirty
j. Odors	Absent (*Note:* Some cultures do not promote use of deodorants.)	Pungent ammonia or fetid breath odors Foul body odors
k. General mannerisms	Client may be quiet, thoughtful, somewhat passive (frightened), or active, moderately talkative, and demonstrative with body language	Tearful, angry, suspicious, questioning, evasive Constant laughter and inappropriate joking Markedly subdued

Continued.

Clinical guidelines—cont'd

The student will:	To identify:	
	Normal	**Deviations from normal**
	Mild to moderate anxiety (may be normal in a health alteration state; following are some common behaviors) 1. Client able to focus on conversation and respond appropriately 2. Increased alertness 3. Some muscle tension (leaning forward, listening intently) 4. Some fidgeting, restlessness 5. Speech more rapid, voice pitch higher 6. Rapid-fire questions and responses 7. Increased eye contact 8. Moderately increased perspiration	Moderate to severe anxiety (common signs and symptoms) 1. Client either very limited or totally unable to focus on present situation 2. Skin cold, clammy; pallor 3. Frequent wetting of lips, tongue 4. Palpitations 5. Breathlessness 6. Dizziness 7. Trembling 8. Chills 9. Urinary frequency 10. Diarrhea 11. Abdominal cramp 12. Tires easily 13. Chest pain Depression (some common behaviors, symptoms, signs) 1. Diminished body movements 2. Slow movements 3. Slouched posture 4. Voice often subdued, low in pitch and volume 5. Eye contact decreased 6. Smile absent or diminished 7. Sighing respirations 8. Tearfulness 9. Indecisive responses 10. Anorexia, weight loss 11. Lack of energy 12. Insomnia (in various forms) 13. Constipation 14. Nagging muscular pains, backaches (*Note:* Some depression is manifested by increased motor activity, agitation, tachycardia, or constant smile.)
	Client shows no acute distress signs Breathing even and moderately slow Facial expression relaxed	Shows acute distress signs, such as dyspnea, pain (client splints, guards a part, limits movement), grimacing, moaning, writhing, coughing, wheezing, marked lethargy, drowsiness

3. Observe mental status
  a. Cognitive functions
    1. Orientation to person, place, and time
	Client can indicate orientation to person, place, and time through discussion of history
	Specific questions should be used only if examiner cannot assess orientation through conversation and general health interview
		Client unable to deliver accurate biographical data (e.g., address, name)
		Client unable to name the agency that he is currently in
		Client unable to identify year, month (*Note:* Many "normal" people cannot recall the day of the month!)

2. Attention span and concentration	Client able to complete entire thought process (e.g., when describing a pain, client can recall location, duration, onset, character, etc. without wandering off subject)	Client unable to complete a thought; may digress in middle of sentence
3. Recent memory	Accurate responses to questions about very recent events (e.g., How did you get to the clinic this morning? What did you have for breakfast?)	Client unable to recall very recent events
4. Remote memory	Client's past medical history delivered accurately	Client unable to recall remote events

The student will:	To identify:	
	Normal	**Deviations from normal**
5. Ability to make judgments	Client usually indicates ability to make judgments when describing personal health care practices and decisions made about maintaining or following health care routines	No indication that client can perceive a particular situation accurately and follow through with appropriate decisions
6. Abstract reasoning (usually tested by asking client to explain proverbs)	Client offers appropriate explanation	Client unable to explain meaning
b. Emotional status, affect, mood	Client responds with smiles alternating with thoughtful or serious facial expressions appropriate to conversation Body behaviors indicate relaxation or mild to moderate anxiety Client describes self as well adjusted, generally happy, or appropriately concerned about present health alteration	Client demonstrates behavior indicating depression or moderate to severe anxiety or indicates through general questions that activities of daily living impeded or altered by mood, that coping capacity inadequate
c. Thought processes and perceptions		
1. Coherency and relevance	Client can complete entire thought (e.g., full symptom analysis description) without losing track of ideas or digressing Answers to examiner's questions direct and appropriate	Ideas run together within sentence or stream of thought Illogical ideas associated
2. Thought content	Consistent, logical, and free-flowing thinking demonstrated as client describes history and self	Thought process interrupted with signs of compulsive or obsessive ideas (going off on a tangent); marked doubting and indecisiveness; phobias; free-floating anxieties; ideas of persecution, delusion; ideas of reference; feelings of unreality
3. Perceptions	Client indicates to examiner, through descriptions of self, a consistent awareness of reality Client perceptions of objects and surroundings consistent with those of examiner Client able to accurately follow all directions: breathe deeply; sit up; walk to the other end of the room; tell me about your last hospitalization; etc.	Illusions Hallucinations interfere with client's flow of perceptions Psychotic client may demonstrate preoccupation with self and little or no interest in examiner activity Affect may be inappropriate Ritualistic, repetitive posturing or gestures may be evident Periods of complete immobility

Clinical strategies

1. The first 5 to 10 minutes of the interview belong to the client. The examiner can begin with a very broad question, such as "What brings you to the clinic today?" This enables the client to talk freely about concerns and priorities and enables the practitioner to observe the client's verbal, nonverbal, and general behavior patterns.

2. Remember that the client is probably observing the examiner with equal intensity. The examiner must be acutely aware of personal behavior so that feelings of concern, caring, concentration, and confidence are conveyed, as well as curiosity.

3. Remember that many clients are anxious when being examined. Normal mild to moderate anxiety may create a number of unusual behaviors—hyperactivity, stammering, excessive perspiration, excessive giggling, or listlessness. All these behaviors are worth noting in the final summary, but the examiner should be cautious about labeling behaviors as abnormal.

Sample recording

The client is a neatly attired, clean-shaven, 42-year-old man. Facial expressions are alert, appropriate to the conversation, and coupled with frequent eye contact with examiner. Varied vocal tones are well modulated, and speech is audible and articulate. Body movements are smooth and coordinated.

General mood is one of seriousness accompanied by mild postural tension and intense listening behaviors while symptoms are discussed. Conversation indicates orientation to time, person, place. Client is able to offer logical and reasonable contributions to the problem and past attempts at dealing with the difficulty.

History and clinical strategies associated with the pediatric client

1. The general and mental assessment of the child is patterned after that of the adult. The examiner must carefully observe the child interacting with the environment, the parents, and the examiner. Depending on the child's age and development the examiner should observe for various normal behaviors. Following is an initial summary. Other areas are further detailed in the data base and subsequent clinical chapters.

   The *newborn* should not mind being undressed or examined but will lie quietly on the examination table or the parent's lap (if not tired or cold) and will cooperatively allow the examiner to collect the appropriate assessment data.

   The examiner should collect history data prior to undressing the infant. During the history collection observe the interaction between parent and child and how the child responds to the parent's techniques. The data base chapter further describes specific information regarding parenting stresses and infant responses to stress.

   The *6-month- to 2-year-old child* is acutely aware of the environment, viewing the parent as protector and the examiner as the enemy. The examiner must evaluate the child with the assistance of the parent in eliciting various responses. During this time observe the parent-child interaction. If the child does not cooperate, how does the parent respond? Does the child have eye contact with the examiner? Does the child separate with difficulty from the parent?

   It is anticipated that the child will respond most favorably if examined while sitting on the parent's lap.

   The *child from ages 2 to 4 years* is curious to find out who the examiner is and what will take place

but still clings to the parent for security. After becoming familiar with the examiner, the child should relax and enter into game playing, conversation, and free expression of giggles and smiles. The examiner should again observe parent-child interactions and the child's ability to communicate and cooperate with the examiner.

The preschool *child from 4 to 6 years of age* will generally cooperate with the examiner and separate with ease from the parent. The examiner should evaluate the child's maturity, eye contact, attention span, and interaction with the parent.

In general, as the child matures, developmental progression, increased attention span, the ability to cooperate with the examiner, and decreased dependence on the parent should be observed. Any deviation from this should stimulate the examiner to develop a thorough behavioral profile for the child based on history and physical data.

2. The examiner must be alert to common behavioral problems in children and common behavioral concerns of parents. Although the actual mental status examination follows the same guidelines as for the adult client, other common problems or concerns that the examiner should screen for follow. In each of these situations the examiner should employ the elements of symptom analysis to develop a situational profile.

   a. Intellectual limitations of the child: the parent may feel the child is not performing up to capacity.

   b. Short attention span: the parent may feel that the child is unable to maintain concentration appropriate for age.

   c. Inability to problem-solve: the parent may express concern that the child is unable to perform tasks or solve problems appropriate for age.

   d. Communication difficulties: the child may have difficulty with speech development, eye contact, or communication with parents or peers.

   e. Variability: the child's mood is unpredictable; one moment happy or organized, the next minute unhappy or disorganized.

   f. Emotional immaturity: the child may lag in development, acting impulsively without thinking through the consequences, even though there has been previous experience with a similar problem.

   g. Hyperactivity: the child demonstrates an inappropriate amount of activity for age; the parent may state that the child has a difficult time sitting still or following through with an activity; may demonstrate a repetitive activity such as finger tapping.

h. Perception difficulties: the child may demonstrate a pattern of inappropriate behaviors that might be a sign of difficulties with perception. Common difficult concepts are the differences between right and left, up and down, in and out, before and after. The child may also demonstrate an inability to complete a puzzle appropriate for age, difficulty learning to tie a shoe, or difficulty screwing or unscrewing the cap on a jar.

i. Aloneness: the preschool or school-age child does not interact with or play with other children.

j. Change in routine: the child may have difficulty with or react violently to a change in routine.

k. Personal contact: the infant or child might not like to be cuddled; does not extend the arms to be picked up; or does not like to be held.

3. Other common stress behaviors that the examiner must note are thumb sucking, nail biting, teeth grinding, rocking, or stuttering.

4. In general, the examiner must assess how the child is developing and coping with the environment. As the examiner collects developmental, psychological, and physical data, patterns or collective signs that indicate how the child is coping with the environment and how the parent is coping with the child must be observed. Areas of the text most likely to facilitate this collective analysis are *adult mental health status* and *pediatric areas* of the data base, musculoskeletal, and neurological chapters.

History and clinical strategies associated with the geriatric client

Elderly clients can be observed and assessed in the same manner as adult clients.

1. It is helpful to remember that elderly individuals are frequently subject to a greater number and intensity of stressors than are many younger people. They invariably suffer losses: loss of friends and loved ones through death, loss of occupation through retirement, and loss of a youthful body and energy. They are frequently subject to changes in living conditions, financial status, and positions of authority and impact previously ensured in work, parenting, and social environments. There is no indication that the number and intensity of stressors can predict the individual's responses; in terms of depression, withdrawal, anxiety, or grieving, however, the examiner must be alert for signals indicating a maladaptive response.

2. The examiner should also be alert for signs of confusion. Many elderly people are confused as a result of physical illness. Confusion may be the first indicator of an altered health state, and its onset is usually sudden. Early indicators of confusion are:

a. Limited attention span (losing track of thought in midsentence or indicating loss of attention through nonverbal behavior such as breaking eye contact during a conversation)

b. Loss of recent memory (remote memory may remain intact)

c. Emotion lability (sudden episodes of tearfulness)

d. Decreased use of judgment (inability to think through a situation and make decisions)

e. Confusion that is exaggerated at night (wandering or sleeplessness) and diminishes or disappears during the day

3. Some physiological states that might be associated with confusion follow:

a. Infectious process

b. Cardiorespiratory disturbances

c. Metabolism disorders

d. Trauma

e. Alcohol or drug abuse

f. Neoplasms

Most often, confusion associated with altered health states is reversible.

This kind of confusion is usually compounded when elderly individuals are admitted to hospitals. Loss of a familiar environment and daily routines creates complex problems.

Mild confusion can sometimes be masked in clients who have well-preserved social skills. They can participate in polite conversations and skirt issues or direct questions that they are unsure of.

Hearing loss or visual impairment can be mistaken for confusion. The examiner should assess early in the interview the client's ability to receive communications.

4. Organic brain syndrome is not a disease. The term describes brain changes that result in a variety of altered client behaviors. The onset is usually slow and can be manifested in an intermittent or progressive fashion. A stable environment and a limited number of stressors can be therapeutic. Altered behaviors associated with this syndrome vary greatly according to the individual clients. Some common behaviors are:

a. Diminished emotional responsiveness

b. Disorientation (especially to time and place)

c. Depression (often in the form of apathy or withdrawal)

d. Confabulation

e. Agitation

f. Paranoic beliefs

g. Loss of interest in appearance
h. Shortened attention span
i. Decreased intellectual skills
j. Decreased ability to make judgments

5. The examiner must assess the client's use of drugs (over the counter and prescribed) and alcohol if confusion or disorientation is suspected.

Vocabulary

1. Affect

2. Catatonic

3. Compulsion

4. Conversion reaction

5. Delusion

6. Dysarthria

7. Dyslexia

8. Dysphasia

9. Dysphonia

10. Echolalia

11. Euphoria

12. Hallucination

13. Illusion

14. Neologism

15. Neurotic

16. Obsession

17. Perseveration

18. Phobia

19. Prognathism

20. Psychotic

21. Rumination

22. Sensorium

23. Sentient

24. Schizoid

25. Schizophrenia

Cognitive self-assessment

1. The holistic nature of humans means:
   - ☐ a. that they are the sum of all their parts
   - ☐ b. that they are dynamic and ever-changing
   - ☐ c. that they constantly interact with their environment
   - ☐ d. that they are sentient beings
   - ☐ e. that they are fluctuating energy fields
   - ☐ f. all the above
   - ☐ g. all except e
   - ☐ h. a, b, and c
   - ☐ i. all except a
2. Name eight general areas of behavior that you would look for while performing a general assessment, beginning with:
   a. posture

   b. movement

   c. appearance

   d. response to examiner

   e. odor

   f. grooming

   g. expression

   h. speech

3. A symptom that a client might exhibit if mildly anxious is:
   - ☐ a. breathlessness
   - ☐ b. dizziness
   - ☑ c. increased alertness
   - ☐ d. abdominal cramps
   - ☐ e. none of the above
4. A sign of severe anxiety is:
   - ☐ a. intense listening
   - ☐ b. increased alertness

☐ c. constipation
☒ d. inability to clearly focus on present situation
☐ e. none of the above

5. Which of the following behavior(s) might be seen with depression?
☐ a. slow body movements
☐ b. indecisive responses
☐ c. constipation
☐ d. b and c
☒ e. a, b, and c

6. When an individual appears to be disoriented, the examiner can validate this suspicion by:
☐ a. asking the client to name the present date
☐ b. asking the client to describe personal feelings
☐ c. asking the client to define words on a vocabulary list
☒ d. all the above
☐ e. none of the above

7. If an individual can follow a series of brief, simple directions without prompting, you know that the client is:
☐ a. intelligent
☒ b. able to control attention span
☐ c. not depressed
☐ d. not hallucinating
☐ e. none of the above

8. Hallucinations:
☐ a. are most often auditory
☐ b. can be visual
☐ c. can be experienced through taste
☐ d. are not always obvious to the observer
☐ e. are always obvious to the careful observer
☒ f. all except e
☐ g. a, b, and e
☐ h. a, b, and d
☐ i. b and d
☐ j. all except d

9. Thought content can be disrupted by:
☐ a. free-floating anxiety
☐ b. phobia
☐ c. obsessive ideas
☐ d. ideas of persecution
☐ e. ideas of reference
☐ f. b, c, and d
☐ g. all except a
☒ h. all the above
☐ i. none of the above
☐ j. a, d, and e

SUGGESTED READINGS
General

American Journal of Nursing, Programmed Instruction: Anxiety: recognition and intervention, **65**:9, Sept., 1965.

Bates, Barbara: A guide to physical examination, ed. 2, Philadelphia, 1979, J. B. Lippincott Co., pp. 359-366.

Jones, Dorothy A., Dunbar, Claire Ford, and Jirovec, Mary Marmoll:

Medical-surgical nursing, New York, 1978, McGraw-Hill Book Co., pp. 3-22.

Malasanos, Lois, Barkauskas, Violet, Moss, Muriel, and Stoltenberg-Allen, Kathryn: Health assessment, St. Louis, 1977, The C. V. Mosby Co., pp. 89-96, 379-387.

Snyder, Joyce Cameron, and Wilson, Margo Foltz: Elements of a psychological assessment, Am. J. Nurs. **77**(2):235-239, Feb., 1977.

Pediatric

Alexander, Mary, and Brown, Marie Scott: Physical examination: the why and how of examination, Nursing '73 **3**:25-28, July, 1973.

DeAngelis, Catherine: Basic Pediatrics for the primary health care provider, Boston, 1975, Little, Brown & Co., pp. 337-378.

Erickson, Marcene: Assessment and management of developmental changes in children, St. Louis, 1976, The C. V. Mosby Co., pp. 1-15.

Pillitteri, Adele: Nursing care of the growing family: a child health

text, Boston, 1977, Little, Brown & Co., pp. 17-22, 710-713, 777-782.

Geriatric

Burnside, Irene Mortenson: Nursing and the aged, New York, 1976, McGraw-Hill Book Co., pp. 136-181.

Caird, F. I., and Judge, T. G.: Assessment of the elderly patient, London, 1977, Pitman Medical Publishing Co., Ltd, pp. 87-98.

Comfort, Alex: Non-threatening mental testing of the elderly, J. Am. Geriatr. Soc. 26(6):216-262, 1978.

Dodd, Marilyn J.: The confused patient: assessing mental status, Am. J. Nurs. **78**(9)1500-1503, Sept., 1978.

Steinberg, Franz U., editor: Cowdry's the care of the geriatric patient, St. Louis, 1976, The C. V. Mosby Co., pp. 321-350.

CHAPTER 3

Assessment of the integumentary system

Cognitive objectives

At the end of this unit the learner will demonstrate knowledge of assessment of the integument by the ability to do the following:

1. Identify relationships and primary functions of the following integumentary components:
   a. Stratum corneum
   b. Epidermis
   c. Dermis
   d. Sebaceous gland
   e. Eccrine sweat gland
   f. Apocrine sweat gland
   g. Subcutaneous tissue
   h. Keratin
   i. Melanin
2. Identify differentiating characteristics of twelve common primary and secondary lesions:
   a. Macule
   b. Papule
   c. Nodule
   d. Vesicle
   e. Bulla
   f. Pustule
   g. Wheal
   h. Scale
   i. Crust
   j. Erosion
   k. Scar
   l. Fissure
3. Identify client conditions or situations that increase the importance of periodic skin assessment.
4. Identify some systemic or local conditions that affect the skin, hair, and nails.
5. Define the terms in the vocabulary section.
6. Identify selected pediatric characteristics of the integumentary examination, including:
   a. Newborn characteristics
   b. Common alterations in pigmentation
   c. Common lesions
   d. Common developmental changes
7. Identify selected common integumentary characteristics of the geriatric client.

Clinical objectives

At the end of this unit the learner will perform a systematic assessment of the integumentary system, demonstrating the ability to do the following:

1. Obtain a pertinent health history from a client.
2. Demonstrate and describe the results of inspection and palpation of the following skin characteristics:
   a. Color
   b. Moisture
   c. Temperature
   d. Texture
   e. Thickness variations
   f. Mobility and turgor
   g. Hygiene
   h. Lesions
3. Demonstrate and describe the results of inspection and palpation of nails for:
   a. Configuration
   b. Consistency
   c. Color
   d. Adherence to nail bed
4. Demonstrate and describe the results of inspection of hair for:
   a. Distribution and configuration
   b. Texture
   c. Color
   d. Quantity
   e. Parasites
5. Summarize results of the assessment with a written description of findings.

Health history related to integumentary assessment additional to data base

1. Is there a family history of skin problems (chronic, allergic, intermittent, or acute in nature)?
2. Does anyone at home (or closely associated with client) have any skin lesions, itching, or infections?
3. Does the client use any lotions, home remedies, or local applications of any kind on the skin?
4. Inquire about the client's assessment of the "delicacy" or "sensitivity" of the skin. Do cuts, bruises, or minor injuries heal fast enough and without complications? Does the client feel diminished or heightened skin sensitivity to discomfort?
5. What are the client's sun exposure circumstances (outdoor work) or sunbathing habits?
6. Facial care: What cosmetics, soaps, or cleansing agents are used? How does the client manage pimples or minor lesions (by squeezing or picking)?
7. Hair care: What shampoos, rinses, coloring, or lubricating agents are used? Have there been any recent changes in hair care patterns?
8. Does the client have difficulty cutting or clipping fingernails or toenails? What instruments are used?
9. Itching (sometimes unaccompanied by rash or redness) should be located. Is it generalized or more intense in certain areas? Is it intermittent; more pronounced at certain times of the day (or night)? How severe is it? Does it interfere with daily activities (especially sleep)? Does the client have problems with scratching?
10. Dry skin: Is it more intense in certain areas of the body or generalized? Does client use bath oils or powder? How would the client estimate the degree of humidity at home or at work (especially in the winter)? Is the skin dryness seasonal, intermittent, constant? Is it associated with itching?
11. If a client has a skin problem, these additional questions are warranted:
    a. Is the problem seasonal?
    b. Is it associated with stress?
    c. Are there occupational hazards (e.g., skin contact materials, radiation, abnormal lighting)?
    d. Inquire again about drugs being taken (prescribed and over the counter), especially recent changes.
    e. Is the problem associated with leisure activities (e.g., weekends, hiking, swimming, yard work, hobbies involving use of special materials)?
    f. How is the client adjusting to the problem (e.g., use of wig or excessive cosmetics to cover up the problem, fear of rejection, fear of infecting others)?
12. Multiple cuts or bruises need to be followed by careful inquiry. The examiner should consider the possibility of abuse. Posing direct or indirect questions about the source of injury will depend on the situation, the condition of the client, the relationship between practitioner and client, and information gathered previously regarding the client and the family.
13. Multiple cuts or bruises might also indicate frequent falls. The underlying cause for the falls should be considered (e.g., dizziness, alcohol or drug abuse, sensorium disturbances).

Clinical guidelines

| | To identify: | |
The student will:	Normal	Deviations from normal
1. Be certain that there is adequate light available		
2. Inspect and palpate the skin for:		
a. Color		
1. General tone (best determined in areas of body not exposed to sun)	Deep to light brown, whitish pink to ruddy pink, olive, and yellow overtones	Diffuse, marked hyperpigmentation
		General pallor (loss of underlying red tones in dark skin)
		Ashen grey appearance
		Yellow tone (jaundice)
		General redness or flush
2. Uniformity	Sun-darkened areas	Localized hyperpigmentation (especially in skinfolds, nail beds, old scars)

Continued.

Clinical guidelines–cont'd

The student will:	To identify:	
	Normal	**Deviations from normal**
	Areas of lighter pigmentation in dark-skinned individuals (palms, nail beds, lips) (Fig. 3-1)	Pigmentation around ankles (Fig. 3-2) Patchy or localized hypopigmentation (associated with inflammation, scaling, atrophy, scarring)

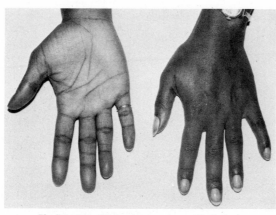

Fig. 3-1. Area of light pigmentation on black skin.

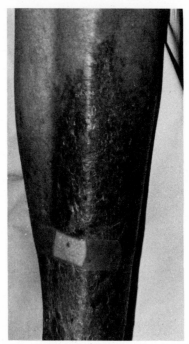

Fig. 3-2. Stasis dermatosis pigmentation.

The student will:	Normal	Deviations from normal
	Labile pigment areas often associated with use of birth control pills or pregnancy (cheeks, forehead, axillae, linea alba, areolae, flexor surface of wrist, genital area) (Fig. 3-3) Crinkled skin areas appear darker (knees, elbows) Calloused areas appear yellowish (palms, soles)	
3. Examine extremities at heart level		Marked pallor or mottling of extremities (especially when elevated) Deep, dusky red color of dependent extremities Cyanosis (dusky, bluish pallor), especially lips, area around mouth, nail beds, extremities
	Dark-skinned (Mediterranean origin) individual may have lips with bluish hue Vascular flush areas (cheeks, neck, upper chest, genital area) may appear red, especially with excitement or anxiety Skin color masking incurred through use of cosmetics, tanning agents	
b. Moisture	Dampness in skinfolds Increased perspiration associated with warm environs or activity Wet palms, scalp, forehead, axillae often associated with anxiety	Excessive dryness and flaking Excessive perspiration Onset of excessive oiliness
c. Surface temperature (examiner's hands should be warm)		Excessive coolness (general or localized), especially extremities Excessive heat (general or localized)
d. Texture: stroke inner aspect of client's arms with finger pads	Smooth, even, soft	Rough, dry, coarse Velvety smooth
e. Thickness	Wide body variation Thickness increases in response to pressure and rubbing (e.g., calluses)	Excessive thickness (generalized change in condition or localized, especially extremities)

	To identify:	
The student will:	**Normal**	**Deviations from normal**

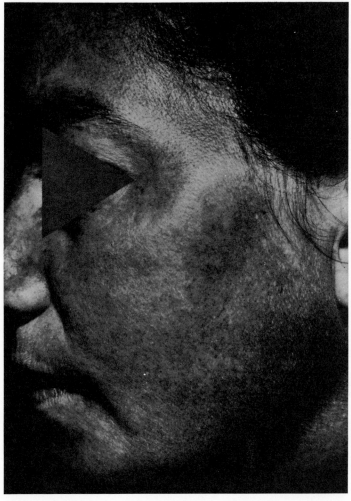

Fig. 3-3. Pigmentation associated with pregnancy. (From Stewart, W., Danto, J., and Maddin, S.: Dermatology: diagnosis and treatment of cutaneous disorders, ed. 4, St. Louis, 1978, The C. V. Mosby Co.)

f. Mobility and turgor: pick up skin under clavicle where there is usually no excess (Fig. 3-4)

Skin moves easily when lifted and returns to place immediately when released

Skin remains in pinched position and returns slowly to place (tenting) (Fig. 3-5)

Decreased mobility with edema (skin appears shiny, taut)

Edema present (legs, feet, fingers, eyelids)

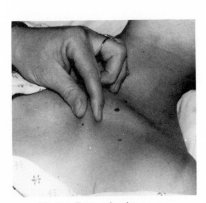

Fig. 3-4. Testing for skin turgor.

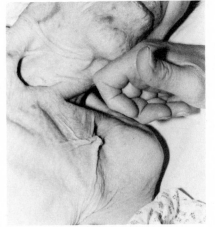

Fig. 3-5. Tenting associated with loss of skin turgor.

Continued.

Clinical guidelines—cont'd

The student will:	To identify:	
	Normal	**Deviations from normal**
g. Hygiene	Skin clean, free of odor	Crusted, dirty Marked body odor
h. Surface alterations or lesions	Striae (stretch marks, usually silver or pinkish) (Fig. 3-6) Freckles (prominent in sun-exposed areas) Some birthmarks Some flat and raised nevi (in various shades of brown, tan, or near skin color) Patchy depigmented areas (vitiligo unassociated with inflammation, scaling, or scarring) (Fig. 3-7)	Macules, papules, nodules, vesicles, bullae, pustules, wheals, scales, crusts, erosions, scars, fissures, erythema Increased vascularity Mixed lesions

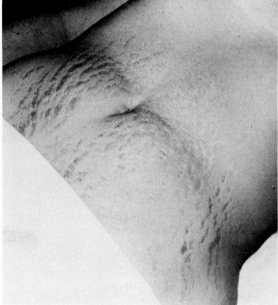

Fig. 3-6. Abdominal striae.

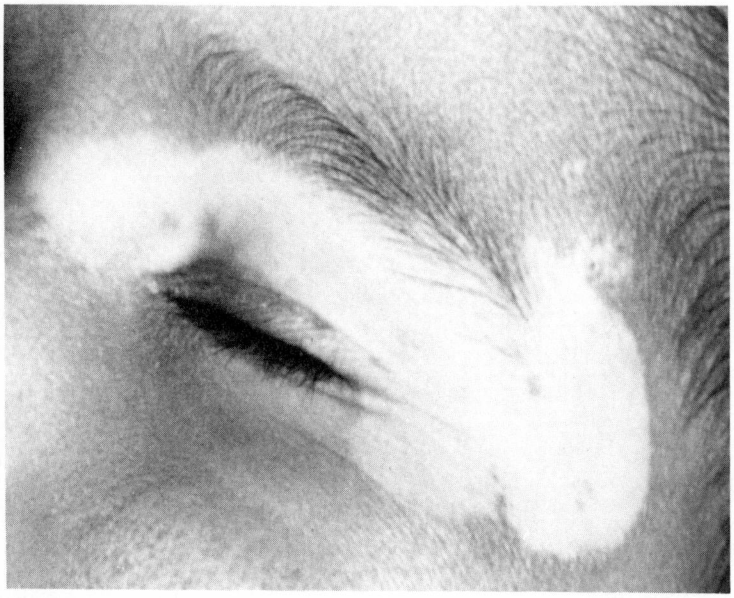

Fig. 3-7. Vitiligo. (From Stewart, W., Danto, J., and Maddin, S.: Dermatology: diagnosis and treatment of cutaneous disorders, ed. 4, St. Louis, 1978, The C. V. Mosby Co.)

i. Trauma-induced surface alterations		Bruises, scabs Lacerations Needle marks
3. Inspect and palpate the nails for:		
a. Configuration	Nail edges smooth and rounded Nail base angle 160° Nail surface flat or slightly curved	Edges bitten, ragged Clubbing Spooning, transverse depressions
b. Consistency	Smooth, hard surface Uniform thickness	Excessive and/or irregular thickening; flaking
c. Color	Variations of pink Dark-skinned individual may have pigment deposits in nail beds	Cyanotic Very pale Splinter hemorrhages Redness at nail bed (paronychia)
d. Adherence to nail bed	Nail base feels firm when palpated	Nail base not firm Nail base tender on palpation
4. Inspect and palpate scalp and hair for:		
a. Surface characteristics	Scalp smooth Hair shiny	Scalp flaky; scaling, reddened, or open lesions Hair dull
b. Distribution and configuration	"Normal" varies with individuals; hair may be present on scalp, lower face, nares, ears, axillae, anterior chest around nipples, arms, legs, back of hands and feet, back, and buttocks	Sudden or marked increase or decrease in body hair

The student will:	To identify:	
	Normal	Deviations from normal
	Female pubic configuration forms inverted triangle (Fig. 3-8) (hairline may extend up linea alba) Male configuration is upright triangle with hair extending up linea alba to umbilicus (Fig. 3-9)	Alteration of pubic configuration appropriate to male or female

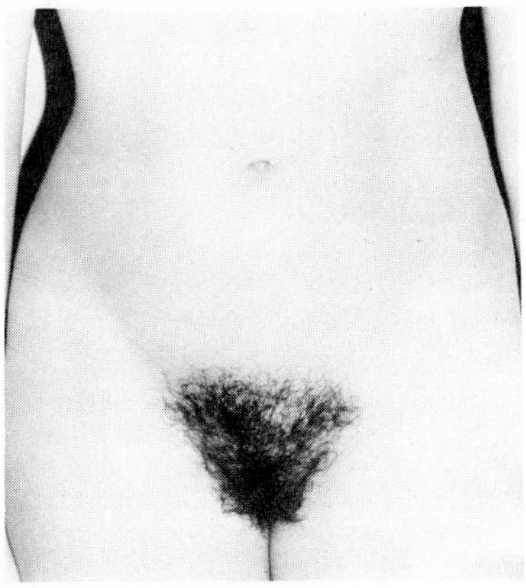

Fig. **3-8.** Normal triangular configuration of female pubic hair.

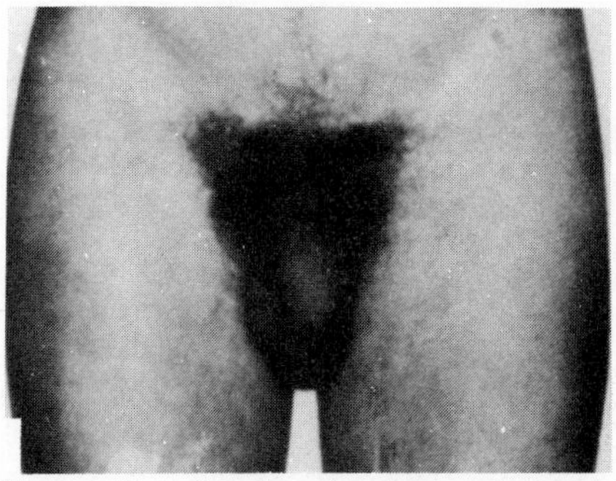

Fig. **3-9.** Normal male pubic hair configuration. (From Tanner, J. M.: Growth at adolescence, ed. 2, Oxford, England, 1962, Blackwell Scientific Publications.)

The student will:	Normal	Deviations from normal
c. Texture	Scalp hair may be fine or coarse Fine hair over body Coarse hair in pubic and axillary areas	Increased coarseness of body hair Dryness, brittleness, or coarseness of scalp hair
d. Color	Wide variation from pale blond to black Color may be masked or changed with rinses, dyes	
5. Inspect hair for: a. Quantity	"Normal" varies according to individuals Gradual symmetrical balding of scalp hair in some men	Excess body hair—hirsutism Female: hair growth intensified on upper lip, chin, cheeks, chest, and from pubic crest to umbilicus Excessive loss of body hair Scalp hair: asymmetrical or patchy balding (alopecia) Marked hair loss
b. Parasites		Body lice (especially in pubic and axillary areas) Head lice and nits in scalp

Clinical strategies

1. Be certain to have the client completely undressed for skin inspection. Examination of face and exposed extremities does not constitute a full assessment. Clients may be unaware of lesions or problems in areas that are inaccessible to them (e.g., the back, under skinfolds, bottom of feet).
2. Be certain to carefully inspect skinfolds (e.g., axillary, groin, area under pendulous breasts). These areas are usually warm and moist and may harbor bacteria, parasites (e.g., scabies), and fungi. Obese people have more skinfolds, so inspecting their skin will probably consume more time.
3. Be certain to remove shoes and socks or stockings to inspect *bottom of feet* and *between toes!* Elderly people and diabetics sometimes manifest decreased sensitivity to pain (especially in extremities). Open, infected, ulcerated lesions can be missed when direct inspection is neglected.

4. Long, jagged, thick toenails should be viewed as a problem. Inquire about the client's attempts to cut them. Sometimes elderly, obese, or disabled people cannot reach their feet to provide self-care.
5. Long toenails can interfere with shoe fit.
6. Skin lesions or surface alterations should be described in terms of the following:
   a. Distribution and location (e.g., confined to face, trunk, extremities, sun-exposed areas, or general distribution with no pattern; or placement on symmetrical body parts)
   b. Surface and color characteristics (e.g., confluent, macular)
   c. Lesion dimension: use metric system; do not compare tumors or nodules to fruits or vegetables
   d. Color and condition of surrounding tissue
7. Wearing gloves is appropriate when examining open lesions. Washing hands is a necessity after any inspection.

<table>
<tr><td>

Sample recording

Skin: Pink, moist, soft, warm, and elastic. No lesions, discolorations, excess thickening, trauma, odor, or edema.

Nails: Pink, smooth, and hard. No clubbing, biting, or thickening or tenderness on palpation.

Body hair: Moderate, uniform distribution. Male pubic configuration.

Scalp and hair: Moderately thick, evenly distributed brown hair. Scalp clean. No flaking, lesions, or tenderness.

</td></tr>
</table>

History and clinical strategies associated with the pediatric client

1. Although assessment of the skin is important at all stages of a child's development, findings can be assigned to one of four categories:
   a. Integumentary characteristics present at birth that are considered deviations within normal limits, including mongolian spots, hemangiomas, café au lait spots, and lanugo
   b. Integumentary characteristics present at birth or shortly thereafter that may indicate disease, including jaundice appearing within 24 hours of birth, cyanosis in the nonchilled infant, tufts of hair over the spine or sacrum, or dermatoglyphics of the palm
   c. Integumentary characteristics that change as the child develops, including appearance of pubic and axillary hair or acne
   d. Integumentary characteristics that occur as either primary or secondary lesions due to local irritations, communicable diseases, or infectious processes, including the following*:
      (1) Primary lesions
         (a) Poor skin turgor due to dehydration
         (b) *Macules* seen in rubella, scarlet fever, or rubeola
         (c) *Papules* seen in ringworm, pityriasis rosea, psoriasis, or eczema
         (d) *Vesicles* seen in poison ivy, chickenpox, and shingles
         (e) *Bullae* seen in burns or on the palms and soles of children with scarlet fever
         (f) *Pustules* seen in impetigo, scabies, or acne
         (g) *Wheals* seen in hives or insect bites
      (2) Secondary lesions, which are alterations in

*Adapted from Alexander, M., and Brown, M. S.: Pediatric physical diagnosis for nurses, New York, 1974, McGraw-Hill Book Co., p. 19.

the skin due to another problem, such as trauma, unclean surface area, or continuous irritation:
   (a) *Scales* seen in very dry skin or cradle cap
   (b) *Crusts* (dried blood, scales, pus) from infected dermatitis, such as impetigo
   (c) *Excoriation* seen in scrapes after falling
   (d) *Erosions or ulcers* seen in infected, sloughing tissue or pressure sores
   (e) *Scars* seen in healing tissue
   (f) *Lichenification* seen over body areas where the child chronically rubs or scratches

2. The integumentary history of the pediatric client should include all the components of the adult history. In addition, the examiner should inquire about the following situations:
   a. Specific exposure to communicable diseases.
   b. Specific exposure to other children with environmentally caused skin problems, such as poison ivy or scabies.
   c. If integumentary signs were present at birth or shortly thereafter, how have these signs changed or progressed since birth or the last visit?
   d. If signs such as cyanosis, pallor, or jaundice are found, an expanded, detailed history should be collected.
   e. Care and cleansing routines for children with conditions such as diaper rash, dry skin, or acne.
   f. Environmental contacts for children with rashes, dry patchy skin, or areas of irritation.
   g. Young children with rashes or skin irritations should have a detailed history taken regarding skin care routines, soap or lotions used, new foods eaten, new detergents or fabrics exposed to, as well as parental treatment techniques.

3. The pediatric client must be completely undressed for the integumentary system to be adequately evaluated. The age and shyness of the child will determine examination techniques.
   a. *Newborns* can easily be undressed to provide a comprehensive integumentary examination. The practitioner must carefully examine all the baby's cracks and crevices, observing skin characteristics, irritations, or rashes. The baby must not be allowed to chill.
   b. *Older babies and toddlers* usually enjoy being undressed, thus making the integumentary examination easy. Special attention should be given to the fat creases, the diaper area, and the scalp.

c. Because of the acquired modesty of *preschoolers and school-age children,* the integumentary examination is more difficult. It may become necessary for the examiner to integrate this examination with other components of the physical assessment, for example, to provide integumentary assessment of the abdominal area while evaluating the abdomen. The hazard of this approach is that subtle skin problems or changes may be missed. At the completion of the examination the examiner must feel confident that total integumentary evaluation has been achieved. Again, this includes all the cracks and crevices.

d. Modesty is perhaps the biggest concern of *older school-age children and adolescents.* Examination criteria are the same as those for the adult client. Special attention should be paid to acne, complexion, and rashes that can develop around the genital area.

4. As the examiner evaluates the skin, signs of child abuse or neglect must not go unnoticed. Examples of problems include multiple bruises above the knees and elbows, multiple bruises at different stages of healing, bruises reflecting belt or electrical cord marks; cigarette burns or burns with even lines of demarcation that could indicate submersion, or any injury that does not coincide with the history. For example, the parent states that her 18-month-old child fell into hot bathtub water, but the clinical observation shows a submersion burn up to the waist with an even line of termination. There is no evidence of splash burns of the hands, face, or chest. A more subtle observation of child neglect involves the parents' nontreatment of obvious integumentary problems, for example, a diaper rash that has been allowed to progress to the point of blistering, infection, and bleeding. These situations require in-depth investigation and referral.

5. If a rash is identified, it is important for the examiner to determine the body surface involved, the rash migration and evolutionary pattern, and home care tried.

Clinical variations associated with the pediatric client

Characteristic or area examined	Normal	Deviations from normal
1. Skin color		
a. General tone	Newborn reddish during first 8 to 24 hours, then pale pink with transparent tone	Cyanosis
		Pallor
	Slight jaundice starting second or third day of life; may last up to a month	Beefy red color that persists beyond 24 hours
		Jaundice within first 24 hours of life
	Mottled appearance of hands and feet in newborn; disappears with warming	Mottled appearance not disappearing with rewarming
	Black newborns: melanotic pigmentation not intense, with exception of nail beds and scrotum	Half of newborn's body reddened and other half pale (harlequin sign)
	Older children: same as adult	
b. Uniformity (Compare color of upper and lower extremities.)	Similar color tones	Increased cyanosis of lower extremities may indicate aortic or congenital heart defect
2. Moisture	Perspiration present in all children over 1 month of age	Perspiration in infant less than 1 month of age
		Excessive sweating, as seen in children with fever, hypoglycemia, hyperthyroidism, or heart disease
3. Texture	Smooth, soft, flexible	Dryness or flakiness in children over 1 month
	Dryness and flakiness of skin in infants less than 1 month of age (shedding of vernix caseosa); may appear as white cheesy skin	
	Presence of *milia*—small white papules over nose and cheeks, which are plugged sebaceous glands that may remain for 2 months	
		Dryness or scaling between fingers or toes (may be from ringworm)
		Scaling over knees, elbows, or behind ears (may be from eczema)
		Scaliness of palms and soles (seen with scarlet fever)

Continued.

Clinical variations associated with the pediatric client–cont'd

Characteristic or area examined	Normal	Deviations from normal
		Dermatoglyphics—straight single folds seen across the upper palm of hands at base of fingers in children with Down syndrome
		Dryness or chafing of diaper area
4. Thickness	Varying degrees of adipose tissue, dimpling of skin over joint areas	Skin dimpling at areas other than over joints
5. Mobility and turgor	Skin rises with pinch but falls quickly when released	Skin remains in pinched position (Fig. 3-10)
a. Pinch large area of skin over lower abdomen		

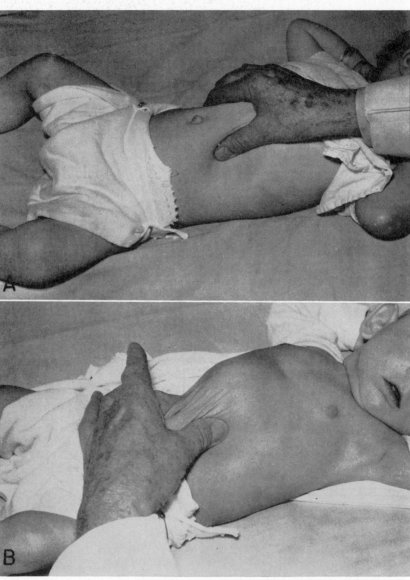

Fig. 3-10. A, Good tissue turgor. **B,** Poor tissue turgor. (From Prior, J. A., and Silberstein, J. S.: Physical diagnosis: the history and examination of the patient, ed. 5, St. Louis, 1977, The C. V. Mosby Co.)

b. Palpate the calf	Full, taut skin	Loose and "extra" skin
		Edema
6. Hygiene	Skin free from odor, clean	Dirty, crusted, or excoriated areas: skinfolds, diaper area, behind ears, neck region; dirty look

Characteristic or area examined	Normal	Deviations from normal
7. Skin surface		
a. Alterations in pigmentation	*Mongolian spots**—irregularly shaped, darkened flat areas over sacral area and buttocks; usually seen in black or darkly pigmented children; may be gone by first or second year Note size and location	Vitiligo—absence of pigmentation in areas
	*Café au lait spots**—light, cream-colored spots found on darkened backgrounds Note size and location	Multiple areas of spots
	*Hemangiomas**—increase in pigmentation with crying I. *Flat capillary* A. Storkbites: small red or pink spots often seen on back of neck, upper lip, or upper eyelid (Fig. 3-11); usually disappear by age 5	
	B. Port wine stain: large, flat, bluish purple capillary area; most frequently found on face along distribution of fifth cranial nerve (Fig. 3-12); usually do not disappear spontaneously	In children with port wine stains, screen for nervous system complications

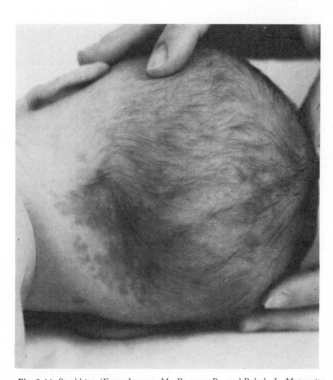

Fig. 3-11. Storkbite. (From Jensen, M., Benson, R., and Bobak, I.: Maternity care, St. Louis, 1977, The C. V. Mosby Co.)

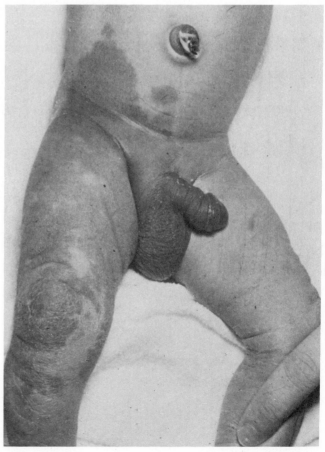

Fig. 3-12. Port wine stain. (From Jensen, M., Benson, R., and Bobak, I.: Maternity care, St. Louis, 1977, The C. V. Mosby Co.)

*These lesions are commonly seen in the pediatric client. Many practitioners consider them a "normal" deviation. Beginners in assessment should consider all pigment alterations as problems until experience enables them to recognize common deviations within normal limits.

Continued.

Clinical variations associated with the pediatric client–cont'd

Characteristic or area examined	Normal	Deviations from normal
	II. *Raised capillary:* strawberry mark, slightly raised, reddened area with sharp demarcation line; may be 2 to 3 cm in diameter; appears at birth or within first few months and usually gone by age 5 (Fig. 3-13)	

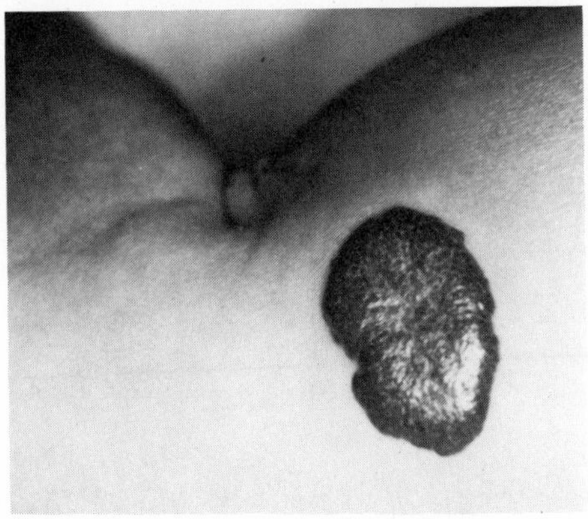

Fig. 3-13. Strawberry mark. (From Shirkey, H.: Pediatric therapy, ed. 5, St. Louis, 1975, The C. V. Mosby Co.)

Characteristic or area examined	Normal	Deviations from normal
	Note size and location	
	III. *Cavernous hemangioma:* reddish blue; round masses of blood vessels; may continue to grow until child is 10 to 15 months old	Some may require surgical removal
	Note size and location	
	Child should be reevaluated frequently	
	IV. *Nevus* (mole): vary in size and number; brown in pigmentation	Large hairy nevi
	Note size, location, and number	Bathing trunk nevi
	Those which are large or in irritating areas must be frequently evaluated for change	
b. Common lesions		*Macules,* as seen in measles, German measles, or drug rash
		Papules, as seen in tinea (ringworm) or psoriasis
		Vesicles (blebs), as seen in chickenpox, herpes zoster, or poison ivy
		Pustules, as seen in impetigo or scabies
		Xanthomas, small yellow plaques seen across nose of newborn
		Miliaria (prickly heat), tiny red irritation
		Hives (wheals or urticaria), as seen in allergic reactions
		Petechial rash, or macular type of rash that does not blanch with palpation or pressure (may indicate meningococcemia, a medical emergency)
		Acne, resulting in blackheads, papules, pustules, and cysts
	Ecchymoses, bruises commonly seen below knees and elbows	*Ecchymoses,* bruises seen elsewhere on body, or multiple bruises seen at different stages of healing
8. Nails		
a. Configuration	Generally longer than wider	Nail beds wider than longer; may be seen in children with Down syndrome or other congenital malformations
b. Consistency	Soft nails in infants and small children; become hardened with age	Pitting of nails, as seen with fungal diseases
	Vernix may be found under nails of newborns	
c. Color	Same as adult	
	Postmature infants may show yellow staining	

Characteristic or area examined	Normal	Deviations from normal
d. Adherence to nail bed	Same as adult	Paronychia, commonly seen infections around nail bed (Fig. 3-14)

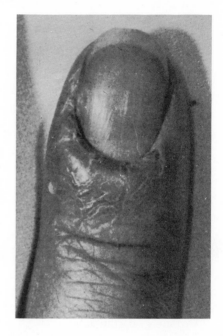

Fig. 3-14. Paronychia. (From Stewart, W., Danto, J., and Maddin, S.: Dermatology: diagnosis and treatment of cutaneous disorders, ed. 4, St. Louis, 1978, The C. V. Mosby Co.)

9. Scalp and hair		
a. Scalp	Smooth, soft	Scaliness of scalp with crusting, seborrheic dermatitis (cradle cap) (Fig. 3-15) Ringworm or eczema of scalp

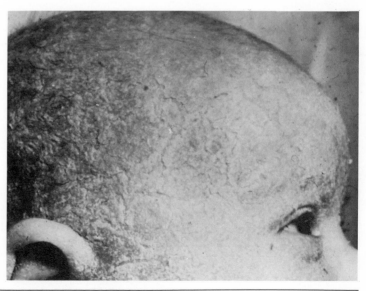

Fig. 3-15. Seborrheic dermatitis (cradle cap). (From Shirkey, H.: Pediatric therapy, ed. 5, St. Louis, 1975, The C. V. Mosby Co.)

Continued.

Clinical variations associated with the pediatric client–cont'd

Characteristic or area examined	Normal	Deviations from normal
b. Scalp hair	Shiny, soft, fine texture; as child grows, hair takes on adult characteristics Irregularity in pigmentation	Brittle hair may be seen in children with hypothyroidism, ringworm of scalp, or other conditions Presence of nits
c. Distribution and configuration of body hair	Newborn displays lanugo, fine hair over body, mostly over shoulders and back; will disappear during first 3 months of life	Hairy trunk may be seen in children with Cushing syndrome Tufts of hair seen anywhere over spine, especially over sacrum (may mark spot of spina bifida)
	Pubic hair begins to develop between 8 and 12 years; smooth hair at first, changing to coarse, curly hair; followed approximately 6 months later by axillary hair; followed approximately 6 months later by facial hair in boys	Absence of secondary hair characteristics

History and clinical strategies associated with the geriatric client

1. Differentiating normal from abnormal skin changes is very difficult when assessing elderly clients. A novice examiner should consult regularly with an experienced clinician.
2. "Normal" lesions must be considered a problem if they are causing client distress (e.g., cosmetic concern, clothing rubbing or irritating lesion).
3. Elderly clients sometimes exhibit a more intense response to skin irritations. The client may feel more pain or more severe itching. Lesions or dermatitis problems may respond more slowly to treatment.
4. Elderly clients may manifest a *reduced* pain response to lesions (especially in extremities): (a) they may be unable to feel pain; (b) they may accept chronic discomfort as part of aging and fail to report it.
5. If a client complains of itching and scratching (a fairly common complaint among elderly clients), assess the fingernails. Dirty, jagged fingernails often contribute to the problem.
6. The integumentary system reflects an individual's relationship to the outer as well as the inner environment. Some of the variables affecting the skin, hair, and nails follow:
   a. Outer environment
      (1) Cold weather conditions: increased sensitivity to cold.
      (2) Humidity and moisture: low humidity (especially in winter) will irritate dry skin; individuals who habitually soak in warm water (to relieve arthritic pain) may develop dry skin.
      (3) Sun: chronic exposure (especially with light-skinned individuals) results in a higher incidence of precancerous and cancerous growths. Sun sensitivity may develop; certain drugs and chemicals contribute to phototoxic reactions: sulfonamides, thiazide diuretics, antibacterial soaps.
      (4) Skin irritants: soaps, detergents, lotions with high alcohol content, disinfectants, and woolen clothing may aggravate dry skin.
      (5) Allergic reactions: occur fairly often; jewelry, dark blue or black dyes in clothing or shoes, chemicals in crease-resistant clothing, and linens or clothing containing residual soap or detergent are some of the more common causative factors.
      (6) Decreased activity (pressure friction) will stress the system.
   b. Internal environment
      (1) Medications (often numerous with the elderly) may create problems (rash, itching).
      (2) Systemic/chronic disease (itching).
      (3) Nutritional deficiencies (e.g., vitamin A deficiency may result in rough, dry skin).
      (4) Decreased circulation lowers skin resistance to infection.

Clinical variations associated with the geriatric client

Characteristic or area examined	Normal	Deviations from normal
1. Skin color		
a. General tone	Caucasian skin appears white	Pallor associated with anemia
b. Uniformity	More freckles, uneven tanning, or pigment deposits in sun-exposed areas (more evident on fair skin) (Fig. 3-16) Hypopigmented patches	Hypersensitivity to sun (marked reddening, eczematous changes)

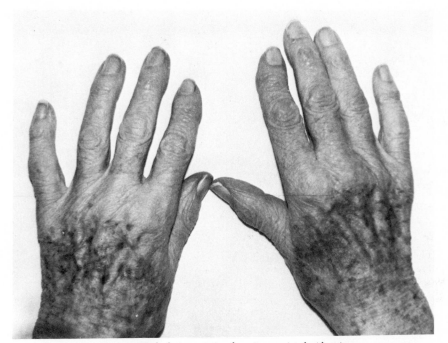

Fig. 3-16. Marked pigmentation deposits associated with aging.

Characteristic or area examined	Normal	Deviations from normal
2. Moisture	Increased dryness (especially extremities) Decreased perspiration	Marked flaking
3. Texture	Flaking, scaling (associated with dry skin, especially over lower extremities)	Scaling associated with dryness, itching, and scratching (erythema, excoriation may be present)
4. Thickness	Thinner skin (especially over dorsal surface of hands and feet, forearms, lower legs, bony prominences such as scapula, trochanter, knees)	
	Other skin areas may be thicker (abdomen, torso)	Torso obesity distribution associated with disease
5. Mobility and turgor	General loss of elasticity; appears lax	

Continued.

Clinical variations associated with the geriatric client—cont'd

Characteristic or area examined	Normal	Deviations from normal
	Increased wrinkle pattern (more marked in sun-exposed areas, in fair skin, in expressive areas of face) (Fig. 3-17)	Marked wrinkling or sagging associated with weight loss (Fig. 3-18) Perlèche—deep wrinkling, fissures or maceration at corners of mouth (associated with ill-fitting dentures or edentulous client) (Fig. 3-19)

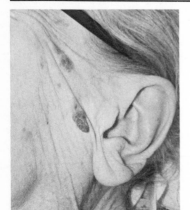

Fig. 3-17. Increased wrinkling and skinfolds associated with aging.

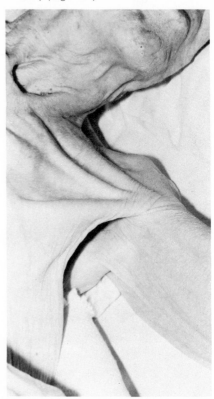

Fig. 3-18. Marked weight loss. Note bony prominences and sagging skinfolds.

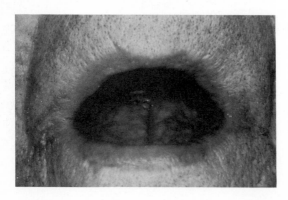

Fig. 3-19. Perleche. (Courtesy Dr. George Blozis, The Ohio State University College of Dentistry.)

Characteristic or area examined	Normal	Deviations from normal
	Pendulous parts sag or droop (skin under chin, earlobes, breasts, scrotum)	Pendulous scrotal tissue may become excoriated or damaged due to client sliding or sitting on it
6. Hygiene		Hard-to-reach areas may be less clean (e.g., feet, axillary area, buttocks, or inguinal skinfolds)
7. Skin surface **a.** Alterations or lesions	Nevi (common moles) often become lighter in color or disappear	Evaluated in same manner as with adult client

Characteristic or area examined	Normal	Deviations from normal
1. Seborrheic keratosis*		Use extra caution in assessing the following:
a. Location	Temples, neck, back, under pendulous breasts	Any lesions or skin changes appearing in chronically sun-exposed areas (especially on face, around ears, neck, lips)
b. Size	2 to 3 cm in diameter	
c. Color	Light tan to black	Any skin changes in lower extremities, reddening or dusky color, blanching, mottling, eczematous appearance
d. Surface characteristics	Appears "stuck on"; lobulated or warty, scaly, thickened	
e. Distribution	Often multiple (Fig. 3-20)	

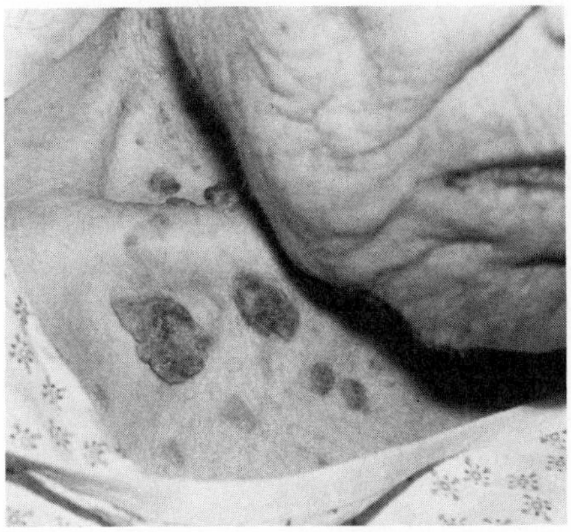

Fig. 3-20. Seborrheic keratosis.

2. Skin tags (acrochordons)*		
a. Location	Side of neck, face, axillary folds	
b. Size	1 mm to 1 cm	
c. Color	Pinkish tan to light brown	
d. Surface	Soft, pedunculated	
e. Distribution	Often multiple, may be singular (Fig. 3-21)	

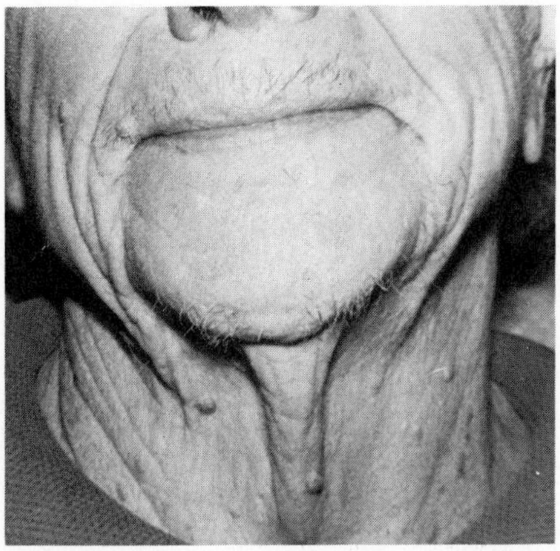

Fig. 3-21. Skin tags in the neck and bristly facial hair.

3. Senile angiomas*		
a. Location	Trunk, proximal extremities, scrotum	Multiple scrotal angiomas associated with systemic vascular problems
b. Size	1 to 5 mm diameter	
c. Color	Purplish or red	
d. Surface	Smooth, soft, dome-shaped. May bleed if traumatized	
e. Distribution	Singular or multiple	
4. Sebaceous hyperplasia* (more common in males)		
a. Location	Forehead, nose, cheeks	
b. Size	2 to 3 mm diameter	
c. Color	Yellow	
d. Surface	Papular, flat, may be umbilicated or lobular	

*These lesions commonly occur in elderly adults. They are described by some authors as "normal," in that the chief concern for the client is cosmetic. Beginners in assessment should consider all lesions as problems until experience enables them to recognize common deviations within normal limits.

Continued.

Clinical variations associated with the geriatric client–cont'd

Characteristic or area examined	Normal	Deviations from normal
e. Distribution	Singular or multiple (Fig. 3-22)	

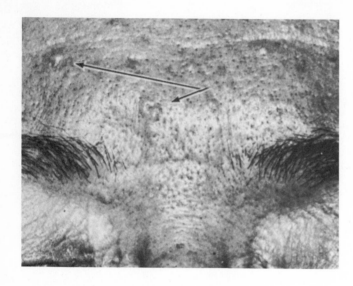

Fig. 3-22. Sebacious hyperplasia. (From Steinberg, F.: Cowdry's the care of the geriatric patient, ed. 5, St. Louis, 1976, The C. V. Mosby Co.)

b. Skin alterations: trauma induced	Bruises, lacerations, excoriations may heal more slowly	Large number of bruises Tearing of thin skin Reddened areas from pressure (bony prominences) Fissures or hyperkeratosis associated with friction (heels, toes, side of foot rubbing against shoe) Evaluated in same manner as with adult client
8. Nails **a.** Configuration	Toenails may be thickened, distorted (toenails treated for fungal infection may not return to normal configuration) (Fig. 3-23)	Toenail thickening associated with fungal infection (yellowish discoloration, granular surface) Uncut toenails curled over foot

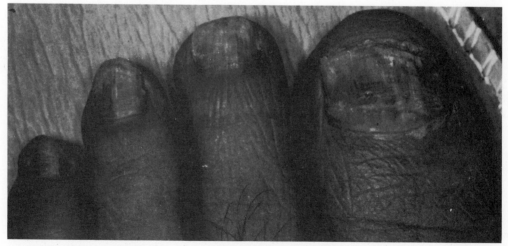

Fig. 3-23. Fungal infection of toenails. (From Stewart, W., Danto, J., and Maddin, S.: Dermatology: diagnosis and treatment of cutaneous disorders, ed. 4, St. Louis, 1978, The C. V. Mosby Co.)

Characteristic or area examined	Normal	Deviations from normal
b. Consistency	Fingernails may be more brittle, may peel	
c. Color	Toenails may lose translucency	
9. Hair and scalp		
a. Surface	Sebaceous hyperplasia may extend into scalp	Evaluated in same manner as with adult client
b. Distribution	Increased facial hair (especially women), bristly quality (Fig. 3-21)	
	Men may have coarse hair in ears, nose, eyebrows	
	Decreased scalp hair (scalp may be visible)	Sudden hair loss
	Symmetrical balding in men (most often frontal or occipital)	Patchy, asymmetrical hair loss
	Decreased pubic and axillary hair	
c. Texture	Facial hair coarse, body hair fine	Sudden change in texture
d. Color	Greying, whitening (hairs that do not lose pigment often become darker)	
e. Quantity	General decrease of body and scalp hair	

Vocabulary

1. Anular   *ringlike*

2. Atrophy

3. Circinate

4. Confluent   *meeting of streams*

5. Crust

6. Desquamation   *shedding of material from surface*

7. Ecchymosis   *escape of blood into tissue*

8. Eczematous   *itching, swelling, blistering, oozing scaling → fissures*

9. Erythematous   *redness 2° capillary engorgement*

10. Excoriation   *superficial loss of substance*

11. Induration   *abnormally hard spot*

12. Ischemia   *↓ blood to part*

13. Keloid

benign tumor/scar

21. Pruritus *itching*

14. Keratosis

formation of horny growth

22. Purpura

15. Lichenification

thickening + hardening of skin

23. Seborrhea

excess discharge from sebaceous glands

16. Melanin

24. Stria

colorless lines

17. Nevus *mole*

25. Telangiectasia

cap. dilatation

18. Paronychia *- infection around nail*

26. Tumor *>1-2cm. nodule*

19. Petechiae

27. Turgor

20. Plaque *patch, flat area papules*

28. Urticaria *hives*

Cognitive self-assessment

Following is a series of statements about integumentary function and formation. Mark each statement "T" or "F."

1. ___T___ Skin without epidermis is freely permeable.
2. ___T___ Corns and calluses are areas of hypertrophied horny epidermis.
3. ___T___ Eccrine sweat glands are widely distributed over the body and contribute to temperature regulation.
4. ___F___ Skin turgor (normal firmness) is determined by the amount of subcutaneous tissue available.
5. ___T___ Calluses may distort normal skin coloration.
6. ___T___ Effective resistance to skin injury is determined, in part, by adequate circulation.
7. ___T___ Effective resistance to skin injury is determined, in part, by the presence of sufficient subcutaneous tissue.

8. _F_ Apocrine sweat glands are widely distributed over the body.
9. _T_ The amount of skin moisture normally varies according to environmental conditions.
10. _T_ Pallor, in dark skin, may be observable by noting the absence of underlying red tones.

For questions 11 through 17, all the statements but one are true. Pick the false one.

11. The stratum corneum:
    - ☐ a. is composed of keratin
    - ☐ b. is part of the epidermis
    - ☐ c. is composed of dead cells
    - ☐ d. absorbs water readily
    - ☒ e. lies under the subcutaneous layer
12. The epidermal layer:
    - ☐ a. is avascular
    - ☒ b. is uniformly paper thin
    - ☐ c. is a barrier to external substances
    - ☐ d. prevents excessive water loss
    - ☐ e. contains melanin
13. Keratin:
    - ☒ a. originates in the dermis
    - ☐ b. is the principal constituent of nails and hair
    - ☐ c. is a tough fibrous protein
    - ☐ d. originates in the epidermis
14. Melanin:
    - ☐ a. produces varying skin shades of yellow, brown, and black
    - ☐ b. is produced in some people in response to ultraviolet rays
    - ☒ c. deposits are usually heavier in the palms, soles, and nail beds
    - ☐ d. acts as a barrier to ultraviolet radiation
    - ☐ e. deposits may normally be patchy or uneven
15. The dermis:
    - ☐ a. is well supplied with blood and lymph vessels
    - ☐ b. contains the peripheral nervous system
    - ☐ c. is freely permeable
    - ☒ d. is nourished by the epidermis
    - ☐ e. contains sebaceous glands
16. Sebum:
    - ☒ a. is an oily secretion produced in the apocrine glands
    - ☐ b. glands are more numerous on the face and scalp
    - ☐ c. production is increased at the time of puberty
    - ☐ d. production is decreased when peripheral circulation is impaired
    - ☐ e. accumulation on the skin can cause skin irritation
17. The subcutaneous layer:
    - ☐ a. stores fat
    - ☐ b. contributes to body heat conservation
    - ☐ c. varies greatly in amounts among individuals
    - ☒ d. supplies melanocytes for pigmentation
    - ☐ e. acts as a cushion
18. Systematic integument evaluation is especially important when the client:
    - ☐ a. is receiving treatments (e.g., topical medications, soaks) that involve the skin
    - ☐ b. has impaired circulation
    - ☐ c. depends on others for physical care or protection (e.g., infants, debilitated, immobilized)

☐ d. has been living under unhygienic circumstances
☐ e. is known to have particularly sensitive or delicate skin
☐ f. a, b, and c
☑ g. all the above
☐ h. all except d
☐ i. all except e

19. Which of the following statements are true?
    ☐ a. Prolonged anoxemia will result in clubbing of the nails.
    ☐ b. Spider angiomas can be associated with pregnancy.
    ☐ c. Hypothyroidism can cause scalp hair to be dry and coarse.
    ☐ d. Acne is likely to be more prominent on the face, scalp, chest, and back.
    ☐ e. Scabies is likely to be more prominent on the wrists, hands, axillae, and inguinal area.
    ☐ f. All except b
    ☐ g. a, d, and e
    ☑ h. All the above
    ☐ i. All except c

Match the definitions in column B with the terms in column A.

Column A	*Column B*
20. _c_ Macule	a. Large, superficial, fluid-containing elevation greater than 0.5 cm
21. _f_ Papule	
22. _g_ Nodule	b. Loss of superficial epidermis, moist but not bleeding
23. _j_ Vesicle	c. Circumscribed, flat, change in skin color
24. _a_ Bulla	d. Thin flakes of exfoliated epidermis
25. _i_ Pustule	e. Deep linear crack in the skin
26. _l_ Wheal	f. Solid elevated mass, usually less than 0.5 cm
27. _d_ Scale	g. Solid mass extending into subcutaneous or dermal tissue
28. _k_ Crust	
29. _b_ Erosion	h. Replacement of skin by fibrous tissue
30. _h_ Scar	i. Elevation containing purulent exudate
31. _e_ Fissure	j. Small superficial elevation, less than 0.5 cm, containing serous fluid
	k. Dried residue of serum, pus, or blood
	l. Flat-topped, superficial, and well-circumscribed elevation

PEDIATRIC QUESTIONS

32. All the following skin color characteristics are normal except one. Pick the statement that indicates an abnormal finding.
    ☐ a. Beefy red color seen in a newborn less than 24 hours old
    ☐ b. Jaundice appearing on the third day of life
    ☐ c. Jaundice of the palms and soles of a toddler who loves carrots
    ☑ d. Jaundice appearing within 24 hours of birth
    ☐ e. Mottled appearance of the hands and feet of a newborn

33. A healthy newborn may show which of the following skin characteristics?
    ☐ a. Flakiness of skin around wrists and ankles
    ☐ b. Milia—small white papules over nose
    ☐ c. Dermatoglyphics—straight lines across upper palms of hands
    ☐ d. Mongolian spots
    ☐ e. Hair over shoulders and upper back
    ☐ f. All except d
    ☐ g. a, b, and d

☐ h. b and c
☒ i. All except c
☐ j. All the above

Mark each statement "T" or "F."

34. ___T___ A "strawberry mark" is a red, raised, and soft capillary hemangioma.
35. ___F___ Tufts of hair found over the spine are generally considered to be a sign of retardation.
36. ___F___ An example of a disease having papules is poison ivy.

GERIATRIC QUESTIONS

For questions 37 through 39, all the statements are true except one. Pick the false statement.

37. A number of epidermal and dermal changes occur with aging.
☐ a. Outer skin moisture and suppleness often directly reflect the amount of moisture available in the environment.
☐ b. Toenails may be thicker and somewhat disfigured.
☐ c. The loss of melanocytes may contribute to a pale appearance in Caucasians.
☒ d. Precancerous lesions are a noted hazard for brown- and yellow-skinned people.
☐ e. Pigment deposits (lentigines) may be more numerous in sun-exposed skin areas.

38. Subcutaneous fat decreases with aging.
☐ a. Bony prominences emerge.
☐ b. Sensitivity to cold weather increases.
☒ c. Sensitivity to warm weather increases.
☐ d. A folded, wrinkled, and lax appearance of the skin increases.
☐ e. The abdomen may remain obese in spite of fat loss over arms and legs.

39. A healthy elderly person might manifest the following integumentary changes.
☐ a. Hyperkeratosis
☐ b. Vitiligo
☐ c. Increased coarsening of facial hair
☐ d. Decrease and thinning of body hair
☒ e. Patchy balding (men)

SUGGESTED READINGS
General

Bates, Barbara: A guide to physical examination, ed. 2, Philadelphia, 1979, J. B. Lippincott Co., pp. 43-51.

Capell, Peter T., and Case, David B.: Ambulatory care manual for nurse practitioners, Philadelphia, 1976, J. B. Lippincott Co., pp. 283-313.

Davis, Mardell: Getting to the root of the problem: hair grooming techniques for black patients, Nursing '77 7(4):60-65, 1977.

Judge, Richard D., and Zuidema, George, editors: Methods of clinical examination: a physiologic approach, Boston, 1974, Little, Brown & Co., pp. 53-60.

Malasanos, Lois, Barkauskas, Violet, Moss, Muriel, and Stoltenberg-Allen, Kathryn: Health assessment, St. Louis, 1977, The C. V. Mosby Co., pp. 367-378.

Nordmark, Madelyn T., and Rohweder, Ann W.: Scientific foundations of nursing, ed. 3, Philadelphia, 1975, J. B. Lippincott Co., pp. 221-238.

Prior, John A., and Silberstein, Jack S.: Physical diagnosis: the history and examination of the patient, ed. 5, St. Louis, 1977, The C. V. Mosby Co., pp. 63-69.

Roach, Lora B.: Color changes in dark skin, Nursing '77 7(1):48-51, 1977.

Sana, Josephine, and Judge, Richard D.: Physical appraisal methods in nursing, Boston, 1975, Little, Brown & Co., pp. 86-97.

Wasson, John, Walsh, Timothy, Thompkins, Richard, and Sax, Harold: The common symptom guide, New York, 1975, McGraw-Hill Book Co., pp. 270-271, 280-284.

Pediatric

Alexander, Mary, and Brown, Marie Scott: Pediatric physical diagnosis for nurses, New York, 1974, McGraw-Hill Book Co., pp. 10-25.

Barness, Lewis: Manual of pediatric physical diagnosis, ed. 4, Chicago, 1972, Year Book Medical Publishers, Inc., pp. 24-39.

Bates, Barbara: A guide to physical examination, ed. 2, Philadelphia, 1979, J. B. Lippincott Co., pp. 381-382.

Brown, Marie Scott, and Murphy, Mary Alexander: Physical examination. Part 3. Examining the skin, Nursing '73 **3**(9):39-43, 1973.

Cohen, Stephen: Skin rashes in infants and children, Programmed Instruction, Am. J. Nurs. **78**(6):1041-1072, 1978.

DeAngelis, Catherine: Basic pediatrics for the primary health care provider, Boston, 1975, Little, Brown & Co., pp. 38-42, 249-264.

Malasanos, Lois, Barkauskas, Violet, Moss, Muriel, and Stoltenberg-Allen, Kathryn: Health assessment, St. Louis, 1977, The C. V. Mosby Co., p. 424.

Geriatric

Burnside, Irene, editor: Nursing and the aged, New York, 1976, McGraw-Hill Book Co., pp. 83-85, 91.

Chinn, Austin B., editor: Clinical aspects of aging, Working with older people: a guide to practice, vol. 4, Rockville, Md., 1971. U.S. Department of Health, Education, and Welfare, pp. 3-27.

Malasanos, Lois, Barkauskas, Violet, Moss, Muriel, and Stoltenberg-Allen, Kathryn: Health assessment, St. Louis, 1977, The C. V. Mosby Co., p. 443.

Palmore, Erdman, editor: Normal aging II: reports from the Duke Longitudinal Studies, Durham, N.C., 1974, Duke University Press, pp. 18-23.

Steinberg, Franz V., editor: Cowdry's the care of the geriatric patient, St. Louis, 1976, The C. V. Mosby Co., pp. 178-190, 310-317.

Uhler, Diana: Common skin changes in the elderly, Am. J. Nurs. **78**(8):1342-1344, 1978.

Wells, Thelma J.: In geriatric patients: that "minor" skin problem could be trouble, R.N. **41**(7):41-46, 1978.

Wright, Edwin T.: Identifying and treating common benign skin tumors, Geriatrics **33**(6):37-44, 1978.

CHAPTER 4

Assessment of the head and neck

Cognitive objectives

At the end of this unit the learner will demonstrate knowledge of assessment of the head and neck by the ability to do the following:

1. Systematically list structures of the head and neck evaluated during the physical examination.
2. Describe the characteristics of a lymph node that must be evaluated.
3. Describe the lymphatic drainage of the head and neck.
4. Describe the significance and methods for examining the thyroid gland and trachea.
5. Define the terms in the vocabulary section.
6. Identify selected elements of the pediatric head and neck examination.
7. Identify selected elements of the geriatric head and neck examination.

Clinical objectives

At the end of this unit the learner will perform a systematic assessment of the head and neck, demonstrating the ability to do the following:

1. Obtain a pertinent health history from the client.
2. Demonstrate and describe the results of inspection and palpation of the following aspects of the head:
   a. Skull for contour and size
   b. Scalp for texture and color
   c. Hair for distribution, quality and quantity
   d. Facies for symmetry, quality, color, expression, and movements
   e. Head movements
3. Demonstrate and describe the results of inspection and palpation of the neck and thyroid gland for:
   a. Symmetry
   b. Muscular development and movement
   c. Landmarks and location of the trachea
   d. Location, size, shape, delineation, mobility, consistency, and surface characteristics of the faciocervical lymph nodes

   e. Placement, symmetry, and characteristics of the thyroid gland
4. Summarize results of the assessment with a written description of findings.

Health history related to head and neck assessment additional to screening history

1. Head injury profile
   a. Events associated with the injury
      (1) Predisposing factors leading to injury, such as epilepsy or seizure disorder, blackout, poor vision, dizziness, light-headedness
      (2) Precipitating factors leading to injury, such as unsafe conditions, wet floors, getting up too fast
   b. If possible, describe the exact details of the injury
      (1) Specifically, what happened?
      (2) How did client appear immediately following injury (loss of consciousness, dazed, crying, convulsion)?
      (3) How was client 5 minutes later (vomiting, complained of headache, appeared fine, same as immediately following, or different)?
      (4) In general, has client gotten progressively worse or better or been unchanged since injury?
   c. Associated symptoms
      (1) State of consciousness: unconscious (momentary vs. prolonged—describe), dazed, sleepy
      (2) Neck or head pain (see headache profile)
      (3) Visual problems: droopy eyes, blurred or double vision
      (4) Vomiting: number of times, associated distress, projectile in nature
      (5) Motor or sensory changes: staggered gait, tremors, numbness of limbs
      (6) Ear or nasal discharge: serous or bloody discharge from nose or ears

(7) Loss of urine or bowel control since injury
(8) Loss of memory: recent or long term
d. Medications
   (1) Those routinely being taken
   (2) Any discontinued within 1 week prior to the injury

2. Headache profile

Because of the vast complexity of headaches, profile questioning will incorporate the analysis of a symptom format presented in Chapter 1.

a. When was client last entirely well?
   (1) When did *this type* of headache start occurring?
   (2) How long has client been bothered with headaches in general?
b. Date of current problem onset: if headache has been going on for some time, try to determine beginning date.
c. Character
   (1) Constant bandlike pressure
   (2) Throbbing, pounding
   (3) Single area pressure
   (4) Single area pain (dull vs. sharp)
   (5) Shooting pains (dull vs. sharp)
   (6) Severity of headache
d. Nature of problem onset
   (1) Slowly over several weeks, days, hours
   (2) Abrupt onset over several minutes
e. Client's hunch of precipitating factors
   (1) Stress
   (2) Sudden movement or exercise
   (3) Alcohol
   (4) Medication
f. Course of problem
   (1) Lasts for minutes, hours, days, weeks before disappearing; relieved by medication
   (2) Lasts for minutes, hours, days, weeks before disappearing; medication not necessary for relief
   (3) Appears in clusters (several over given time period), then disappears for extensive period before returning
g. Location of problem
   (1) Occipital region
   (2) Frontal region
   (3) Temporal region
   (4) Neck region
   (5) Maxillary sinus region
   (6) Behind eyes

   (7) Unilateral or bilateral
   (8) Generalized or specific
h. Relation to other entities
   (1) Visual changes ($\downarrow$ acuity or blurring, tearing)
   (2) Nausea and vomiting (which came first, headache or nausea and vomiting?)
   (3) Nasal stuffiness and discharge
   (4) Muscle aches and pains
   (5) Cough, sore throat
   (6) Neck pain and/or stiffness
   (7) Fever
   (8) Change in level of consciousness as headache increases
   (9) Movement aggravates headache symptoms
i. Patterns
   (1) Timing
      (a) Worse in AM or PM
      (b) Occurs only during sleep
      (c) Worse or better as day progresses
   (2) Duration
      (a) Episodes getting closer together and worse
      (b) Getting worse but no closer together
      (c) Lasting longer
j. Efforts to treat
   (1) Physician help sought for headache
   (2) Current medications taken, prescription and over the counter
   (3) Body positions that help headache
   (4) Other remedies that help headache
k. How do headaches interfere with client's activities of daily living?

3. Complaints of neck pain
a. Head or neck injury or strain
b. Swelling of neck
c. Limitations of neck movement (continuous vs. sporadic)
d. Does neck movement aggravate or alleviate neck pain?
e. Radiation patterns to arms, shoulders, hands, down back

4. If the client complains of dizziness, it is important to determine exactly what is meant. The term *dizziness* means the inability to maintain equilibrium. In the objective type the room spins; in the subjective type the client is moving.

Clinical guidelines

The student will:	To identify:	
	Normal	Deviations from normal
1. Ask client to sit and remove wigs or hairpieces **2.** Inspect and palpate: **a.** Skull 1. Contour	Rounded and symmetrical with frontal, parietal, and bilateral occipital prominences	Lumps, marked protrusions, depressions

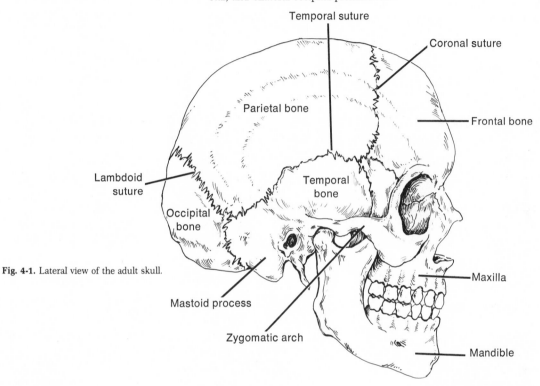

Fig. 4-1. Lateral view of the adult skull.

Temporal suture

Coronal suture

Parietal bone

Frontal bone

Temporal bone

Lambdoid suture

Occipital bone

Maxilla

Mastoid process

Zygomatic arch

Mandible

2. Size	Wide variety of sizes	Greatly enlarged Abnormally small Protruding mandible
b. Scalp 1. Texture	Skin intact	Lesions, scabs Tenderness Scaliness Superficial nodules

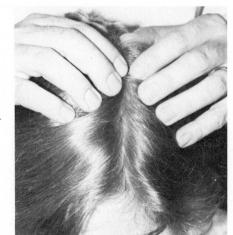

Fig. 4-2. Scalp palpation.

Continued.

Clinical guidelines–cont'd

The student will:	To identify:	
	Normal	**Deviations from normal**
2. Color	Pigmentation will vary depending on race	Reddened areas Areas of increased or decreased pigmentation
c. Hair		
1. Foreign bodies		Flaking Nits
2. Distribution	Even Bilateral, symmetrical balding (Fig. 4-3, *A*)	Patchy, asymmetrical alopecia (Fig. 4-3, *B*)

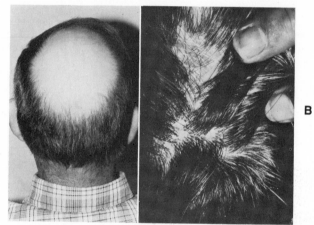

Fig. 4-3. A, Normal balding pattern. **B,** Abnormal balding pattern. (From Stewart, W. D., Danto, J. L., and Maddin, S.: Dermatology: diagnosis and treatment of cutaneous disorders, ed. 4, St. Louis, 1978, The C. V. Mosby Co.)

3. Quantity	Thick, thin, sparse	Excessive loss
4. Quality	Shiny, smooth	Dull, brittle Excessive coarseness or dryness
5. Hygiene	Clean	Odor; matted, dirty
d. Face		
1. Symmetry	Symmetrical placement and shape of eyes, ears, mouth, eyebrows, nasolabial folds	Marked asymmetry
2. Quality	Facial qualities vary according to race and body build (Note slight facial asymmetry in photograph on left.)	Edema (especially of eyelids) Exceptionally coarse features Puffiness Excessive perspiration Waxy pallor Lesions Lip lesions, fissures, swelling Acne, scarring

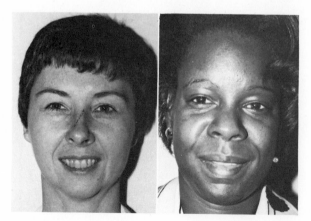

	To identify:	
The student will:	**Normal**	**Deviations from normal**
3. Color	Pigmentation varies with race	Jaundice Cyanosis (especially around lips) Pigmentation variations
4. Expression	Alert; response appropriate to conversation	No responsiveness Tense, drawn muscles Inappropriate expression
5. Movements	Controlled, smooth	Involuntary
3. Evaluate head and neck movements		
a. Instruct client to:		
1. Move chin to chest	Controlled and smooth throughout series of movements	Ratchety movement
2. Move head back so that chin is pointing toward ceiling	Movement of neck from neutral upright position	Bounding (up and down), synchronizes with pulse
	Chin toward chest, 45° flexion	
	Chin upward toward ceiling, 55° extension	
3. Move head so that ear is moved toward shoulder (do not allow client to move shoulder up to ear)	Lateral bending, 40° each way Rotation 70° for both right and left directions	Rhythmic movement or tremor
4. Move head and neck in lateral rotation so that while head is upward and looking forward, the client's chin is placed on first one shoulder and then the other	No discomfort or limitation of movement (Fig. 4-4)	Pain throughout movement Pain at particular points during movement Spasms or tics Limited range of motion Unable to touch points (as indicated)

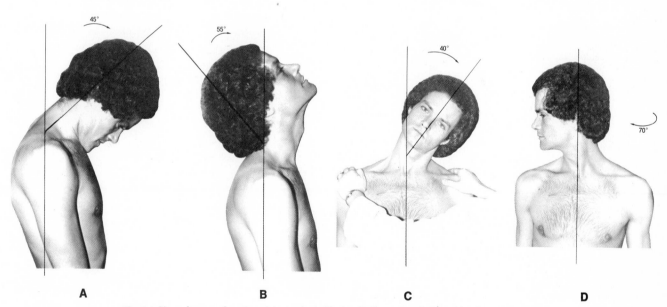

Fig. 4-4. Normal range of motion of the neck. **A,** Flexion. **B,** Extension. **C,** Lateral bending. **D,** Rotation.

b. Neck range of motion may be evaluated by one single rotary movement incorporating the four touch points

Continued.

Clinical guidelines–cont'd

The student will:	To identify:	
	Normal	**Deviations from normal**
c. Neck symmetry (Fig. 4-5)	Head position centered Bilateral symmetry of trapezius and sterno- cleidomastoid muscles	Head tilted Muscle shortening, waste Tenderness on palpation Masses, scars

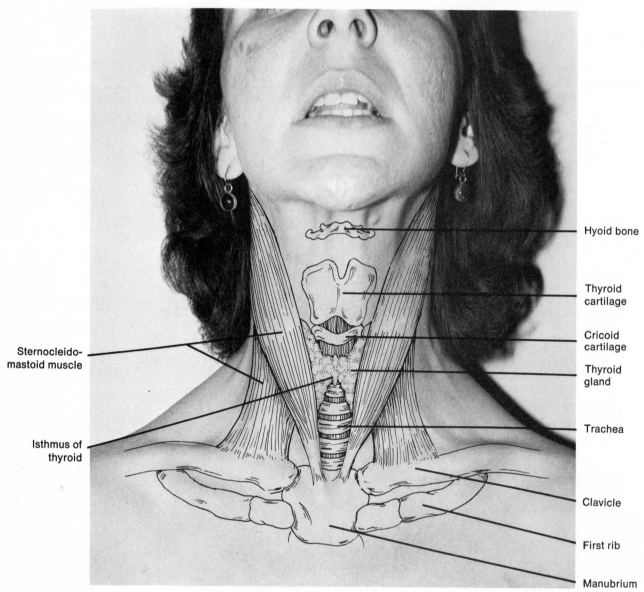

Sternocleido-
mastoid muscle

Isthmus of
thyroid

Hyoid bone

Thyroid
cartilage

Cricoid
cartilage

Thyroid
gland

Trachea

Clavicle

First rib

Manubrium

Fig. 4-5. Anatomical structure of the neck.

4. Palpate trachea (easiest just above suprasternal notch)		
a. Location	Central placement	Lateral displacement Tenderness on palpation
b. Landmarks	Tracheal rings Cricoid cartilage Thyroid cartilage	

	To identify:	
The student will:	**Normal**	**Deviations from normal**

5. Inspect thyroid

  a. Instruct client to:

    1. Put chin up as if drinking from glass

    2. Swallow

  b. Note symmetry and placement — Gland usually not visible — Unilateral or bilateral lobe enlargement* (Fig. 4-6)

  c. Plapate thyroid

    1. Stand behind client

    2. Instruct client to flex head slightly

    3. Tilt chin slightly toward side you are examining

    4. Place your fingers anteriorly with finger pads over client's trachea

    5. Instruct client to swallow periodically so that you may locate identifying landmarks, including:

      a. Thyroid cartilage — Smooth / Centrally located

      b. Cricoid cartilage — Smooth ringlike structure

      c. Isthmus — Smooth tissue found approximately 1 cm below cricoid cartilage / May not be felt / With swallowing may feel smooth tissue slide under skin

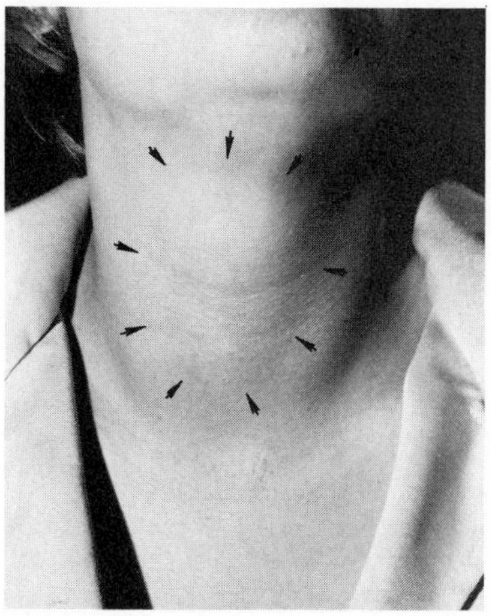

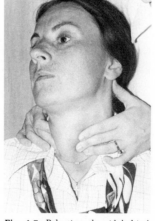

Fig. 4-6. Minimal thyroid enlargement encroaching on the sternocleidomastoid muscle. Note full appearance of the neck.

      d. Thyroid lobes on lateral border of gland

        (1) Right lobe felt with chin slightly to right — Lobes may not be felt / If lobes felt, they are small, smooth, rise freely with swallowing, nontender — Enlarged lobes / Palpated easily without swallowing / Nodular or irregular lobe consistency / Tender to palpation / Gland not freely moving with swallowing

        (2) Place right fingertips directly behind sternocleidomastoid muscle

        (3) Fingertips of left hand slightly displace trachea to right

        (4) Instruct patient to swallow (Fig. 4-7) — Right lobe larger than left

      e. Main body of gland

        (1) Right lobe felt with chin slightly to right

        (2) Place right fingertips directly in front of sternocleidomastoid muscle

        (3) Fingertips of left hand slightly displace trachea to right

        (4) Instruct patient to swallow (Fig. 4-8)

      f. Reverse procedure for left lobe evaluations

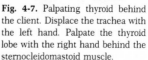

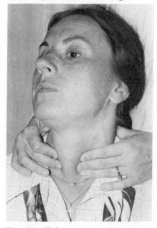

Fig. 4-7. Palpating thyroid behind the client. Displace the trachea with the left hand. Palpate the thyroid lobe with the right hand behind the sternocleidomastoid muscle.

Fig. 4-8. Palpating the thyroid behind the client. Displace the trachea with the left hand. Palpate the thyroid lobe with the right hand in front of the sternocleidomastoid muscle.

---

*Auscultate the thyroid gland if enlargement is found (use bell of stethoscope). Evidence of abnormality is systolic bruit or continuous venous hum in supraclavicular areas.

Continued.

Clinical guidelines–cont'd

The student will:	To identify:	
	Normal	Deviations from normal

6. Lymphatic nodes
   a. Inspect lateral neck (Fig. 4-9)

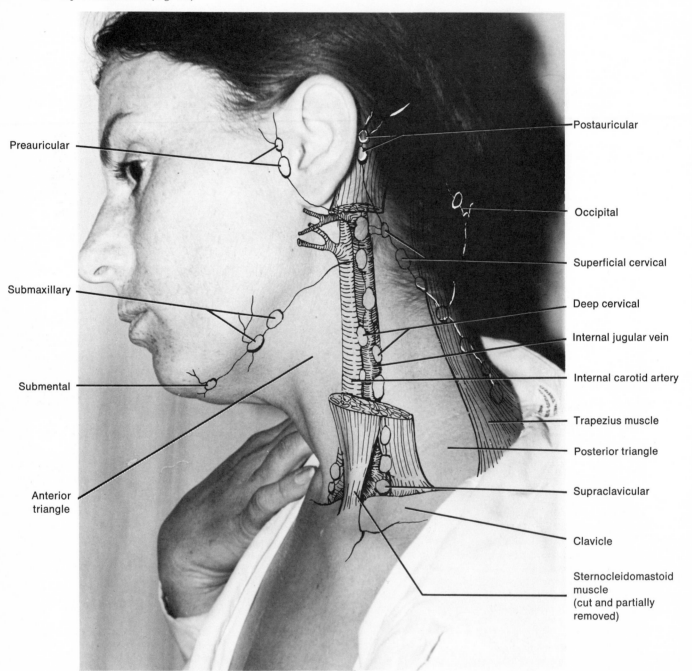

Preauricular

Postauricular

Occipital

Superficial cervical

Submaxillary

Deep cervical

Internal jugular vein

Submental

Internal carotid artery

Trapezius muscle

Posterior triangle

Supraclavicular

Anterior
triangle

Clavicle

Sternocleidomastoid
muscle
(cut and partially
removed)

Fig. 4-9. Lateral view of anatomical lymph structures of the neck with nodes.

The student will:	To identify:	
	Normal	**Deviations from normal**

b. Palpate the following nodes:
 1. Preauricular (Fig. 4-10)
 2. Postauricular and occipital (Fig. 4-11)
 3. Tonsillar, submaxillary, and submental (Fig. 4-12)
 4. Superficial and deep cervical (Fig. 4-13)
 5. Posterior cervical (Fig. 4-14)
 6. Supraclavicular (Fig. 4-15)

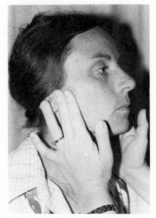

Fig. 4-10. Palpating preauricular lymph nodes.

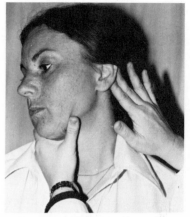

Fig. 4-11. Palpating posterior auricular chain of lymph nodes.

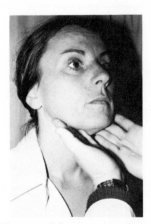

Fig. 4-12. Palpating submaxillary lymph nodes.

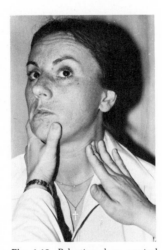

Fig. 4-13. Palpating deep cervical chain of lymph nodes.

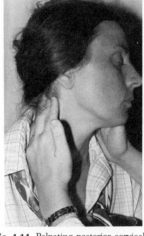

Fig. 4-14. Palpating posterior cervical chain of lymph nodes.

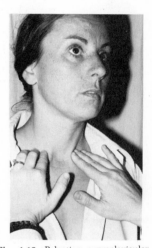

Fig. 4-15. Palpating supraclavicular chain of lymph nodes.

The student will:	Normal	Deviations from normal
c. Size (cm) and shape	Usually not palpable If palpable, small, mobile, discrete, nontender nodes	Palpable Large, round, cylindrical, irregular
d. Delimitation		Multiple discrete or matted nodes
e. Mobility		Fixed to underlying tissue Fixed to overlying tissue Induration
f. Consistency		Hard, firm; soft, spongy
g. Surface characteristics		Smooth, nodular
h. Tenderness		Tender on palpation
i. Heat		Present
j. Erythema		Present

Note: Inspection and palpation of the jugular vein and carotid arteries and auscultation of the carotid arteries are described in Chapter 9.

Clinical strategies

1. Abnormal hair or scalp texture or quantity should be carefully explored with the client. Most clients are aware of recent or marked changes in texture. Thinning hair, loss of elasticity, or changing pigmentation may be part of the normal aging process. Change in hair care habits can contribute to hair texture changes.

2. Nits can be confused with dandruff. Nits are creamy, yellowish, ovoid, and smooth. They cling to a strand of hair. Dandruff flakes will shake away from scalp or hair and are irregularly shaped.

3. When palpating the skull/scalp, use the palmar surface of distal fingers. Some beginning examiners tend to use the distal tips of the fingers instead of the distal finger pads. The finger pads are much more sensitive to subtle changes.

4. Have client flex neck slightly forward for thyroid and trachea palpation. This permits muscle relaxation in this area so that the examiner's fingers can probe more effectively.

5. When palpating the neck and thyroid, have the client comfortably seated so that the neck is relaxed. Some examiners actually encourage the client to rest the back of the head against the examiner's chest.

6. Some textbooks present both anterior and posterior thyroid palpation. Posterior position thyroid palpation is presented here because it is the easiest technique for the beginner to master.

7. There are many teaching techniques for cervical lymph node palpation. Each text the beginning student reads locates these nodes in slightly different places with slightly different names. The important points for the student to remember follow:

   a. Find the text you believe best describes node locations and stick to that text for memorization and practice.

   b. Although general anatomical node positions are described in texts, individual locations vary.

   c. When palpating for lymph nodes, the examiner must screen the *entire area* of the anticipated nodes before summarizing clinical findings.

   d. *Light* palpation is necessary to pick up smaller, more superficial nodes.

   e. At times it is helpful for the examiner to place one hand on the client's head and to palpate with the other. In this way the client's head can be moved into any desired position.

8. If the examiner finds identifiable lymph nodes, he must evaluate the findings, noting:

   a. Node size, shape, perimeters, mobility, consistency, and tenderness.

   b. Systemic symptoms that may be related to node enlargement. Table 1 is helpful in evaluations of this type. It describes node locations and the areas of the body drained by them.

Sample recording

Skull: Normocephalic. No tenderness.
Hair: Normal female hair distribution. Dark brown natural color with beginning graying.
Facies: Symmetrical. No involuntary movements.
Neck: Symmetrical; trachea midline; thyroid not palpable. No palpable nodes or masses. Full and strong range of motion without pain.

Table 1. Lymphatic drainage pattern for cervical lymph nodes

Node	Location	Receives drainage from
Preauricular	In front of tragus of external ear	Scalp, external auditory canal, forehead or upper facial structures, lateral portion of eyelids
Postauricular	Behind ear on mastoid process	Parietal region of scalp, external auditory canal
Occipital	Midway between external occipital protuberance and mastoid process	Parietal region of scalp
Tonsillar	At angle of mandible	Tonsils, posterior palate, thyroid, floor of mouth
Submaxillary	Halfway between angle and tip of mandible	Tongue, submaxillary glands, mucosa of lips and mouth
Submental	In midline behind tip of mandible	Tongue, mucosa of lips and mouth, floor of mouth
Superficial cervical	Superficial to sternocleidomastoid muscle	Skin of neck, ear
Posterior cervical chain	Along anterior edge of trapezius muscle	Posterior scalp, thyroid, posterior skin of neck
Deep cervical chain	Under sternocleidomastoid muscle; includes four separate chains extending over larynx, thyroid gland, and trachea	Larynx, thyroid, trachea, ear, and upper part of esophagus
Supraclavicular	Deep in angle formed by sternocleidomastoid muscle and clavicle	Upper abdomen, lungs, breast, arm

History and clinical strategies associated with the pediatric client

1. The head and neck examination of a child is easy to do because it is not considered an intrusive procedure; it is difficult, however, because the size of the examiner's hands may be too large to accurately assess the tiny structures of a child's head and neck.

   a. The fontanels usually present no difficulty in palpation. The examiner must remember that even though babies are born with six fontanels, generally only the frontal and occipital fontanels are palpated. The examiner must have a firm understanding of normal findings so that there may be early identification of deviations.

   b. Head circumference should be evaluated on every child, during every visit until the age of 2 years. Because cloth tape measures can stretch, the examiner should use either a metal or paper tape measure. The tape measure should be placed in front at midforehead level and in the back at the level of the occipital protuberance.

   c. For successful evaluation of the child's cervical lymph nodes, the neck muscles must be relaxed. We have found it most helpful to palpate both sides of the child's neck at the same time. This permits comparison of unilateral or bilateral findings.

   d. The techniques for evaluating the thyroid are the same as those for the adult. The examiner should use only two fingers of each hand as the tracheal stabilizer and lobe palpator, as opposed to all four fingers on an adult client.

   e. Because of the lack of neck muscle stability in the infant, the examiner may elect to evaluate the thyroid from an anterior position with the infant supine.

2. Lymph node presence in children seems to be the norm rather than the exception. The important point is to draw a relationship between the presence of lymph nodes and the general wellness or illness of the child. Barness states: "Shotty, discrete, movable, cool, nontender nodes up to 1 cm in the cervical region are normal when found in the child under 12 years of age."[*]

3. When examining the child's head and neck, evaluate also the range of motion of the neck. Although an older child is instructed to perform this maneuver, younger children and infants should be passively moved through the ranges of neck motion.

4. Before remarking on the "funny looking" facial characteristics of a child, be sure to take a good look at the parents.

5. Risk factors for the pediatric client follow:

   a. Child whose fontanels close earlier than scheduled or those which remain open longer than scheduled

   b. Fontanels with diameters larger than 4 or 5 cm

   c. Child with overriding suture lines or prolonged separated suture lines

   d. Child whose head and chest circumferences are disproportionate prior to age 2

   e. Any bulge areas noted on the scalp or skull

   f. Child with multiple lymph nodes palpated (unexplained presence)

   g. Child with any supraclavicular nodes palpated

   h. Child whose neck does not seem to be growing in proportion to the body

   i. Any neck stiffness or crying with range of motion exercise

   j. Child who maintains a tonic neck reflex beyond 3 to 5 months

   k. Infant unable to hold head up by 2 months

   l. Infant, when in sitting position, unable to hold head steady by 4 months

[*]Barness, Lewis: Manual of pediatric physical diagnosis, ed. 4, Chicago, 1974, Year Book Medical Publishers, Inc., p. 39.

Clinical variations associated with the pediatric client

Characteristic or area examined	Normal	Deviations from normal
1. Head		
a. Contour	Symmetry noted with frontal, parietal, and bilateral occipital prominences	Asymmetry, marked depressions or protrusions
	Long heads in Nordic children	Flattening of part of head
	Broad heads in Oriental children	Odd-shaped heads that do not follow racial heritage
		Frontal bulging
b. Size (Measure during every visit until age 2 years.)	At birth the head measures between 32 and 38 cm; head is normally about 2 cm larger than the chest; by age 2 years both chest and head circumferences are same size;	Any sudden increase in head size
		Failure of head to grow

Continued.

Clinical variations associated with the pediatric client—cont'd

Characteristic or area examined	Normal	Deviations from normal
	during childhood chest becomes 5 to 7 cm larger than head	
2. Sutures and fontanels (Fig. 4-16)	Suture ridges may be palpated until approximately 6 months	Sutures that are overriding or remain open beyond 6 months

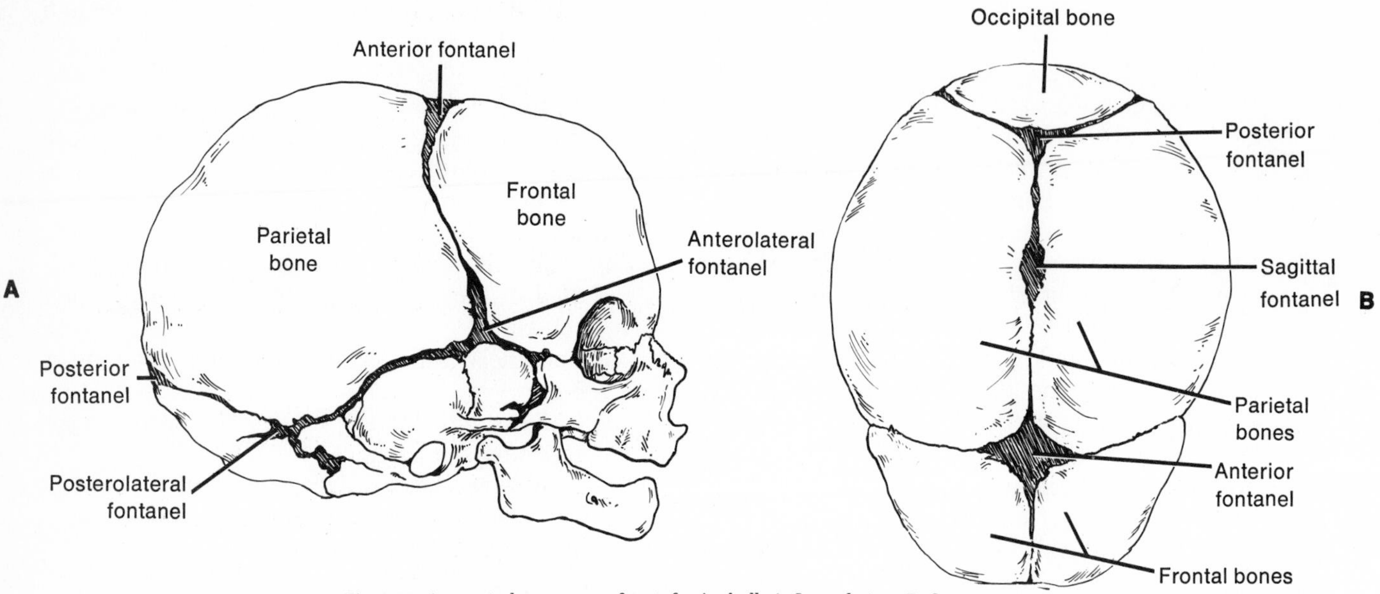

Fig. 4-16. Anatomical structures of an infant's skull. **A,** Lateral view. **B,** Superior view.

Characteristic or area examined	Normal	Deviations from normal
	Anterior fontanel: small or absent at birth, then enlarges to average 2.5 × 2.5 cm; normally closes between 9 months and 2 years	Late closure of fontanel beyond age 2 years
	Posterior fontanel: may or may not be able to palpate at birth; usually closes between 1 and 2 months	
a. Palpate fontanel for quality (Infant should be sitting and *not* crying; lying or crying may give fontanel a full or bulging appearance.)	No bulging Slight depression normal Slight palpitations	Bulging or significant depression Bounding palpitations
3. Scalp texture	Skin intact	Crusting Lesions, scabs Tenderness Scaliness Ringworm patches Superficial nodules
4. Hair		White streaks from forehead toward crown (Waardenburg syndrome symptom) Lack of hair pigment
a. Foreign bodies		Flaking Nits
b. Distribution	Even	Patchy, asymmetrical alopecia
c. Quantity	Thick, thin, sparse	Excessive loss
d. Quality	Shiny, smooth	Dull, brittle Excessive coarseness or dryness
e. Hygiene	Clean	Odor; matted, dirty
5. Face		
a. Symmetry	Eyes same level Symmetrical placement and shape of eyes, ears, mouth, eyebrows, nasolabial folds	Wide-set or close-set eyes Marked asymmetry Wide bulge at base of nose

Characteristic or area examined	Normal	Deviations from normal
b. Quality		Edema (especially of eyelids)
		Markedly coarse features
		Puffiness
		Excessive perspiration
		Waxy pallor
		Lesions
		Lip lesions, fissures, swelling
		Acne, scarring
c. Color	Pigmentation will vary with race	Jaundice
		Cyanosis (especially around lips)
		Pigmentation variations
d. Expression	Alert; response appropriate to conversation	No responsiveness
		Tense, drawn muscles
		Inappropriate expression
e. Movements	Controlled, smooth	Involuntary
6. Head and neck movements		
a. Passive range of motion with infants	Able to hold head up by 2 months from prone position	Unable to hold head up by age 2 months
	Infants younger than 3 months have head lag when pulled into sitting position	Head lag present beyond 3 months
	Tonic neck reflex up to 5 months	Tonic neck beyond 5 months
	Infant in sitting position able to hold head steady by 4 months	Unable to hold head steady
b. Active range of motion with older children	Controlled and smooth throughout series of movement	Ratchety movement
	No discomfort or limitations of movement	Bounding (up and down), synchronizes with pulse
		Pain throughout movement
		Pain of particular points during movement
		Spasms or tics
		Limited range of motion
		Unable to touch points
7. Neck		
a. Symmetry	Head position centered	Head tilted
	Bilateral symmetry of trapezius and sternocleidomastoid muscles	Muscle shortening, waste
		Masses, scars
		Webbing (seen as extra folds of skin)
b. Palpate (Slightly extend chin upward to expose as much anterior neck as possible.)		
1. Location	Central placement	Lateral displacement
		Tenderness on palpation
2. Landmarks	Tracheal rings	
	Cricoid cartilage	
	Thyroid cartilage	
8. Thyroid (Palpate; should be done using two or three fingers; evaluation will depend on cooperation of child.)		
a. Thyroid cartilage	Smooth	
	Centrally located	
b. Cricoid cartilage	Smooth ringlike structure	
c. Isthmus	Smooth tissue found below cricoid cartilage	
	May not be felt	
	With swallowing may feel smooth tissue slide under skin	
d. Thyroid lobes	Lobes may not be felt	Enlarged lobes
	If lobes are felt, they are small, smooth, rise freely with swallowing, nontender	Palpated easily without swallowing
		Nodular or irregular lobe consistency
		Tender on palpation
		Gland not freely moving with swallowing
9. Lymphatic nodes		

Continued.

Clinical variations associated with the pediatric client–cont'd

Characteristic or area examined	Normal	Deviations from normal
a. Palpate the following nodes: 1. Preauricular 2. Postauricular 3. Occipital 4. Tonsillar 5. Submaxillary 6. Submental 7. Superficial cervical 8. Posterior cervical 9. Deep cervical 10. Supraclavicular		
b. Size and shape	Usually not palpable or Small, mobile, discrete, nontender nodes Single nodes up to 1 cm, may appear as shotty, discrete, movable, cool, and nontender	Palpable Large, round, cylindrical irregular Multiple discrete or matted nodes Similar findings in children over 12 years of age
c. Mobility		Fixed to underlying or overlying tissue Induration
d. Consistency		Hard, firm, soft, spongy
e. Surface characteristics		Smooth, nodular
f. Tenderness		Tender on palpation
g. Heat		Present
h. Erythema		Present

History and clinical strategies associated with the geriatric client

1. Mild tremors (rhythmic) of the head are reported by some authors as normal for some elderly people. However, beginning examiners should report any finding of this nature on the problem list.
2. Head and neck range of motion should be assessed slowly and carefully. The single rotary movement recommended in the adult section for this assessment should not be performed with elderly individuals. Each movement should be evaluated separately for the following symptoms:
   a. Pain on movement
   b. Limited movement
   c. Jerky or "cogwheel" motion
   d. Dizziness accompanying or resulting from movement
   e. Crepitation
   f. Tension of muscles in neck during movement
3. If neck pain and/or limitation of movement is a complaint, be certain to get full information about the following:
   a. Duration of problem
   b. Association of problem with trauma (e.g., from lifting, falling)
   c. Any additional discomfort or sensation (e.g., pain radiating to shoulders, arms, chest, or numbness in fingers or hands)
   d. Aggravating factors (e.g., necessity for stooping, lifting at home or work)
   e. Interference with activities of daily living (e.g., housework, driving automobile, discomfort during sleep, inability to look down while climbing or descending stairs)
4. Complaints of dizziness associated with head and neck movement can pose a serious safety problem for the client. Inquire about client's ability to drive an automobile and to move about in the home and community safely.
5. In palpating for nodes or swellings under the mandible, the examiner is usually able to palpate the submandibular parotid glands. They are rather large, soft, and symmetrical and lie approximately midway between the chin and the mandible angles on either side.
6. Occasionally a client may complain of sudden (i.e., within 10 to 30 minutes) swelling under the mandible (usually just anterior to the ear). This may be associated with parotid gland response to obstruction of a duct, duct spasm, or a stone in the duct. Be certain to clarify the timing of onset of swelling, duration (swelling may subside within 30 to 60 minutes), and whether swelling is associated with eating (during or immediately following). The gland may remain enlarged or may swell periodically. This should be considered a problem for referral, but the aforementioned information assists with final differential diagnosis.
7. Refer to the adult section for additional history and clinical strategy considerations.

Clinical variations associated with the geriatric client

Characteristic or area examined	Normal	Deviations from normal
1. Skull		
a. Contour	Rounded and symmetrical with frontal, parietal, and bilateral occipital prominences	Lumps, marked protrusions, depressions Lateral expansion of skull
b. Size	"Normal" encompasses a wide variety of sizes	Markedly enlarged Abnormally small Protruding mandible
2. Scalp	Skin intact and smooth	Lesions, scabs Tenderness
a. Surface characteristics		Scaliness Superficial nodules
b. Color	Pigmentation varies depending on race	Reddened areas Areas of increased or decreased pigmentation
3. Hair		
a. Foreign bodies	None present	Flaking Nits, pediculi
b. Distribution	Even Bilateral, symmetrical balding Women may exhibit increased facial hair over upper lip or on chin	Patchy, asymmetrical alopecia
c. Quantity	Often less hair; appears thin or sparse	Sudden or excessive loss
d. Quality	Smooth; may have less luster than younger adult	Brittle Excessive coarseness or dryness
e. Hygiene	Clean	Odor; matted, dirty
4. Face		
a. Symmetry	Usually symmetrical; however, dentures or loss of some teeth may alter facial arrangement	Marked asymmetry (especially eyelids, nasolabial folds, smile pattern)
b. Quality	Expression is alert, responsive Wrinkling of skin, especially at forehead, mouth, eyes	Flat or expressionless (limited eye blinking) Edema (especially of eyelids) Markedly coarse features Puffiness Excessive perspiration Waxy pallor Lesions Lip lesions, fissures Swelling Cachectic Acne, scarring
c. Color	Pigmentation varies with race Color evenly distributed	Jaundice Cyanosis (especially around lips) Pigmentation variations
d. Expression	Alert; eye contact in response to conversation	Tense, drawn Inappropriate expression
e. Movements	Controlled, smooth	Tremors, twitches, tics, involuntary (e.g., grinding motion of jaws, tremors either localized to lips or eyes or over entire head)
5. Head and neck position		
a. Observe head and neck while client is relaxed and looking straight ahead	The head, neck, and lower jaw may be thrust slightly forward (particularly if client manifests a kyphotic stance)	Head and neck held rigidly (diminished or absent cervical concavity); inability to normally thrust head forward
b. Involuntary movements	None present	Tremors (coarse or fine) Bounding (up and down) Synchronizes with pulse
c. Instruct client to:		
1. Move chin to chest (examiner places one hand over back of neck)	Many elderly clients with cervical arthritis cannot touch chin to chest No discomfort or marked limitation	Pain with movement Crepitation (felt by examiner) Gross limitation of movement or jerky motion
2. Move chin toward right shoulder	Movement smooth and easily controlled Smooth, easy motion	Client experiences pain, dizziness with side movements
3. Move chin to left shoulder (do not permit client to shrug or elevate shoulders)	No gross limitation (movement approximately 70° from straight-ahead gaze in both directions)	Crepitation or limitation

Continued.

Clinical variations associated with the geriatric client–cont'd

Characteristic or area examined	Normal	Deviations from normal
4. Move head toward right shoulder (so that client's ear directed toward shoulder)	Client should be able to move head 40° from midline in either direction	Pain, grossly limited movement Crepitation
5. Move head toward left shoulder		
6. Move head back so chin points toward ceiling	30° back from straight-up position	Pain, grossly limited movement Crepitation
6. Neck		
a. Symmetry	Head position centered	Head tilted
	Bilateral symmetry of trapezius and sternocleidomastoid muscles	Muscle asymmetry or shortening
b. Surface	Neck veins prominent; loss of subcutaneous fat	Marked muscle wasting or tension
	Overlying skin is thin	
	Smooth, symmetrical, & nontender on palpation	Tenderness, masses
7. Trachea		
a. Location	Central placement	Lateral displacement Tenderness on palpation
b. Landmarks	Tracheal rings Cricoid cartilage Thyroid cartilage	
8. Thyroid		
a. Symmetry	Gland usually not visible	Unilateral or bilateral lobe enlargement
b. Palpate along trachea for:	Smooth	
1. Thyroid cartilage	Centrally located	
2. Cricoid cartilage	Smooth ringlike structure	
3. Isthmus	Smooth tissue found approximately 1 cm below cricoid cartilage	
	May not be felt	
	With swallowing may feel smooth tissue slide under skin	
4. Thyroid lobes	Lobes may not be felt	Enlarged lobes
	If lobes are felt, they are small, smooth, rise freely with swallowing	Palpated easily without swallowing Nodular or irregular lobe consistency
	Nontender	Tender to palpation
		Gland not freely moving with swallowing
9. Lymphatic nodes		
a. Inspect and palpate the following nodes:		
1. Preauricular		
2. Postauricular		
3. Occipital		
4. Tonsillar		
5. Submaxillary		
6. Submental		
7. Superficial cervical		
8. Posterior cervical		
9. Deep cervical		
10. Supraclavicular		
b. Size and shape	Usually not palpable	Palpable
c. Delimitation		Large, round, cylindrical, irregular Multiple discrete, or matted nodes
d. Mobility		Fixed to underlying or overlying tissue Induration
e. Consistency		Hard, firm, soft, spongy
f. Surface characteristics		Smooth, nodular
g. Tenderness		Tender on palpation
h. Heat		Present
i. Erythema		Present

Vocabulary

1. Alopecia

2. Anterior triangle (neck)
   between midline &
   scm

3. Cricoid cartilage

4. Fontanel

5. Frontal bone

6. Goiter

7. Hirsutism

8. Hyoid   *bone at base of tongue*

9. Isthmus

10. Lymphadenitis

11. Lymphoma

12. Manubrium   *uppermost portion of sternum*

13. Mastoid process

14. Occipital bone

15. Parietal bone

16. Posterior triangle (neck)
    between scm & trapezius

17. Ramus (mandible)
    above angle of mandible

18. Scalene triangle

19. "Shotty" nodes

20. Sternocleidomastoid muscle

21. Thyroid bruit

23. Trapezius muscle

22. Thyroid cartilage

24. Zygomatic bone

cheekbone

Cognitive self-assessment

1. Which *one* of the following statements about cervical lymph nodes is *not* true?
   - ☐ a. The deep cervical chain is largely obscured by the sternocleidomastoid muscle.
   - ☐ b. Normally, faciocervical lymph nodes are not palpable in an adult.
   - ☐ c. Lymphatics from the thorax drain up to the supraclavicular nodes.
   - ☒ d. Deep, firm palpation is necessary to effectively reach the tonsillar nodes.
   - ☐ e. Nodes enlarged as a consequence of prior inflammation are frequently palpable.
2. An ear infection might involve all the following lymph nodes except one. Identify the *one not involved*.
   - ☐ a. Preauricular
   - ☐ b. Superficial cervical
   - ☒ c. Posterior cervical chain
   - ☐ d. Deep cervical chain
   - ☐ e. Postauricular
3. An infected tooth might involve all the following lymph nodes except one. Identify the *one not involved*.
   - ☒ a. Posterior cervical
   - ☐ b. Submental
   - ☐ c. Submaxillary
   - ☐ d. Tonsillar
   - ☐ e. Deep cervical
4. The anterior triangle of the neck includes all but one of the following structures. Identify the *one not included*.
   - ☐ a. Thyroid gland
   - ☐ b. Anterior cervical nodes
   - ☐ c. Trachea
   - ☐ d. Carotid artery
   - ☒ e. Omohyoid muscle
5. The largest endocrine gland in the body is the:
   - ☐ a. adrenal gland
   - ☐ b. parotid gland
   - ☒ c. thyroid gland
   - ☐ d. ovary
   - ☐ e. submaxillary gland
6. Swallowing causes the lateral parts of the thyroid tissue to __ against the examiner's fingers.
   - ☐ a. fall
   - ☒ b. rise
   - ☐ c. bulge
   - ☐ d. remain stationary

7. The thyroid isthmus is most easily palpated:
   □ a. just above the cricoid cartilage
   ☑ b. just below the cricoid cartilage
   □ c. just below the thyroid cartilage
   □ d. just above the thyroid cartilage
   □ e. just below the hyoid bone

Identify the lymph nodes in the accompanying illustration.

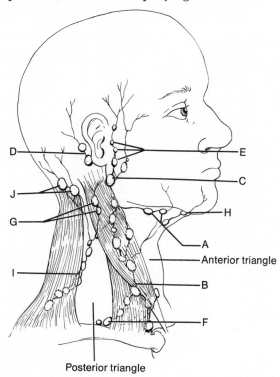

Anterior triangle

Posterior triangle

8. __E__ Preauricular
9. __J__ Occipital
10. __C__ Tonsillar
11. __D__ Postauricular
12. __H__ Submental
13. __A__ Submaxillary
14. __G__ Superficial cervical
15. __B__ Deep cervical
16. __I__ Posterior cervical
17. __F__ Supraclavicular

PEDIATRIC QUESTIONS

18. When palpating the skull of a 4-month-old child, the examiner would *expect* the following *normal findings.*
    □ a. Skull size 36 cm
    □ b. Sagittal suture palpated
    □ c. Coronal suture palpated
    □ d. Anterior fontanel approximately 2 cm × 2 cm; soft, not full
    □ e. Posterior fontanel approximately 1 cm × 1 cm; soft, not full
    □ f. All except b
    □ g. All except c
    □ h. All except a
    ☑ i. All except e
    □ j. All the above

19. All the following statements about lymph node palpation in the child are true except *one*. Identify the false statement.
    ☐ a. Multiple palpable lymph nodes less than 1 cm in diameter may be normal.
    ☐ b. Single palpable lymph nodes less than 3 mm in diameter may be normal.
    ☐ c. Palpable supraclavicular nodes are considered abnormal regardless of size.
    ☑ d. Shotty nodes are considered "red flags" for possible systemic infections.
    ☐ e. Because of a child's fat or short neck, it may be impossible to palpate any cervical lymph nodes.

GERIATRIC QUESTIONS

20. When assessing an elderly client for head and neck range of motion:
    ☐ a. a single rotary motion is a good screening mechanism
    ☐ b. assess for dizziness associated with movement
    ☐ c. crepitation may be felt by the examiner
    ☐ d. assess for jerky motions
    ☐ e. ask client to shrug shoulders to complete full range of motion testing
    ☐ f. all the above
    ☑ g. b, c, and d
    ☐ h. a, c, and e
    ☐ i. all except b

21. Painful limited head and neck motion:
    ☐ a. can be accompanied by pain radiating to shoulders and arms
    ☐ b. can impose safety risks on client
    ☐ c. can always be resolved with proper exercises and rest
    ☐ d. all the above
    ☑ e. a and b

SUGGESTED READINGS
General

American Journal of Nursing: Examination of the head and neck, **75**(5):1-24, 1975.

Bates, Barbara: A guide to physical examination, ed. 2, Philadelphia, 1979, J. B. Lippincott Co., pp. 45-48.

Malasanos, Lois, Barkauskas, Violet, Moss, Muriel, and Stoltenberg-Allen, Kathryn: Health assessment, St. Louis, 1977, The C. V. Mosby Co., pp. 132-142, 167-173.

Prior, John A., and Silberstein, Jack S.: Physical diagnosis: the history and examination of the patient, ed. 5, St. Louis, 1977, The C. V. Mosby Co., pp. 70-97.

Pediatric

Barness, Lewis: Manual of pediatric physical diagnosis, ed. 4, Chicago, 1972, Year Book Medical Publishers, Inc., pp. 39-40, 41-50, 92-96.

Brown, Marie Scott, and Alexander, Mary: Physical examination. Part 4. The lymph system, Nursing '73 **3**(10):49-52, 1973.

Brown, Marie Scott, and Alexander, Mary: Physical examination. Part 6. The head, face, and neck, Nursing '74 **4**(1):47-50, 1974.

Geriatric

Caird, F. I., and Judge, T. G.: Assessment of the elderly patient, London, 1977, Pitman Medical Publishing Co. Ltd., pp. 53-55, 59-61.

Chinn, Austin B., editor: Clinical aspects of aging, Working with older people: a guide to practice, vol. 4, Rockville, Md., 1971, U.S. Department of Health, Education, and Welfare, Public Health Service, pp. 156, 164, 165.

CHAPTER 5

Assessment of the nose, paranasal sinuses, mouth, and oropharynx

Cognitive objectives

At the end of this unit the learner will demonstrate knowledge of assessment of the nose, paranasal sinuses, mouth, and oropharynx by the ability to do the following:

1. List inspection criteria and processes for evaluating the external and internal nose, including nasal structure, turbinates, meatuses, and septum.
2. List inspection and palpation criteria for evaluating the maxillary and frontal sinuses.
3. Discuss a systematic method to test intactness of the olfactory nerve (CN I).
4. Identify the anterior and posterior boundaries of the mouth.
5. Identify characteristics of the lips, gums, tongue, teeth, and buccal mucosa that are relevant to assessment.
6. Identify characteristics of the oropharynx that are relevant to assessment.
7. Identify selected common physical variations with pediatric and geriatric clients.
8. Define the terms in the vocabulary section.

Clinical objectives

At the end of this unit the learner will perform a systematic assessment of the nose, paranasal sinuses, mouth, and oropharynx by demonstrating the ability to do the following:

1. Obtain a pertinent health history from a client.
2. Demonstrate and describe results of inspection and palpation of the following:
   a. External and internal nose for structure, septum position, patency, turbinates, and meatuses
   b. Frontal and maxillary sinuses
   c. Temporamandibular joint for mobility, tenderness, crepitus, referred pain, and occlusion
   d. Lips for color, symmetry, moisture, and surface characteristics

   e. Gingivobuccal fornices and buccal mucosa for color, landmarks, and surface characteristics
   f. Gums for color and surface characteristics
   g. Teeth for number, color, form, surface characteristics, and insertion
   h. Tongue for symmetry, movement, color, surface characteristics, and texture
   i. Floor of mouth for color and surface
   j. Hard and soft palates for color and surface
3. Demonstrate and describe results of inspection and observation of mouth odor and the oropharynx for landmarks, color, and surface.
4. Summarize results of the assessment with a written description of the findings.

Health history related to assessment of nose, paranasal sinuses, mouth, and oropharynx additional to data base

1. If client states that the nose is "stopped up" or obstructed, ask the following questions:
   a. History of nasal surgery?
   b. History of blow or injury to nose?
   c. Are both nares usually obstructed, or just right or left naris?
   d. Often necessary to breathe through the mouth (especially at night)?
   e. History of discharge followed by crusting and localized pain? Is nose picking or scratching contributing to the problem?
   f. Nose drops or nasal spray used? Clarify type, amount, frequency, and how long client has used medication.
2. If client has a history of nosebleeds, ask the following questions:
   a. Bleeding usually from both nostrils, or just right or left naris?
   b. Is bleeding aggravated by crusting; pain followed by picking or scratching?
   c. Do full symptom analysis with this complaint.

87

3. History of repeated sinusitis? General treatment?
4. History of chronic postnasal drip? Is it associated with seasons or weather changes?
5. If mouth or dental problems are observed, the following inquiries are appropriate:
   a. Do you experience pain? If so, how severe and how often? Do you treat the pain? What medications? How often? Do you apply anything locally to teeth or gums? What and how often?
   b. Do your mouth problems interfere with or alter food intake? Describe foods that you can no longer eat.
   c. Are other members of the family having dental or mouth problems?
6. If lesions are observed on mouth or lips, inquire about:
   a. Efforts to treat (medications or local applications).
   b. Whether lesions disappear and reappear. Identify pattern, if possible, associated with foods, stress, seasons, fatigue.
   c. Whether others close to client have lesions.
   d. Whether client smokes a pipe.
7. If client wears dentures, inquire about their effectiveness. Are they worn all the time? Just for meals? Do they permit the eating and chewing of all foods? Are they loose or wobbly? Do they click or whistle or interfere with talking? Does client use any adhesive to retain dentures in place? Ask about denture cleaning habits. Are gums or palate ever irritated or tender? Does client feel that the dentures are cosmetically satisfactory?
8. If client complains of or offers a history of sore throat, ask the following questions:
   a. Are others in your home ill at present time, or do others close to you often have colds or sore throats?
   b. Do you have to inhale dust or fumes at work?
   c. Does it feel as though you have a lump in your throat?
   d. Does it hurt to swallow?
   e. Is the sore throat associated with fever, cough, headache, decreased appetite?
   f. Is your nose obstructed ("stopped up"); do you have to breathe through your mouth?
   g. Is your throat more tender in the morning? Evening?
   h. Is your home dry (humidity level)?
   i. Is sore throat associated with hoarseness?
   j. Treatment (medications, gargling)?
9. If client complains of a hoarse voice (either acute, intermittent, or chronic), ask:
   a. Do you use your voice a lot?
   b. Is hoarseness associated with fever, sore throat, or cold symptoms?
   c. Does the weather affect your voice?
   d. In addition to hoarseness, has your voice changed (e.g. weak, husky, higher or lower pitch)?
   e. Do you have a constant urge to clear your throat?

Clinical guidelines

The student will:	To identify:	
	Normal	**Deviations from normal**
1. Assemble necessary equipment: **a.** Penlight **b.** Otoscope with broad-tipped nasal speculum or nasal speculum		
2. Inspect general appearance of nose **a.** Surface/skin	Smooth, intact Skin color same as face	Lesions, warty appearance Redness, discoloration Vascularization
b. Contour	External alignment symmetrical (or nearly symmetrical)	Marked asymmetry Swelling or hypertrophy (bulbous appearance)
c. Nares	Symmetrical Dry, no crusting No flaring or narrowing associated with breathing	Marked asymmetry Discharge present, crusting Narrowing on inspiration (associated with chronic obstruction and mouth breathing)
3. Press finger on side of client's nose to occlude one naris, and ask client to close mouth and breath through opposite side to test for patency; repeat with other naris	Noiseless, free exchange of air through each naris	Breathing noisy or obstructed

The student will:	To identify:	
	Normal	**Deviations from normal**

4. Palpate external nose for:
  a. Stability
  b. Tenderness
5. Evaluate olfactory nerve (CN I): ask client to close eyes and mouth; occlude one naris at a time and hold aromatic substance (lemon extract, coffee) under each nostril for odor identification
6. Inspect internal nasal cavity using nasal speculum: hold speculum in left hand and stabilize with index finger against side of nose; insert approximately 1 cm and dilate outer naris as much as possible (Fig. 5-1); use right hand to adjust client's head and to hold penlight, or use otoscope with nasal speculum attached; observe naris:
	Firm
	Nontender
	Client able to identify odor
		Unstable
		Tender on palpation; masses
		Incorrect identification of odor

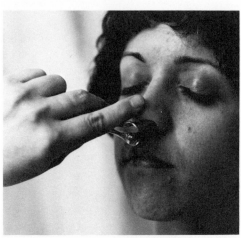

Fig. 5-1. Nasal speculum insertion.

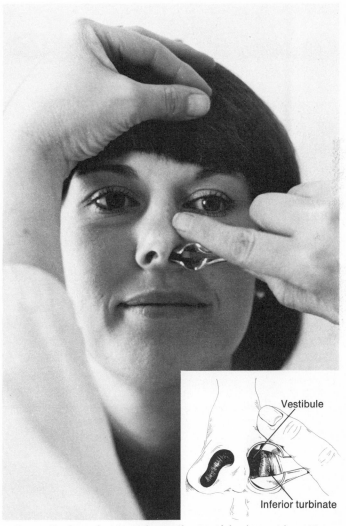

Vestibule

Inferior turbinate

Fig. 5-2. Nasal speculum inserted; view of naris with head in upright position.

a. With client's head erect (Fig. 5-2)	Floor of nose (vestibule) Inferior turbinate Nasal hairs present Mucosa slightly darker (redder) than oral mucosa	Furuncle (most often present in vestibule) Tenderness Marked redness Crusting, discharge Lesions or masses

Continued.

Clinical guidelines—cont'd

The student will:	To identify:	
	Normal	Deviations from normal
b. With client's head back (Fig. 5-3)	Middle meatus Middle turbinate Turbinates same color as surrounding nasal mucosa Film of clear discharge (small amount)	Sinus drainage Polyps, masses Turbinates appear pale, swollen (allergic responses) Mucosa markedly red with copious discharge Yellow, thick, green discharge
c. With client's head to side (Fig. 5-4); repeat with opposite naris	Lower third is vascular area (Kiesselbach's area) Septum midline and straight	Bleeding, crusting Tenderness Lesions Marked deviation of septum

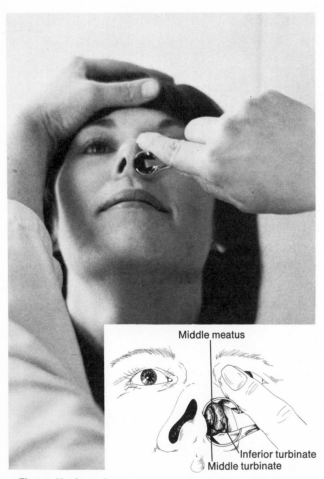

Fig. 5-3. Nasal speculum inserted; view of naris with head tilted back.

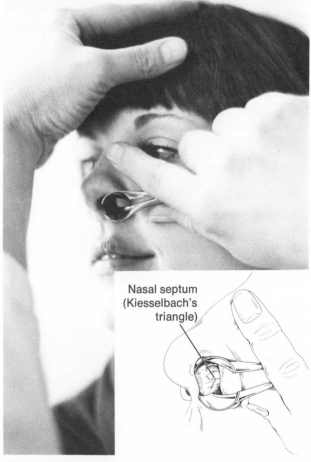

Fig. 5-4. Nasal speculum inserted; view of naris with head turned to side.

The student will:	To identify:	
	Normal	Deviations from normal
d. Inspect and palpate paranasal sinuses for tenderness and swelling 1. Frontal (Fig. 5-5) 2. Maxillary (Fig. 5-6)	Nontender No swelling	Tender on palpation Swelling of soft tissue over sinus area

7. Assemble equipment for examination of mouth and pharynx:
  a. Penlight
  b. Two tongue blades
  c. Two 4 × 4-inch gauze sponges
  d. Gloves or finger cots

8. Inspect, palpate, and maneuver temporomandibular joint: place fingers in front of each ear and ask client to open and close mouth slowly (Fig. 5-7)

Fig. 5-5. Palpating frontal sinuses.

Fig. 5-6. Palpating maxillary sinuses.

Fig. 5-7. Palpating the temporomandibular joint.

a. Mobility	Smooth jaw excursion, 3.5 to 4.5 cm (1⅓ to 1¾ inches)	Limited excursion
b. Tenderness	Absent on palpation	Present on palpation
c. Crepitus	Absent	Present
d. Referred pain	Absent	Present (especially on closure of jaw)

9. Inspect closed mouth: ask client to clench teeth and smile

a. Occlusion	Top back teeth rest directly on lower teeth; upper incisors slightly override lowers (Fig. 5-8)	Protrusion of upper incisors Protrusion of lower incisors

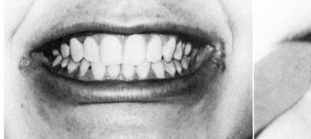

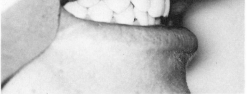

Fig. 5-8. Normal occlusion. **A,** Front view. Note vesicular and ulceration patterns at the corners of the mouth. **B,** Lateral view.

Continued.

Clinical guidelines—cont'd

The student will:	To identify:	
	Normal	**Deviations from normal**
		Upper incisors do not overlap lowers on closure (Fig. 5-9) Lateral displacement of teeth; back teeth do not occlude

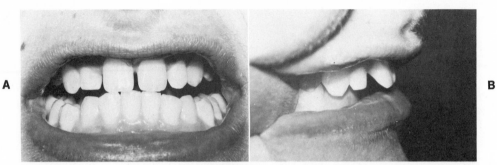

Fig. 5-9. Example of malocclusion. **A,** Front view. **B,** Profile.

10. Inspect and palpate lips for:		
a. Color	Pink	Pale, cyanotic, reddened
b. Symmetry	Vertical and lateral symmetry at rest or on movement	Swelling (general or localized), induration
c. Moisture	Smooth and moist	Dry, flaking, cracked
d. Surface characteristics	Slight vertical linear markings	Lesions: plaques, vesicles (Fig. 5-10), nodules, ulcerations Inflamed fissures at corners

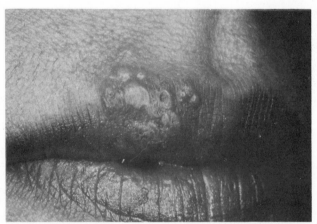

Fig. 5-10. Herpes simplex I. (Courtesy Dr. George Blozis, The Ohio State University College of Dentistry.)

11. Ask client to remove any dental appliances and to open mouth partially; inspect and palpate inner lips and upper and lower gingivobuccal fornices; ask client to open wide to inspect buccal mucosa; use tongue blade and penlight		
a. Color	Pale coral, pink Increased pigmentation (general or localized) with dark-skinned individuals	Pale, cyanotic, reddened Local deposits of brown pigmentation

The student will:	To identify:	
	Normal	**Deviations from normal**
b. Landmarks	Parotid duct (pinpoint red marking); may be slightly elevated (Fig. 5-11)	
c. Surface characteristics	Smooth Where teeth meet, occlusion line may appear on adjacent mucosa (Fig. 5-11) Clear saliva over surface	Ulcers White patches White plaques Swelling (local/general) Bleeding Excessively dry mouth Excessive salivation

Parotid duct

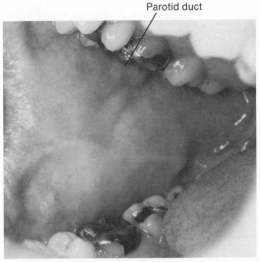

Fig. 5-11. Occlusion line on buccal membrane. Note parotid (Stensen) duct. (Courtesy Dr. George Blozis, The Ohio State University College of Dentistry.)

12. Inspect and palpate gums for: **a.** Color **b.** Surface characteristics	Pink, coral Slightly stippled (Fig. 5-12) Clearly defined, tight margin at tooth Patchy brown pigmentation (usually with dark-skinned individuals)	Reddened, pale Swelling (stippling disappears) Bleeding with slight pressure Enlarged crevice between teeth and gums Pockets containing debris at tooth margin (Fig. 5-13)

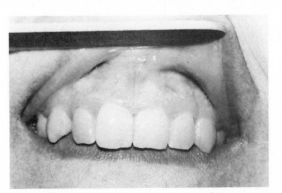

Fig. 5-12. Slightly stippled gum surface is a normal characteristic.

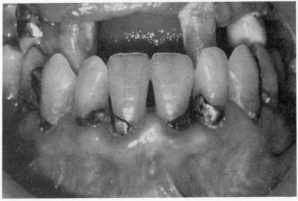

Fig. 5-13. Pockets containing debris at tooth margin.

Continued.

Clinical guidelines—cont'd

The student will:	To identify:	
	Normal	**Deviations from normal**
	Hypertrophy may appear at puberty or during pregnancy (Fig. 5-14)	Ulcers, epulis
	If inflammation (gingivitis) appears, client should be referred for appraisal by dentist	Blue-black line at gum margin
		Marked enlargement (Fig. 5-15)
		Tenderness on palpation
		White patches (especially with edentulous clients)

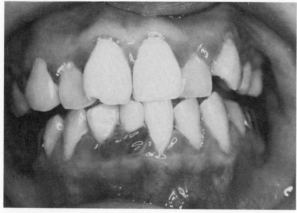

Fig. 5-14. Pregnancy gingivitis with hypertrophy. (Courtesy Dr. George Blozis, The Ohio State University College of Dentistry.)

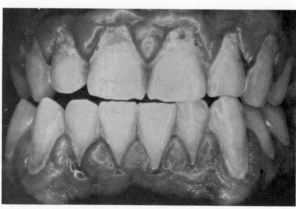

Fig. 5-15. Marked enlargement of gums. (Courtesy Dr. Leonard K. Ebel, The Ohio State University College of Dentistry.)

The student will:	Normal	Deviations from normal
13. Inspect teeth for:		
a. Number	Thirty-two (full adult)	Missing teeth
	Upper and/or lower third molars sometimes congenitally absent	
b. Color	White, yellowish, or grayish hues	Darkened, stained (individual teeth or all)
c. Form	Smooth edges	Central incisor notching
		Irregular notching
		Broken
		Peglike
d. Surface characteristics	Smooth	Debris present (especially at gum line)
	Dental restorations present	Caries (Fig. 5-16)
		Much tooth neck exposed, with receding gums

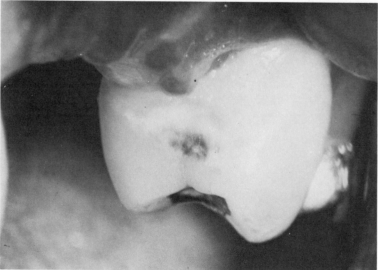

Fig. 5-16. Early tooth decay with surface intact. (Courtesy Dr. George Blozis, The Ohio State University College of Dentistry.)

The student will:	To identify:	
	Normal	**Deviations from normal**
14. Maneuver teeth for tightness	No movement or slight movement	Marked movement (generalized or localized)
15. Inspect and palpate tongue: ask client to protrude tongue		
a. Symmetry and movement	Forward thrust smooth and symmetrical Appearance of tongue symmetrical	Unilateral atrophy Lateral movement Fasciculation
b. Color	Pink	Red
c. Surface characteristics	Dorsal and lateral: Moist, glistening coating Papillae present Elongated vallate papillae Fissures present (Fig. 5-17)	Papillae absent Lesions

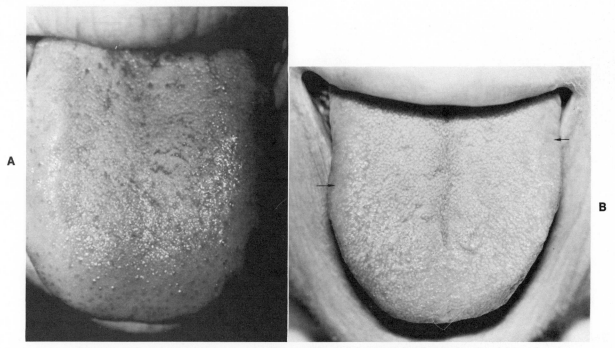

Fig. 5-17. A, Normal dorsal surface of tongue. Note papillae, small fissures, and scalloped effect along left lateral border, a normal deviation caused by adjacent teeth. **B,** Dorsal surface on elderly individual's tongue. Arrows indicate smoothness (papillary atrophy) on lateral borders.

16. Grasp tongue with 4 × 4-inch gauze pad and palpate all sides for texture	Smooth, even tissue	Lumps, nodules Induration

Clinical guidelines—cont'd

The student will:	To identify:	
	Normal	**Deviations from normal**
17. Ask client to put tongue to roof of mouth; inspect and palpate ventral surface and floor of mouth for:	Pink and smooth, with large veins (Fig. 5-18)	Lesions, patches

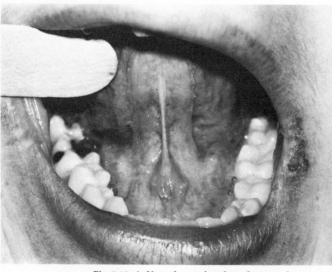
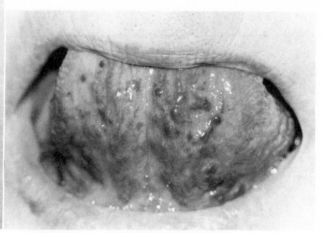

A

B

Fig. 5-18. A, Normal ventral surface of tongue showing vessels, septum, and floor of mouth. **B,** Ventral surface of elderly individual's tongue. Note engorged and nodular vessels.

a. Color	Pale, coral, pink	Pallor; redness
b. Surface characteristics	Frenulum (centered)	Lesions, lumps
	Submaxillary duct opening	
18. Inspect and palpate hard and soft palates for:		
a. Color	Hard palate: pale	Reddened
	Soft palate: pink	Pallor; redness
b. Surface characteristics	Hard palate immovable, with irregular transverse rugae	Patches, lesions
		Petechiae
	Midline exostosis (torus palatinus) may be present (Fig. 5-19)	
	Soft palate movable	Lesions
	Symmetrical elevation	
	Smooth	

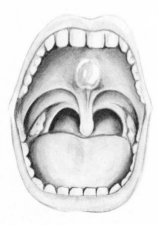

Fig. 5-19. Midline exostosis (torus palatinus).

The student will:	To identify:	
	Normal	**Deviations from normal**
19. Observe for mouth odor	Absent or sweet	Fetid, musty, or acetonic
20. Inspect oropharynx for:		
a. Landmarks	Anterior and posterior pillars symmetrical	
	Uvula midline	Pulled laterally
	Tonsils (may be partially or totally absent); may also be called tonsil tag (Fig. 5-20)	Hypertrophied (adult)
b. Color	Posterior wall pink	Reddened
c. Surface characteristics	Smooth	Lesions, plaques
	Tonsils may be cryptic (Fig. 5-20)	Increased vascularity
	Posterior wall: slight vascularity may be present	Crypts inflamed or filled with debris or exudate
		Vertical reddened lines or general redness
		Swelling, exudate
		Grayish membrane

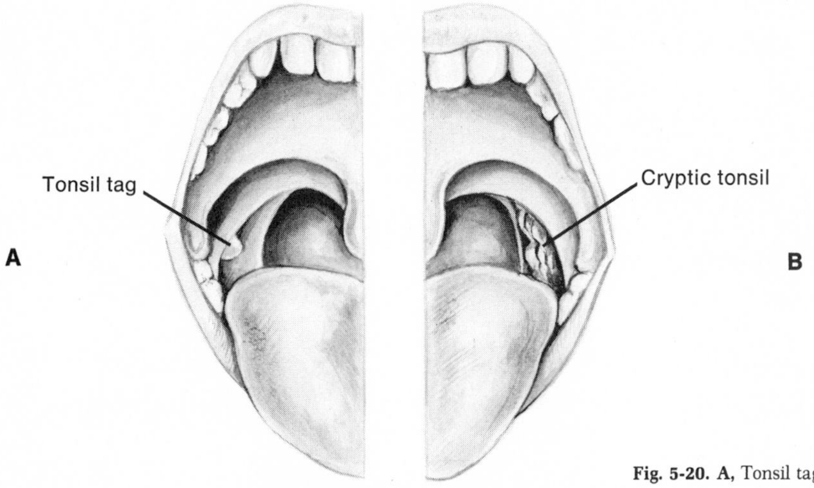

Fig. 5-20. **A,** Tonsil tag. **B,** Cryptic tonsil.

Note: Gag reflex is tested at this time (CN IX, CN X). This is covered in the neurological assessment (Chapter 15).

Clinical strategies

1. A prolonged nose or mouth examination should be accompanied by client comfort. The head needs to be supported. Having the client lie down may be easiest for both of you. (Remember that the head must be tilted at various angles for viewing the nose.)

2. To visualize the lower and middle turbinates, the examiner must insert the nasal speculum at least 1.3 cm (½ inch) into the nares.

3. Stabilize the nasal speculum with the index finger against the side of the patient's nose to avoid jiggling the speculum unnecessarily while it is in the naris.

4. The nasal speculum (if otoscope not in use) is to be inserted with the blades up and down to avoid pressure of the speculum blades against the septum, which can cause much discomfort. Open the blades as wide as possible for optimum viewing.

5. Watch out for hair in the nose. Be careful not to pinch hair as you remove the speculum.

6. For oral examination some practitioners use angled mouth mirrors. They are helpful for viewing posterior angles.

7. Early dental caries cannot be recognized without the use of radiography. An examination of teeth with the use of a penlight, mirror, and tongue blade does not constitute adequate screening for dental caries.

8. Open, crusted lesions on the lips or in the mouth should be palpated with a gloved hand.

9. The tongue blade on the posterior dorsal surface of the tongue will usually cause a gag reflex. For the majority of the examination the tongue blade,

when used, should rest lightly on the anterior part of the tongue.

10. Many clients can elevate their soft palate and depress their own tongue for viewing of the pharyngeal wall, so that the examiner does not have to use a tongue depressor.

11. Explain your procedure to the client *before* beginning (especially when grasping the tongue).

Sample recording

Nose: Appears straight and symmetrical with nostrils patent. Odors properly identified. Nasal mucosa pink, moist, with no discharge or lesions. Sinuses nontender on palpation.

Mouth and pharynx

Temporomandibular joint fully mobile, without tenderness or crepitus.

Lips pink, moist, without lesions.

Buccal mucosa gingivae and hard and soft palates pink, with no lesions, inflammation, patches, or swelling.

Teeth: twenty-eight (all third molars absent). Firmly seated, with five gold restorations. No debris, staining, obvious caries. No inflammation at gingivae.

Tongue: midline, symmetrical. No lesions or fasciculations.

Floor of mouth without lesions

Uvula midline, tonsils absent. Pharyngeal wall pink with no lesions, exudate, or swelling. Mouth odor faintly sweet.

History and clinical strategies associated with the pediatric client

1. It is important to assess individually the nose, mouth, teeth, and oropharynx of all children. The frontal and maxillary sinuses are routinely palpated in children over 8 years of age.

2. Because of the intrusive nature of these examinations, the examiner should delay assessment until the end of the entire examination.

3. Although it is desirable to assess the nose, mouth, and throat while the child is sitting, a young or uncooperative child will need to be firmly restrained. Following are examination strategies:

   a. Infants to 1 year are usually restrained in a supine position with child's arms extended over the head and secured in position by parent or helper.

   b. Toddlers may be restrained in either a supine position as just described or when sitting on parent's lap. If the second method is used, the child's legs are trapped between the parent's knees, and the arms and chest are restrained with one of the parent's arms while the other

hand is used to restrain the child's head firmly against the chest (Fig. 5-21).

   c. For preschoolers, spend time getting to know the child, allow him to play with the tongue blade during the examination, and play smiling and "aah" games as a buildup to the actual mouth and throat examination. Although these techniques may work for some children, others will need to be restrained with one of the techniques just described. Regardless of the technique used for the throat examination, we have discovered that it may be helpful to divide the examination of the mouth and throat into two phases and evaluate each at different times during the total assessment. The mouth evaluation is easily done early in the examination process. If the examiner simply approaches the sitting child with a flashlight and

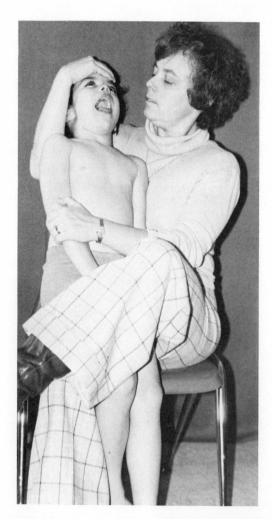

Fig. 5-21. Technique to restrain child for mouth examination.

asks the child to show lips, teeth, and tongue, an initial assessment can be made. A more thorough evaluation of unexposed spots and the throat should be postponed until the end of the examination (Fig. 5-22).

    d. School-age children are usually cooperative and willing to show off their new teeth or the absence of their teeth. The mouth and throat are easiest to evaluate if the child is sitting upright on the cart.

4. It is a universal problem to attempt to open the mouth of an uncooperative child whose teeth are clenched tight. Although not every technique will work on every child, the following might be helpful. Slowly advance the tongue blade along the lips to the posterior teeth. Carefully ease the blade between the teeth toward the pharynx. If possible, maintain a downward motion on the tongue blade so that the tongue is pushed forward and the base of the tongue is pressed downward. The child will suddenly gag, and the mouth will open wide. During what appears to be a split second of visibility the examiner must view all the structures therein. Repeated practice is necessary to develop the inclusive scanning view required during mouth and throat evaluation.

5. Several techniques can be used to facilitate the posterior pharynx viewing while avoiding the gag reflex. A common one is to instruct the child to pant like a puppy while sticking the tongue far forward. This technique lowers the posterior tongue and raises the uvula. The second technique requires placing the tongue blade along the lateral aspect of the tongue instead of down the middle.

6. Whenever the nose is inspected or whenever there is a history of unilateral nasal drainage or a "strange" odor about the child's head or mouth, a foreign body in the nose must be considered.

7. Bruising or lacerations about the lips, gums, frenulum, or buccal mucosa of an infant or young child must be further evaluated as a possible sign of child abuse. Forced feedings by either a bottle or spoon may cause such bruising.

8. It is important to inquire about tooth brushing from the time the first tooth appears. Brushing habits as well as who brushes the child's teeth are important.

9. In young children with extensive caries of the central upper teeth, the examiner should inquire about the child's continuing use of a bottle, especially as a nighttime routine.

10. When inspecting the child's occlusion, instruct the child to bite down as if chewing food. If the examiner instructs the child to show his teeth, a purposeful malocclusion might be noted.

11. The clinical evaluation of the pediatric client's sinuses differs from that of the adult. Because of the difficulty and reliability of clinical assessment, the frontal and maxillary sinuses are not normally evaluated until about age 8. From that age on the technique of evaluation is the same as for the adult client, testing for disorders such as puffiness or tenderness to palpation.

12. Because of the smallness of the subject and the difficulty in adult technique instrumentation, the nasal evaluation may best be done using the otoscope with the nasal speculum.

13. In trying to evaluate the patency or possibility of a naris obstruction, the examiner may either listen for patency by using a stethoscope at the naris opening or by using a small mirror to detect spot fogging during exhalation.

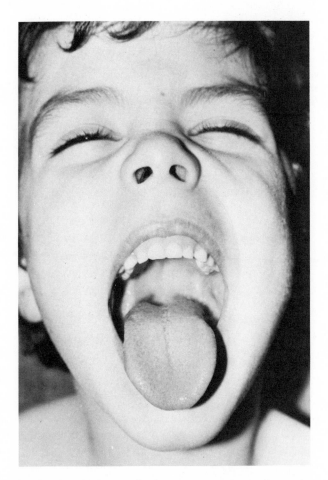

Fig. 5-22. Cooperative preschooler participating in mouth examination.

14. Risk factors of the pediatric client include the following:
    a. History of recurrent nosebleeds
    b. Obvious nasal septal deviation following trauma
    c. Obvious malocclusion
    d. History of thumb sucking, especially as secondary teeth erupt
    e. "Bottle babies," those who routinely have access to a bottle especially after teeth erupt; continue to evaluate for caries.
    f. Children with poor hygiene habits or those who do not routinely seek preventive dental care
    g. Recurrent mouth infections, thrush, gingivostomatitis, or canker sores
    h. Recurrent tonsil infections
    i. Noted bruising to the gums, lips, or hard palate
    j. No teeth by age 12 months

Clinical variations associated with the pediatric client

Characteristic or area examined	Normal	Deviations from normal
1. Nose		
a. Outer surface	Smooth, intact	Lesions
	Skin color same as face	Eczema
	Newborns may show milia	Acne
	May have some redness around nares openings if child has a cold	
b. Contour	External alignment symmetrical or nearly symmetrical	
c. Form	Some children with allergies may show transverse ridge from chronic upward wiping of nares (called the "allergic salute")	Flaring with inhalation
d. Patency of nares	Noiseless, free exchange of air through each naris	Breathing noisy or obstructed
		Unilateral patency (evaluate for foreign body or polyps)
e. Evaluation of olfactory nerve (CN I) not normally conducted in the pediatric client		
2. Internal nasal cavity—observe nares:		Septal deviation
		Septal perforation (noted by viewing spot of light in other naris)
a. With client's head erect	Floor of nose (vestibule)	Furuncle (most often present in vestibule)
	Inferior turbinate	Tenderness
	Nasal hairs present	Marked redness
	Mucosa slightly darker (redder) than oral mucosa	Crusting, discharge
		Lesions or masses
b. With client's head back	Middle meatus	Sinus drainage
	Middle turbinate	Polyps, masses
	Turbinates same color as surrounding nasal mucosa	Turbinates appear pale, swollen (allergic responses)
		Mucosa markedly red with copious discharge present
	Film of clear discharge (small amount)	Yellow, thick, green discharge
c. With client's head to side	Septum	Bleeding, crusting
	Lower third is vascular area (Kiesselbach's area)	Tenderness
		Lesions
	Septum midline and straight	Marked deviation of septum
3. Frontal and maxillary sinuses (see clinical strategy no. 11)	Nontender	Tender on palpation
	No swelling	Swelling of soft tissue over sinus area

Characteristic or area examined	Normal	Deviations from normal
4. Temporomandibular joint (to be evaluated if the child is cooperative)		
a. Mobility	Smooth jaw excursion	Limited excursion
b. Tenderness	Absent on palpation	Present on palpation
c. Crepitus	Absent	Present
d. Referred pain	Absent	Present (especially on closure of jaw)
5. Occlusion	Top back teeth rest directly atop lower teeth; upper incisors slightly override lowers	Protrusion of upper incisors Protrusion of lower incisors Upper incisors do not overlap lowers on closure Lateral displacement of teeth
6. Jaw size	Appears appropriate for face size	Very *small* or *large* mandible, seen in numerous congenital diseases
7. Lips		
a. Color	Pink	Pale, cyanotic Cherry pink Marked circumoral pallor
b. Symmetry	Vertical and lateral symmetry at rest or on movement	Swelling (general or localized), induration, twisting, drooping clefts
c. Moisture	Smooth and moist	Dry, flaking, cracking, corners are especially common (evaluate for impetigo)
d. Surface characteristics	Slight vertical linear markings Breast- or bottle-fed babies may develop a sucking tubercle in the middle of the upper lip	Fissures Lesions: plaques, vesicles, nodules, ulcerations
8. Inner lips and buccal mucosa		
a. Color	Pale coral, pink Increased pigmentation (general or localized) with dark-skinned individuals	Pale, cyanotic, reddened Local deposits of brown pigmentation Blackish, blue areas
b. Landmarks	Parotid duct (pinpoint red marking) may be slightly elevated	Puffy, reddened area
c. Surface characteristics	Smooth Fine grayish ridge Where teeth meet, occlusion line may appear Salivation in children between 3 months and 2 years may be normal If child also appears ill, salivation should be considered abnormal until proved otherwise	Ulcers White patches (*Candida albicans,* or thrush) where scraped off patches are reddened and tend to bleed White plaques Swelling Bleeding Excessively dry mouth (observe for other signs of dehydration, fever, or possible atropine ingestion) Excessive salivation may be seen in gingivostomatitis (child appears ill and usually drools) or in child with multiple caries
9. Gums		
a. Color	Pink, coral	Reddened, pale
b. Surface characteristics	Slightly stippled Sharp margin at tooth Patchy brown pigmentation (usually with dark-skinned individuals) Hypertrophy may appear at puberty May see downward extension of alveolar frenulum as child's central incisors separate; should self-correct Small pearly white cysts (Epstein's pearls) may be seen along gums of infants; usually disappear by age 2 or 3 months; called Bohn's nodules when on midpalate	Swelling (stippling disappears) Bleeding (with slight pressure) Enlarged crevice between teeth and gums Pockets containing debris at tooth margin Ulcers, epulis Blue-black line at gum margin Marked hypertrophy Tenderness on palpation Hypertrophy of gum tissue may be indicative of mouth breathers, vitamin deficiency, or phenytoin (Dilantin) ingestion

Continued.

Clinical variations associated with the pediatric client—cont'd

Characteristic or area examined	Normal	Deviations from normal
10. Teeth		
a. Number: note eruption timing, sequence of eruption, and positioning of teeth	See Fig. 5-23 for normal number of teeth at given age	No teeth by age 1 year Missing teeth inappropriate for age
b. Color	White, yellowish, or grayish hues	Darkened teeth Brownish teeth (may indicate decay) Mottled or pitted permanent teeth (may indicate decreased fluoride or tetracycline ingestion) Green or black teeth (iron ingestion; will go away on withdrawal)
c. Surface characteristics	Smooth, regularly formed teeth	Excessive smoothness (may indicate grinding of teeth) Debris present, especially at gum line Caries

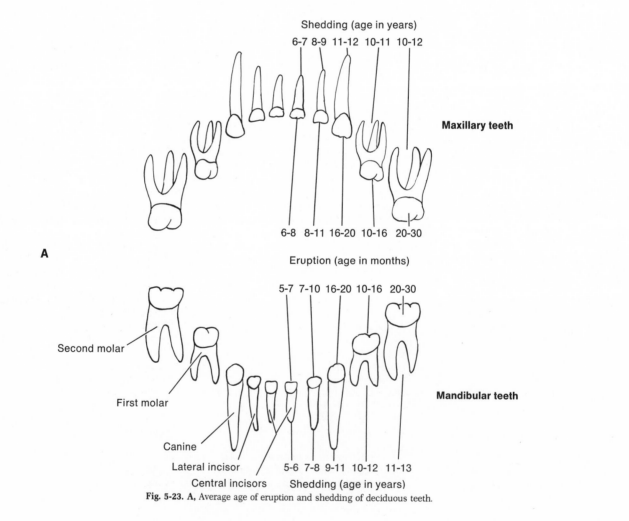

Fig. 5-23. A, Average age of eruption and shedding of deciduous teeth.

Characteristic or area examined	Normal	Deviations from normal

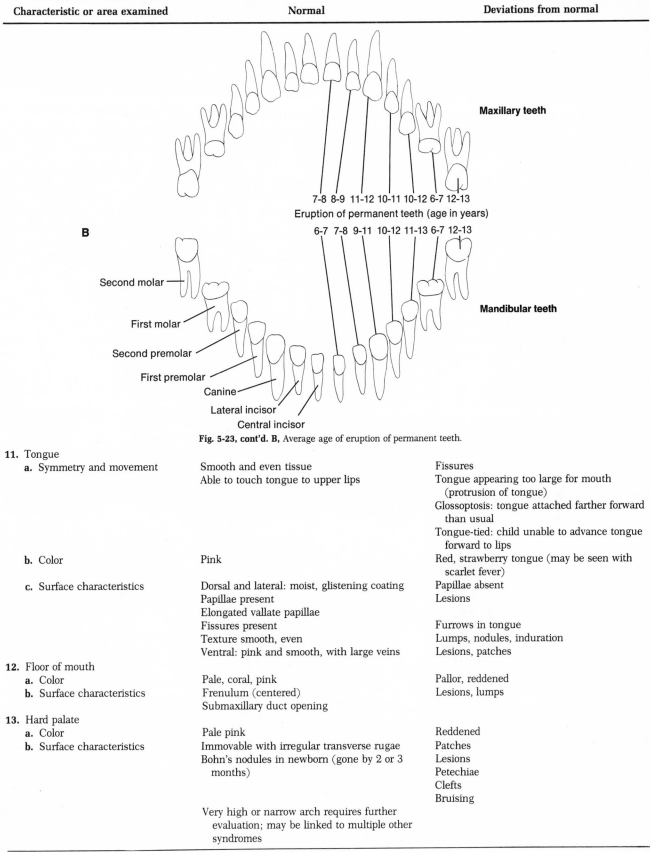

Maxillary teeth

7-8 8-9 11-12 10-11 10-12 6-7 12-13
Eruption of permanent teeth (age in years)
6-7 7-8 9-11 10-12 11-13 6-7 12-13

Second molar
First molar
Second premolar
First premolar
Canine
Lateral incisor
Central incisor

Mandibular teeth

Fig. 5-23, cont'd. B, Average age of eruption of permanent teeth.

Characteristic or area examined	Normal	Deviations from normal
11. Tongue		
a. Symmetry and movement	Smooth and even tissue	Fissures
	Able to touch tongue to upper lips	Tongue appearing too large for mouth (protrusion of tongue)
		Glossoptosis: tongue attached farther forward than usual
		Tongue-tied: child unable to advance tongue forward to lips
b. Color	Pink	Red, strawberry tongue (may be seen with scarlet fever)
c. Surface characteristics	Dorsal and lateral: moist, glistening coating	Papillae absent
	Papillae present	Lesions
	Elongated vallate papillae	
	Fissures present	Furrows in tongue
	Texture smooth, even	Lumps, nodules, induration
	Ventral: pink and smooth, with large veins	Lesions, patches
12. Floor of mouth		
a. Color	Pale, coral, pink	Pallor, reddened
b. Surface characteristics	Frenulum (centered)	Lesions, lumps
	Submaxillary duct opening	
13. Hard palate		
a. Color	Pale pink	Reddened
b. Surface characteristics	Immovable with irregular transverse rugae	Patches
	Bohn's nodules in newborn (gone by 2 or 3 months)	Lesions
		Petechiae
		Clefts
		Bruising
	Very high or narrow arch requires further evaluation; may be linked to multiple other syndromes	

Continued.

Clinical variations associated with the pediatric client—cont'd

Characteristic or area examined	Normal	Deviations from normal
14. Soft palate		
a. Color	Pink	Reddened
		Pallor
b. Surface characteristics	Movable	Discharge
	Symmetrical elevation	Edema
	Smooth	Patches
		Lesions
15. Mouth odor	Absent	Fetid, musty (further investigate poor hygiene, local or systemic infections, sinusitis, mouth breathers)
		Foreign body in nose
		Acetonic or very sweet smell
16. Oropharynx		
a. Landmarks	Anterior and posterior pillars symmetrical	Lateral deviation
		Bifid uvula
	Uvula midline	Uvula with lateral deviation
	Tonsils pink	Reddened; pus, coating, exudate present
	Size may vary from barely visible to very large (Fig. 5-24)	Tonsils occluding swallowing or breathing
		White or yellow follicles filling crypts
	Cryptic	Ulcerative
b. Color	Posterior wall pink	Reddened
c. Surface characteristics	Posterior wall may show slight vascularity	Vertical reddened lines or general redness
		Swelling, exudate, grayish membrane

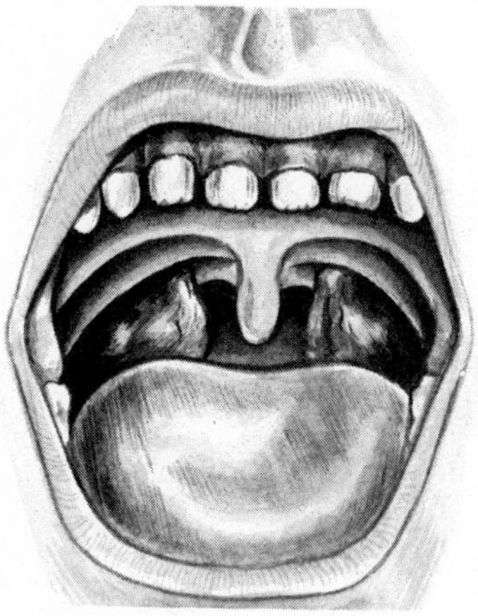

Fig. 5-24. Large tonsils in a child.

History and clinical strategies associated with the geriatric client

1. A number of variables contribute to mouth problems in elderly adults.
   a. Bone resorption is considered a normal aging process, but it can be escalated by systemic disease or local factors within the mouth.
   b. The diminished flow of saliva decreases the self-cleaning process within the mouth.
   c. Slower healing processes decrease the oral tissue's potential for repairing minor trauma from food, cold, or other assaults from the external environment.
   d. The presence of systemic disease (more common with geriatric clients) often manifests local changes or problems in the mouth.
   e. Physical disability (especially loss of manual dexterity or visual problems) decreases the individual's potential for a high level of self-care.
   f. Time itself has an effect: (1) old dental restorations deteriorate; (2) tooth enamel becomes calcified and harder; (3) gingival tissue becomes less elastic and more vulnerable to trauma; and (4) poor dental hygiene habits result in gingival deterioration that becomes increasingly apparent as the individual grows older.
   g. Other problems sometimes associated with aging interfere with mouth care: nutritional deficiency, emotional or mental changes, financial concerns.

2. The practitioner must take a careful history of self-care habits, frequency of visits to the dentist, and client's concerns about problems that interfere with self-care. (See history in adult section for specific history questions related to nose, sinus, mouth, and throat assessment.)

3. Below is a list of risk factors that can serve as a "red flag" to examiners as they assess the oral cavities of elderly clients.
   a. Confused clients (even transient confusion or a shortened attention span can drastically alter self-care habits)
   b. Physically disabled clients (unable to provide adequate self-care)

c. Poor eating habits: no intake of "cleaning" foods, high sugar content, limited intake of foods that require chewing
d. Chronic mouth breathing (increases vulnerability of oral tissue to trauma, inflammatory response)
e. History of chronic smoking (associated with higher incidence of oral cancer)
f. History of chronic use of alcohol (higher associated incidence of cancer)
g. Systemic diseases (only a sample of relevant diseases included)
  (1) Osteoporosis (associated with bone resorption)
  (2) Cirrhosis of liver (higher associated incidence of cancer of mouth)
  (3) Any disease disrupting protein metabolism
  (4) Anemia; blood dyscrasias
  (5) Diabetes mellitus
h. Illness that creates general disability (e.g., fatigue, weakness) and thus interferes with self-care
i. Local irritants chronically assaulting oral tissues (e.g., pipe smoking, chewing tobacco)
j. History of poor dental care habits

Clinical variations associated with the geriatric client

Characteristic or area examined	Normal	Deviations from normal
1. General appearance of nose		
a. Surface/skin	Smooth, intact	Lesions, warty appearance
	Skin color same as face	Redness, discoloration
		Vascularization
b. Contour	External alignment symmetrical (or nearly symmetrical)	Marked asymmetry
		Swelling or hypertrophy (bulbous appearance)
c. Nares	Symmetrical	Marked asymmetry
	Dry, no crusting	Discharge present, crusting
	No flaring or narrowing associated with breathing	Narrowing on inspiration (associated with chronic obstruction and mouth breathing)
	Increase in bristly hairs (especially men)	
d. Patency	Noiseless, free exchange of air through each naris	Patency may be occluded due to nose drying out and crusting; associated with inflammatory response
		Breathing noisy or obstructed
e. Stability	Firm	Unstable
f. Tenderness	Nontender	Tender on palpation; masses
2. Sense of smell and odor identification	Sense of smell somewhat decreased with aging, but client should be able to identify strong odor	Unable to identify strong odor
3. Internal nasal cavity—observe nares:		
a. With client's head erect	Floor of nose (vestibule)	Furuncle (most often present in vestibule)
	Inferior turbinate	Tenderness
	Nasal hairs present	Marked redness
	Mucosa slightly darker (redder) than oral mucosa	Crusting, discharge
		Lesions or masses
b. With client's head back	Middle meatus	Sinus drainage
	Middle turbinate	Polyps, masses
	Turbinates same color as surrounding nasal mucosa	Turbinates appear pale, swollen (allergic responses)
	Mucosa tends to be dryer	Increased friability of tissues
		Increased vulnerability to inflammatory response
		Mucosa markedly red with copious discharge present
c. With client's head to side	Film of clear discharge (small amount)	Yellow, thick, green discharge
	Septum	Bleeding, crusting
	Lower third is vascular (Kiesselbach's area)	Tenderness
	Septum midline and straight	Lesions
		Marked deviation of septum
4. Sinuses (frontal and maxillary)	Nontender	Tender on palpation
	No swelling	Swelling of soft tissue over sinus area

Continued.

Clinical variations associated with the geriatric client—cont'd

Characteristic or area examined	Normal	Deviations from normal
5. Temporomandibular joint		
a. Mobility	Smooth jaw excursion, 3.5 to 4.5 cm (1⅓ to 1¾ inches)	Joint may dislocate when mouth opened wide (associated with loss of elasticity of joint ligaments)
		Limited excursion
b. Tenderness	Absent on palpation	Present on palpation
c. Crepitus	Absent	Present
d. Referred pain	Absent	Present (especially on closure of jaw)
6. Occlusion	May be changed due to missing teeth	Protrusion of upper incisors
	Marked overclosure of jaws may be associated with edentulous client	Protrusion of lower incisors
	Individuals who stoop and thrust head forward tend to habitually protrude lower jaw	Upper incisors do not overlap lowers on closure
		Lateral displacement of teeth; back teeth do not occlude
7. Lips		
a. Color	Pink	Pale, cyanotic, reddened
b. Symmetry	Vertical and lateral symmetry at rest or on movement	Swelling (general or localized), induration
c. Moisture	Decreased supply of saliva may contribute to dryer lips	Dry, flaking, cracked
d. Surface	Increased vertical markings	Marked, deep wrinkling and fissures at corner of mouth (perléche) associated with inflammatory response to severe overclosure or vitamin deficiency)
	"Purse-string" appearance associated with edentulism or overclosure of jaws	Lesions at vermilion border (Fig. 5-25) or development of indistinct border
		Fissures radiating across lip border
		Lesions: plaques, vesicles, nodules, ulcerations
		Inflamed fissures at corners

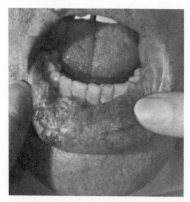

Fig. 5-25. Squamous cell carcinoma. (From Stewart, W. D., Danto, J. L., and Maddin, S.: Dermatology: diagnosis and treatment of cutaneous disorders, ed. 4, St. Louis, 1978, The C. V. Mosby Co.)

8. Ask client to remove any dental appliances; inner lips and buccal mucosa		
a. Color	Pale coral, pink	Pale, cyanotic, reddened
	Increased pigmentation (general or localized) with dark-skinned individuals	Local deposits of brown pigmentation
b. Landmarks	Parotid duct (pinpoint red marking); may be slightly elevated	

Characteristic or area examined	Normal	Deviations from normal
c. Surface characteristics	Mucosa becomes thinner and less vascular; may appear shinier than in younger adult Fordyce's granules common (Fig. 5-26)	White or gray patches (Fig. 5-27) Monilial patches fairly common problem Hyperkeratotic response (whitish areas, may be raised, rough); might be normal response to trauma but should be referred for validation Petechiae Swelling (local/general) Bleeding Ulcers Excessively dry mouth Excessive salivation

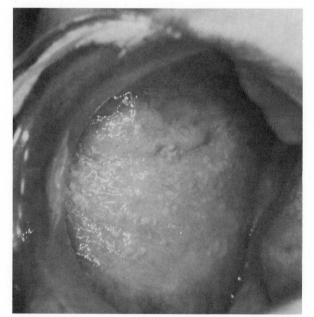

Fig. 5-26. Fordyce granules on buccal mucosa. (Courtesy Dr. George Blozis, The Ohio State University College of Dentistry.)

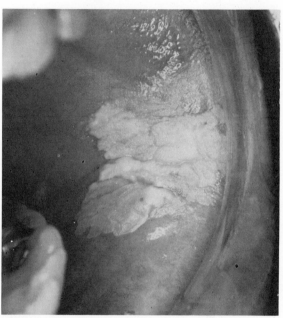

Fig. 5-27. Leukoplakia. (Courtesy Dr. George Blozis, The Ohio State University College of Dentistry.)

9. Gums 　**a.** Color 　**b.** Surface characteristics	May appear slightly paler Stippling may be somewhat decreased	Reddened, excessively pale Increased friability of gums; bleeding with slight pressure Lesions, redness, uneven ridges, spurs, white patches, or tenderness of edentulous gums Marked pallor (fibrotic changes) of gums
	Clearly defined, tight margin at tooth Patchy brown pigmentation (usually with dark-skinned individuals)	Enlarged crevices between teeth and gums Pockets containing debris at tooth margin
10. Teeth 　**a.** Number	Thirty-two (full adult) Third molars, upper and/or lower, sometimes congenitally absent	Missing teeth
b. Color	May appear more yellowish or slightly darker (uniformly)	Darkened, stained (individual teeth or all)
c. Form and surface characteristics	Teeth may appear elongated (increased root surface or neck of tooth exposure associated with resorption of supporting bone) (Fig. 5-13)	Enamel of old teeth may display cracks with stains (Fig. 5-13) Old dental restorations may be deteriorated (especially at the margins)

Continued.

Clinical variations associated with the geriatric client—cont'd

Characteristic or area examined	Normal	Deviations from normal
		Dentin surface may appear abraded
		Occlusal surfaces markedly worn down (leaving hollow surface appearance)
		Cusps of teeth may break off
d. Maneuverability	No movement or slight movement	Loosening of teeth a special hazard, associated with periodontal disease, bone resorption
11. Tongue		
a. Symmetry and movement	Forward thrust smooth and symmetrical	Unilateral atrophy
		Lateral movement
		Fasciculation
	Appearance of tongue is symmetrical	Tongue lies limp on floor of mouth
b. Color	Pink	Red
c. Surface characteristics	Dorsal and lateral:	Papillae absent
	Moist, glistening coating	Lesions
	Papillae may appear slightly smoother, shinier (Fig. 5-17, *B*)	Very smooth tongue (associated with vitamin deficiency)
	Fissures present	
d. Texture	Smooth, even tissue	Lumps, nodules
		Induration
	Ventral:	Lesions, patches
	Epithelium thin and loosely attached	
	Veins often varicosed (Fig. 5-18, *B*)*	
12. Floor of mouth		
a. Color and surface	Pale coral, pink	Pallor, redness
	Frenulum (centered)	Lesions, lumps
	Submaxillary duct opening	Watch for retention cysts at salivary duct opening
13. Hard and soft palates		
a. Color	Hard palate pale	Reddened
	Soft palate pink	Pallor, redness
b. Surface characteristics	Hard palate immovable, with irregular transverse rugae	Patches, lesions
		Petechiae
	Midline exostosis (torus palatinus) may be present	Watch for injuries, lesions related to denture trauma
	Soft palate movable	· Mucosal glands may become inflamed in heavy smokers
	Symmetrical elevation	
	Smooth	
14. Mouth odor	Absent or sweet	Fetid, musty, or acetonic
15. Oropharynx		
a. Landmarks	Anterior and posterior pillars symmetrical	
	Uvula midline	Pulled laterally
	Tonsils may be partially or totally absent may also be called tonsil tag	Hypertrophied (adult)
b. Color	Posterior wall pink	Reddened
c. Surface characteristics	Smooth	Lesions, plaques
	Tonsils may be cryptic (Fig. 5-20, *B*)	Increased vascularity
	Slight vascularity may be present on posterior wall	Crypts inflamed or filled with debris or exudate
		Vertical reddened lines or general redness
		Swelling, exudate
		Grayish membrane

---

*Varicosities should be considered a problem for consultation by the beginning examiner.

Note: Gag reflex is tested at this time (CN IX, CN X). This is covered in the neurological assessment (Chapter 15).

Vocabulary

1. Aphthous ulcer

   whitish canker sore

2. Buccal

   inner cheeks

3. Choanae

   post. cavity of nose

4. Epistaxis

   fibrous tumor of gingiva

5. Epulis

   local gingival enlargement

6. Exostosis

   benigh new growth from bone

7. Fordyce's spots

   yellowish white papules on oral mucosa

8. Fornices (fornix)

   archlike structure

9. Frenulum

10. Gingiva *- gum*

11. Glossitis

    inflammation of tongue

12. Laryngopharynx

13. Leukoplakia

    thick white patches

14. Meatus

15. Moniliasis

    thrush

16. Nares

17. Nasopharynx

18. Oropharynx

19. Papillae

20. Periodontitis

    inflammation of tissue around tooth

21. Ptyalism

excessive secretion of saliva

22. Rhinorrhea

Copious mucous D/C

23. Sinuses
    a. Ethmoidal

    b. Frontal

    c. Maxillary

    d. Sphenoidal

24. Stoma

25. Torus palatinus

midline exostosis

26. Turbinates

27. Vermilion

lip

28. Xerostomia

dryness of mouth from ↓ secretion

Cognitive self-assessment

1. The function of the nasal turbinates is to:
   - ☐ a. warm the air
   - ☐ b. detect odors
   - ☐ c. provide humidity
   - ☐ d. stimulate tear formation
   - ☐ e. all the above
   - ☐ f. b, c, and d
   - ☐ g. b and d
   - ☐ h. a, c, and d
   - ☑ i. a and c
2. With a nasal speculum and penlight, an examiner is able to view:
   - ☐ a. vestibule
   - ☐ b. anterior septum
   - ☐ c. inferior turbinate
   - ☐ d. middle turbinate
   - ☐ e. a and c
   - ☐ f. b, c, and d
   - ☐ g. a, b, and d
   - ☑ h. all the above
3. A nasal speculum is inserted:
   - ☐ a. 0.5 cm (1/5 inch)
   - ☑ b. 1 cm (1/3 inch)
   - ☐ c. 2 cm (3/4 inch)

4. It is then opened:
   - ☐ a. transversely
   - ☑ b. vertically
   - ☐ c. transversely, initially; then vertically
5. The _____ of the nose is bone.
   - ☑ a. upper third
   - ☐ b. upper two thirds
   - ☐ c. lower half
   - ☐ d. entire middle partition
6. The paranasal sinuses directly evaluated are:
   - ☐ a. sphenoid
   - ☑ b. frontal
   - ☐ c. splanchnic
   - ☐ d. ethmoid
   - ☑ e. maxillary
   - ☐ f. a, c, and d
   - ☐ g. c and e
   - ☐ h. b and c
   - ☑ i. b and e
   - ☐ j. b, c, and d
7. About 90% of all nosebleeds originate from:
   - ☐ a. inferior turbinate
   - ☐ b. middle concha
   - ☐ c. dorsum nasi point
   - ☑ d. Kiesselbach's area
8. One sign by which allergies may be distinguished from a common cold is that in allergies:
   - ☐ a. the nasal mucosa is red, inflamed, and swollen
   - ☑ b. the nasal mucosa is comparatively pale
   - ☐ c. the discharge is clear and watery at the beginning
   - ☐ d. the presence of nasal congestion is prominent
9. The paranasal sinuses drain into:
   - ☐ a. the superior turbinate
   - ☐ b. the middle turbinate
   - ☑ c. the middle meatus
   - ☐ d. the vestibule
10. The anterior and posterior boundaries of the mouth are:
    - ☐ a. the gingivobuccal fornices and the posterior pharyngeal wall
    - ☑ b. the lips and the soft palate and uvula
    - ☐ c. the teeth and the laryngopharynx
    - ☐ d. none of the above
11. Which statement(s) is/are true about the lips?
    - ☐ a. Overclosure of the mouth can cause fissuring at the mouth angles.
    - ☐ b. A chancre on the lip might resemble a carcinoma or a cold sore.
    - ☐ c. There is a rich blood and lymphatic supply to the lips.
    - ☐ d. Aging tends to diminish the pattern on the vermilion surface.
    - ☐ e. Herpetic vesicles of the lip are common.
    - ☑ f. All the above
    - ☐ g. All except d
    - ☐ h. b, c, and e
    - ☐ i. All except b
12. Which statement(s) is/are true about the gums?
    - ☐ a. The gums are composed of fibrous tissue covered with mucous membrane.

- ☐ b. The most common irritant to gums are calculus deposits around the necks of teeth.
- ☐ c. Stippling of gums is an early indicator of periodontal disease.
- ☐ d. *Interdental papillae* is a term describing the gums between the teeth.
- ☐ e. Gingival enlargement (hypertrophy) can occur in healthy as well as disease states.
- ☐ f. All except 5
- ☐ g. b, c, and d
- ☐ h. a, b, and e
- ☑ i. All except c
- ☐ j. a and b

13. Which statement(s) is/are true about the buccal mucosa?
- ☐ a. Fordyce spots are an early indicator of rubeola.
- ☐ b. Aphthous ulcers are painless and might be precancerous lesions.
- ☐ c. Leukoplakia may be a precancerous lesion.
- ☐ d. Wharton's duct opens into the buccal membrane opposite the second molar.
- ☐ e. Cheek biting can result in a hyperkeratotic reaction.
- ☑ f. c and e
- ☐ g. b, d, and e
- ☐ h. All except b
- ☐ i. None of the above
- ☐ j. a, b, and d

14. Which statement(s) is/are true about the tongue?
- ☐ a. A whitish coating of the tongue is associated with vitamin B deficiency.
- ☐ b. Carcinoma of the tongue first appears on the posterior dorsal surface.
- ☐ c. Tongue fissures may appear with aging.
- ☐ d. Tongue functions include speech, mastication, taste, and swallowing.
- ☐ e. The lingual frenum attaches the ventral surface of the tongue to the mandibular gingivae.
- ☐ f. All the above
- ☐ g. d only
- ☑ h. c, d, and e
- ☐ i. a, b, and d
- ☐ j. All except e

15. Which statement(s) is/are true about the teeth?
- ☐ a. The crowns of teeth may become reduced in length by attrition.
- ☐ b. Teeth are firmly anchored in the gingivae except during pregnancy or puberty.
- ☐ c. The biting surface of incisors may become abraded by opening bobby pins.
- ☐ d. Radiography is necessary for early detection of caries.
- ☐ e. Teeth can darken because of some systematic medications, local exposure (e.g., smoking), or trauma.
- ☐ f. All except a
- ☐ g. All the above
- ☐ h. b, c, and d
- ☑ i. All except b

16. Which statement(s) is/are true about the oropharynx?
- ☐ a. Smoking may result in a generalized redness of the oropharynx.

□ b. Malignant tumors may arise from the tonsils.
□ c. Benign tumors may arise from the tonsils.
□ d. Tonsils may be enlarged without being infected.
□ e. Streptococcal pharyngeal infection produces classic signs and is easily diagnosed.
□ f. All except b
□ g. a, b, and d
☑ h. All except e
□ i. a and d
□ j. None of the above

PEDIATRIC QUESTIONS

17. Transverse creasing across the bridge of a child's nose is most often indicative of:
    □ a. chromosomal abnormality
    ☑ b. an allergic child
    □ c. child with Down syndrome
    □ d. trauma to the nose
    □ e. a birth defect

18. Normally, salivation in the child is noted about age:
    □ a. birth
    □ b. 1 month
    ☑ c. 3 months
    □ d. 5 months
    □ e. none of the above

19. Which of the following findings indicate an abnormality requiring additional assessment and referral?
    □ a. Pink tonsils extending almost to midline of throat; no difficulty swallowing or breathing
    □ b. Cryptic tonsils
    ☑ c. Transverse tongue fissures
    □ d. Epstein pearls
    □ e. None of the above

20. Any child with a strange mouth odor must be evaluated for:
    □ a. possible ingestion
    □ b. poor hygiene habits
    □ c. certain diseases including diphtheria and diabetes
    □ d. foreign object in nose
    □ e. multiple caries
    □ f. a, b, and e
    □ g. b, c, and d
    □ h. all but c
    ☑ i. all the above
    □ j. none of the above

21. Which of the following is not routinely evaluated in the pediatric client?
    □ a. Tongue
    □ b. Nares
    ☑ c. Olfactory nerve
    □ d. Gums
    □ e. Hard palate

GERIATRIC QUESTIONS

22. Some studies show that the most common reason for loss of teeth with elderly clients is:

    ☐ a. dental caries

    ☐ b. root canal problems

    ☐ c. soft enamel

    ☑ d. periodontal disease

23. Lesions commonly found in the mouth of geriatric clients are:

    ☐ a. Fordyce granules

    ☐ b. hyperkeratosis

    ☐ c. petechiae

    ☐ d. purpura

    ☐ e. all except d

    ☑ f. a and b

    ☐ g. a and c

    ☐ h. all except c

24. Xerostomia:

    ☐ a. is caused by bone resorption

    ☐ b. is rare and occurs in people over 80 years of age

    ☑ c. interferes with self-cleaning of the mouth

    ☐ d. only occurs following poor oral self-care habits

25. Some of the risk factors that could alert a practitioner to potential mouth or dental problems are:

    ☐ a. cirrhosis of the liver

    ☐ b. use of chewing tobacco

    ☐ c. severe arthritis of the hands

    ☐ d. osteoporosis

    ☐ e. chronic heavy smoking

    ☑ f. all the above

    ☐ g. all except d

    ☐ h. a, b, and e

    ☐ i. b and e

SUGGESTED READINGS
General

American Journal of Nursing: Programmed Instruction, Patient assessment: examination of the head and neck, **75**:5 May, 1975.

Bates, Barbara: A guide to physical examination, ed. 2, Philadelphia, 1979, J. B. Lippincott Co., pp. 60-62, 78-82, 103-110.

DeGowin, Elmer, and DeGowin, Richard: Bedside diagnostic examination, ed. 3, New York, 1976, Macmillan Publishing Co., Inc., pp. 126-139.

Judge, Richard D., and Zuidema, George, editors: Methods of clinical examination: a physiologic approach, Boston, 1974, Little, Brown & Co., pp. 81-91.

Keough, Gertrude, and Niebel, Harold N.: Oral cancer detection, Am. J. Nurs. **73**(4): 684-686, April, 1973.

Malasanos, Lois, Barkauskas, Violet, Moss, Muriel, and Stoltenberg-Allen, Kathyrn: Health Assessment, St. Louis, 1977, The C. V. Mosby Co., p. 65, pp. 124-131.

Prior, John A., and Silberstein, Jack S.: Physical diagnosis: the history and examination of the patient, ed. 5, St. Louis, 1977, The C. V. Mosby Co., pp. 162-171, 179-186.

Sana, Josephine, and Judge, Richard D.: Physical appraisal methods in nursing, Boston, 1975, Little, Brown & Co., pp. 97-98, 100-101, 136-141.

Pediatric

Barness, Lewis: Manual of pediatric physical diagnosis, ed. 4, Chicago, 1972, Year Book Medical Publishers, Inc., pp. 74-92.

Bates, Barbara: A guide to physical examination, ed. 2, Philadelphia, 1979, J. B. Lippincott Co., pp. 399-403.

Brown, Marie Scott, and Alexander, Mary: Physical examination. Part 9. Examining the nose, Nursing '74 **4**(7):35-38, 1974.

Brown, Marie Scott, and Alexander, Mary: Physical examination. Part 10. Mouth and throat, Nursing '74 **4**(7):57-61, 1974.

DeAngelis, Catherine: Basic pediatrics for the primary health care provider, Boston, 1975, Little, Brown & Co., pp. 46-50.

Prior, John A., and Silberstein, Jack S.: Physical diagnosis: the history and examination of the patient, ed. 5, St. Louis, 1977, The C. V. Mosby Co., pp. 460-461.

Geriatric

Chinn, Austin B., editor: Clinical aspects of aging, Working with older people: a guide to practice, vol. 4, Rockville, Md., 1971, U.S. Department of Health, Education, and Welfare, Public Health Service, pp. 337-353.

Langer, Anselm: Oral signs of aging and their clinical significance, Geriatrics **31**(12):63-69, Dec., 1976.

Steinberg, Franz, V., editor: Cowdry's the care of the geriatric patient, ed. 5, St. Louis, 1976, The C. V. Mosby Co., pp. 300-309.

CHAPTER **6**

Assessment of the ears and auditory system

Cognitive objectives

At the end of this unit the learner will demonstrate knowledge of assessment of the ear and auditory system by the ability to do the following:

1. Systematically list examination criteria for evaluating the external ear, including:
   a. Anatomical positioning
   b. Surface characteristics of the external ear and ear canal
   c. Tympanic membrane (TM)
2. Describe the technique of manipulating the external ear and canal for otoscopic examination of the adult and the child.
3. List six methods to screen for hearing problems, three for the adult client and three for the pediatric client.
4. Identify selected common variations for pediatric and geriatric clients.
5. Differentiate testing methods to evaluate conductive and perceptive hearing loss. Describe the Rinne and Weber tests and discuss normal and abnormal findings for each.
6. List descriptors for evaluating the TM. Describe normal findings and the suggested significance of deviations from normal.
7. Demonstrate knowledge by defining the terms in the vocabulary list.

Clinical objectives

At the end of this unit the learner will perform a systematic assessment of the ear and auditory system, demonstrating the ability to do the following:

1. Obtain a pertinent health history from a client.
2. Demonstrate inspection of the external ear and relate findings concerning:
   a. Ear position, size, and symmetry
   b. Skin color, intactness, deformities, and lesions
   c. Patency of external canal

3. Demonstrate palpation of the external ear and mastoid process, and relate findings relevant to skin texture, tenderness, nodules, and swelling.
4. Demonstrate inspection of the external canal and TM and relate findings concerning:
   a. Color of canal tissue, evidence of tissue intactness, discharge, deformities, masses or lesions, cerumen presence, and characteristics
   b. Landmark identification, including umbo, malleus, light reflex, pars tensa, pars flaccida, anulus
   c. Color of the TM
   d. Tension of the TM
   e. Intactness, scars, or deformities of the TM
5. Demonstrate ability to evaluate the client's auditory system by using screening techniques, including the Rinne and Weber tests, and interpret findings.
6. Summarize results of the assessment with a written description.

Health history related to ear and auditory system additional to data base

1. Is there a family history of hearing problems or hearing loss?
2. Is there history of frequent ear problems or infections during childhood? Describe typical treatment techniques and course of the problem.
3. Is there history of any ear injury or hearing problems related to trauma?
4. If client complains of painful ears, the examiner should collect descriptive data using the analysis of a symptom format. In addition, the possibility of trauma to the ears either by foreign body, harsh cleaning, or environmental noise must be investigated; and related complaints including recent problems with mouth, teeth, paranasal sinuses, or throat must be inquired about.

115

5. Medication history is especially important if the client has any complaints of tinnitus or extra noise in the ears. Special emphasis should be to collect information about ototoxic drugs, including acetylsalicylic acid, quinine, streptomycin, neomycin, gentamicin, or nitrofurantoin.
6. If the client complains of dizziness or vertigo, the examiner must collect detailed information to describe the exact nature of the problem.
   a. Vertigo is the sensation of whirling motion: with eyes open, the client states that the surroundings are moving; with eyes closed, the client feels himself in motion. Dizziness is the disturbed sense of relationship to space.
   b. How does the sensation change with the client's change in position, e.g., lying down, bending, standing?
   c. Is the client taking medications or is there a systemic disease?
   d. Does the symptom (e.g., falling, losing balance)

interfere with the client's activities of daily living?
7. If the client complains of a hearing loss, the examiner should inquire about the following:
   a. Sudden or slow onset of hearing problem
   b. Environmental factors such as factory noise
   c. Specific types of sounds or tones that the client has difficulty hearing, such as a telephone ringing or conversation
   d. To what degree the hearing problem interferes with the client's activities of daily living; whether it causes a problem on the job, in television viewing, phone conversations, etc.
   e. What types of corrective devices the client has tried; where and from whom they were obtained
8. If environmental or employment noise is a problem, what precautions, if any, are taken? Head sets or ear plugs? What is the extent of the environmental exposure?

Clinical guidelines

The student will:	To identify:	
	Normal	Deviations from normal
1. Collect equipment: **a.** Otoscope with bright light, several sizes of ear specula, pneumatic bulb **b.** Tuning fork (500 to 1000 cps) **2.** Perform physical assessment of the ear **a.** Inspect both ears for alignment and configuration	Ears of equal height and size Located so that pinna on line with corner of eye Ear within 10° angle of vertical position	Abnormal configuration Low-set or unequal positioning
b. Inspect external ear (anterior and posterior bilateral and mastoid areas) (Fig. 6-1)	Skin color pink, uniform Skin intact	Redness Swelling Deformities, lesions, nodules such as Darwin's tubercle

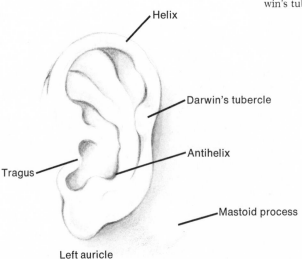

Left auricle

The student will:	To identify:	
	Normal	**Deviations from normal**
		Tophi (Fig. 6-2) Cauliflower ear (Fig. 6-3) Furuncles

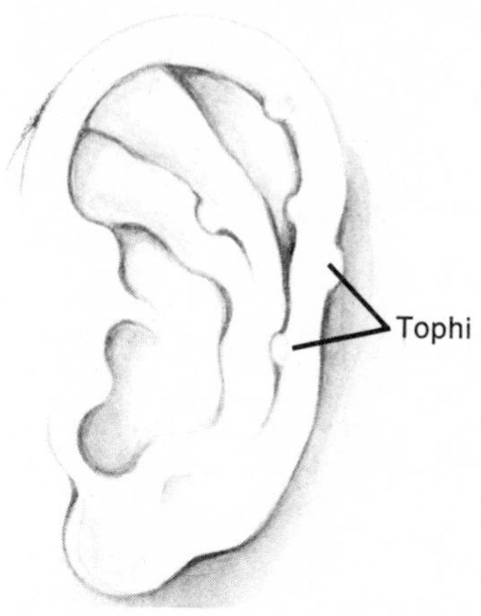

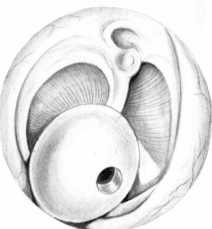

Fig. 6-2. Tophi.

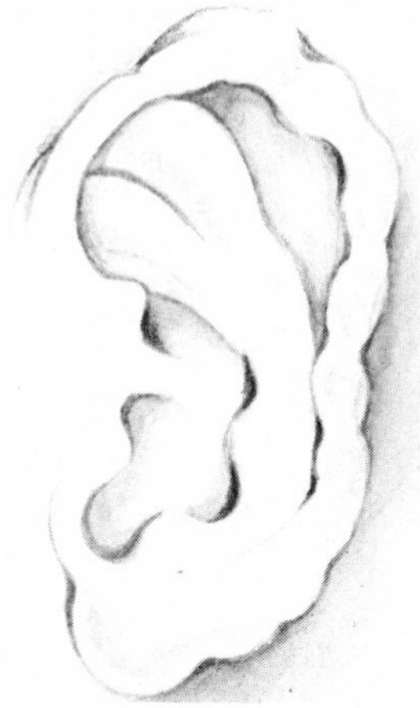

Fig. 6-3. Cauliflower ear.

The student will:	Normal	Deviations from normal
c. Palpate external ear (auricles and mastoid areas)	Intact Smooth, nontender	Tenderness Pain Swelling Nodules
d. Use otoscope to examine: 1. External auditory canal (see clinical strategies for technique)	Cerumen present; note color (may vary: black to brown to creamy pink), texture (may vary from moist waxy to dry flaky or hard texture); no odor Hair present (Fig. 6-4) Canal skin intact Uniform pink color Tenderness with deep speculum insertion	Cerumen impacting ear canal; unable to visualize canal or TM (Fig. 6-5) Lesions, bleeding, discharge (note appearance and odor), foreign bodies (Fig. 6-6), inflammation, growths (Fig. 6-7), pain, tenderness, swelling, infection Partial occlusion of auditory canal due to improper retraction of auricle; can usually be remedied by correct traction (Fig. 6-8)

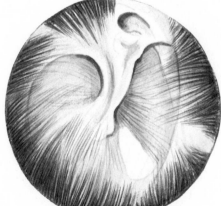

Fig. 6-4. Hairy ear canal.

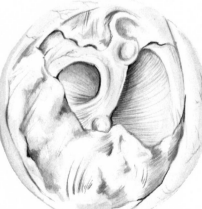

Fig. 6-5. Cerumen in ear canal.

Fig. 6-6. Foreign object in ear canal.

Continued.

Clinical guidelines–cont'd

The student will:	To identify:	
	Normal	Deviations from normal

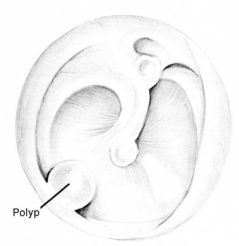

Polyp

Fig. 6-7. Polyp in external canal.

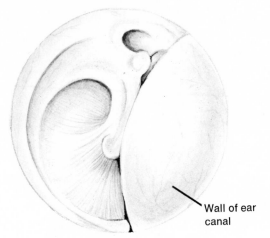

Wall of ear canal

Fig. 6-8. Wall of ear canal obstructing view.

2. Tympanic membrane (TM)
   (Fig. 6-9)

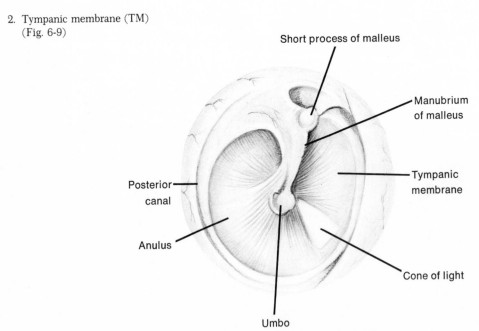

Short process of malleus

Manubrium of malleus

Tympanic membrane

Cone of light

Posterior canal

Anulus

Umbo

Fig. 6-9. Tympanic membrane landmarks.

The student will:	To identify:	
	Normal	**Deviations from normal**
a. Characteristics	Drum intact	Membrane not intact (Fig. 6-10) or showing scarring (Fig. 6-11)
	Slight fluctuation present when swallowing	Fixed, nonfluctuating or jerky fluctuation

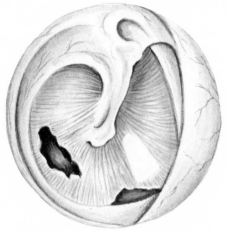

Fig. 6-10. Perforated membrane.

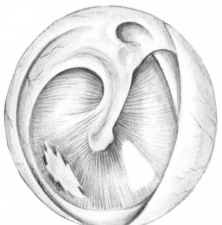

Fig. 6-11. Scarring.

b. Color	Shiny, pearly gray, translucent appearance	Other TM colors indicating abnormality: Serum—yellow-amber Blood—blue or deep red Pus—chalky white Infection—red or pink Fibrosis—dull surface
c. Landmarks: follow anulus around periphery of pars tensa	Cone of light (pars tensa) Umbo Handle of malleus Short process of malleus Malleolar folds Pars flaccida	Diffuse or spotty light Obliteration of some or all landmarks Increased vascularization (injection) Accentuated landmarks (indicating negative pressure behind TM) Bulging membrane (indicating buildup of pressure behind TM)
3. Perform screening evaluation of auditory function		
a. Whispered voice: stand 30 to 60 cm (1 to 2 feet) from client, mask client's opposite ear, exhale, then whisper in very low voice; increase intensity until client responds correctly at least 50% of time; use both monosyllabic and bisyllabic words; repeat other side	Able to hear softly whispered words at distance of 30 to 60 cm (1 to 2 feet) Bilaterally equal response	Unilateral response or bilaterally unequal response Unable to repeat words until whispered voice is louder
b. Watch tick: place ticking watch 2 to 5 cm (1 to 2 inches) from ear; mask opposite ear; repeat other side	Able to hear ticking watch at distance of 2 to 5 cm (1 to 2 inches)	Clients with high-frequency hearing loss unable to hear ticking
c. Tuning fork		
1. Rinne test: softly strike tuning fork and place on client's mastoid process; when	Air-conducted sound heard twice as long as bone conducted (AC 2:BC 1); called "positive result"	Bone-conducted sound heard as long as or longer than air conducted

Continued.

Clinical guidelines–cont'd

	To identify:	
The student will:	**Normal**	**Deviations from normal**

client no longer able to hear tone, remove tuning fork and place it in front of same ear; tone should be heard approximately twice as long in this position (Fig. 6-12)

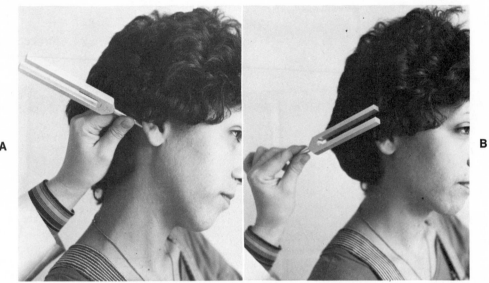

Fig. 6-12. Rinne test. **A,** Behind ear, on mastoid process. **B,** In front of ear.

2. Weber test: softly strike tuning fork and place on midline of forehead (Fig. 6-13)

Bilaterally equal sound

If client has conductive loss, sound lateralizes to poorer ear

If client has sensorineural loss, sound lateralizes to good ear

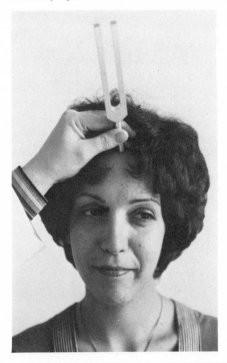

Fig. 6-13. Weber test. Tuning fork is placed on forehead.

The student will:	To identify:	
	Normal	Deviations from normal
4. Evaluate vestibular portion of auditory nerve (CN VIII) (labyrinth system) **a.** Test for nystagmus	Slow movement of eyes in one lateral direction until they reach their limit; steady gaze in that position	Rapid compensatory rhythmic movement of eyes in opposite direction (Fig. 6-14)

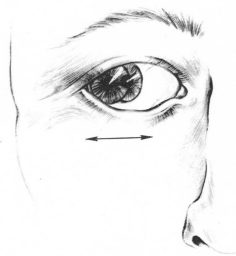

Fig. 6-14. Nystagmus associated with CN VIII vestibular malfunction.

b. Test for falling (Romberg sign): client stands with feet together, eyes closed, arms to side; watch for steadiness of stance; (stand close by in case client loses balance) (Fig. 6-15)	Swaying but able to maintain body and feet positioning	Unable to maintain positioning Need to widen base support Unable to keep from falling

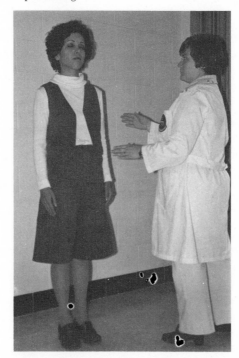

Fig. 6-15. Romberg test.

Clinical strategies

1. Hearing evaluation should begin from the moment you meet the client. Note how the individual responds to your speaking; *note posturing of head or types of words that need repeating.*

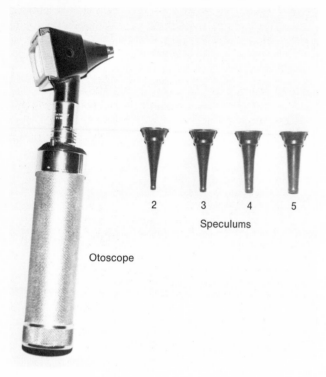

Fig. 6-16. Ostoscope with all sizes of available specula.

2. When using the otoscope, consider the following guidelines:
   a. Use the largest speculum that will fit into the ear canal comfortably (Fig. 6-16).
   b. The otoscope must have good batteries or adequate illumination of the landmarks of the ear will be impossible. (Batteries should give off white, *not* yellow, light.)
   c. The adult client should be sitting with the head tilted toward the opposite shoulder.
   d. Hold the otoscope between the palm and first two fingers of one hand.
   e. With the other hand, grasp the pinna with the thumb and fingers and pull out, up, and back to straighten the canal (Fig. 6-17).
   f. Remember, the inner two thirds of the external ear canal are bony. It will *hurt* if the speculum is pressed against either side (Fig. 6-18). If the examiner is having difficulty seeing the TM, a combination of repositioning the head, pulling the auricle in a slightly different position, and reangling the otoscope should be attempted.
   g. When placing the speculum in the client's ear, make sure to steady your hand against the client's head by extending one or two fingers from the hand holding the otoscope.
3. A cerumen spoon or irrigation may be used to remove cerumen from the external canal. The examiner must see the TM in anyone with a history suggestive of hearing or ear problems.

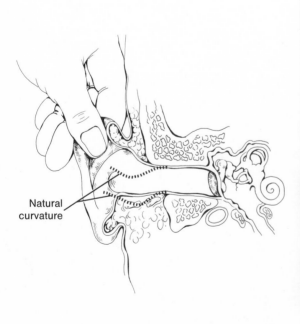

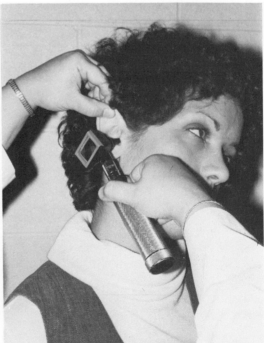

Fig. 6-17. Straighten external canal of adult ear by pulling helix up and out.

4. If, because of bone structure or excessive hair in the ear canal, only about half of the TM is visualized, and if that half appears healthy and without disease, it can be assumed that the other half is also healthy.

5. When striking a tuning fork, be careful not to make the tone too loud. If this happens, it will take so long to quiet the tone enough for auditory testing that the client may become tired of waiting. It is best to just lightly tap the tuning fork on the back of your hand.

6. During the whisper test, make sure to position yourself so that the client cannot read your lips.

7. The technique of masking is very important. The examiner should simply instruct the client to insert a finger into the ear that is not being tested and then wiggle it back and forth slightly to occlude hearing in that ear. The technique is reversed during examination of the opposite ear.

History and clinical strategies associated with the pediatric client

1. The basic evaluation of a child's ear is exactly like that of an adult's ear. For screening purposes the vestibular component is not evaluated.

2. The examiner must evaluate the same anatomic structures in both an adult's and a child's ears. It is important for the examiner to scale down expectations to maintain a gentle approach (Fig. 6-19). Consequently, insert the speculum into the canal between 0.6 and 1.2 cm (¼ and ½ inch).

3. Another difference in examining a child's ear is the curvature of the external canal (Fig. 6-20). Because of the upward canal curvature, the examiner

---

Sample recording

Ear: Positioning bilaterally symmetrical; smooth auricles without lesions or discharge.
External canal, small smount of dark cerumen noted.
Tympanic membrane intact; all landmarks clearly identified.
Auditory: Can hear low whisper at 60 cm (2 feet).
Rinne: AC > BC.
Weber: equal lateralization.
Vestibular: CN VIII intact.

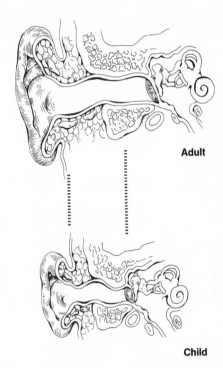

Fig. 6-19. Anatomical comparison of adult's and child's ear.

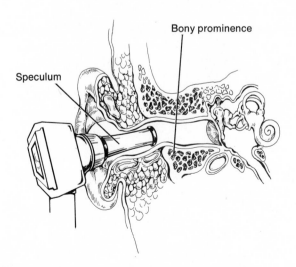

Fig. 6-18. Relationship of speculum insertion and bony prominence.

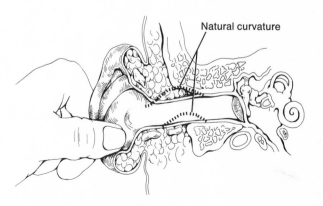

Fig. 6-20. Pull ear down and out to straighten ear canal.

must grasp the lower portion of the child's auricle and retract the ear downward and outward to straighten the canal.

4. Because young children can be "squirmy," we have found it best to examine the child's ear canal and TM in the following manner:
   a. Place child in either prone position with head to side and arms downward (Fig. 6-21), or
   b. Place child in supine position on cart with arms extended overhead and secured by the parent (Fig. 6-22).
   c. Hold the otoscope like a pencil, with the handle extending upward toward the top of the child's head. Brace the otoscope and your hand against the child's head by extending one or two fingers as securing forces (Fig. 6-21). This will allow your hand and instrument to go along with any sudden movements.
   d. The child *must* be securely immobilized during the ear examination.

5. Because of the sensitive nature of the ear examination, it is best left until the last part of the physical examination. Should the child become upset, this will permit immediate return to the parent for cuddling.

6. During the tympanic membrane evaluation the examiner should use a pneumatic bulb attached to the head of the otoscope to pump small puffs of air against the TM (Fig. 6-23). Slight fluctuation of the membrane is a normal response; no movement or jerky movement is abnormal. For the test to be performed, the examiner must choose the largest speculum that will fit into the child's canal. The secure, tight fit will allow air pressure to move the TM.

7. Every child should have an ear evaluation. If the ear canal is occluded with wax, the examiner must use one of the common techniques to remove it. If the child is ill or running a fever, examination of the TM is an absolute must!

8. History questions specifically related to the pediatric client include the following:
   a. Recurrent infections of the throat or ears? Number during past 6 months? Usual treatment?
   b. Are ear problems becoming more frequent and/or severe?
   c. History of ear surgery? If so, what and when?
   d. Does child play with his ears frequently or have tendency of putting objects in his ears?

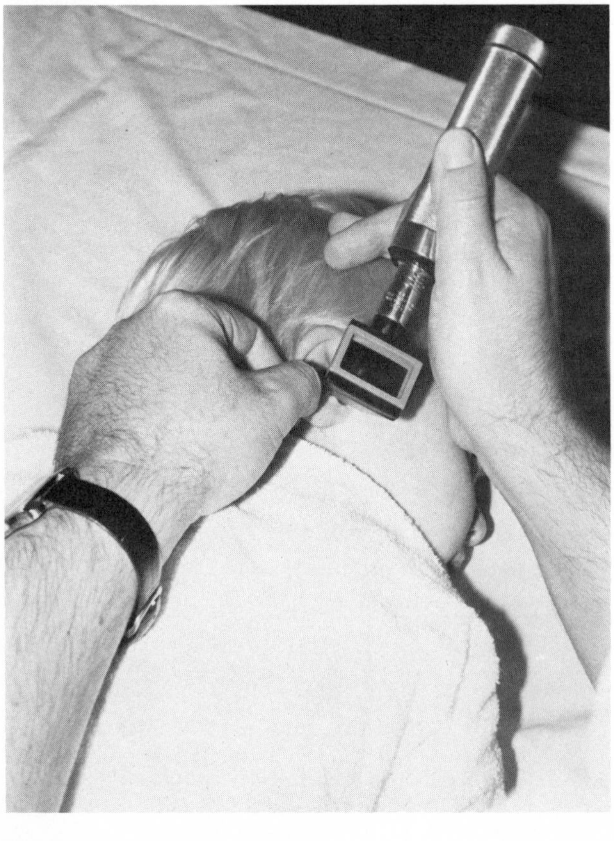

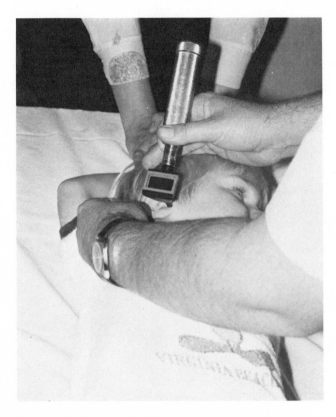

Fig. 6-21. Examination of child in prone position with arms to side.

Fig. 6-22. Examination of child in supine position with arms overhead.

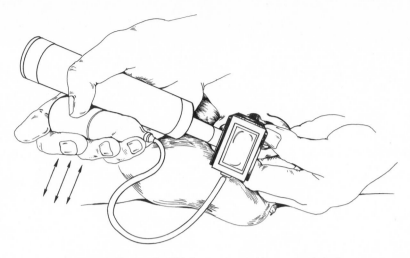

Fig. 6-23. Testing for TM fluctuations with pneumatic bulb.

e. History of foreign body in ears?

f. How does the parent clean the child's ears?

g. Has child ever had his ears tested? If so, by whom and where?

h. If the child has low-set ears, question extensively about kidney or other congenital problems.

i. If a child has symptoms of ear or auditory dysfunction, it is specifically important to inquire about any past disease or drug usage that is considered potentially ototoxic. High-risk children are those who have had measles, mumps, otitis media, any disease with high fever, or drugs including streptomycin, kanamycin, and neomycin.

Clinical variations associated with the pediatric client

Characteristic or area examined	Normal	Deviations from normal
1. External ear **a.** Alignment	Ears of equal height and size Located so that pinna on line with corner of eye Ear within 10° angle of vertical position	Low-set or unequal positioning

b. Configuration		Abnormal configuration
		  Deformities, lesions, nodules such as Darwin's tubercle
		  Tophi
		  Cauliflower ear
		  Furuncles

2. External canal **a.** Color and surface	Skin color pink, uniform Skin intact Hair present Canal skin intact Tenderness with deep speculum insertion	Redness Swelling Lesions, bleeding, discharge (note appearance and odor), foreign bodies, inflammation, growths, pain, tenderness, swelling, infection Partial occlusion of auditory canal due to improper retraction of auricle; can usually be corrected with traction
	Smooth, nontender	Tenderness Pain Swelling Nodules
b. Cerumen	Cerumen present; note color (may vary: black to brown to creamy pink), texture (may vary from moist waxy to dry flaky or hard texture); no odor	Cerumen impacting ear canal; unable to visualize canal or TM

Continued.

Clinical variations associated with the pediatric client–cont'd

Characteristic or area examined	Normal	Deviations from normal
3. Tympanic membrane		
a. Characteristics	Drum intact Presence of myringotomy tube (Fig. 6-24) in selected clients	Membrane not intact or showing scarring

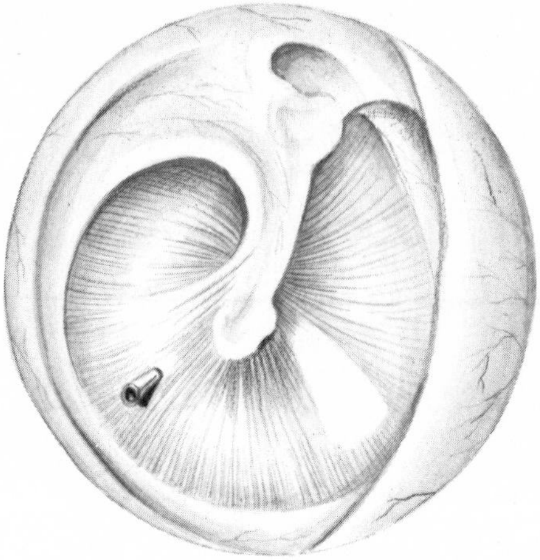

Fig. 6-24. Drainage tube inserted following myringotomy.

b. Tension: use pneumatic or squeeze bulb to evaluate TM fluctuation	Slight fluctuation of drum with air puffs	Fixed, nonfluctuating or jerky fluctuation
c. Color	Shiny, pearly gray, translucent appearance	Other TM colors indicating abnormality: Serum: yellow-amber Blood: blue or deep red Pus: chalky white Infection: red or pink Fibrosis: dull surface
d. Landmarks	Cone of light (pars tensa) Umbo Handle of malleus Short process of malleus Malleolar folds Pars flaccida	Diffuse or spotty light Obliteration of some or all landmarks Increased vascularization (injection) Accentuated landmarks (indicating negative pressure behind TM) Bulging membrane (indicating buildup of pressure behind TM)
4. Auditory function		
a. Newborn: at distance of approximately 30.5 cm (12 inches), and so that infant does not see, snap fingers loudly or ring bell (may need to repeat several times)	Startle reflex or eye blink	No response
b. 2 to 3 months: at distance of approximately 30.5 cm (12 inches), and so that infant does not see, snap fingers loudly or ring bell	Eye blink, or stopping movement to listen for sound	No response
c. 3 months and older: at distance of approximately 30.5 cm (12 inches), and so that infant does not see, snap fingers loudly or ring bell	Turns head toward noise	No response
d. Older infants and toddlers: have child sit on parent's lap; stand behind parent; at first on one side and then the other, either ring bell, whisper "s" or "sh" words, or call child's name	Turns head toward noise	No response

Characteristic or area examined	Normal	Deviations from normal
e. Preschool and school age: should receive audiometric testing; for preschool and school-age client, if audiometry unavailable, use same screening as for adult client:	Able to hear 1000, 2000, 4000, and 6000 cps at 25 dB	Unable to hear recommended levels
1. Whispered voice	Able to hear whispered voice at 30 to 60 cm (1 to 2 feet)	Unilateral or unequal response Unable to repeat words until whispered voice is louder
2. Watch ticking	Able to hear ticking watch at distance of 2 to 5 cm (1 to 2 inches)	Unable to hear ticking
3. Tuning fork: Rinne test Weber test	AC2:BC1 Bilaterally equal sound	AC = BC Lateralization of sound

History and clinical strategies associated with the geriatric client

1. Formal hearing screening should be delayed until near the end of the assessment. Client anxiety or insecurity about ability to perform may exist at the beginning of the examination and may interfere with accurate assessment.
2. Informal hearing screening should occur at the beginning and throughout the assessment. Noting whether the client is able to respond appropriately to questions or conversation, with and/or without direct eye contact, is an important clue for assessment of hearing acuity.
3. Other clues or "red flags" indicating possible hearing difficulty follow:
   a. Client watches examiner's face and mouth movements closely.
   b. Client's speech volume control is erratic or constantly pronounced.
   c. Client's tone of voice is monotonous, unvaried.
   d. Client's speech is distorted (especially with use or omission of vowel sounds).
4. Fairly extensive hearing loss can occur before the client complains about it or reports it as a problem.
5. If hearing loss is offered as a complaint, the following questions should be asked:
   a. Is the loss in both ears or one ear?
   b. Was the onset sudden or gradual? (*Note:* A sudden onset is a "red flag" for immediate referral to a physician.) "Sudden" should be clarified in terms of instant loss (may be indicative of vascular disruption) vs. a loss that occurred over a few hours or days (may indicate a viral disorder).
   c. Is all hearing diminished or just certain types

of sounds (e.g., does conversation sound garbled, can you hear the telephone)?
   d. Do outside or environmental noises interfere with or distort your hearing (e.g., is it more difficult to understand conversation if a lot of people are talking at once)?
   e. Do you have a history of exposure to loud or continuous noises? (e.g., the whine of machinery on the job)?
   f. Have you ever had any auditory training?
   g. Does your hearing loss interfere with your daily life (e.g., responses of family or friends to loss, general social or family relationships, ability to function at work or at home)?
   h. Have you ever used or do you now use a hearing aid?
6. If a hearing aid is used, the following questions should be asked:
   a. Do you feel it is effective?
   b. How often do you wear it? All the time, social occasions, rarely, never?
   c. Do you have any difficulty operating it or using it (e.g., pushing small switches or buttons, inserting batteries, fastening aid to clothing, inserting earmold, untangling wires)?
   d. Do you have difficulty keeping it in good repair, or are you concerned about expenses related to repair?
   e. Do you have difficulty cleaning it? (*Note:* Cerumen or other debris can plug the tiny hole that carries sound through the earmolds.)
   f. When was it purchased? Who prescribed it?
7. Tinnitus may be interpreted as a ringing, cracking, whistling, or buzzing sound by the client. In addition to full symptom analysis, be certain to clarify the quality of the sound.
8. Vertigo must be differentiated from unsteadiness,

which is fairly common with elderly people. If vertigo is established as a complaint, ask if it is associated with head or neck movement (in addition to full symptom analysis).

9. Ear pain or feeling of "fullness" may reflect a problem related to temporomandibular joint movement.
10. Following is a list of risk factors that can alert the examiner to possible hearing deficiency potential:
    a. History of long exposure to loud or continuous noise
    b. History of chronic nasal allergy
    c. Systemic disease (some of the more commonly associated diseases: cardiovascular disease, diabetes mellitus, nephritis)
    d. Sensitivity to some medications (see list in adult history section of this chapter)
    e. Chronic cigarette smoking
    f. General physical or emotional disability (some authors state there is a correlation between impaired physical and/or emotional well-being and diminished hearing acuity)
11. See adult history in this chapter for further questions.

Clinical variations associated with the geriatric client

Characteristic or area examined	Normal	Deviations from normal
1. External ear		
a. Alignment	Ears of equal height and size	Low-set or unequal positioning
	Located so that pinna on line with corner of eye	
	Ear within 10° angle of vertical position	
b. Configuration	Earlobes may appear pendulous	Abnormal configuration
c. Surface characteristics	Skin color pink, uniform	Redness
	Skin intact	Swelling
		Deformities, lesions, nodules such as Darwin's tubercle
		Tophi
		Cauliflower ear
		Furuncles
	Smooth, nontender	Tenderness
		Pain
		Swelling
		Nodules
2. External canal		
a. Color, surface characteristics, discharge	Canal skin intact	Lesions, bleeding, discharge (note appearance and odor), foreign bodies (Fig. 6-6), inflammation, growths (Fig. 6-7), pain, tenderness, swelling, infection
	Uniform pink color	
	Tenderness with deep speculum insertion	
	Cerumen present; note color (may vary from black to brown to creamy pink) and texture (may vary from moist waxy to dry flaky or hard texture)	Be alert for sebaceous cysts, furuncles, dermatosis or increase in granulation tissue (*Note:* Earmolds—part of hearing aids—may cause irritation of canal, especially if they do not fit well)
	Impacted cerumen usually contains more keratin and may be more difficult to remove	
	Hair present	
3. Tympanic membrane		
a. Characteristics	Drum intact	Membrane not intact (Fig. 6-10) or showing scarring (Fig. 6-11)
	Slight fluctuation present with swallowing	Fixed, nonfluctuating or jerky fluctuation
b. Color	Shiny, pearly gray, translucent appearance	Other TM colors indicating abnormality:
		Serum: yellow-amber
		Blood: blue or deep red
		Pus: chalky white
		Infection: red or pink
		Fibrosis: dull surface
c. Landmarks: follow anulus around periphery of pars tensa	Cone of light (pars tensa)	Diffuse or spotty light
	Umbo	Obliteration of some or all landmarks
	Handle of malleus	Increased vascularization (injection)
	Short process of malleus	Accentuated landmarks (indicating negative pressure behind TM)
	Malleolar folds	

Characteristic or area examined	Normal	Deviations from normal
	Pars flaccida Landmarks may appear slightly more pronounced with atrophic or sclerotic tympanic changes	Bulging membrane (indicating buildup of pressure behind TM)
4. Screening evaluation of auditory function		
a. Whispered voice	Able to hear softly whispered words at distance of 30 to 60 cm (1 to 2 feet) Bilaterally equal response	Unilateral response or bilaterally unequal response Unable to repeat words until whispreed voice is louder
b. Watch tick	Able to hear ticking watch at distance of 2 to 5 cm (1 to 2 inches)	Clients with high-frequency hearing loss unable to hear ticking
c. Tuning fork		
1. Rinne Test	Air-conduction sound heard twice as long as bone conduction (AC 2:BC 1); called a positive result	Bone-conduction sound heard as long as or longer than air conduction
2. Weber test	Bilaterally equal sound	If client has conductive loss, sound will lateralize to poorer ear If client has sensorineural loss, sound will lateralize to better ear
5. Vestibular portion of auditory (CN VIII) (evaluates labyrinth system)		
a. Test for nystagmus	Slow movement of eyes in one lateral direction until they reach their limit; steady gaze in that position	Rapid compensatory rhythmic movement in eyes in opposite direction (Fig. 6-14)
b. Test for falling (Romberg sign): client stands with feet together, eyes closed, arms to side; watch for steadiness of stance; stand close by in case client loses balance	Swaying but able to maintain body and feet positioning	Unable to maintain positioning Need to widen base support Unable to keep from falling

Vocabulary

1. Auricle

2. Cerumen ear wax

3. Cochlea contains organ of hearing

4. Darwin's tubercle

5. Dizziness disturbed sense of relationship to space

6. Eustachian tube connects tympanum & NP ⊖ pressure on sides of drum

7. Helix

8. Incus middle ossicle; anvil

9. Injection

10. Labyrinth   inner ear
    cochlea + vestibule +
        semicircular canals

11. Malleus
    hammer; largest ossicle

12. Mastoid
    part of temporal bone
        behind ear

13. Nystagmus

14. Otalgia
    ear pain

15. Otitis
    inflammation of ear

16. Otitis externa

17. Otitis media
    middle ear

18. Pars flaccida

19. Pinna
    auricle

20. Presbycusis
    ↓ hearing ī age

21. Stapes
    innermost ossicle
    stirrup

22. Tinnitus
    noise in ears
    ringing, buzzing, roaring

23. Tophi
    uric acid crystal deposits

24. Tragus
    cartilaginous projection
    anterior to meatus of ear

25. Umbo

26. Vertigo
    sensation of whirling motion

27. Vestibule

Cognitive self-assessment

1. The eardrum divides:
   - ☐ a. the external ear from the inner ear
   - ☐ b. the middle ear from the inner ear
   - ☑ c. the external ear from the middle ear

2. When looking at the right tympanic membrane, the quadrant farthest away from the examiner is the:
   - ☑ a. anteroinferior
   - ☐ b. posteroinferior
   - ☐ c. anterosuperior
   - ☐ d. posterosuperior

3. One of the most likely spots to find perforations of the eardrum is:
   - ☐ a. along the malleus
   - ☐ b. at the light reflex
   - ☑ c. along the anulus
   - ☐ d. at the pars faccida

4. When choosing a tuning fork for testing auditory function, pick one with frequencies between:
   - ☐ a. 200 and 500 cps
   - ☐ b. 400 and 800 cps
   - ☑ c. 500 and 1000 cps
   - ☐ d. 1000 and 2000 cps

5. Functions of the middle ear are to:
   - ☑ a. transmit sounds across the ossicle chain to the inner ear
   - ☐ b. transmit stimuli to the cochlear branch of the auditory nerve
   - ☐ c. maintain balance
   - ☑ d. protect the auditory apparatus from intense vibrations
   - ☐ e. equalize air pressure
   - ☐ f. a, c, and e
   - ☐ g. b, d, and e
   - ☐ h. a, c, d, and e
   - ☑ i. a, d, and e
   - ☐ j. all the above

6. The cochlear branch of the auditory nerve responsible for hearing is:
   - ☐ a. CN II
   - ☐ b. CN IV
   - ☑ c. CN VIII
   - ☐ d. CN IX
   - ☐ e. None of the above

7. Which statements are true concerning the Rinne test?
   - ☐ a. It is a test of bone conduction only.
   - ☑ b. It is a test of bone conduction and air conduction.
   - ☐ c. The sound is referred to the better ear because the cochlea or auditory nerve is functioning more effectively.
   - ☑ d. A normal response would be that if the tuning fork were placed on the mastoid process until it were no longer heard and then placed in front of the auditory meatus, the sound would continue to be heard.
   - ☐ e. A normal response would be that if the fork were placed in the middle of the forehead, the sound would radiate bilaterally and equally.
   - ☐ f. a and d
   - ☐ g. b, c, and d
   - ☐ h. a, c, and e
   - ☑ i. b and d
   - ☐ j. None of the above

8. The structures of the inner ear include:
   - ☐ a. stapes
   - ☐ b. anulus
   - ☑ c. vestibule
   - ☑ d. organ of Corti
   - ☐ e. ecderon
   - ☐ f. a, b, and e
   - ☐ g. b, c, and e
   - ☐ h. b and d
   - ☐ i. c, d, and e
   - ☑ j. c and d

9. When examining the adult client's ear, the examiner should:
   - ☐ a. instruct the client to sit with head erect
   - ☑ b. instruct the client to sit with head tilted toward the opposite shoulder
   - ☐ c. pull the auricle out
   - ☐ d. pull the auricle out and down
   - ☑ e. pull the auricle out and up
   - ☐ f. a and c
   - ☐ g. a and e
   - ☐ h. a and d
   - ☐ i. b and d
   - ☑ j. b and e

PEDIATRIC QUESTIONS

10. The external ear of the child:
    - ☐ a. is normally at a position lower than the corner of the eye, but by the child's first birthday it is at its normal adult position
    - ☐ b. is slanted backward at about a 10° angle
    - ☐ c. is normally above the position of the corner of the eye, but by the child's first birthday it is at its normal adult position
    - ☐ d. is directly vertical to the position of the head
    - ☑ e. is normally at the same level as the corner of the eye
    - ☐ f. a and b
    - ☐ g. b and c
    - ☑ h. b and e
    - ☐ i. c and d
    - ☐ j. d and e

11. A child considered at high risk for auditory dysfunction is one who has:
    - ☐ a. had measles
    - ☐ b. had chickenpox
    - ☐ c. had mumps
    - ☐ d. been taking streptomycin
    - ☐ e. been taking kanamycin
    - ☐ f. all but e
    - ☐ g. all but c
    - ☑ h. all but b
    - ☐ i. all but a
    - ☐ j. all the above

Mark each statement "T" or "F."

12. __F__ The best time to examine the child's ear is at the beginning of the examination to "get it over with."

13. __T__ While looking at the TM the examiner sees a dull nonglistening spot. This is most likely a scar.

14. __F__ The best method to remove dry, hard wax is with a cerumen spoon.
15. __F__ The normal curvature of an infant's ear canal is downward.
16. __F__ A child who received audiometry scoring at 1000, 2000, 4000 and 6000 at 60 dB has normal hearing.

GERIATRIC QUESTIONS

17. Pick the false statement. Presbycusis:
    - ☐ a. is a progressive, bilaterally symmetrical hearing loss
    - ☑ b. can often be relieved with surgical repair
    - ☐ c. often involves auditory loss of high tones initially
    - ☐ d. when advanced may cause speech to sound garbled or distorted
    - ☐ e. can exist to a fairly advanced degree before a client will report it as a symptom
18. Pick the false statement. Tinnitus:
    - ☐ a. might be caused by cerumen impaction
    - ☐ b. can be associated with temporomandibular joint malfunction
    - ☐ c. can be associated with chronic emotional upset
    - ☑ d. is an early symptom of presbycusis
    - ☐ e. might occur with an arthritis client who is taking regular doses of an analgesic

Mark each statement T or F.

19. __T__ Speech can eventually become distorted with a client who has a prolonged severe hearing loss.
20. __F__ A sudden hearing loss in an elderly client usually indicates mechanical obstruction and subsides quickly (within 3 days).
21. __T__ Loss of general physical well-being may affect the client's auditory effectiveness.
22. __F__ Earmolds (part of hearing aids) should fit very loosely when inserted into the canal to avoid friction or pressure irritation.

SUGGESTED READINGS
General

American Journal of Nursing: Programmed Instruction, Patient assessment: examination of the ear, **75**(3), 1975.

Bates, Barbara: A guide to physical examination, ed. 2, Philadelphia, 1979, J. B. Lippincott Co., pp. 58-59, 76-78, 100-102.

DeGowin, Elmer, and DeGowin, Richard: Bedside diagnostic examination, ed. 3, New York, 1976, Macmillan Publishing Co., Inc., pp. 178-193.

Malasanos, Lois, Barkauskas, Violet, Moss, Muriel, and Stoltenberg-Allen, Kathryn: Health assessment, St. Louis, 1977, The C. V. Mosby Co., pp. 118-123.

Prior, John A., and Silberstein, Jack S.: Physical diagnosis: the history and examination of the patient, ed. 5, St. Louis, 1977, The C. V. Mosby Co., pp. 151-162.

Sana, Josephine, and Judge, Richard D.: Physical appraisal methods in nursing, Boston, 1975, Little, Brown and Co., pp. 121-132.

Pediatric

Alexander, Mary, and Brown, Marie Scott: Pediatric physical diagnosis for nurses, New York, 1974, McGraw-Hill Book Co., pp. 71-85.

Barness, Lewis: Manual of pediatric physical diagnosis, ed. 4, Chicago, 1972, Year Book Medical Publishers, Inc., pp. 66-74.

Bates, Barbara: A guide to physical examination, ed. 2, Philadelphia, 1979, J. B. Lippincott Co., pp. 394-399.

Brown, Marie Scott, and Alexander, Mary: Physical examination. Part 7. Examining the ear, Nursing '74 **4**(2): 48-51, 1974.

Brown, Marie Scott, and Alexander, Mary: Physical examination. Part 8. Hearing acuity, Nursing '74 **4**(4):61-65, 1974.

DeAngelis, Catherine: Basic pediatrics for the primary health care provider, Boston, 1975, Little, Brown Co., pp. 79-82, 185-190.

Malasanos, Lois, Barkauskas, Violet, Moss, Muriel, and Stoltenberg-Allen, Kathryn: Health assessment, St. Louis, 1977, The C. V. Mosby Co., pp. 428-429.

Geriatric

Chinn, Austin B., editor: Clinical aspects of aging, Working with older people: a guide to practice, vol. 4, Rockville, Md., 1971, U.S. Department of Health, Education, and Welfare, Public Health Service, pp. 38-44.

Palmore, Erdman, editor: Normal aging II, Durham, N.C., 1974, Duke University Press, pp. 32-41.

Steinberg, Franz V., editor: Cowdry's the care of the geriatric patient, ed. 5, St. Louis, 1976, The C. V. Mosby Co., pp. 380-392.

CHAPTER 7

Assessment of the eyes and visual system

Cognitive objectives

At the end of this unit the learner will demonstrate knowledge of assessment of the eyes and visual system by the ability to do the following:

1. Identify the purposes for measuring distant and near visual acuity.
2. Appropriately interpret the readings reporting distant visual acuity measurement.
3. Identify the purposes for testing the corneal light reflex.
4. Identify potential abnormal results when using confrontation method for testing vision fields.
5. Identify the purpose of the cover-uncover test.
6. Identify the cranial nerves responsible for eyeball movement in the six fields of gaze.
7. Identify the physiological events that occur with direct and consensual pupillary response.
8. Identify the characteristics of normal anatomical structures of the external eye, including:
   a. Eyelids and lashes
   b. Spherical body in position within the socket
   c. Lacrimal apparatus
   d. Conjunctiva
   e. Cornea
   f. Iris and pupil
   g. Anterior chamber
9. Identify proper and effective techniques for handling the ophthalmoscope.
10. Identify the characteristics of normal anatomical structures of the internal eye, including:
    a. Layers covering the eyeball
    b. Red reflex
    c. Retinal structures
       (1) Disc and physiological cup
       (2) Vessels
       (3) Retina surface
       (4) Macula and fovea centralis
11. Identify selected common variations of pediatric and geriatric clients.
12. Define the terms in the vocabulary section.

Clinical objectives

At the end of this unit the learner will perform a systematic assessment of the eyes and visual system, demonstrating the ability to do the following:

1. Obtain a pertinent health history from the client.
2. Demonstrate the correct procedures for testing a client for the following:
   a. Distant vision acuity
   b. Near vision acuity
   c. Visual fields (confrontation method)
   d. Extraocular movement control and parallel eye positioning by means of:
      (1) Corneal light reflex
      (2) Six fields of gaze
      (3) Cover-uncover test
   e. Corneal reflex
   f. Direct and consensual pupillary response
3. Demonstrate and describe the results of inspection and palpation of the following:
   a. Eyebrows for hair quality and distribution, skin surface and bilateral movement
   b. Eyelids and lashes for height and bilateral dimension of palpebral fissures, lash formation and distribution, lid closure, blinking, tenderness, and surface characteristics
   c. Eyeball position in bony socket
   d. Lacrimal apparatus for puncta appearance and response to pressure at inner canthus
   e. Conjunctiva for color, tenderness, discharge, and surface characteristics
   f. Cornea: transparency, surface characteristics
   g. Anterior chamber and iris for transparency, iris color, surface and shape, and clearance between iris and cornea
   h. Pupil for shape and bilateral size
4. Demonstrate proper use of the ophthalmoscope.
5. Demonstrate a systematic inspection of the internal eye, including the following:
   a. Red reflex for color and shape
   b. Clear media of eye for transparency

c. Optic disc for margin, shape, size, color, and physiological cup

d. Retinal vessels for artery size, color, caliber, and distribution; vein size, color, caliber, and distribution

e. Retinal surface for color and surface characteristics or alterations

f. Macula and fovea centralis for color and surface characteristics

6. Summarize results of the assessment with a written description.

Health history related to the eyes and visual system additional to data base

1. History of eye surgery, injury or trauma? Describe what and when.

2. Currently taking or using any medications for eye problems? If so, describe. (*Note:* Eyedrops or ointments may not be reported as part of list of medications taken in original data base.)

3. Is client subject to work or environmental conditions that could irritate or injure the eyes (e.g., irritating fumes, dust, smoke, flying sparks, or particles in air)? If so, does client wear goggles? If client rides a motorcycle, are goggles worn?

4. Does client engage in any contact sport that creates problems with wearing corrective lenses or increases risk for eye injury?

5. If client wears contact lenses, the following questions should be asked:

   a. When prescribed? By whom?

   b. Any difficulty with pain (mild, acute), burning, excessive tearing, photophobia (mild or severe), feeling of dryness, foreign body sensation, eye infections, swelling of eyelids or eyes (conjunctiva)?

   c. Does client wear soft or hard lenses?

   d. How often are lenses checked by physician?

   e. What are client's habits concerning the wearing of lenses?

      (1) Duration (in a given day)?

      (2) Ever sleep with lenses in place?

      (3) Worn every day or just for special occasions?

      (4) Lenses alternated with glasses?

      (5) Removed for special activities (e.g., contact sports, swimming)?

   f. Ask client to describe:

      (1) Insertion/removal procedure

      (2) Cleaning/storage procedure

   g. Following are risk factors for contact lens wearers (or candidates):

      (1) Disorganized life-style (difficulty storing, cleaning, wearing for appropriate periods)

      (2) Swimming, contact sports

      (3) Poor hygiene habits

      (4) Susceptibility to infections (especially eye infections)

      (5) Severe allergy (sneezing, eye watering)

      (6) Limited or reduced manual dexterity

      (7) Limited motivation to endure adjustment to new lenses or to tolerate foreign body in eye

      (8) History of seizures

      (9) Environment or work situation where fumes, smoke, or eye irritants exist

      (10) Traveling (lens care and transport habits need to be considered, especially for soft lenses)

   h. Does client have any special problems with lenses? Keeping surface clean, free of scratches, lenses popping out, etc.?

6. *Note:* If client complains of *sudden onset* of any eye or visual symptoms (e.g., pain, loss of peripheral vision, blind spot, floaters, or any visual change), consider this an emergency for referral.

7. If client complains of blurring:

   a. Does it involve one or both eyes?

   b. Is it constant or transient?

   c. Can it be cleared by blinking several times?

   d. Does client have sensation that something is obstructing vision (e. g., cloudy or foggy interference) or are images out of focus?

   e. Do images appear bent or warped?

   f. Does squinting or frowning help to reduce blur?

   g. Is blurring related to fatigue or eye strain?

8. If client complains of eye strain, ask for a definition in terms of pain (localized in one or both eyes), headache (do symptom analysis), visual changes, association with time of day, use of corrective lenses, reading or other vision use demands.

9. If client complains of floaters or moving spots:

   a. Is the onset sudden (recent) or is this a chronic problem?

   b. Are there large numbers, just a few, or do they occur singly?

   c. Are they seen in one or both eyes?

10. If client complains of redness, watering, or discharge around eyes:

    a. Is there a history of allergies? Is problem seasonal, associated with sports activities, swimming?

    b. Does anyone else in family or others in close contact with client have similar problems?

    c. Any environmental factors that could serve as irritants?

11. If client complains of diplopia (double vision):
    a. Is the onset sudden or gradual?
    b. Does it persist all the time?
    c. Does it occur with both eyes open? Right eye closed? Left eye closed?
12. If client complains of blind spot or peripheral vision loss:
    a. Is the onset sudden or gradual?
    b. Does blind spot move with eye movement (i.e., does it remain in a constant position in relation to direction of gaze)?

13. Does client have any unusual or different eye symptoms or sensations (e.g., flashes of light, distortion of color such as brownish green or yellowish hues, confusion about differentiating colors, haloes around lights)?
14. If client has a vision problem, how does this interfere with activities of daily living (e.g., getting around the house or community, caring for self, family, belongings, ability to read, driving a car, difficulty visualizing steps and curbs, difficulty maintaining job)?

Clinical guidelines

The student will:	To identify:	
	Normal	**Deviations from normal**
1. Gather equipment necessary to perform eye and vision assessment: **a.** Snellen chart **b.** Jaeger chart or newsprint for testing near vision **c.** Cover card (opaque) **d.** Penlight **e.** Cotton wisp **f.** Cotton-tipped applicator **g.** Ophthalmoscope		
Acuity and function		
1. Perform measurement of distant vision (CN II) **a.** Stabilize Snellen chart* on wall in well-lighted room **b.** Seat client comfortably 6 m (20 feet) from chart **c.** Ask client to cover one eye with cover card **d.** Ask client to repeat each letter as you point to it; begin pointing at letters in line where client is most comfortable reading—usually 20/30 or 20/20 line **e.** Urge client to read as many of smallest letters as possible, even if unable to complete a particular line **f.** Repeat procedure with other eye		
g. Clients who wear corrective lenses for far vision should be tested first while wearing glasses and then without†	20/20 O.D. and 20/20 O.S.	O.D. or O.S.: any letters missed in 20/20 line or above
h. Observe reading pattern and facial expression during acuity test	Reading pattern smooth, without hesitation Eyes remain open without frowning or squinting	Behaviors indicating reading difficulty: frowning, squinting, "cheating," leaning forward, head tilting, hesitancy or difficulty naming letters

*A "Block E" chart may be used with clients who do not read English or are illiterate.
†*Note:* Reading glasses should not be used for testing far vision.

The student will:	To identify:	
	Normal	**Deviations from normal**

2. Perform measurement of near vision
  a. Seat client comfortably
  b. Ask client to hold Jaeger chart or newsprint 35 cm (14 inches) from face

Jaeger chart:
  14/14 O.D.
  14/14 O.S.
Newsprint read without hesitancy or attempt to position reading material closer or farther away

Unable to read letters at 35-cm (14-inch) distance
Pushes reading material farther away

  c. Ask client to read aloud letters or words in sentence
  d. If client wears corrective lenses for reading, perform test with glasses on

Eyes remain open without excessive blinking or facial distortions

Behaviors indicating difficulty: frowning, squinting, hesitancy, pulling reading material closer

3. Test for peripheral visual fields
  a. Examiner and client sit directly facing each other at distance of 60 to 90 cm (2 to 3 feet)
  b. Client covers one eye with cover card
  c. Examiner covers own eye directly opposite client's covered eye
  d. Client and examiner stare directly at each other's open eye
  e. Examiner holds pencil or penlight in hand and extends it to farthest periphery (Fig. 7-1) temporally and gradually brings object closer to midline point (equal distance between client and examiner)

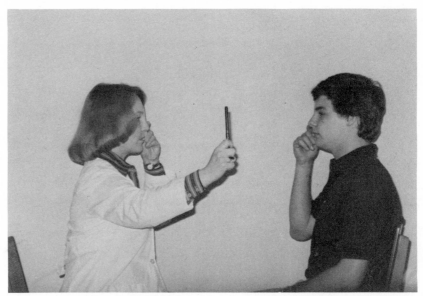

Fig. 7-1. Visual field testing; examiner holding object at midline.

  f. Client asked to report when object first seen
  g. Procedure repeated upward, nasalward, and downward
  h. Ask client to repeat entire procedure with other eye covered; examiner also covers other eye

Client and examiner report seeing object at approximately same time as it approaches from periphery; test assumes examiner has normal peripheral vision, described as:
Temporal peripheral—90°
Upward—50°
Nasalward—60°
Downward—70°

Client fails to report sighting object at same time as examiner in any one or in all directions (peripheral visual loss may involve both eyes or one eye)

4. Test for extraocular muscle function
  a. Assess corneal light reflex
    1. Ask client to stare straight ahead with both eyes open
    2. Shine penlight, held at midline and directed toward corneas

Light reflection appears symmetrically in both pupils

Light reflections appear at different spots (asymmetrically) in each eye

Continued.

Clinical guidelines–cont'd

	To identify:	
The student will:	**Normal**	**Deviations from normal**

b. Test movement of eyes in six cardinal fields of gaze (CN III, IV, VI) (Fig. 7-2)
1. Client stabilizes head, looking directly ahead at examiner
2. Client asked to move *eyes only* to follow object in examiner's hand
3. Examiner moves object from center position to upper and outer extreme (hold in position momentarily), back to center, and then to lower and inner extreme (Fig. 7-3)

Fig. 7-3. Field testing position no. 1.

4. Examiner moves object to temporal-nasal extremes, holding object in extreme positions momentarily (Fig. 7-4)

Fig. 7-4. Field testing position no. 2.

5. Examiner moves object to opposite upper and outer extreme and back to opposite lower and inner extreme (Fig. 7-5)

Fig. 7-5. Field testing position no. 3.

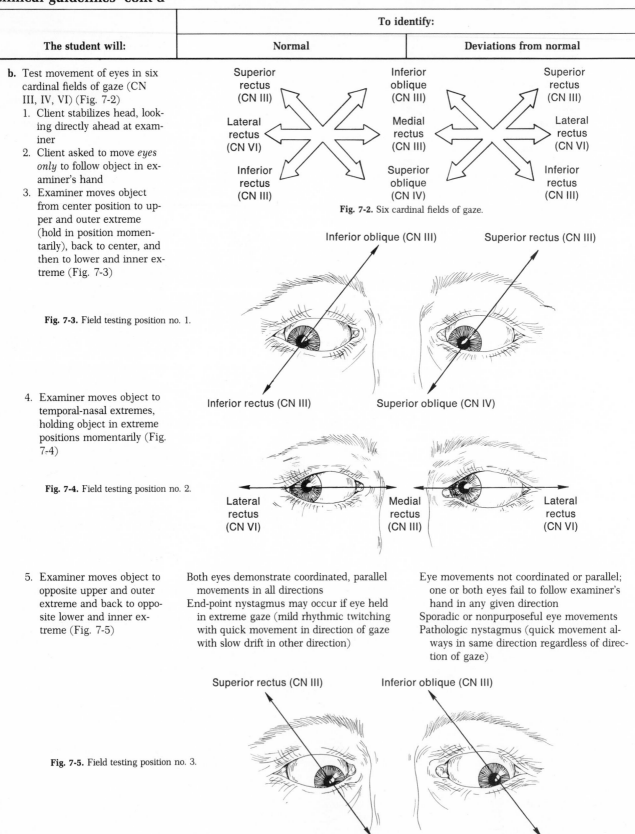

Superior rectus (CN III)   Inferior oblique (CN III)   Superior rectus (CN III)
Lateral rectus (CN VI)   Medial rectus (CN III)   Lateral rectus (CN VI)
Inferior rectus (CN III)   Superior oblique (CN IV)   Inferior rectus (CN III)

Fig. 7-2. Six cardinal fields of gaze.

Inferior oblique (CN III)   Superior rectus (CN III)
Inferior rectus (CN III)   Superior oblique (CN IV)

Lateral rectus (CN VI)   Medial rectus (CN III)   Lateral rectus (CN VI)

Both eyes demonstrate coordinated, parallel movements in all directions
End-point nystagmus may occur if eye held in extreme gaze (mild rhythmic twitching with quick movement in direction of gaze with slow drift in other direction)

Eye movements not coordinated or parallel; one or both eyes fail to follow examiner's hand in any given direction
Sporadic or nonpurposeful eye movements
Pathologic nystagmus (quick movement always in same direction regardless of direction of gaze)

Superior rectus (CN III)   Inferior oblique (CN III)
Superior oblique (CN IV)   Inferior rectus (CN III)

	To identify:	
The student will:	**Normal**	**Deviations from normal**
c. Perform cover-uncover test 1. Client asked to stare straight ahead at fixed point 2. Examiner covers one eye with cover card and observes uncovered eye for movement to focus on designated point	Uncovered eye does not move as examiner places card over other eye	Uncovered eye moves to focus on designated point (Fig. 7-6)

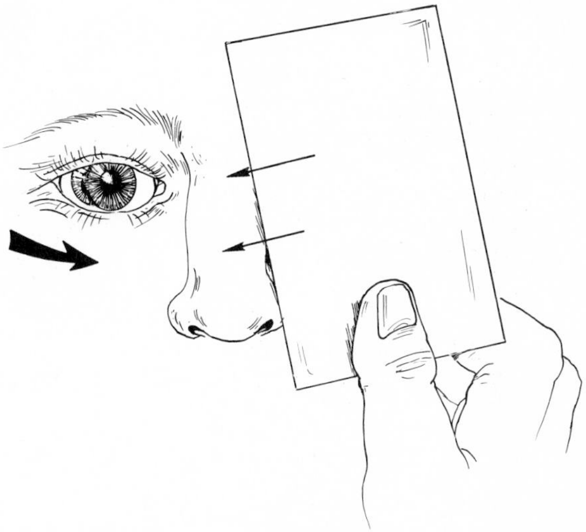

Fig. 7-6. Cover test for right eye demonstrating abnormal shift from lateral to central gaze.

3. Examiner removes card from same eye and observes newly uncovered eye for movement to focus 4. Repeat steps (2) and (3) with other eye	Newly uncovered eye does not move	Newly uncovered eye moves to focus on designated point (Fig. 7-7)

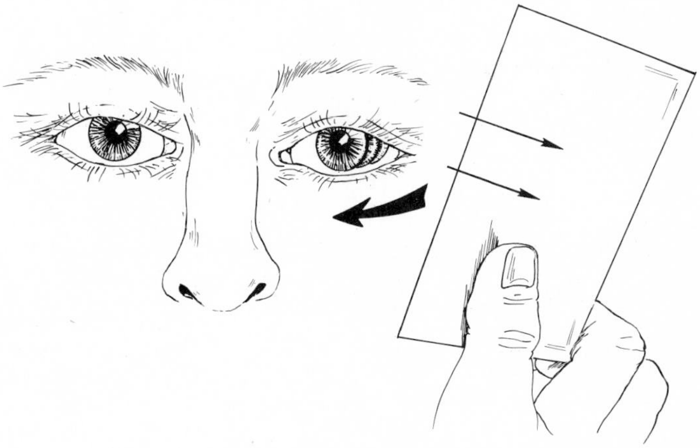

Fig. 7-7. Uncover test for left eye demonstrating abnormal shift from lateral to central gaze.

5. Test corneal reflex (CN V) **a.** Ask client to keep both eyes open and to look up **b.** Examiner approaches from side with wisp of cotton **c.** Examiner lightly touches cornea (not conjunctiva) with cotton **d.** Repeat procedure with other eye		
	Lids of both eyes close when either cornea touched*	Lids of one or both eyes fail to respond
6. Evaluate pupillary response (CN II, III) **a.** Evaluate direct and consensual reactions to light 1. Room should be partially darkened		

*Note: Contact lenses will interfere with results.

Continued.

Clinical guidelines–cont'd

The student will:	To identify:	
	Normal	Deviations from normal
2. Client holds both eyes open and fixes gaze straight ahead 3. Examiner approaches with penlight beam from side and shines light on pupil 4. Repeat procedure with other eye	Illuminated pupil constricts (direct response) Other eye (pupil) constricts simultaneously (consensual response) Speed of constrictive response (bilateral) may vary among clients	Unequal (in size or speed) reflex responses or absent response
b. Test for accommodation 1. Client fixes gaze at object directly ahead at distant point 2. Examiner holds up object about 10 to 12 cm (4 or 5 inches) from client's nose 3. Ask client to adjust focus of gaze from distant object to object in front of nose	Pupils converge and constrict as eyes focus on near object Symmetrical response (Fig. 7-8) Client reports object in focus	Pupils fail to constrict or converge Asymmetrical response

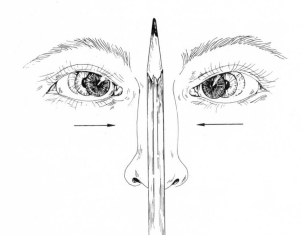

Fig. 7-8. Test for accomodation, with convergence of eyes and pupil constriction.

External ocular structures

1. Have client seated at eye level **2.** Inspect eyebrows, noting hair quality and distribution, skin quality, movement	Skin intact, without hair loss Equal alignment and movement	Flakiness, loss of hair, scaling Unequal alignment or movement
3. Inspect eyelids and lashes, noting the following: **a.** Height of palpebral fissures **b.** Lid positioning	Bilaterally equal in position With eyes opened lid margins overlay cornea at both superior and inferior borders	Asymmetrical positioning Sclera visible between upper lid(s); covers part of the pupil
c. Lid closure **d.** Blinking	Complete, with smooth, easy motion Frequent involuntary, bilateral movements (average 15 to 20 blinks per minute)	Incomplete, or closure with difficulty or pain Rapid blinking Monocular blinking Absent or infrequent blinking
e. Surface characteristics	Skin intact, without discharge Lid margins flush against eyeball surface	Lesions, nodules, redness, flaking, crusting, excessive tearing, discharge

The student will:	To identify:	
	Normal	Deviations from normal

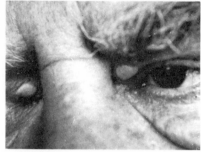

| | Lashes equally distributed and curled slightly outward | Cream or yellowish plaques (xanthelasma) (Fig. 7-9)
Lid edema or deformity (pulled away from eyeball or turned inward)
Lashes absent
Lashes turned inward |

Fig. 7-9. Xanthelasma. (From Stewart, W., Danto, J., and Maddin, S.: Dermatology: diagnosis and treatment of cutaneous disorders, ed. 4, St. Louis, 1978, The C. V. Mosby Co.)

4. Observe position of globe in bony socket	Caucasians: eyeball does not protrude beyond supraorbital ridge of frontal bone Negroes: eyeball may protrude slightly beyond supraorbital ridge	Asymmetrical placement Forward displacement (exophthalmos) Backward displacement (enophthalmos)
5. Inspect and palpate lacrimal apparatus (puncta) and eyelids		
a. Examiner presses index finger against lower orbital rim near inner canthus (Fig. 7-10); pressure slightly everts lower lid	Puncta seen on tiny elevations on nasal side of upper and lower lid margins Mucosa pink and intact with no response to pressure	Puncta red, swollen, with response of tenderness to pressure Fluid or purulent material discharged from puncta in response to pressure

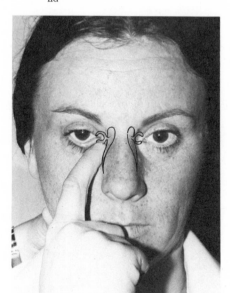

Fig. 7-10. Palpating the lacrimal puncta.

b. Gently palpate upper and lower lids for tenderness and nodules Exert minimal pressure over eyeball with examining finger*	No tenderness or nodules	Tenderness, nodules, or irregularities

*If client complains of scratching or localized tenderness of eye, do not palpate over lid.

Continued.

Clinical guidelines–cont'd

The student will:	To identify:	
	Normal	**Deviations from normal**
6. Inspect bulbar conjunctiva and sclera and palpebral conjunctiva	Bulbar conjunctiva clear; tiny red vessels may be visible	Blood vessels dilated
a. Separate lids widely with thumb and index finger, exerting pressure over bony orbit surrounding eye; ask client to look up, down, and to both sides	Sclera appears white	Conjunctiva reddened
	Tiny black dots (pigmentation) may appear near limbus (in dark-skinned individuals)	Lesions or nodules
		Sclera yellow (jaundice) or significantly bluish
	Slight yellowish cast (in dark-skinned individuals)	Foreign body
		Tenderness (especially on eye movement)
b. Pull down and evert lower lid and ask client to look up	Palpebral conjunctiva pink, intact, without discharge	Redness, lesions, nodules, discharge, tenderness, crusting
c. Eversion of upper lid not ordinarily performed in screening examination; if indicated, the following steps should be performed*:	No tenderness or itching	

c. Eversion of upper lid not ordinarily performed in screening examination; if indicated, the following steps should be performed*:

1. Explain entire procedure to the client before beginning
2. Ask the client to look down but to keep his eyes slightly open. This relaxes the levator muscle, whereas closing the eyes contracts the orbicularis muscle, preventing lid eversion.
3. Gently grasp the upper eyelashes and pull gently downward. Do not pull the lashes outward or upward; this, too, causes muscle contraction.
4. Place a cotton-tipped applicator about 1 cm above the lid margin on the upper tarsal border and push gently downward with the applicator while still holding the lashes. This everts the lid.
5. Hold the lashes of the everted lid against the upper ridge of the bony orbit, just beneath the eyebrow, never pushing against the eyeball.
6. Examine the lid for swelling, infection, a foreign object, and so on.
7. To return the lid to its normal position, move the lashes slightly forward and ask the client to look up and then to blink. The lid returns easily to a normal position.

7. Inspect cornea, using oblique lighting; slowly move light reflection over corneal surface and check for:

*Points 2 through 7 from Malasanos, Lois, Barkauskas, Violet, Moss, Muriel, and Stoltenberg-Allen, Kathryn: Health assessment, St. Louis, 1977, The C. V. Mosby Co., p. 153.

The student will:	To identify:	
	Normal	**Deviations from normal**
a. Transparency **b.** Surface characteristics	Transparent Smooth Clear, shiny	Opacities Irregularities appearing in light reflections on surface Lesions, abrasions Foreign body Arcus senilis (younger clients) Tissue growth from periphery toward corneal center (pterygium)
8. Inspect anterior chamber using oblique lighting for: **a.** Transparency **b.** Iris surface **c.** Chamber depth	 Transparent Iris flat Adequate clearance between cornea and iris	 Cloudiness or any visible material, blood Iris bulging toward cornea (crescent-shaped shadow may appear on far side of iris) Chamber appears shallow
9. Inspect iris for: **a.** Shape **b.** Color and consistency	 Round Consistent coloration	 Irregular shape Inconsistent coloration in one eye or between two eyes
10. Inspect pupil for: **a.** Shape **b.** Bilateral size	 Round Equal in size	 Other than round Unequal in size

Internal eye

The student will:	Normal	Deviations from normal
1. Use the ophthalmoscope (see clinical strategies for technique) to observe: **a.** Red reflex from about 30 cm (1 foot) away, at 0 setting **b.** Cornea, anterior chamber, and lens (+15 to +20) **c.** Vitreous body (moving from +15 to +20 *back* to 0) **d.** Retinal structures (lens at 0) (Fig. 7-11)	 Bright, round, red-orange glow seen through pupil Clear Clear Transparent	 Decreased redness or roundness of reflex Dark spots or any opacities Cloudy or any visible materials Blood Cloudy Floating particles

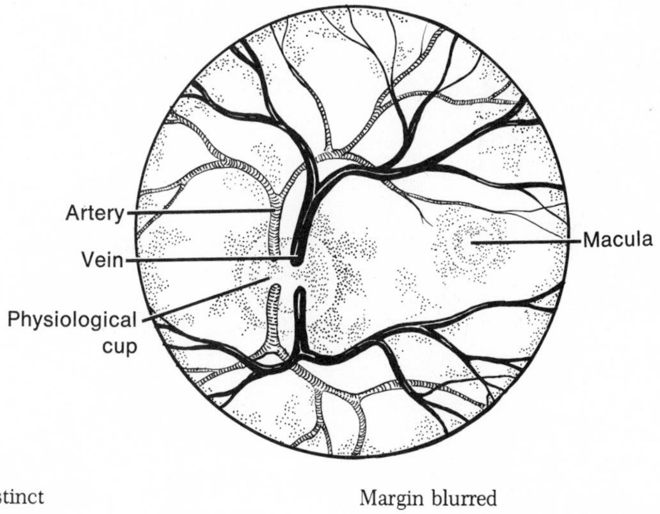

Fig. 7-11. Retinal structures of the left eye.

The student will:	Normal	Deviations from normal
1. Optic disc margin a. Shape b. Size	Regular, distinct Sharp outline Scattered or dense pigment deposits may be visualized at border Grayish crescent may appear at temporal border Round or slightly vertically oval Approximately 1.5 mm diameter (appears magnified fifteen times to examiner)	Margin blurred Irregular Shape and size of discs not equal in both eyes

Continued.

Clinical guidelines–cont'd

The student will:	To identify:	
	Normal	**Deviations from normal**
c. Color	Marked myopic refractive errors may make disc appear larger Hyperopic errors may make it appear smaller Creamy pink Lighter than retina Tiny vessels may be visible on disc surface	Diffuse pallor or pallor of section of disc, which always extends from center of disc to border Hyperemic disc with engorged, tortuous vessels on surface
d. Physiological cup	Small depression just temporal of center of disc, does *not* extend to disc border Usually appears paler than disc, sometimes grayish Usually occupies four tenths to five tenths of diameter of disc Vessels entering disc may drop abruptly into cup or may appear to fade gradually (Discs more pronounced in some clients than others)	Cup extends to border of disc Cup occupies more than five tenths of diameter of disc Cup size or placement not equal in both eyes
2. Retinal vessels: follow from disc to periphery, dividing retina into four quadrants		
a. Arteries	Usually about 25% narrower than veins (²/₃ or ⁴/₅ ratio; size varies with the number of branches) Narrow band of light may appear at center Light red	Arteries become narrow (²/₄ or ³/₅ ratio or less) Width of light reflex increases to cover over one third of artery Opaque or pale
b. Veins	Larger than arteries No light reflection Darker in color Venous pulsations may be visible	Veins become larger
c. Distribution and pattern (*Note:* Vessel abnormalities are not evenly distributed; scan all quadrants in orderly fashion for observation.)	Vessel caliber should be regular and uniformly decreasing in size as it branches and moves toward periphery Artery/vein crossings should not alter (or pinch) caliber of underlying vessel	Irregularities of caliber; dilation or constriction Neovascularization (appears as compact patches of tortuous, narrow vessels) Indentations or nicks of vessels at artery/vein crossing
3. Retinal background: scan the four quadrants in orderly fashion		
a. Color and surface characteristics	Fine granular texture Pink, usually uniform throughout Negroid fundi often heavily pigmented and uniformly dark Choroidal vessels may be visible through retinal layer (appear as linear, light orange streaks) Movable light reflections may appear on retinal surface (more prominent in young persons)	Pallor of fundus (general or localized) Hemorrhage (may be linear, flame-shaped, round, dark or red, large or small) Microaneurysms (appear as discrete tiny red dots) Soft or hard exudates (fuzzy or well-defined white patches)
4. Macula and fovea centralis (located 2 disc diameters [DD] temporal to disc)		
a. Color and surface	Appears slightly darker than remainder of retina Fovea may appear as tiny bright light in center of macula Tiny vessels may appear on surface Fine pigmentation and granular appearance may be visible	Any abnormalities or lesions described for remainder of retinal surface

Clinical strategies

1. When testing with the Snellen chart, remember the following:
   a. Always use an opaque card for covering the client's eyes (in lieu of client's hand).
   b. Client "cheating" may not be deliberate; it may be an unconscious attempt to resolve the frustration of not being able to perform the test.
   c. Be certain that the client can read or identify the letters. An illiterate client may simply indicate an inability to see the letters.
   d. Proceed slowly enough to permit the client sufficient time to follow directions.
   e. Far vision errors should be recorded in the following manner. If the client misses two letters in the 20/20 line with the left eye: O.S. 20/20 − 2; if the client reads only one letter correctly in the 20/20 line with the right eye: O.D. 20/25 + 1.
2. When testing by confrontation for visual fields, hold the object in the *midline* between you and client. Beginning students often extend the object too far toward the client (this enables the examiner to spot the object first); or they hold the object too far back (Fig. 7-12). This gives the client the advantage in spotting the object.
3. When using the ophthalmoscope, the following procedures are helpful:
   a. Turn the diaphragm dial so that the small, round white light can be used. Turn on light to maximum brightness (old or defective batteries will reduce lighting).
   b. Client should be comfortably seated. Either stand or be seated facing the client.
   c. Client and examiner remove glasses. Removal of client's contact lenses is optional. It might help to reduce light reflection.
   d. The room should be darkened.
   e. Ask the client to hold both eyes open and to direct gaze slightly upward and straight ahead. Gaze should be fixed on some distant object and maintained even if the examiner's head gets in the way.
   f. For examination of the client's right eye, hold the ophthalmoscope in your right hand, over your right eye. Stand slightly to the right, at about a 15° angle (temporally) from the client.
   g. The ophthalmoscope is held with the index finger on the lens wheel. Rotate the lens wheel to 0 diopter setting (a lens that neither converges nor diverges light rays) (Fig. 7-13).
   h. Place left hand over client's right eye, with thumb on upper brow.
   i. Hold the ophthalmoscope firmly against your head and approach to within 30 cm (1 foot) of the client (Fig. 7-14). Direct ophthalmoscope light into the pupil. Continue approach, and red reflex will appear. Try to keep both eyes open.

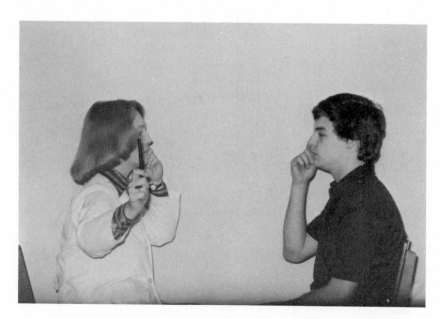

Fig. 7-12. Visual field testing; examiner fails to hold object at midline.

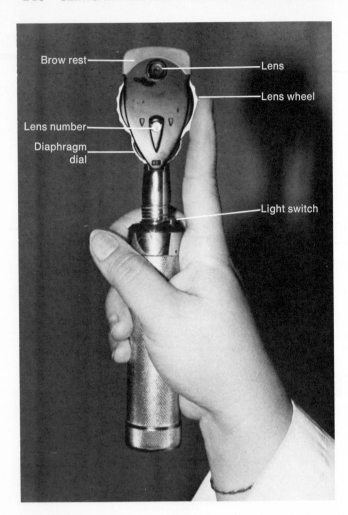

Brow rest

Lens

Lens wheel

Lens number

Diaphragm dial

Light switch

Fig. 7-13. Ophthalmoscope. Index finger is on lens wheel.

j. Continue approach until 3 to 5 cm (1 to 2 inches) from client's eye (Fig. 7-15). Turn the lens wheel so that it is between +15 and +20. This should bring the cornea and anterior chamber into focus.

k. Slowly move the dial from +20 back to 0. As the black numbers become smaller, the structures farther away from your eye come into focus (i.e., lens, vitreous body, fundus) (Fig. 7-16).

l. As the ophthalmoscope lens approaches 0, the retina should come into clear view. Clear focus can be established by looking closely at a vessel to see if the borders are sharp. Adjustments can be made for refractive errors. The hyperopic (far-sighted) eye requires more plus spheres for clarity, and the myopic (near-sighted) eye requires minus spheres for clarity.

m. The examiner may not initially focus on the disc. It is helpful to follow vessel bifurcations that lead toward the disc.

n. After inspection of the disc, follow the vessels peripherally in each of four directions. Light must always be shown through the pupil as the examiner directs the ophthalmoscope in various directions.

o. Inspect the retinal background and the macula (2 DD temporal to the disc).

p. Now change to the left eye. Stand at patient's left, holding the ophthalmoscope with the left hand over your left eye.

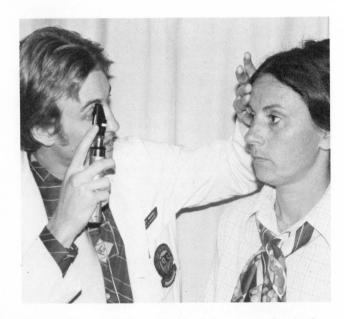

Fig. 7-14. Distance: 30.5 cm (12 inches); focus on pupil; red reflex visualized.

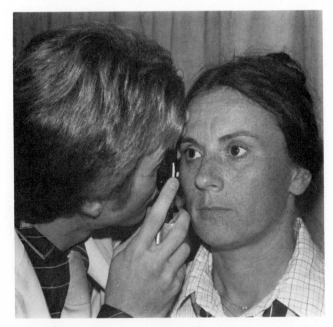

Fig. 7-15. Distance: 3 to 5 cm; lens wheel setting moves from +20 to 0; focuses from cornea to retina.

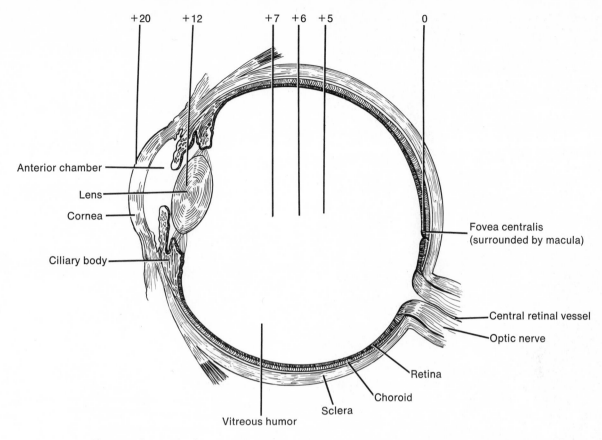

Fig. 7-16. Longitudinal cross section of eye showing focused ophthalmoscope lens setting.

q. *Note:* Clients who talk during the examination often tend to blink and move their eyes more often.

r. *Note:* Absence of the red reflex may indicate an abnormal eye, an improperly positioned ophthalmoscope, or that the client moved his eyes. If the red reflex is lost, back away and start over.

s. *Note:* It is extremely important that you consider your head and the ophthalmoscope as a unit. Be certain that the instrument is stabilized against your brow and cheek.

History and clinical strategies associated with the pediatric client

1. When examining a newborn who was vaginally delivered, the practitioner should carefully inquire about vaginal infections the mother may have had prior to delivery. This is of particular importance if the baby shows conjunctival irritation, pus, redness, or granular development.

Sample recording

Distant vision: 20/20 O.U.; near vision: 14/14 O.U., no glasses.

Visual fields intact (by confrontation).

Parallel corneal light reflex, EOM intact, no nystagmus.

Eyes symmetrical without deviation of gaze with cover test.

Brows, lids, and lashes intact without deformity, ptosis, or lesions.

Conjunctiva/sclera clear; puncta patent; no discharge.

Cornea smooth and clear.

Iris flat, round, PERRLA.

Funduscopy

Full bilateral red reflex, discs round, cream color, well-defined margins.

Vessels—2:3 (A/V ratio); arteries light red with narrow light reflex and even caliber.

Retina uniform red-orange without exudates or lesions.

Maculae 2 DD from discs; no lesions.

2. The practitioner should inquire about the developmental maturation of the child's visual system. Table 2 indicates developmental milestones. Numerous studies have shown that mothers are *most commonly* the ones who identify vision problems in their children.

3. There is much controversy regarding novice practitioners using the ophthalmoscope with small children. We encourage the beginning examiner to attempt its use with all children. Although the findings may not equal the effort, repeated practice will increase the examiner's skill so that when there is a child who needs a funduscopic examination, the likelihood of seeing the internal structures will be increased. Following is a list of suggested techniques for infants and small children:

   a. Babies up to about 18 months should be lying on their backs on the examining table. The overhead examination room lights should be off, but some type of sideroom lighting should be on.

   b. Hold a penlight or lighted object at arm's length (using left hand) above the baby's head to attract his focus while using the right hand on the ophthalmoscope to perform the internal eye examination. Assistance will be necessary to immobilize the baby's head or to hold the light.

   c. Do not attempt to pry the child's eye open. If this technique is necessary, the child will not cooperate by focusing during the funduscopy examination.

   d. Older children are likely to assist in the funduscopy examination if the examiner offers proper instructions and actually involves the child in the participation. This may include:

   (1) Letting the child know in advance that the room lights will be turned out but that some small light will be left on

   (2) Informing the child during the time the light is out that the examiner will be using a small flashlight to look into the child's eyes

   (3) Reassuring him that the procedure will not hurt

   (4) Instructing the child to look at a particular picture on the wall, or providing the child with a penlight to shine onto a picture on the wall and then look at the "lighted picture"

   (5) Remembering that older children prefer to sit

   e. The findings of the ophthalmoscopic examination for a child are very similar to those for an adult. The primary difference is the length of time the examiner has to survey the internal structures. The comparison is several seconds for the adult to split seconds for the child. During this time the examiner should at least attempt to do the following:

   (1) Focus on the retina (most likely for children under 6 years old the lens wheel will be between 0 and -5).

   (2) Observe disc and note flatness and sharpness of disc edges.

   (3) Note color and gross characteristics of the retina.

4. Vision screening begins informally with the newborn examination as the examiner notes the child's following and fixation capabilities. This should continue during each physical assessment period. Although there is some disagreement about the exact age children should receive

Table 2. Sequence of visual development*

Age	Characteristics of development
Birth	Pupils react to light
	Moderate photophobia
	Eyes usually kept closed
	Blink reflex in response to light stimulus
	Corneal reflex in response to touch
	Retinoscopy indicates 1 to 3 diopters of hyperopia
	Nystagmus may be present
	Rudimentary fixation on objects with ability to follow to midline
	Visual acuity approximately 20/300
2 to 4 weeks	Fixation ability advances; stares at light source
	Follows to midline more readily
	Tear glands begin to function

*Based on Chinn, Peggy, and Leitch, Cynthia: Child health maintenance: a guide to clinical assessment, ed. 2, St. Louis, 1979, The C. V. Mosby Co., p. 75.

Age	Characteristics of development
4 to 12 weeks	Infant becoming alert to moving objects but convergence and following are jerky and inexact Fascination for light objects and bright colors Tear glands begin to display response to emotion Binocular fixation established Follows moving object with head and eyes through 180°
12 to 20 weeks	Infant inspects hands One-inch colored cubes stimulate immediate fixation within 60 cm (2 feet) of eyes Accomodative convergence reflexes organizing Able to fixate on objects more than 90 cm (3 feet) distant Foveal pit becomes distinguishable as macula development proceeds Pigmentation of fundus not developed; appearance of fundus pale Visual acuity 20/200
20 to 28 weeks	Color preference for bright reds and yellows develops Ciliary muscle function begins and accomodation convergence reflexes start to organize Coordination between hand and eye developing True blinking appears Binocular fixation clearly established Ultimate color of iris can now be determined Able to rescue dropped block
28 to 44 weeks	About 36 weeks, depth perception begins development Very interested in small objects, can accurately pick up 7 mm pellet Follows in both vertical and horizontal planes Tilts head backward to see upward Visual acuity exceeds 20/200
44 weeks to 12 months	Central acuity approaches 20/100 Readily discriminates simple geometrical forms and gazes intently at facial expressions Transverse diameter of cornea is 12 mm, the adult size Full binocular vision developed Amblyopia may develop with lack of binocularity
12 to 15 months	Keen interest in pictures Can identify forms and associate simple visual experience Associates with visual experiences Able to scribble on paper Convergence becomes well established Depth perception remains crude
18 months to 2 years	Depth perception still immature Accomodation well developed Visual acuity 20/40
2 to 3 years	Convergence smooth Fixation on small objects or pictures should approach 50 seconds Able to recall visual images Visual acuity 20/30
3 to 5 years	Acuity appears well established, but amblyopia can occur from disuse Able to copy geometrical figures Reading readiness may be present
5 years	Only small potential for reduction of acuity from disuse (amblyopia development unlikely) Color recognition well established
6 years	Central acuity unconditionally established Physiological hyperopia decreases Visual acuity approaches 20/20 Gross attention span lengthened to 20 minutes, and detailed attention will last about 2 minutes Color shading can be differentiated Depth perception fully developed

Table 3. Vision screening schedule

Age	Screening	Anticipated results	Referral criteria
Newborn	General vision ability	Should follow short distance	No recognition or blink
3 months	Strabismus screen	May be positive	
6 months to 1 year	Strabismus screen	Should be negative	Positive screen
3 years	"E" test	20/30 to 20/40	Grossly abnormal results
4 years	Color vision screening for boys (Ishihara test if possible)	Normal color identification	Abnormal color identification
	Visual field-confrontation screening	Sees objects at same time as examiner	Grossly abnormal results
5 to 8 years (test each year)	"E" test or Snellen test	20/30 to 20/40	20/40 results after two screening periods
			Unequal results (e.g., 20/20 O.D., 20/40 O.S.)
9 to 11 years (test each year)	Snellen test	20/20 to 20/30	20/30 results after two screening periods
			Unequal results

formalized vision screening, Table 3 serves as a guide.

5. Although it is impossible to perform an accurate vision screening on a newborn, the examiner must perform some method of visual screening to rule out gross vision problems. For example, use a penlight at a distance of about 25 cm (10 inches), blink it on and off several times, and then move it around slightly. The infant should indicate recognition of the light and should follow it momentarily. No recognition or following requires further vision evaluation.

6. When using either the Snellen "E" chart or the Snellen alphabet chart with children, it is necessary to have two examiners, one to show the various lines of the chart and to point to the desired item, and the other to assist the child to stand or sit in the correct spot and correctly cover the eye not being tested.

7. The alphabet chart is by far the most accurate, and whenever possible it should be used. Directions for using the Snellen chart have been previously discussed.

8. The mechanics of the "E" chart are generally the same as with the alphabet chart. The child is instructed to point with his finger and entire arm to the direction which the "legs of the table" are pointing. This evaluates not only the ability to see the letter but also the ability to comprehend the idea of direction.

9. If the child wears glasses, vision screening should be done with glasses both on and off.

10. Problems with strabismus or heterophoria should be carefully evaluated in every child over the age of 6 months. Babies under 6 months may have intermittent eye crossing, which can be normal. Such a finding in any child over the age of 6 months is considered abnormal, and the client should be referred. The two techniques for evaluating the situation in which the child's eyes do not focus to transmit good coordinated binocular vision are the cover test and the corneal light reflex test. Both have been previously described; they should be evaluated at near point (35 cm [14 inches]) and far point (6 m [20 feet]) distances. The age and cooperation of the child will determine the success of the evaluation.

11. The importance of color vision screening is disputed among authorities. We believe it can be easily incorporated into a well child examination and should therefore be done. Because color blindness is extremely rare among girls, only the boys need to be tested. Before beginning the evaluation, the examiner must first evaluate the child's knowledge and correct recognition of colors. Color testing needs to be done only once.

12. The eyesight of a child is so precious that the examiner should refer any questionable finding to a physician for further evaluation.

Clinical variations associated with the pediatric client

The overall success of this evaluation depends on the cooperation of the child. It is desirable to evaluate each component during every well child visit. If the child is uncooperative, the examiner must decide whether to postpone the component being evaluated until later during the examination or to wait until the child's next visit.

There are five components of the pediatric vision screening examination that are most important, including visual acuity, testing for farsightedness, strabismus screening, color vision screening, and visual field evaluation. These five components are incorporated into the following clinical guidelines.

Characteristic or area examined	Normal	Deviations from normal
Acuity and function		
1. Distant vision (CN II) in children over age 3 years	3 years: 20/20 to 20/40 5 to 8 years: 20/30 to 20/40 9 to 11 years: 20/20 to 20/30	20/40 results after two screening periods or unequal results in either eye (5 to 8 years) 20/30 results after two screening periods or unequal results in either eye (9 to 11 years)
2. Near vision: not routinely used until *older school-age evaluation;* when used, directions are same as for adult	Jaeger chart: 14/14 O.D. 14/14 O.S. Newsprint read without hesitancy or attempt to pull it closer or push it farther away Eyes remain open without excessive blinking or facial distortions	Client unable to read letters at 35-cm (14-inch) distance Note any other behaviors indicating difficulty (frowning, squinting, hesitancy, pulling reading material closer)
3. Peripheral visual fields: should be evaluated from age 3 years on or as soon as child is able to cooperate by maintaining *his position* throughout procedure	Client and examiner report seeing object at approximately same time as it approaches from periphery; this test assumes that the examiner has normal peripheral vision Another affirmative response is exact second child changes head position to gaze toward object, indicating that child did see object coming into view (Examiner must be alert to judge if this is same instance he saw object.) Temporal peripheral vision: 90° Upward: 50° Nasalward: 60° Downward: 70°	Client fails to report sighting object at same time as examiner, in any one direction or in all directions (peripheral visual loss may involve both eyes or one eye)
4. Extraocular muscle function (also a test for strabismus); eye muscle coordination not fully mature until 1 year; at this time it shows mature adult function		
a. Corneal light reflex Because infants unable to cooperate, examiner must use penlight to attract infant's attention; while infant focuses on light, examiner must evaluate light reflection position	Light reflection appears symmetrically in pupils If child under 6 months of age, asymmetry of image may be normal	Light reflections appear at different spots (asymmetrically) in each eye Refer for further evaluation if child over 6 months
b. Movement of eyes in six cardinal fields of gaze: test in children over 2 years of age; examiner may need to stabilize child's chin with hand to prevent entire head movement	Both eyes demonstrate coordinated, parallel movements in all directions End-point nystagmus may occur if eye is held in extreme gaze (mild rhythmic twitching with quick movement in direction of gaze with slow drift in other direction)	Eye movements not coordinated or parallel One or both eyes fail to follow examiner's hand in any given direction Sporadic or nonpurposeful eye movements Pathological nystagmus (quick movement always in same direction regardless of direction of gaze)
c. Cover-uncover test: performed on all children 3 months and older until school age; test should be done with child looking at object about 35 cm (14 inches) away and then repeated as he views object approximately 6 m (20 feet) away	Uncovered eye does not move as examiner places card over other eye Newly uncovered eye does not move	Uncovered eye moves to focus on designated point Newly uncovered eye moves to focus on designated point Refer if child over 6 months of age
5. Corneal reflex (CN V): not routinely tested in preschool children; When tested, technique is same as for adult	Lids of both eyes close when either cornea touched	Lid(s) of one or both eyes fail to respond
6. Pupillary response: direct and consensual reaction to light	Pupil with light shining on it constricts (direct response)	Unequal (in size or speed) reflex responses or absent response

Continued.

Clinical variations associated with the pediatric client–cont'd

Characteristic or area examined	Normal	Deviations from normal
	Other eye (pupil) constricts simultaneously (consensual response)	
	Pupils converge and constrict as eyes focus on near object	Pupils fail to constrict or converge
	Response symmetrical	Asymmetrical response
7. Color vision: use Ishihara test if possible; single line testing for preschool boys	Able to correctly differentiate colors	Unable to correctly differentiate colors
External ocular structures		
1. Have client seated at eye level		
2. Eyebrows		
a. Hair quality/distribution and skin quality	Skin intact, without hair loss	Flakiness, loss of hair, scaling
b. Movement	Equal alignment and movement	Unequal alignment or movement
3. Eyelids and eyelashes		
a. Height of palpebral fissures	Bilaterally equal in position	Asymmetrical positioning
b. Lid positioning	With eyes opened lid margins overlay cornea at both superior and inferior borders	Sclera visible between upper lid(s) and part of iris
c. Lid closure	Complete with smooth, easy motion	Incomplete, or closure with difficulty or pain
d. Blinking	Frequent involuntary, bilateral movements (average 15 to 20 blinks per minute)	Rapid blinking Monocular blinking Absent or infrequent blinking
e. Surface characteristics	Skin intact, without discharge Lid margins flush against eyeball surface Lashes equally distributed and curled slightly outward	Lesions, nodules, redness, flaking, crusting, excessive tearing, discharge Cream or yellowish plaques (xanthelasma) Lid edema, lid deformity (pulled away from eyeball or turned inward) Lashes absent Lashes turned inward
	Epicanthal folds: vertical folds of skin covering inner canthus of eye; should disappear by age 10 years	Epicanthal folds present past age 10, unless Oriental child Any sign of ptosis needs referral
4. Position of globe in socket	Caucasians: eyeball does not protrude beyond supraorbital ridge of frontal bone Negroes: may protrude slightly beyond supraorbital ridge	Forward displacement (exophthalmos) Backward displacement (enophthalmos) Sunken eyes may need further dehydration or malnutrition evaluation
5. Lacrimal apparatus	No tearing during first month	Excessive tearing before 3 months No tearing by second month
a. Examiner presses index finger against lower orbital rim near inner canthus; pressure slightly everts lower lid	Puncta seen on tiny elevations on nasal side of upper and lower lid margins Mucosa pink and intact with no response to pressure	Puncta red, swollen, with tenderness on pressure Fluid or purulent material discharged from puncta in response to pressure
b. Gently palpate upper and lower lids for tenderness and nodules; exert minimal pressure over eyeball with examining finger	No tenderness or nodules	Tenderness, nodules, or irregularities
6. Bulbar conjunctiva and sclera	Infant sclera may have blue tinge due to its thinness Bulbar conjunctiva clear; tiny red vessels may be visible Sclera appears white Tiny black dots (pigmentation) may appear near limbus in dark-skinned persons Some pigmented deposits may appear Slight yellowish cast in dark-skinned persons	Darker blue sclera Blood vessels dilated Conjunctiva reddened Lesions or nodules Sclera yellow (jaundice) Foreign body Tenderness (especially on eye movement)
a. Lower lid eversion: not routinely performed in children unless examiner expects irritation, infection, or foreign body	Palpebral conjunctiva pink, intact, without discharge No tenderness or itching	Redness, lesions, nodules, discharge, tenderness, crusting
b. Upper lid eversion: not ordi-		

Characteristic or area examined	Normal	Deviations from normal
narily performed in screening examination unless examiner expects irritation, infection, or foreign body; when performed, techniques are same as for adult		
7. Cornea (using oblique lighting)		
a. Transparency	Transparent	Opacities
b. Surface characteristics	Smooth	Irregularities appearing in light reflections on surface
	Clear, shiny	Lesions, abrasions
		Foreign body
		Arcus senilis
		Tissue growth from periphery toward corneal center (pterygium)
		Corneal ulcerations
8. Anterior chamber: child must be old enough to cooperate		
a. Transparency	Transparent	Cloudiness or any visible material, blood
b. Iris surface	Iris flat	Iris bulging toward cornea (crescent-shaped shadow may appear on far side of iris)
c. Chamber depth	Adequate clearance between cornea and iris	Chamber appears shallow
9. Iris		
a. Shape	Round	Irregular shape
b. Color and consistency	Coloration from newborn to 6 months may be blue	Inconsistency of coloration (in one eye or between two eyes)
	Generally between 6 and 9 months permanent color determined	
	By 1 year all children should have permanent iris color	
10. Pupil		
a. Shape	Round	Other than round
b. Bilateral size	Equal in size	Unequal in size
Internal eye (See both adult and pediatric clinical strategies for techniques)		
1. Red reflex	Bright, round, red-orange glow seen through pupil (even in infants)	Decreased redness or roundness of reflex
		Dark spots or any opacities
2. Cornea, anterior chamber, and lens: lens wheel setting will vary with age of child; should be approximately +8 to +15	Clear	Cloudy or any visible materials
		Blood
3. Vitreous body (approximately +8 to +15 back to 0 to −5)	Clear	Cloudy
	Transparent	Floating particles
4. Retinal structures (lens at −5 to 0)		
a. Optic disc margin	Regular, distinct	Margin blurred
	Sharp outline scattered or dense pigment deposits may be visualized at border	
	Grayish crescent may appear at temporal border	
1. Shape	Round or slightly vertically oval	Irregular
2. Size	Approximately 1.5 mm diameter (appears magnified fifteen times to examiner)	Shape and size of discs not equal in both eyes
	Marked myopic refractive errors may make disc appear larger	
	Hyperopic errors may make it appear smaller	
3. Color	Creamy pink	Diffuse pallor or pallor of section of disc, which always extends from center of disc to border
	Lighter than retina	
	Tiny vessels may be visible on disc surface	Hyperemic disc (with engorged, tortuous vessels on disc surface)

Continued.

Clinical variations associated with the pediatric client–cont'd

Characteristic or area examined	Normal	Deviations from normal
4. Physiological cup	Small depression just temporal of center of disc; does *not* extend to disc border Usually appears paler than disc, sometimes grayish Usually occupies four-tenths to five-tenths of diameter of disc Vessels entering disc may drop abruptly into cup or may appear to fade gradually Discs more pronounced in some people than others	Cup extends to border of disc Cup occupies more than five-tenths of diameter of the disc Cup size of placement not equal in both eyes
b. Retinal vessels: follow from disc to periphery, dividing retina into four quadrants		
1. Arteries	Usually about 25% narrower than veins (2:3 or 4:5 ratio; size varies with number of branches) Narrow band of light may appear at center Light red	Arteries become narrow (2:4 or 3:5 ratio or less) (hypertension) Width of light reflex increases to cover over one third of artery Opaque or pale in color
2. Veins	Larger than arteries No light reflection Darker in color Venous pulsations may be visible	Veins become larger
3. Distribution and pattern (*Note:* Vessel abnormalities are not evenly distributed; scan all quadrants in orderly fashion for observation.)	Vessel caliber should be regular and uniformly decreasing in size as it branches and moves toward periphery Artery/vein crossings should not alter (or pinch) caliber of underlying vessel	Irregularities of caliber; dilation or constriction Neovascularization (appears as compact patches of tortuous, narrow vessels) Indentations or nicks of vessels at artery/vein crossing
c. Retinal background: scan four quadrants in orderly fashion		
1. Color and surface characteristics	Pink, usually uniform throughout Negroid fundi often heavily pigmented or uniformly dark Choroidal vessels may be visible through retinal layer (appear as linear, light orange streaks) Movable light reflections may appear on retinal surface (more prominent in young persons)	Pallor of fundus (general or localized) Hemorrhage (may be linear, flame-shaped, rounded, dark or red, large or small) Microaneurysms (appear as discrete tiny red dots) Soft or hard exudates (fuzzy or well-defined white patches)
d. Macula and fovea centralis: not fully mature until end of first year		
1. Color and surface	Appears slightly darker than remainder of retina Fovea may appear as tiny bright light in center of macula Tiny vessels may appear on surface Fine pigmentation and granular appearance may be visible	Any abnormalities or lesions described for remainder of retinal surface

History and clinical strategies associated with the geriatric client

1. Glaucoma symptoms and information follow:
   a. Open-angle, or chronic simple, glaucoma is the most common type of glaucoma in elderly clients.
   b. Early symptoms are absent or subtle:
      (1) Vague loss of peripheral vision (which client may not notice or just attribute to aging)
      (2) Aching or discomfort around eyes
      (3) Difficulty adjusting to darkness (a common complaint *not* associated with glaucoma, due to normal pupillary decrease in size)
   c. May be familial (tonometry screening should be performed with other family members)

d. Usually bilateral
e. Noncompliancy with treatment prescribed for glaucoma may be a problem because:
    (1) The disease itself is often asymptomatic, and the miotic drops create difficulty in adjusting to darkness.
    (2) Clients may have difficulty administering medication.
f. Clients with acute closed-angle glaucoma have acute symptoms, and it is regarded as an emergency medical problem. The symptoms are:
    (1) Severe eyeball pain and headache
    (2) Colored haloes around lights
    (3) Sudden decrease in visual acuity
    (4) Nausea, vomiting
g. Clients with closed-angle (or narrow-angle) glaucoma can also have acute intermittent attacks alternating with remissions.

2. Cataract symptoms and information follow:
    a. The extent of client visual loss or blurring may not correlate with the extent of opacity viewed by the examiner.
    b. Opacities may be nuclear (central), which tend to interfere with central vision, peripheral, or scattered.
    c. Lens opacities increase glare (e.g., lights at night, bright sunlight, highly polished floors). This should be considered a safety problem.
    d. Cataracts are usually bilateral; however, they can progress at different rates in each eye.
    e. Common symptoms accompanying cataracts are:
        (1) General darkening of images
        (2) Glare
        (3) Sense of dimness
        (4) Image distortion
    f. If the cataracts have been removed and corrective lenses are worn, the client may have good central vision, but images appear closer and larger than they really are. Peripheral vision will be diminished. Safety concerns such as using stairs, learning to turn head to side to view peripheral images, maneuvering in traffic, and adjusting to visual change should be covered.
    g. Corneal contact lenses can be prescribed for individuals who have had cataracts removed. Peripheral vision is more accurate with these lenses. However, adjustment to wearing lenses is difficult (see adult history section for some details).
    h. Intraocular lens implantation is being performed increasingly for post–cataract removal clients. The implantation offers more normal central and peripheral vision. Miotic eyedrops are prescribed to ensure that the lens remains in place.

3. The examiner will probably be working with clients who are chronically visually handicapped. Some common problems follow:
    a. Blurred or diminished vision acuity
    b. Decreased ability to perceive depth
    c. Difficulty adjusting to darkness; light, in general, appears dimmer
    d. Increased glare
    e. Diminished peripheral vision
    f. Loss of color perception acuity (lens becomes more yellowish with aging, and objects appear more yellow; difficulty differentiating blue/green hues)

4. The problems just mentioned may be perceived by the client as mild inconveniences or as major problems. The practitioner must take an adequate history to cover safety concerns and successful and satisfactory performance of activities of daily living (see original data base screening, Chapter 2, for details). Particular safety and convenience concerns to inquire about follow:
    a. Sufficient lighting available in home (dark hallways, stairways, night light)
    b. Sufficient lighting for close work (reading, sewing, writing)
    c. Safety concerns at night or in the dark (driving, walking on irregular surfaces)
    d. Reduction of glare and excess lighting ("cool" lighting contributes to glare), windows without curtains, highly polished floors
    e. If depth perception altered, concerns about using stairs, stepping off curbs
    f. If necessary, client access to special materials available for visually handicapped (e.g., large-print books, magazines and calendars, special dials for telephone)
    g. Resources available for help (e.g., relatives, neighbors, local community agencies)
    h. Difficulty with administration of medication
    i. Adequacy of *total* sensory input with visually handicapped clients (e.g., is client alone for long periods; able to use television or radio as a means of receiving information?)

5. When interviewing visually handicapped clients, the following behaviors are helpful:
    a. Remember that this individual is probably in a strange environment and is receiving a multitude of sensory stimuli. New sounds, odors, environmental temperatures, and a busy, crowded environment may overload a client whose vision is diminished to the extent that he

cannot accommodate. Privacy, a quiet area, and the use of touch to communicate is helpful.

b. Questions should be worded distinctly and slowly, allowing client sufficient time to respond.

c. The examiner must explain every activity *before* it happens.

6. Review history and clinical strategies in the adult section of this chapter for additional information related to eye and visual examination.

7. *Note:* Testing for intraocular pressure with the use of the tonometer has not been covered in this chapter. It is considered a necessary component of regular eye/vision screening for adults over 40 years of age.

Clinical variations associated with the geriatric client

Characteristic or area examined	Normal	Deviations from normal
Visual acuity and function		
1. Distant vision measurement (CN II)	20/20 to 20/30 O.D., O.S. (with corrective lenses)	O.D. or O.S.: any letters missed in 20/20 to 20/30 line or above*
a. Reading patterns	Smooth, without hesitation Eyes remain open without frowning or squinting	Behaviors indicating difficulty reading (frowning, squinting, "cheating," leaning forward, head tilting, hesitancy or difficulty naming letters)
2. Near vision measurement	One author states that average individual over 60 cannot focus more closely than 3 feet without corrective lenses With corrective lenses: 14/14 O.D. 14/14 O.S.	Inability to read newsprint or Jaeger chart at 35 cm (14 inches) with corrective lenses Tendency to push reading material farther away
a. Reading patterns	Newsprint or chart read without hesitancy or attempt to pull it closer or push it farther away Eyes remain open without excessive blinking or facial distortions	Note any other behaviors indicating difficulty (frowning, squinting, hesitancy, pulling reading material closer)
3. Peripheral visual fields (confrontation method)	Client and examiner report seeing object at approximately same time as it approaches from periphery; this test assumes that the examiner has normal peripheral vision Normal described as: Temporal peripheral vision: 90° Upward: 50° Nasalward: 60° Downward: 70°	Client fails to report sighting object at same time as examiner in any one direction or in all directions (peripheral visual loss may involve both eyes or one eye)
4. Extraocular muscle function		
a. Corneal light reflex	Light reflection appears symmetrically in the two pupils	Light reflection appears at different spots (asymmetrically) in each eye
b. Movement of eyes in six cardinal fields of gaze (CN III, IV, VI)	Both eyes demonstrate coordinated, parallel movements in all directions End-point nystagmus may occur if eye is held in extreme gaze (mild rhythmic twitching with quick movement in direction of gaze with slow drift in other direction)	Eye movements not coordinated or parallel One or both eyes fail to follow examiner's hand in any given direction Sporadic or nonpurposeful eye movements Pathological nystagmus (quick movement always in same direction regardless of direction of gaze) *Note:* Clients with Parkinson disease tend to manifest a restriction of conjugate upward gaze
c. Cover-uncover test	Uncovered eye does not move as examiner places card over other eye Newly uncovered eye does not move	Uncovered eye moves to focus on designated point Newly uncovered eye moves to focus on designated point
5. Corneal reflex (CN V)	Lids of both eyes close when either cornea touched	Lid(s) of one or both eyes fail to respond

*Several authors state that distant visual acuity begins to decrease in the 60s, and that only about 15% of the individuals over 80 years measure at 20/20. However, for screening purposes any measurement less than 20/20 to 20/30 is considered a problem for referral regardless of client age.

Characteristic or area examined	Normal	Deviations from normal
6. Pupillary response (CN II, CN III)		
a. Direct and consensual reaction to light	Constriction response (bilateral) somewhat delayed: pupil with light shining on it constricts (direct response); other pupil constricts simultaneously (consensual response)	Unequal (in size or speed) reflex response or absent response
b. Accommodation	Pupil constriction remains intact in response to accommodation	Pupils fail to constrict
	Client will probably report that near object out of focus (near vision reading test measures client's ability to focus on near objects)	Asymmetrical response
External ocular structures		
1. Eyebrows		
a. Hair quality and distribution, skin quality	Skin intact, without marked or patchy hair loss	Flaking, scaling, lesions
	Moderate thinning of brows (especially at temporal side)	Marked or patchy hair loss
	Brows in equal alignment	Unequal alignment
b. Movement	Equal (bilateral)	Asymmetrical
2. Eyelids/lashes		
a. Height of palpebral fissures	Bilaterally equal in position	Asymmetrical positioning
b. Lid positioning	Upper lids may droop to greater extent than in young adult (lids overlie cornea at both superior and inferior borders)	Lids droop to extent of interfering with vision
		Sclera visible between upper and/or lower lid margins and iris
c. Lid closure	Complete with smooth, easy motion	Incomplete, or closure with difficulty or pain
d. Blinking	Frequent involuntary, bilateral, movements (average 15 to 20 blinks per minute)	Rapid blinking
		Monocular blinking
		Absent or infrequent blinking
e. Surface characteristics	Numerous wrinkles, thin skinfolds	Flaking, crusting
	Skin intact, without discharge	Lesions (basal cell carcinoma most commonly found in this area)
	Lower lid margins may droop slightly away from eyeball surface	Ectropion, with tearing (Fig. 7-17) (may become infected)
	Lashes curled outward (lashes may be sparse)	

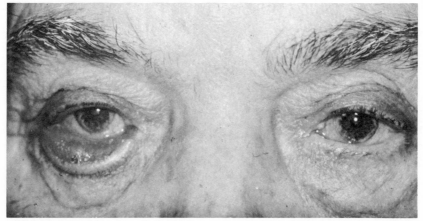

Fig. 7-17. Ectropion. (From Steinberg, F.: Cowdry's the care of the geriatric patient, ed. 5, St. Louis, 1976, The C. V. Mosby Co.)

	Creamy yellowish plaques (sometimes raised) may appear (especially near inner canthus) (xanthelasma, Fig. 7-9)	Entropion (may become infected), lashes curled inward or absent
3. Position of globe in socket	Globe sinks deeper into socket (loss of fat cushion)	Forward displacement (exophthalmos)
		Marked backward displacement (enophthalmos)
		Asymmetrical placement

Continued.

Clinical variations associated with the geriatric client–cont'd

Characteristic or area examined	Normal	Deviations from normal
4. Lacrimal apparatus		
a. Puncta and eyelids (on palpation)	Puncta seen on tiny elevations on nasal side of upper and lower lid margins	Puncta red, swollen with tenderness on pressure
	Mucosa pink and intact with no response to pressure	Fluid or purulent material discharged from puncta in response to pressure
	Occasionally lacrimal gland can be viewed if upper eyelid is raised or everted (loss of circumorbital fat)	
b. Upper and lower lids	No tenderness or nodules	Tenderness, nodules, or irregularities
5. Bulbar conjunctiva, sclera, palpebral conjunctiva	Bulbar conjunctiva may appear somewhat dry, lacking luster of younger adult	Profuse tearing
	Bulbar conjunctiva clear; tiny red vessels may be visible	Blood vessels dilated
	Sclera appears white	Conjunctiva reddened
	Tiny black dots (pigmentation) may appear near limbus in dark-complexioned persons	Lesions or nodules
	Some pigmented deposits may appear	Sclera yellow (jaundice) or significantly bluish
	Slight yellowish cast in dark-complexioned persons	Foreign bodies
		Tenderness (especially on eye movement)
	Palpebral conjunctiva pink, intact, without discharge	Redness, lesions, nodules, discharge, tenderness, crusting
	No tenderness or itching	
6. Cornea (use oblique lighting)		
a. Transparency	Transparent	Opacities
b. Surface characteristics	Smooth	Irregularities appearing in light reflections on surface
	Clear, shiny	Lesions, abrasions, foreign body
	Arcus senilis (deposit of white-yellow material around periphery of cornea; may be slightly elevated)	Tissue growth from periphery toward corneal center (pterygium)
7. Anterior chamber (use oblique lighting)		
a. Transparency	Transparent	Cloudiness or any visible material, blood
b. Iris surface	Iris flat	Iris bulging toward cornea (crescent-shaped shadow may appear on far side of iris)
c. Chamber depth	Chamber becomes shallower with aging, however, clearance between cornea and iris maintained	Marked shallowness
8. Iris		
a. Shape	Round (wedge or portion of iris may be absent in clients who have had cataract removal)	Irregular
b. Color and consistency	May be some irregularity of density of pigmentation (bilateral)	Inconsistency of coloration between eyes
	Normal pigment replaced by pale brownish coloration	
9. Pupil		
a. Shape and size	Round (shape may appear somewhat irregular or square with intraocular lens implant following cataract surgery)	Irregular shape
	Aged pupils often smaller in size (sometimes markedly so)	
	Elderly client receiving topical miotic agents (for glaucoma) will have constricted pupils	
b. Bilateral size	Equal	Unequal
Internal eye		
1. Red reflex	Bright, round, red-orange flow seen through pupil	Opacities or decreased redness or roundness of reflex
	Increasing opacities of lens viewed as part of normal aging; examiner may commonly see various patterns of dark spots or clouds	

Characteristic or area examined	Normal	Deviations from normal
	(either central, peripheral or scattered) in the aged reflex	
	However, for screening purposes all opacities should be viewed as problem for referral	
2. Cornea, anterior chamber, lens	Clear	Cloudy or any visible materials, blood
3. Vitreous body	Clear	Cloudy
	Transparent	Floating particles
4. Retinal structures		
a. Optic disc margin	Regular, distinct	Margin blurred
	Sharp outline scattered or dense pigment deposits may be visualized at border	
	Grayish crescent may appear at temporal border	
1. Shape	Round or slightly vertically oval	Irregular
2. Size	Approximately 1.5 mm diameter (appears magnified fifteen times to examiner)	Shape and size of discs not equal in both eyes
	Marked myopic refractive errors may make disc appear larger	
	After cataract extraction, disc appears very small	
	Hyperopic errors may make it appear smaller	
3. Color	Creamy pink	Diffuse pallor or pallor of section of disc, which always extends from center of disc to border
	Lighter than retina	
	Tiny vessels may be visible on disc surface	Hyperemic disc (with engorged, tortuous vessels on disc surface)
4. Physiological cup	Small depression just temporal of center of disc; does *not* extend to disc border	Cup extends to border of disc
	Usually appears paler than disc, sometimes grayish	
	Usually occupies four tenths to five tenths of diameter of disc	Cup occupies more than five tenths of diameter of disc
	Vessels entering disc may drop abruptly into cup or may appear to fade gradually	Cup size or placement not equal in both eyes
	Discs more pronounced in some clients than others	
b. Retinal vessels		
1. Arteries	Arteriolar reflex slightly widened	Arteries become narrow (2:4 or 3:5 ratio or less) (hypertension)
	Arteriolar column may appear slightly narrower, straighter with slight irregularities in caliber (Fig. 7-18)	Width of light reflex increases to cover over one third of artery

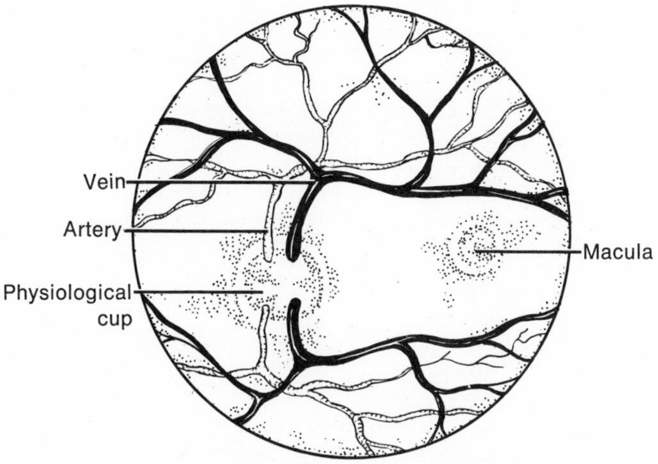

Fig. 7-18. Retinal changes in the aging eye. The arteriolar columns are slightly narrower, with slight irregularities in caliber; it may appear more opaque.

Continued.

Clinical variations associated with the geriatric client–cont'd

Characteristic or area examined	Normal	Deviations from normal
	Arteries may appear more opaque, grayish	Opaque or pale in color
	Adult arteries usually about 25% narrower than veins (2:3 or 4:5 ratio; size varies with number of branches)	
	Narrow band of light may appear at center	
	Light red	
2. Veins	Larger than arteries	Veins become engorged
	No light reflection	
	Darker in color	
3. Distribution and pattern	Vessel caliber should be regular and uniformly decreasing in size as it branches and moves toward periphery	Irregularities of caliber; dilation or constriction
	Artery/vein crossings should not alter (or pinch) caliber of underlying vessel	Neovascularization (appears as compact patches of tortuous, narrow vessels)
		Indentations or nicks of vessels at artery/vein crossing
c. Retinal background		
1. Color and surface characteristics	Fine granular surface	Pallor of fundus (general or localized)
	Pink, usually uniform throughout	White choroid and vessels clearly visible through thinned or absent retina
	Negroid fundi often heavily pigmented and uniformly dark	Hemorrhage (may be linear, flame-shaped, rounded, dark or red, large or small)
	Choroidal vessels may be visible through retinal layer (appear as linear, light orange streaks)	Microaneurysms (appear as discrete, tiny red dots)
	Movable light reflections may appear on retinal surface (more prominent in young clients)	Drusen commonly seen (usually located symmetrically in both eyes)
		Any fuzzy or well-defined white or yellow patches
d. Macula and fovea centralis	Appears slightly darker than rest of retina (slight dispersion of granular pigment)	Macular degeneration manifests small areas or clumps of black pigment in and around macula (degree of pigmentation does not always correlate with visual loss symptoms)
	Foveal (light) reflex may be less bright than young adult	
	Tiny vessels may appear on surface	May be hemorrhage visible in area

Vocabulary

1. Accommodation – A for distance
   reflex – pupil constricts
   eyes converge
   lens ↑ convex

2. Amblyopia
   dimness of vision not
   2° organic/refractive error

3. Arcus senilis
   opaque line inside limbus

4. Asthenopia
   ↓vision c̄ neck eye pain
   head
   cillary muscle, Eomstram

5. Astigmatism
   refractive error 2° differences in
   curvature of cornea + lens

6. Blepharitis
   inflammation of edges of eyelid
   margins

7. Bulbar conjunctiva
   over sclera

8. Cardinal fields of gaze

9. Cataract

lens opacity

10. Chalazion

eyelid cyst a° infection
of sebaceous gland

11. Choroid

vascular coat c̄ brown
pigment to ↓ light diffusion +
reflection

12. Diplopia

13. Ectropion

eversion of lid

14. Enophthalmos

sunken eyeball

15. Entropion

inverted lid

16. Exophthalmos

protruding eyeball

17. Glaucoma

↑ intraocular pressure

18. Hordeolum

sty; hair follicle
inflammation

19. Hyperopia = presbyopia
farsighted
light falls behind
retina

20. Hyphemia

anterior chamber hemorrhage

21. Macula

cones
maximal acuity, central
vision

22. Myopic

nearsighted
light in front of retina

23. Nicking

24. Nystagmus

involuntary rhythmic oscillation
of eyeball

25. O.D.

Ⓡ eye

26. Optic disc

head of optic nerve

27. O.S.

Ⓛ eye

28. O.U.

both

29. Palpebral conjunctiva

inside lids

30. PERRLA

pupils Ⓔ round
reactive to light +
accomodation

31. Photophobia

35. Red reflex

32. Presbyopia

loss of lens elasticity
hyperopia of aging

36. Strabismus

deviation of eye
visual axes uncoordinated

33. Pterygium

patch of thickened conjunctiva
over bulbar conjunctiva, cornea

37. Visual acuity

34. Ptosis

drooping of lid

38. Xanthelasma

tumor like deposit of
fatty substances

Cognitive self-assessment

1. Distance visual acuity measurement:
   - ☐ a. is used in a screening examination only when a refractive error is suspected
   - ☐ b. is not necessary for individuals over 40 years of age
   - ☑ c. tests, to some extent, the adequacy of macular vision
   - ☐ d. may be improved if the client wears prescribed reading glasses
   - ☑ e. tests the functioning of the nerve fibers from the macula to the occipital cortex
   - ☐ f. a and d
   - ☐ g. a and b
   - ☑ h. c and e
   - ☐ i. c and d
2. Distance visual acuity results are reported in fraction form. Mrs. Jones' medical record states that she measured 20/40 O.D. and 20/40 O.S. This means:
   - ☐ a. that she was standing 40 feet from the eye chart and could read the line that someone with normal vision could read standing 20 feet from the chart
   - ☑ b. that she was standing 20 feet from the chart and could read the line that someone with normal vision could read standing 40 feet from the chart
   - ☐ c. that she was able to read twenty out of the forty letters on the chart
   - ☐ d. that she has presbyopia
   - ☐ e. none of the above
3. Near vision acuity measurement:
   - ☐ a. is not necessary if the client masters the Snellen chart screening
   - ☑ b. tests for presbyopia
   - ☑ c. tests for loss of flexibility of the lens of the eye
   - ☑ d. tests for loss of accomodation
   - ☐ e. tests for amblyopia
   - ☐ f. a and e
   - ☐ g. b and e

    ☒ h. b, c, and d
    ☐ i. a and d
    ☐ j. none of the above

4. The corneal light reflex:
    ☒ a. tests for alignment of the anteroposterior axes of the two eyes
    ☐ b. tests for corneal reflex
    ☐ c. demonstrates bilateral pupillary convergence
    ☒ d. might indicate a weak extraocular muscle if asymmetry is present
    ☒ e. will help to differentiate epicanthus and crossed eyes
    ☐ f. c and e
    ☒ g. a, d, and e
    ☐ h. all except b
    ☐ i. none of the above

5. Visual field defects:
    ☒ a. may occur unilaterally
    ☒ b. may occur bilaterally
    ☐ c. may occur in the form of a blind spot
    ☒ d. may involve temporal field loss of both eyes
    ☒ e. may involve temporal field loss of one eye and nasal field loss of the other eye
    ☐ f. a and c
    ☐ g. b, d, and e
    ☐ h. all except a
    ☐ i. all except d
    ☒ j. all the above

6. The cover-uncover test:
    ☐ a. is a test for nystagmus
    ☐ b. when successfully performed, demonstrates that CN VIII is intact
    ☒ c. is a test for maintenance of parallel eyes
    ☐ d. is a test to demonstrate near vision acuity
    ☐ e. none of the above

7. Eye orbit movement is controlled by six muscles and three cranial nerves. The cranial nerves involved are:
    ☐ a. the optic (CN II), oculomotor (CN III), and abducens (CN VI)
    ☒ b. the oculomotor (CN III), trochlear (CN IV), and abducens (CN VI)
    ☐ c. the oculomotor (CN II), trigeminal (CN V), and facial (CN VII)
    ☐ d. the optic (CN II), trigeminal (CN V), and abducens (CN VI)

8. The pupil of the eye:
    ☒ a. normally constricts in response to a bright light
    ☐ b. dilates in response to accomodation for near objects
    ☐ c. may normally be slightly irregular in shape
    ☒ d. tends to be larger in myopic clients
    ☐ e. constricts in response to parasympathetic stimulation of the iris muscles
    ☐ f. all the above
    ☒ g. a, d, and e
    ☐ h. b and d
    ☐ i. all except c

9. Consensual pupillary response:
    ☒ a. occurs because the afferent part of the optic nerve from either eye transmits pupillary reflex
    ☐ b. occurs because the efferent pupil constriction stimulus is sent to ciliary nerves in both eyes

- ☐ c. occurs when a lesion is present in the optic chiasm
- ☑ d. will not occur if a blind eye (severed optic nerve) is stimulated
- ☐ e. is a "red flag" for early glaucoma
- ☑ f. a, b, and d
- ☐ g. a and d

10. The eyelids:
- ☑ a. when open, normally cover a small portion of the iris
- ☑ b. are lined with palpebral conjunctiva
- ☑ c. when open, form the palpebral fissure, the distance between the lid margins
- ☑ d. contain the meibomian glands, which secrete an oily substance
- ☑ e. are normally flush against the eyeball when open
- ☑ f. all the above
- ☐ g. c and e
- ☐ h. a, b, and d
- ☐ i. all except b
- ☐ j. all except c

11. The eyeball is a sphere suspended within a bony orbit by means of:
- ☑ a. muscles
- ☑ b. ligaments
- ☑ c. fat cushion
- ☐ d. scleral tissue
- ☐ e. nasolacrimal ducts
- ☐ f. all the above
- ☑ g. a, b, and c
- ☐ h. a, c, and d
- ☐ i. b and e

12. When examining the lacriminal apparatus, only one portion is actually observed; this is the:
- ☐ a. lacrimal gland
- ☑ b. puncta
- ☐ c. lacrimal sac
- ☐ d. nasolacrimal duct

13. The conjunctiva:
- ☑ a. is the transparent lining of the eyelids
- ☑ b. is the transparent covering of the anterior portion of the eyeball
- ☐ c. is the white, porcelain covering of the eyeball
- ☑ d. normally contains a few visible vessels
- ☑ e. surfaces are kept moist and clean by a film of tears
- ☐ f. a and e
- ☐ g. c and d
- ☐ h. a, b, and e
- ☐ i. all except b
- ☑ j. all except c

14. The cornea:
- ☑ a. is normally transparent
- ☐ b. may normally show a somewhat irregular surface
- ☐ c. covers the pupil and meets the conjunctival layer at the pupillary border
- ☑ d. surface, when touched, transmits the sensation through CN V (trigeminal nerve)
- ☑ e. abrasions can often be detected through oblique light reflections on its surface
- ☐ f. all the above

☐ g. a, b, and e
☐ h. c and e
☑ i. a, d, and e
☐ j. all except b

15. You are holding the ophthalmoscope 4 cm from the client's eye. You want to examine the anterior chamber of the lens. You should set the lens wheel at __ for the best focus.
    ☐ a. −3
    ☐ b. 0
    ☐ c. −10 to −15
    ☐ d. +5 to +2
    ☑ e. +15 to +20

16. When using the ophthalmoscope:
    ☑ a. approach the client about 15° temporally
    ☐ b. move the ophthalmoscope forward and backward in front of your eye until the red reflex comes into focus
    ☑ c. stabilize the client's head with your free hand
    ☐ d. ask the client to look at the ophthalmoscope light
    ☐ e. keep the client talking to distract him from the examination
    ☐ f. all the above
    ☐ g. b, c, and d
    ☑ h. a and c
    ☐ i. a, d and e
    ☐ j. all except d

17. Three layers of tissue cover the eyeball. Which of the following statements are true?
    ☑ a. The sclera is the external layer.
    ☑ b. The choroid layer is vascular, and these vessels can sometimes be viewed through the retina.
    ☐ c. The choroid contains many nerve cells that react to light.
    ☐ d. The iris, part of the middle layer, is muscular in function.
    ☑ e. The retina, the innermost layer, is visible to the examiner when using the ophthalmoscope.
    ☐ f. All the above
    ☐ g. b, c, and e
    ☐ h. a and d
    ☑ i. All except c
    ☐ j. All except b

18. Absence or diminishment of the red reflex may be an indication of:
    ☐ a. xanthelasma
    ☑ b. opacity
    ☐ c. CN III malfunction
    ☐ d. glaucoma
    ☐ e. hypertension

19. The normal color of the optic disc is:
    ☑ a. creamy pink
    ☐ b. pinkish red
    ☐ c. pale gray
    ☐ d. bluish gray

20. The physiological depression (cup) within the disc:
    ☑ a. is just temporal of the center of the disc
    ☐ b. may normally extend to the disc border with hyperopic clients
    ☑ c. normally appears paler than the disc
    ☑ d. usually occupies approximately half the diameter of the disc

- ☐ e. may normally be more pronounced in one eye
- ☐ f. all the above
- ☐ g. a and d
- ☐ h. b and e
- ☐ i. all except e
- ☒ j. a, c, and d
21. Normal retinal arteries visible to the examiner are:
    - ☒ a. about 25% narrower than the veins
    - ☐ b. darker in color than the veins
    - ☐ c. opaque in appearance
    - ☐ d. about 50% narrower than the veins
    - ☐ e. none of the above
22. Normal retinal veins visible to the examiner:
    - ☐ a. are about 25% narrower than the arteries
    - ☐ b. are lighter in color than the arteries
    - ☐ c. often manifest a band of light at the center of the vessel
    - ☐ d. are over twice as wide as the arteries
    - ☒ e. none of the above
23. The normal retinal surface visible to the examiner:
    - ☒ a. may show a fine granular texture
    - ☒ b. may show marked dark-pigmented spots
    - ☒ c. may show light orange streaks (choroidal vessels)
    - ☐ d. a and b
    - ☒ e. a and c
24. The macula:
    - ☒ a. is about 1 DD in size
    - ☒ b. is nourished by the choroid layer vessels
    - ☐ c. is 2 DD nasalward from the disc
    - ☒ d. a and b
    - ☐ e. a and c

PEDIATRIC QUESTIONS

25. Which of the following findings alone indicate referral of the child for further physician evaluation?
    - ☐ a. Four-month-old child whose eyes periodically cross
    - ☐ b. Four-year-old child whose visual acuity was 20/40 both eyes
    - ☒ c. Six-year-old child whose visual acuity was 20/30 O.D., 20/40 O.S.
    - ☒ d. Ten-month-old child who demonstrates right eye drifting with cover test
    - ? ☐ e. Five-year-old boy who excessively blinks but who shows no signs of corneal irritation or infection
    - ☐ f. All except b
    - ☐ g. b and c
    - ☐ h. a, d, and e
    - ☒ i. c and d
    - ☐ j. None of the above
26. All the following are true but one. Identify the *false* statement.
    When performing vision screening on kindergarten children using the Snellen "E" chart, the examiner should:
    - ☐ a. test each eye separately
    - ☐ b. test both eyes together
    - ☒ c. evaluate only those children who have never been tested before
    - ☐ d. place the child 20 feet from the chart
    - ☐ e. retest any child who scores over 20/40

27. If you were to develop a 4-year-old vision screening program, which of the following techniques would you include?
   ☑ a. Peripheral visual field testing
   ☑ b. Cover test
   ☐ c. Near vision screening
   ☑ d. Snellen visual acuity testing using either alphabet or "E" chart
   ☑ e. Color vision screening using Ishihara test; test boys only
   ☐ f. All the above
   ☐ g. a, c, and d
   ☐ h. b, d, and e
   ☑ i. All except c
   ☐ j. All except e

GERIATRIC QUESTIONS

28. Cataracts
   ☐ a. are inherited
   ☐ b. are chiefly associated with diabetic clients
   ☐ c. do not create any visual problems until they become "ripe"
   ☐ d. all the above
   ☑ e. none of the above

29. Glaucoma:
   ☐ a. is readily recognized in elderly clients because of the associated acute symptoms
   ☐ b. can be diagnosed in its early stages by careful examination of the optic disc
   ☑ c. is usually bilateral
   ☐ d. all the above
   ☐ e. none of the above

30. Presbyopia:
   ☐ a. is synonymous with hyperopia
   ☑ b. affects most individuals over 60 years of age
   ☐ c. does not occur if the individual is myopic
   ☐ d. is rare
   ☐ e. none of the above

31. If an elderly client complains of difficulty adjusting to darkness, this might mean:
   ☑ a. that his pupil is smaller and admits less light to the retina
   ☐ b. advanced macular degeneration
   ☐ c. optic atrophy
   ☐ d. retinal detachment

SUGGESTED READINGS
General

American Journal of Nursing: Programmed instruction, patient assessment: examination of the eye, Part I, **74**(11):1974.

American Journal of Nursing: Programmed instruction, Patient assessment: examination of the eye, Part II, **75**(1):1975.

Bates, Barbara: A guide to physical examination, ed. 2, Philadelphia, 1979, J. B. Lippincott Co.

Boyd-Monk, Heather: Taking a closer look at contact lenses, Nursing '78 **8**(10):38-43, Oct., 1978.

Judge, Richard D., and Zuidema, George, editors: Methods of clinical examination: a physiologic approach, Boston, 1974, Little, Brown & Co., pp. 61-80.

Malasanos, Lois, Barkauskas, Violet, Moss, Muriel, and Stoltenberg-Allen, Kathryn: Health assessment, St. Louis, 1977, The C. V. Mosby Co., pp. 143-163.

Nordmark, Madelyn T., and Rohweder, Ann W.: Scientific foundations of nursing, ed. 3, Philadelphia, 1975, J. B. Lippincott Co., pp. 261-264.

Prior, John A., and Silberstein, Jack S.: Physical diagnosis: the history and examination of the patient, ed. 5, St. Louis, 1977, The C. V. Mosby Co., pp. 98-146.

Sana, Josephine, and Judge, Richard C., editors: Physical appraisal methods in nursing, Boston, 1975, Little, Brown & Co., pp. 105-120.

Pediatric

Alexander, Mary, and Brown, Marie Scott: Physical examination, Part 5. Examining the eye, Nursing '73 **3**(12):41-46, Dec., 1973.

Barness, Lewis: Manual of pediatric physical diagnosis, ed. 4, Chicago, 1972, Year Book Medical Publishers, Inc., pp. 50-66.

Brown, Marie Scott, and Murphy, Mary Alexander: Ambulatory pediatrics for nurses, New York, 1975, McGraw-Hill Book Co., pp. 201-214.

Chinn, Peggy, and Leitch, Cynthia: Child health maintenance: a guide to clinical assessment, ed. 2, St. Louis, 1979, The C. V. Mosby Co.

DeAngeles, Catherine: Basic pediatrics for the primary health care provider, Boston, 1975, Little, Brown & Co., pp. 44-45, 82-84, 191-196.

Geriatric

Burnside, Irene, editor: Nursing and the aged, New York, 1976, McGraw-Hill Book Co., pp. 380-392.

Caird, F. I., and Judge, T. G.: Assessment of the elderly patient, London, 1977, Pitman Medical Publishing Co., Ltd., pp. 56-59.

Chinn, Austin B., editor: Clinical aspects of aging, Working with older people: a guide to practice, vol. 4, Rockville, Md., 1971, U.S. Department of Health, Education, and Welfare, Public Health Service, pp. 28-37.

Jones, Dorothy, Dunbar, Claire Ford, and Jirovec, Mary M.: Medical-surgical nursing: a conceptual approach, New York, 1978, McGraw-Hill Book Co., pp. 1257-1274.

Marmor, Michael: The eye and vision in the elderly, Geriatrics **32**(8):63-67, Aug., 1977.

Steinberg, Franz: Cowdry's the care of the geriatric patient, ed. 5, St. Louis, 1976, The C. V. Mosby Co., pp. 351-363.

CHAPTER **8**

Assessment of the thorax and lungs

Cognitive objectives

At the end of this unit the learner will demonstrate knowledge of assessment of the respiratory system by the ability to do the following:

1. Systematically list the elements included in inspection of the respiratory system.
2. Correctly locate or diagram landmarks of the anterior thorax, including:
   a. Suprasternal notch
   b. Second rib
   c. Costochondral junctions
   d. Manubrium of sternum
   e. Costal angle
   f. Sternal angle
   g. Clavicle
   h. Midsternal line
   i. Midclavicular line
   j. Anterior axillary line
3. Correctly locate or diagram landmarks of the posterior thorax, including:
   a. C_7
   b. T_1
   c. Scapula
   d. Inferior angle of scapula T_6 and seventh rib
   e. Vertebral line
   f. Midscapular line
   g. Posterior axillary line
4. Describe the qualities of the following breath sounds and indicate the location in which they are normally heard in adults and children.
   a. Bronchial
   b. Bronchovesicular
   c. Vesicular
5. Describe the significance of each of the sounds in no. 4 when heard in areas other than their normal locations.
6. Describe the normal respiratory rates for children and adults.
7. Describe the following respiratory patterns:
   a. Kussmaul respirations
   b. Cheyne-Stokes breathing
   c. Sighing respirations
   d. Biot breathing
   e. Tachypnea
   f. Bradypnea
   g. Air trapping
8. Systematically list the elements included in palpating the thorax.
9. Describe the techniques for palpating expansion of the thorax.
10. Identify the following:
    a. One condition that increases lung expansion
    b. Four conditions that limit lung expansion
    c. One condition that results in asymmetrical expansion
11. Describe identifying characteristics of the following adventitious sounds:
    a. Rales
    b. Rhonchi
    c. Wheeze
    d. Pleural friction rub
12. Define the significance of and describe procedures for eliciting:
    a. Tactile fremitus
    b. Bronchophony
    c. Egophony
    d. Whispered pectoriloquy
    e. Diaphragmatic excursion
13. State a rationale for palpating for tenderness of the costovertebral angle.
14. Describe a systematic method for percussing the thorax.
15. Describe four percussion tones elicited throughout the body and state their normal locations.
16. Identify selected common variations with pediatric and geriatric clients.
17. Define the terms in the vocabulary list.

Clinical objectives

At the end of this unit the learner will perform systematic assessment of the thorax and lungs by demonstrating the ability to do the following:

1. Obtain a pertinent health history from client.
2. Demonstrate inspection of the thorax and relate findings relevant to:
   a. General body build
   b. Thorax configuration
   c. Skin, nail, and lip color
   d. Chest movement
   e. Pattern of respiration, including type of breathing, rate, and depth
3. Demonstrate palpation of the thorax and relate findings relevant to:
   a. Chest expansion
   b. Tenderness or pulsations
   c. Skin texture and lesions
   d. Subcutaneous structures or masses
   e. Tactile fremitus in symmetrical areas of the chest
   f. Position of the trachea
4. Demonstrate percussion of the thorax and relate findings relevant to:
   a. Characteristics of percussion tones heard in various areas of the thorax
   b. Intensity, pitch, quality, and duration of tones heard
   c. Diaphragmatic excursion
5. Demonstrate the ability to identify and differentiate lung sounds, including vesicular, bronchovesicular, bronchial, rales, rhonchi, and friction rub.
6. Demonstrate systematic auscultation of the lungs and relate findings relevant to:
   a. Characteristics of auscultatory sounds heard throughout the lungs
   b. Checking abnormal findings by using tests for bronchophony, egophony, and whispered pectoriloquy
7. Summarize findings of the assessment with a written description.

Health history related to thorax and lungs additional to data base

1. Coughing is basically caused by either internal or external stimuli. Internal stimuli include allergic responses or response to an inflammatory process. External stimuli include irritants such as smoke, dust, or gas. When compiling history data from a client complaining of a cough, collect as much descriptive information as possible. The data should include the following:
   a. Duration of the coughing problem
   b. Frequency of the cough; whether it is related to time of day
   c. Type of cough: hacky, dry, bubbly, throaty, barky, hoarse, congested
   d. Sputum production vs. nonproductive cough
   e. If sputum is produced, describe characteristics: mucoid vs. purulent, color, odor, blood-tinged (note that some medications, such as those containing catecholamines, may cause pink-tinged sputum), amount
   f. Circumstances related to cough, such as activity, time of day, client position (lying vs. sitting), anxiety, talking
   g. Whether activity makes cough better or worse (sitting, walking, exercise)
   h. History of allergies in client or others in family (see data base allergy profile)
   i. Is client's cough currently being treated? By whom? With what: over-the-counter medications, prescription medications, other techniques such as a vaporizer?
   j. Client's concern about cough
   k. Is cough tiring?
2. If client complains of shortness of breath or dyspnea on exertion:
   a. Does cough or diaphoresis accompany dyspnea?
   b. What is the onset of breathing problems? Describe severity, duration, efforts to treat
   c. Is breathing problem associated with pain or discomfort?
   d. How does different positioning affect the dyspnea (lying vs. sitting)?
   e. Time of day when dyspnea is likely to occur
   f. Does dyspnea interfere with, alter, or slow down any daily activities?
   g. How much walking creates shortness of breath (number of steps, flights of stairs, or blocks)?
   h. Are there stairs at home or work? How often must they be climbed each day? How does this interfere with breathing problem?
   i. How much walking or other types of exertion must the client do each day? How does this interfere with breathing problem?
3. If client complains of difficulty breathing or breathlessness:
   a. History of asthma, bronchitis, emphysema, or tuberculosis? (Have client describe what these mean personally and to the family.)
   b. Does breathing problem cause lips or fingernails to become cyanotic?
   c. During a "breathing attack" what does the client do (positioning, breathing aids such as medications or oxygen)?
   d. How does the breathing problem interfere with the client's activities of daily living or work?
   e. Client's view of breathing problem

f. Does client think the overall breathing problem is getting worse or staying about the same?

4. Has client had any previous respiratory illnesses, hospitalizations, or surgeries for lung or breathing problems? Describe what and when

5. When was the client's last chest x-ray examination, tuberculosis test, or pulmonary function test? What were the results?

6. Is the client currently taking any medications for breathing or allergy problems? If so, describe

7. Is the client subject to work or environmental conditions that could irritate the respiratory system (e.g., chemical plants, dry-cleaning fumes, coal mines)? If so, what does the client do for protection or monitoring the exposure conditions (e.g., masks, frequent pulmonary function tests or chest x-ray examinations, or ventilatory systems in factory with chemical exposure analysis)?

8. Certain "fumes" cause specific respiratory or systemic irritation. If the client reports a pollution exposure history as well as these symptoms, the examiner must be alert to their interrelationship:
   a. Carbon monoxide may cause dizziness, headache, or fatigue.
   b. Sulphur oxide may cause irritation to the respiratory tract, resulting in a cough or congestion.
   c. Nitrogen oxides may irritate the mucous membranes, resulting in a cough or congestion.

9. If client smokes:
   a. What does he smoke?
   b. How long has client smoked?
   c. How much each day does client smoke?
   d. Does client inhale?
   e. Does client have cough related to smoking?
   f. When did cough begin? Has cough gotten worse since that time?
   g. Does client desire to quit smoking?
   h. If so, what techniques has client used in an attempt to stop?
   i. If client has tried to quit but has failed, what does he see as the reason for failure?

10. If client formerly smoked but has quit:
    a. What had client been smoking?
    b. How long did client smoke?
    c. How much each day did client smoke?
    d. Why did he quit?

Clinical guidelines

The clinical guidelines have been developed to simulate the clinical setting. Total assessment of the thorax and lungs can be carried out with the client in a sitting position. The sequence of assessment techniques is inspection, palpation, percussion, and auscultation. A detailed discussion of the techniques of percussion and auscultation can be found in *clinical strategies* in this chapter.

Inspection of the anterior and posterior chest should be carried out first. Following inspection the examiner should perform palpation, percussion, and auscultation of the posterior chest; then the examiner palpates, percusses, and auscultates the anterior chest. This places the examiner in front of the client to proceed to cardiovascular assessment.

The student will:	To identify:	
	Normal	**Deviations from normal**

1. Secure equipment needed for assessment of thorax and lungs, including:
   a. Stethoscope
   b. Ruler
   c. Marker
2. Instruct client to undress to waist so that thorax may be examined (Females will need anterior cover during posterior examination.)

Inspection of anterior and posterior chest

1. Instruct client to sit on edge of examination table for general inspection of anterior and posterior chest (gown should be removed) (Fig. 8-1)

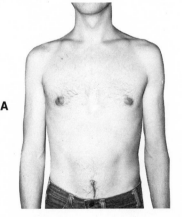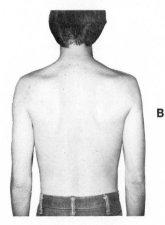

Fig. 8-1. A, Inspection of anterior chest. **B,** Inspection of posterior chest.

Continued.

Clinical guidelines–cont'd

The student will:	To identify:	
	Normal	**Deviations from normal**
2. Observe:		
a. Skin color of thorax and lips	Pink, well oxygenated	Cyanosis, pallor
		Spider nevi
b. Nail beds and nail configuration	Smooth	Clubbing of nail and distal finger
c. General appearance	Flat surface	
	Relaxed posture	Apprehensive
		Tense forward posture
		Restless
		Nostrils flaring
		Supraclavicular retractions
		Intercostal retractions
		Use of accessory muscles during breathing
d. Chest wall configuration	Symmetrical	
1. Imagine topographical landmarks of thorax (Fig. 8-2)	Equal muscular development	

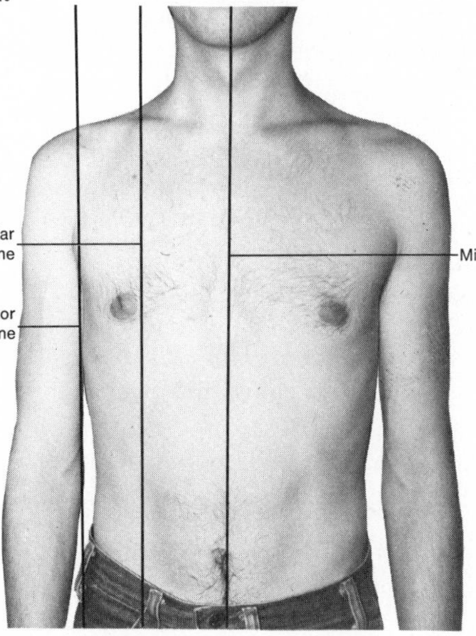

Fig. 8-2. **A,** Topographical landmarks of anterior thorax. **B,** Topographical landmarks of posterior thorax. **C,** Topographical landmarks of thorax (lateral view).

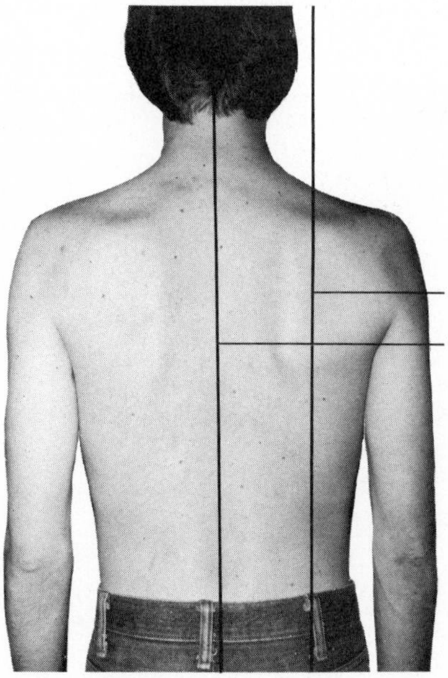

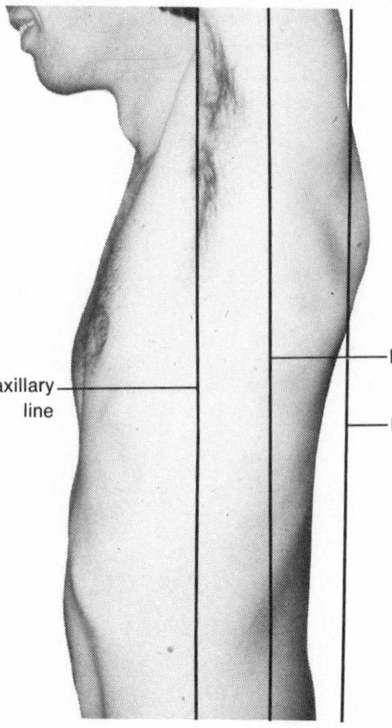

The student will:	To identify:	
	Normal	**Deviations from normal**
2. Imagine underlying structures of thorax (Fig. 8-3)		

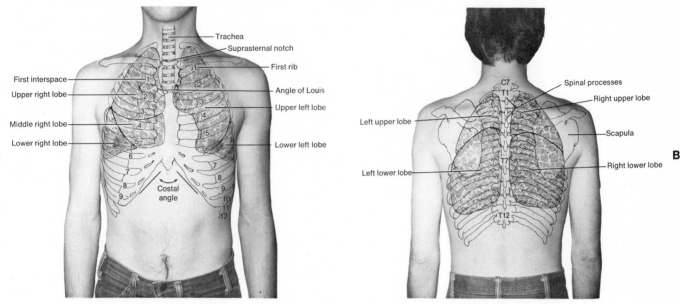

Fig. 8-3. A, Anterior view of anatomy of thorax. **B,** Posterior view of anatomy of thorax.

3. Anteroposterior (AP) diameter of chest	1:2 to 5:7 (AP: transverse diameter) flat connections of rib cartilage with sternum	Barrel chest (Fig. 8-4) Pectus carinatum Pectus excavatum

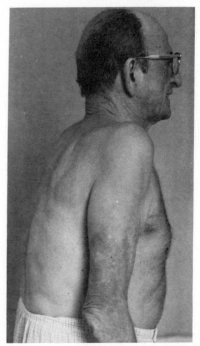

Fig. 8-4. Barrel chest. Note increased anteroposterior diameter.

Continued.

Clinical guidelines—cont'd

The student will:	To identify:	
	Normal	**Deviations from normal**
e. Symmetry of chest	Bilaterally equal musculature (may be slightly more muscle development on client's dominant side) Straight spinal processes (C_7, T_1 through T_{12}) Symmetrical scapular placement Downward and equal slope of ribs Costal angle 90° or less	Atrophy, tremors Asymmetry Loss of or accentuated spinal curvature, scoliosis, kyphosis, deformities Asymmetrical scapular placement Horizontal ribs Costal angle greater than 90°
f. Breathing pattern	Diaphragmatic (male) Thoracic (female) Smooth, even breathing Passive breathing 12 to 20 per minute; ratio of respiratory to pulse rate 1:4	Abnormal, irregular breathing Cheyne-Stokes
	Even pattern 	Increase in rate and depth Hyperpnea > 20 per minute
		Decrease in rate Bradypnea < 12 per minute
	Occasional sighing respirations 	Increase in rate and depth > 20 per minute Kussmaul respirations
	During inspiration chest expands, costal angle increases, and diaphragm descends and flattens	Many sighing respirations accompanied by other characteristics of anxiety Biot breathing: shallow breathing followed by periods of apnea (may also be seen in some healthy persons)
		Air trapping breathing in clients with pulmonary disease: because of obstructive process, air becomes trapped in lungs

	To identify:	
The student will:	**Normal**	**Deviations from normal**

Palpation of posterior chest

1. Use one or two hands to palpate skin and thorax of posterior chest; examiner should use palmar surface of hand, including palmar base of fingers (Fig. 8-5)

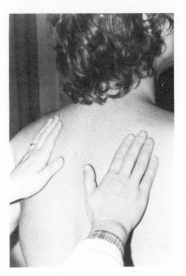

Fig. 8-5. Palpating posterior thorax.

2. Evaluate and/or identify: **a.** Skin texture and temperature, spinal process	Smooth, warm skin	Dry or moist skin Poor skin turgor
b. C_7, T_1	Straight spine, nontender	Crepitation Curved spine Scoliosis, kyphosis
c. Scapulae and surrounding musculature	Symmetrical location with developed musculature	Unequal musculature development
d. Chest wall	Stable ribs, nontender	Unstable chest wall Masses Tenderness Subcutaneous emphysema
3. Use palmar surface of one hand to assess vocal fremitus: examiner should place hand over equal positions of right and left lung fields and instruct client to repeat "one, two, three" or "how now brown cow" (Fig. 8-6); technique should be continued down posterior and posterolateral chest wall, comparing response of one side to other; do not test over bone areas	Varies from person to person due to intensity and pitch of voice Bilaterally equal mild vibratory sensation Most intense area to feel vibration is upper posterior chest wall medial to scapulae	*Increased fremitus* or increased vibratory sensation as seen in pneumonia or consolidation of lung *Decreased fremitus* or decreased vibratory sensation seen when there is decreased production of sound (air blockage) or increase in space vibration must pass before it reaches skin surface; example is chronic obstructive pulmonary disease *Unequal fremitus*

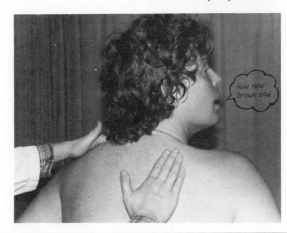

Fig. 8-6. Palpating for fremitus.

Continued.

Clinical guidelines—cont'd

The student will:	To identify:	
	Normal	**Deviations from normal**
4. Palpate lateral chest wall excursion during deep respirations: examiner should place hands on lower posterior chest wall at about tenth rib level; examiner's thumbs should almost touch at spinal process; fingertips should wrap laterally around ribs (Fig. 8-7); instruct client to take several deep breaths; evaluate outward expansion	Bilaterally equal expansion of ribs during deep inspiration; thumbs move equally away from spine Nonpainful breathing No coughing	Unequal excursion or pain with deep inspiration

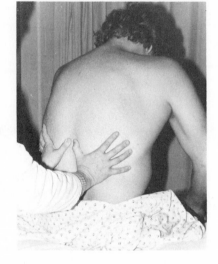

Fig. 8-7. Hand position for measuring respiratory excursion.

The student will:	Normal	Deviations from normal
5. Percuss posterior chest: instruct client to sit and pull shoulders forward by crossing arms; this technique will spread scapulae and permits more lung area for evaluation (Fig. 8-8) (See clinical strategies for percussion techniques.)	*Resonance* throughout lung fields Intensity: loud Pitch: low Duration: long Quality: hollow (Fig. 8-9)	*Hyperresonance* found over emphysematous lung Intensity: very loud Pitch: very low Duration: longer Quality: booming

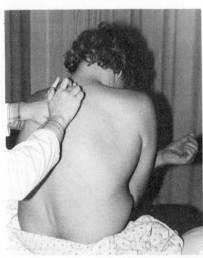

Fig. 8-8. Posture of posterior chest for percussion.

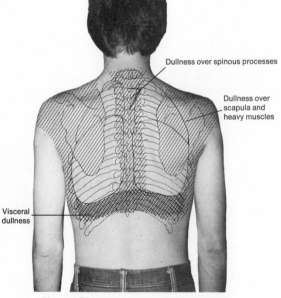

Dullness over spinous processes

Dullness over scapula and heavy muscles

Visceral dullness

Fig. 8-9. Percussion tones of the posterior chest.

The student will:	To identify:	
	Normal	**Deviations from normal**
	Flat sound over bone or heavy muscle such as shoulder or scapula, spinal processes Intensity: soft Pitch: high Duration: short Quality: extreme dullness *Dull sound* over viscera and liver border Intensity: medium Pitch: medium high Duration: medium Quality: thudlike *Tympany sound* over stomach and gas bubble in intestine Intensity: loud Pitch: high Duration: medium Quality: drumlike	*Dullness* over lung field occurs when fluid or solid tissue replaces normal lung tissue or fluid in pleural space
6. Percuss down posterior chest, comparing one side to other; avoid percussing over bone surface (Fig. 8-10) 　**a.** During percussion listen and feel for intensity, pitch, duration, and quality of each percussed sound		

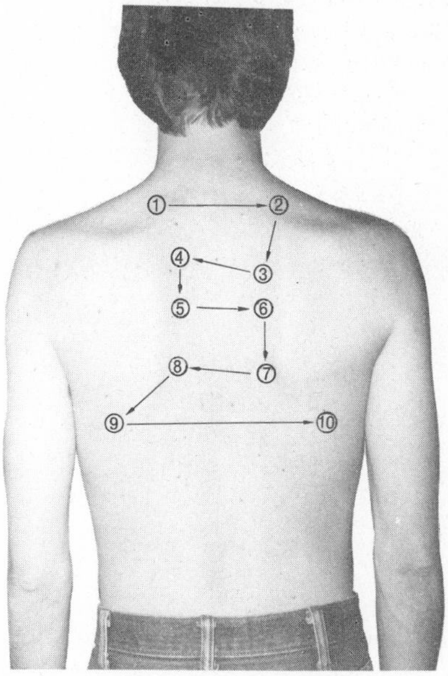

Fig. 8-10. Sequence for the systematic percussion of the posterior thorax.

The student will:	Normal	Deviations from normal
7. Percuss diaphragmatic excursion of posterior lungs; client sits upright and breathes several times, then takes deep breath and holds it 　**a.** At this time percuss down posterior chest, starting at apex of scapulae 　**b.** Percussion continues downward until tone changes; mark that point with marker; then instruct client to breathe several times, exhale completely, and hold breath 　**c.** Again, percuss down line of apex of scapulae until tone changes; mark that point with marker 　**d.** Instruct client to breathe again	Resonance should be heard first; this tone becomes *dull* at bottom of lungs Indicates level of diaphragm Should occur around tenth rib Higher diaphragm level may be present in pregnant women; may also have slightly narrower excursion volume	Unusually high level may accompany pleural effusion or atelectasis
8. Repeat procedure on other side of posterior chest	Equal response on both sides	Unequal responses

Continued.

Clinical guidelines–cont'd

	To identify:	
The student will:	**Normal**	**Deviations from normal**
9. With ruler, measure and record distance between two lines (Fig. 8-11) (The purpose of this technique is to determine client's lung expansion capabilities.)	4 to 6 cm (1½ to 2½ inches) downward excursion	Less than 4 cm (1½ inches) downward excursion

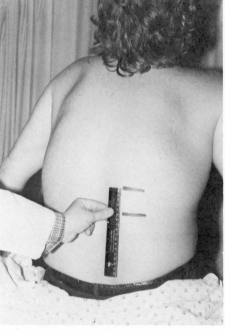

Fig. 8-11. Measurement of respiratory excursion.

Auscultation of posterior chest

1. Auscultate posterior chest from apex to base; client should be seated; diaphragm of stethoscope should be used for breath sound auscultation (Fig. 8-12)

Vesicular breath sounds heard over almost all of posterior lung fields

Low pitch, soft expirations

Bronchial breath sounds over peripheral lung

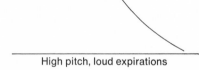

High pitch, loud expirations

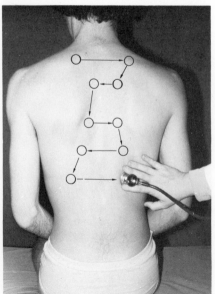

Fig. 8-12. Auscultatory pattern of posterior thorax with the stethoscope.

The student will:	To identify:	
	Normal	**Deviations from normal**

2. Instruct client to take slow, deep breaths in and out of mouth during auscultation; demonstrate breathing style for client

3. Slowly move stethoscope from one spot to next; compare sounds of one side of posterior chest to other; make sure to remain in one spot long enough to clearly analyze both inspiratory and expiratory sounds. (Fig. 8-13)

Bronchovesicular breath sounds over right upper posterior lung field

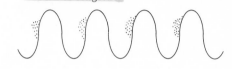

Medium pitch, medium expirations

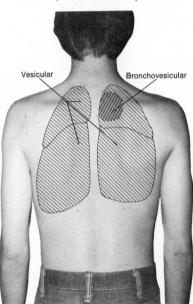

Fig. 8-13. Auscultatory sounds of the posterior chest.

Bronchovesicular breath sounds over peripheral lung

Adventitious sounds, including rales and fine rales, high-pitched crackling sound, heard toward end of inspiration; indicates inflammation or congestion

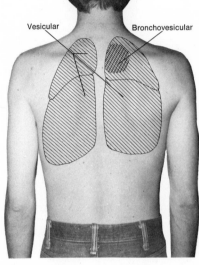

a. If abnormal sound heard, instruct client to cough, then reexamine to evaluate if adventitious sound has changed or disappeared

Medium rales: lower, more moist sound, heard about halfway through inspiration
Found in clients with pneumonia or pulmonary edema (not cleared by cough)

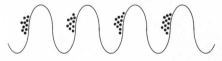

Coarse rales: loud, bubbly noise, heard during inspiration
Found in clients with pneumonia (not cleared by coughing)

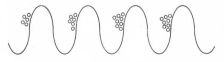

Rhonchi: small airway noise
Sibilant rhonchi (wheeze): musical noise like squeak
May occur during inspiration or expiration, but usually louder during expiration

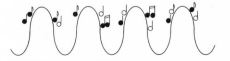

Continued.

Clinical guidelines–cont'd

The student will:	To identify:	
	Normal	**Deviations from normal**
		Sonorous rhonchi (wheeze): low, loud, coarse sound like snore; may occur at any point of inspiration or expiration; usually means obstruction of trachea or large bronchi (coughing may clear sound)
		Pleural friction rub: dry, rubbing or grating sound usually due to inflammation of pleural surfaces; heard throughout inspiration and expiration; loudest over lower anterior lateral surface
4. Evaluate vocal resonance of spoken voice if any abnormalities in tactile fremitus; use one of following techniques:		
a. Bronchophony: use stethoscope (diaphragm) to listen throughout posterior chest as client says "ninety-nine"	Muffled response: "nin-nin"	Sound increased in loudness and clarity: "ninety-nine" Found in consolidation or compression of lung
b. Whispered pectoriloquy: client instructed to whisper "one, two, three"; use stethoscope to listen throughout posterior chest	Muffled sounds: "one, two, three"	Clarity and loudness of sounds: "one, two, three" Found in consolidation or compression of lung
c. Egophony: use stethoscope to listen to posterior chest; ask client to say "e-e-e"	Muffled sound: "e-e-e"	Change in intensity and pitch of sound: "a-a-a" Due to consolidation

Palpation of anterior chest

The student will:	Normal	Deviations from normal
1. Move anterior to client to evaluate anterior thorax and lungs		
2. Use one or two hands to palpate skin and thorax of anterior chest		
3. Evaluate:		
a. Skin texture and temperature, manubrium, suprasternal notch, sternal angle, second rib, body of sternum, costochondral junctions, costal angle, ribs, and chest wall stability	Smooth, warm skin Stable, nontender chest wall and landmarks Well-developed musculature	Dry or moist skin Poor skin turgor Crepitation Thorax deformities Pectus excavatum (funnel chest) characterized by depression deformity of lower sternum May impair breathing or cause compression of heart Pectus carinatum (pigeon chest) characterized by outward deformity of sternum Increase in AP diameter Unequal muscle development, unstable chest wall, masses, tenderness
b. Tracheal position	Midline	Lateral tracheal deviation

The student will:	To identify:	
	Normal	**Deviations from normal**
4. Use palmar surface of one hand to assess vocal fremitus; examiner should place hand over equal positions of both lung fields of superior anterior chest and the anterolateral chest wall (Avoid areas with heavy breast tissue.)	Varies from person to person due to intensity and pitch of voice Bilaterally equal Mild vibratory sensation Most intense area of vibratory sensation should be upper medial chest area, lateral to sternum	Increased fremitus Decreased fremitus Unequal fremitus
5. Instruct client to repeat "one, two, three" or "how now brown cow"		
Percussion of anterior chest		
1. Instruct client to pull shoulders backward and to sit straight while anterior chest is percussed		
2. Percuss downward, comparing one side to other; avoid percussion over breast tissue or bony surface (Fig. 8-14) (If the examiner has difficulty percussing anterior chest while client is sitting, defer this part of examination until client is lying down.)	Resonance throughout lung fields Flat sounds over sternum or heavy breast tissue Dull sounds over heart or liver Tympany over stomach (Fig. 8-15)	Hyperresonance Dullness over lung field

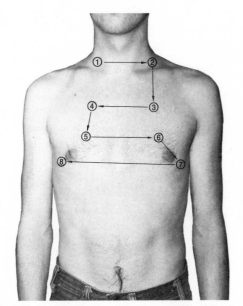

Fig. 8-14. Sequence for the systematic percussion of the thorax.

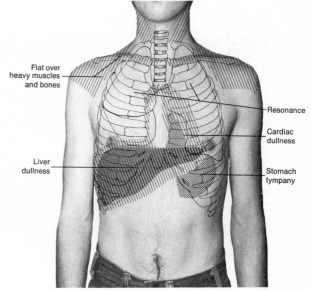

Flat over heavy muscles and bones

Resonance

Cardiac dullness

Liver dullness

Stomach tympany

Fig. 8-15. Percussion tones of the anterior chest.

Auscultation of anterior chest

1. Auscultate anterior chest from apex to base; client may be sitting or lying; use same techniques as for posterior thorax auscultation	Vesicular breath sounds over anterior peripheral lung fields Bronchial breath sounds over trachea	Bronchial breath sounds over peripheral lung fields Bronchovesicular breath sounds over peripheral lung fields

Continued.

Clinical guidelines—cont'd

The student will:	To identify:	
	Normal	**Deviations from normal**
	Bronchovesicular breath sounds over large bronchioles (Fig. 8-16)	Adventitious sounds, including rales (fine, medium, coarse), rhonchi (sonorous, sibilant), and pleural friction rub

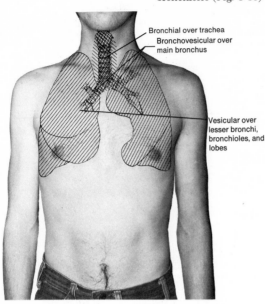

Bronchial over trachea
Bronchovesicular over main bronchus
Vesicular over lesser bronchi, bronchioles, and lobes

Fig. 8-16. Auscultatory sounds of the anterior chest.

2. Evaluate anterior chest resonance of spoken voice if any abnormalities in tactile fremitus; use same techniques as for posterior chest

    a. Bronchophony: instruct client to say "ninety-nine"; evaluate with stethoscope — Muffled response: "nin-nin" — Sound increased in loudness and clarity: "ninety-nine"

    b. Whispered pectoriloquy: instruct client to whisper "one, two, three"; evaluate with stethoscope — Muffled response: "one, two, three" — Clarity and loudness of sounds: "one, two, three"

    c. Egophony: instruct client to say "e-e-e" — Muffled response: "e-e-e" — Change in intensity and pitch of sounds: "a-a-a"

Evaluation of lateral thorax and lungs

1. Instruct client to abduct arm overhead so that lateral chest may be percussed and auscultated (Fig. 8-17)

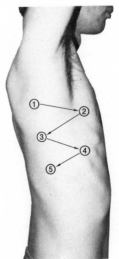

Fig. 8-17. Lateral percussion and auscultation position.

The student will:	To identify:	
	Normal	Deviations from normal
2. Percuss down each lateral thorax	Resonance over lung area Dull sound as percussion reaches liver (on right) and spleen (on left)	Hyperresonance or dullness over lung fields
3. Auscultate down each lateral thorax	Vesicular breath sounds	Bronchovesicular or bronchial breath sounds No breath sounds

Clinical strategies

1. For evaluation of the thorax and lungs, the client must be undressed. This means bra or undershirt off. When inspecting overall respiratory response, the individual should be sitting with the gown dropped to the waist.

2. During inspection first stand back and observe the client. It has been stated that once the examiner touches the client, the client's observable details are no longer seen. This is an essential concept and deserves foremost consideration. During observation carefully analyze the client's posture, breathing difficulties, breathing style, audible sounds, and any other factors that reflect the client's breathing attempts. For example, a client with breathing difficulties may lean forward to breathe (Fig. 8-18).

3. Although inspection of the front and back is done together, the other assessment techniques—palpation, percussion, and auscultation—are first done in the back and then in the front (or reverse, if you prefer).

4. When palpating, use both hands simultaneously: one hand on the right chest wall and the other on the left chest wall. The purpose is to check symmetry, comparing the findings on one side with findings on the other.

5. Any abnormalities identified must be described and defined by intercostal space and distance from sternum, spine, axillary lines, etc.

6. The techniques of percussion are the same whether one is percussing the thorax, the heart, the liver, or the abdomen. The tones elicited in those areas are different. As the beginning examiner learns the technique of percussion, it will require considerable practice until the five tones (resonance, hyperresonance, dullness, flatness, and tympany) are easily recognized. Only after the examiner has memorized the tones and their normal location is there hope of identifying abnor-

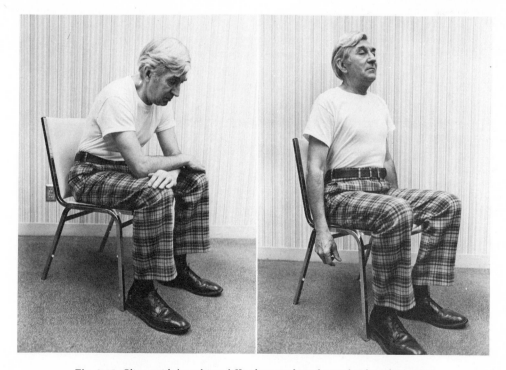

Fig. 8-18. Client with breathing difficulty may lean forward to breathe easier.

mal findings. Following is a description of current percussion techniques:

a. Place left hand flat on posterior chest wall and slightly spread fingers. The distal phalanx of the middle (pleximeter) finger should be firmly pressed on the chest wall. The other fingers should very gently rest on the thorax.

b. The middle finger of the right hand becomes the hammer (plexor), which taps the interphalangeal joint of the pleximeter.

c. The success of the technique of percussion depends on several elements, including the following (Fig. 8-19):

   (1) The downward snap of the plexor *must* be sharp and rapid.

   (2) The downward snap of the plexor *must* be a wrist action and *not* a forearm or shoulder motion.

   (3) The *tip* of the plexor finger *must* be used, not the finger pad.

   (4) Once the plexor has struck the pleximeter, quickly remove the plexor (this ensures pure quality of tone).

   (5) One location should be tapped several times to ensure clear interpretation of the tone elicited.

   (6) *Short* fingernails are essential. Otherwise the examiner is more likely to use the finger pad of the plexor and not the fingertip.

   (7) Loudness of the tone does not ensure good quality. The examiner should practice the percussion techniques until a light percussion tapping elicits an appropriate tone.

7. When percussing the back, it is helpful to have the client sit with the shoulder drooping slightly forward. This pulls the scapulae laterally and allows increased access to the lung field.

8. When percussing the anterior chest wall, have the client sit with the shoulders pulled back. For women with large breasts, percuss anterosuperior lung fields with the client sitting, then have her recline to a 45° angle with hands up and behind the head. This positioning allows percussion access to the inferoanterior lung fields (Fig. 8-20).

9. When percussing for excursion on the posterior chest wall, it is helpful for the examiner as well as the client to hold their breath.

10. Auscultation requires the use of a stethoscope. Because there are many different types of stethoscopes, the ability to accurately assess auscultatory sounds depends partially on the quality of the instrument. Following are characteristics of quality stethoscopes and auscultatory techniques:

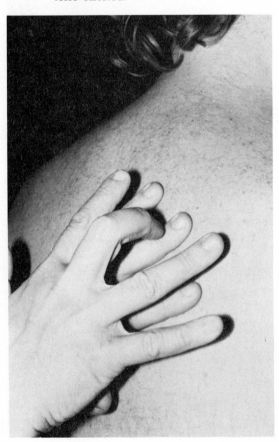

Fig. 8-19. Percussion technique.

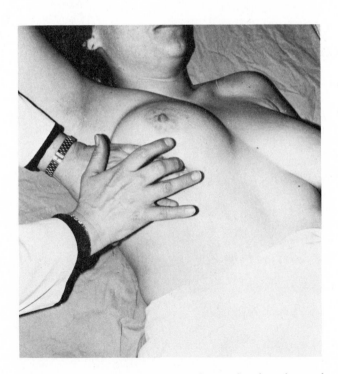

Fig. 8-20. Anterior thorax percussion technique for a large-breasted woman.

a. Characteristics of quality stethoscopes:
   (1) Use a diaphragm that will pick up high-pitched (breath) sounds and a bell that will pick up low-pitched sounds (heart murmurs).
   (2) The diaphragm and bell should have enough weight to lay firmly on the chest wall when placed there.
   (3) The diaphragm should be covered with a factory manufactured diaphragm cover, not a piece of x-ray film.
   (4) The bell should have a small rubber or plastic ring around its tip to ensure a secure fit against the chest wall.
   (5) The tubing may be in one or two pieces. The human ear is unable to detect sound difference between one-tubing and two-tubing stethoscopes. Thick, stiff, and heavy tubing conducts sound better than thin, elastic, or very flexible tubing. Do not use hospital tubing.
   (6) The length of the stethoscope tubing should be between 30.5 and 46 cm (12 and 18 inches).
   (7) Earpieces can make the difference between hearing or not hearing a sound. The examiner should choose the largest earpieces that will snugly fit into the ears. The ability of the earpieces to occlude outside noise is the important consideration.

b. Auscultory techniques:
   (1) The earpieces should point toward the examiner's nose to snugly fit in the auditory canal.
   (2) The examiner should try not to touch or allow the tubing to touch rubbing surfaces during auscultation. This will cause extra noise.
   (3) The examiner should hold the head of the stethoscope between the index and middle fingers to stabilize it during auscultation (Fig. 8-21).
   (4) When using the diaphragm, exert firm pressure to ensure solid contact with the chest wall.
   (5) When using the bell, care must be taken not to flatten the underlying skin by pressing the bell too firmly. The bell must be lightly and evenly placed on the skin. There must be total skin contact around the bell edge. The bell functions by picking up vibratory sensations of the surface tissue in response to the visceral vibrations. If the tissue is stretched too much by firm pressure, vibrations are inhibited and the bell actually converts to a diaphragm.

11. Prior to auscultating the breath sounds, it is appropriate to give instruction on how to breathe. The client should breathe deeply and slowly through the mouth. Stand in front and demonstrate. Nasal breathing is not encouraged because nasal turbulence interferes with clear auscultation of the thorax.

12. When auscultating the posterior chest, again have client sit with the shoulders drooping slightly forward. When listening for breath sounds, move from apices to bases. Compare one side with the other as you move down the posterior wall. Avoid auscultation over bone. Be sure to listen to each spot for at least two inspirations and expirations. This will ensure a clearer interpretation of the sound heard.

13. When auscultating the anterior chest, the client should be sitting straight. Auscultation is begun above the clavicle and should again move down the chest wall while you are comparing one side with the other. For large-breasted women the breasts can be displaced upward and laterally for access to the lower anterior lung fields.

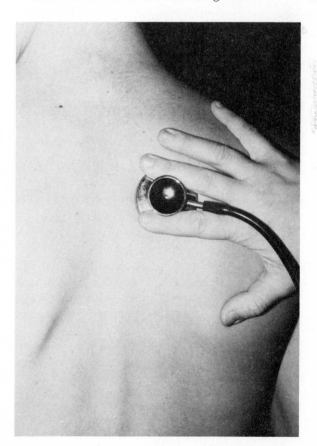

Fig. 8-21. Proper technique for holding the stethoscope.

14. When auscultating the chest, evaluate quality of breath sound, compare inspiration length with expiration length, and listen for any abnormalities. Describe what you hear.
15. If you hear adventitious sounds on auscultation, instruct client to cough. See if they are cleared by a cough.
16. Do not forget to palpate, percuss, and auscultate the lateral chest walls. Compare one side with the other.

Sample recording

Respiration rate 14; regular rhythm without noted difficulty.
Diaphragmatic breathing.
Bilaterally equal excursion.
Client sitting erect, slight kyphosis noted.
Skin intact and warm; no bulging, retractions, tenderness, or asymmetry of chest wall noted.
Thorax oval; AP diameter < lateral diameter.
Tactile fremitus bilaterally equal.
Diaphragmatic excursion 4 cm (1½ inches) bilaterally.
Resonant percussion tone throughout.
Vesicular breath sounds bilaterally throughout.
Few fine basilar rales heard on right, which did not clear with cough.

History and clinical strategies associated with the pediatric client

1. Because many childhood illnesses frequently invade the respiratory system, the thorax and respiratory function of children deserve thorough evaluation.
2. The techniques of pediatric evaluation are the same as for the adult. The results of assessment will depend on cooperation from the child and the examiner's ability to gently assess the child.
3. Coughs and colds seem to accompany the growing child. History data should be gathered about the same elements as discussed for the adult client. An allergic history should also be gathered. If the child is less than 2 years of age and is beginning to eat new foods, the examiner should gather a thorough nutritional history as well.
4. Children with asthma or bronchitis histories should be questioned with regard to the overall progression of that condition. Data should be gathered regarding:
   a. Frequency and duration of the problem
   b. Current care techniques
   c. Precipitating factors
   d. Current medications
   e. Relationship of problem to activities and playing
   f. How does child view the problem?
   g. What does child think is possible in terms of self-help?
5. Any child presenting with a sudden onset of coughing or choking should be expected to have aspirated a foreign object until proved otherwise. The examiner should inquire about the child's playing activities prior to the current problem (e.g., was he playing with *toys* such as beads, a car with removable wheels, or pieces of a game that could have been put into his mouth). *Great* skill must be employed to gather the information needed without the child becoming frightened and answering "no" to every question asked.
   Food aspiration is another cause for sudden coughing or breathing problems. Common aspirated objects are peanuts, popcorn, carrot pieces, hot dogs, or peas. All these tend to block and not dissolve if accidently aspirated. Although it is difficult to determine, some parents may admit that they were force feeding a child prior to the coughing episode or that the child had food and was playing or running around the house prior to the coughing period.
6. The respiratory rate of children is obviously faster than that of the adult. Sometimes the parent may bring the child for evaluation because "he is breathing funny." If this occurs, the examiner must collect a detailed history including a thorough evaluation of the possibility of poisoning or ingestion of a toxic substance. Many times the presenting complaint of salicylate poisoning is a child with rapid, panting respirations.
7. For examination the child should be naked to the waist and sitting on the parent's lap or the examining table. Infants are laid on the examination table.
8. The child must be breathing quietly for breath sounds to be evaluated. As soon as the child is old enough to cooperate, he should be instructed to breathe deeply through his mouth. One technique to facilitate this is to instruct the child to take a deep breath and "blow out" the examiner's penlight while the examiner listens to the child's chest with the stethoscope in the other hand.
9. There has been much written about stridor and retraction evaluation in children. We want to stress that the emphasis of this text is the clinical assessment of "normal" for both children and adults. If the examiner identifies retractions, wheezing, stridor, or persistent coughing, the child should be referred to a physician for further evaluation.

Clinical variations associated with the pediatric client

Characteristic or area examined	Normal	Deviations from normal
1. Anterior and posterior chest		
a. Skin color, thorax, and lips	Pink, well oxygenated Babies' skin may become mottled if they are chilled	Cyanosis, pallor Spider nevi Dilated veins over lower thorax
b. Nail beds, nail configuration	Smooth Flat surface	Clubbing of nail and distal finger
c. General appearance	Relaxed posture	Apprehensive Tense forward posture Restless Nostrils flaring Supraclavicular retractions Intercostal retractions Use of accessory muscles during breathing
d. Chest wall configuration	Symmetrical Equal muscular development	
e. AP diameter of chest	Newborns have rounded chest wall configuration where AP diameter equals transverse diameter By age 6 years AP and lateral diameter ratio should reach toward adult normal of 1:2 or 5:7	Children with rounded rib cage after age 6 years (may be found in children with cystic fibrosis or asthma)
f. Chest wall configuration		
1. Anterior	Symmetrical Flat sternum 45° costal angle Harrison's groove may be normally found in some children: horizontal groove at level of diaphragm; with breathing there may be slight flaring below groove Bilaterally equal musculature Shoulders equal Clavicles equal	Pectus carinatum (pigeon breast) Pectus excavatum (funnel breast) Costal angle larger than 45° or 50° Harrison's groove, with marked flaring below groove, should be considered abnormal Asymmetry Asymmetry Asymmetry
2. Posterior	Straight spinal processes (C_7, T_1 through T_{12}) Symmetrical scapulae Downward and equal slope of ribs	Spinal curvature Scoliosis Kyphosis (humpback) Asymmetry
2. Breathing pattern	Abdominal and nasal breathing during infancy Gradual change until age 6 or 7 years; then girls become mostly thoracic breathers and boys become abdominal breathers Newborn may demonstrate Cheyne-Stokes breathing; this should normally disappear by age 4 weeks	Seesaw breathing where thorax and abdomen alternate during breathing Respiratory grunting Abnormal, irregular breathing pattern Cheyne-Stokes
3. Rate of respiration	Ratio of respirations to pulse 1:4 Newborn: 30 to 50 resp/min 6 months: 20 to 40 resp/min 1 year: 20 to 40 resp/min 3 years: 20 to 30 resp/min 6 years: 16 to 22 resp/min 10 years: 16 to 20 resp/min 17 years: 14 to 20 resp/min	Any respiration rates that fall short of or exceed stated normal rates
4. Depth of respirations (This is an important quality to evaluate in children.)	Respiratory depth guide to be used when child lying supine: examiner takes hand and holds it in front of child's nose; breathing normally felt at following distances*: *Child's age* *Depth of respiration* 1 month 2 inches	Breathing may become deeper and labored in cases of metabolic acidosis such as Kussmaul respirations Breathing becomes evident during metabolic alkalosis as body conserves carbon dioxide

*From Barness, L. A.: Manual of pediatric physical diagnosis, ed. 4. Copyright© 1972 by Year Book Medical Publishers, Inc., Chicago. Used by permission.

Continued.

Clinical variations associated with the pediatric client–cont'd

Characteristic or area examined	Normal	Deviations from normal
	Child's age *Depth of respiration* 3 months 3 inches 6 to 12 months 4 inches 2 years 6 inches 3 to 4 years 8 inches 5 to 6 years 9 inches 8 to 10 years 10 inches	Decreased depth could also be evidence of airway obstruction
5. Posterior chest palpation (May need to use one or two fingers instead of all fingers.) **a.** Skin	Smooth, warm	Dry or moist skin Poor skin turgor
b. Bone, muscle structure **c.** Chest wall stability	Symmetrical, straight spine, nontender Stable ribs, nontender	
6. Vocal fremitus: instruct child to speak as adult was instructed or evaluate when child is crying	Varies from person to person due to intensity and pitch of voice Bilaterally equal mild vibratory sensation Most intense area to feel vibration is upper posterior chest wall medial to scapulae	*Increased fremitus* or increased vibratory sensation as seen in pneumonia or consolidation of lung *Decreased fremitus* or decreased vibratory sensation when there is decreased production of sound (air blockage) or increase in space vibration must pass before it reaches skin surface
7. Lateral chest wall excursion	Bilaterally equal expansion of ribs during deep inspiration; thumbs move equally away from spine Nonpainful breathing No coughing	Unequal excursion or pain with deep inspiration
8. Posterior chest wall percussion: requires lighter pressure than adult technique **a.** "Direct" single finger tapping percussion may elicit clearer tone in very small child	More resonant than adult Some children may display hyperresonant tone Older children: *resonance* Flat sound over bone or heavy muscle Dull sound over viscera or liver	Hyperresonance in older child Dullness over lung field
9. Diaphragmatic excursion percussion: not routinely done in small child; when done in older child, use same technique as for adult	Resonance should be heard first; changes to a *dull* tone at bottom of lungs Indicates level of diaphragm Should occur around tenth rib Amount of downward excursion will depend on size of child	Unusually high level may be present in pleural effusion or atelectasis
10. Posterior chest auscultation: use either *small* diaphragm or *small* rubber-edged bell stethoscope; all edges of either must have "good" contact with child's chest wall; use same technique as for adult	Louder than adult *Bronchovesicular* breath sounds normally heard in infant and small child because of thin chest wall with poorly developed musculature Vesicular breath sounds like adult's as child grows older	Bronchial breath sounds Bronchovesicular breath sounds in older child (over age 6 or 7 years) Adventitious sounds such as fine rales, medium rales, coarse rales, sibilant rhonchi, sonorous rhonchi, and pleural friction rub
11. Vocal resonance: Not routinely evaluated in children; when evaluation is desired, use same technique as for adult		
12. Anterior chest palpation **a.** Skin	Smooth warm skin	Dry or moist skin Poor skin turgor Cold or hot skin Crepitation
b. Bone, muscle structure **c.** Chest wall stability	Stable, nontender chest wall and landmarks Well-developed musculature	Thorax deformities: pectus excavatum (funnel chest) characterized by depression deformity of lower sternum; may impair breathing or cause compression of heart Pectus carinatum (pigeon chest) characterized by outward deformity of sternum

Characteristic or area examined	Normal	Deviations from normal
d. Tracheal position	Midline	Lateral tracheal deviation
13. Vocal fremitus palpation	Varies from person to person due to intensity and pitch of voice	Increased fremitus
	Bilaterally equal	Decreased fremitus
	Mild vibratory sensation	
	Most intense area of vibratory sensation should be upper medial chest area, lateral to sternum	Unequal fremitus
14. Anterior chest percussion: may use direct or indirect palpation technique	More resonant than adult; some small children may demonstrate hyperresonant tone	Hyperresonance in older children or dullness over lung fields
	Dull sound over heart and liver; liver starts at approximately fifth interspace on right at midclavicular line	
	Tympany over stomach	
15. Anterior chest auscultation	Bronchovesicular breath sounds normally heard throughout peripheral lungs of smaller child	Bronchial breath sounds over periphreal lung
	Vesicular breath sounds throughout peripheral lungs of older child	Bronchovesicular over peripheral lung fields in older child
	Bronchial breath sounds heard over trachea	
	Bronchovesicular breath sounds heard over large bronchioles	Adventitious sounds such as fine, medium, and coarse rales, sibilant and sonorous rhonchi, and pleural friction rub
16. Vocal resonance of anterior chest (Not normally evaluated in children.); when evaluation desired, use same techniques as for adult		
17. Lateral thorax and lungs	Resonance over lung area	Hyperresonance or dullness over lung fields
	Dull sound as percussion reaches liver (on right) and spleen (on left)	
	Vesicular breath sounds	Bronchovesicular breath sounds
		No breath sounds

History and clinical strategies associated with the geriatric client

1. The examiner should not assume that aging is automatically accompanied by respiratory disease. The literature reports that physical changes occur with aging; however, the "normal," healthy elderly individual is usually free of chronic respiratory symptoms. Many of the changes that occur may not be clinically remarkable or may not alter or interfere with the clients' life-style. Following are some major changes that occur:
   a. Decrease in muscular strength of the chest wall muscles
   b. Possible stiffening and decreased expansion of chest wall (calcification at the rib articulation points may be involved)
   c. Decrease in elastic lung recoil (and increased lung distensibility); alveoli and bronchioles stretched (enlarged)
   d. Decrease in vital capacity and increase in residual capacity
   e. Underventilation of the alveoli in the lower lung fields
   As with all other changes, these alterations take place at different rates with different individuals. Physical conditioning and general physical health are two very important variables that affect the efficiency of respiratory function. Obese, sedentary, or immobilized individuals have less opportunity to maintain physical fitness and are more vulnerable to respiratory disability.

   In summary, it often takes more energy for the older individual to expand the chest wall to carry through the function of respiration. Many elderly clients do not experience dyspnea unless they exceed the ordinary mild to moderate exertion demands that they are accustomed to. Sudden intense activity can result in shortness of breath. Heavy or unusually demanding exercise can create problems. With aging changes a diminished functional reserve occurs, creating a higher vulnerability to respiratory distress or infection. Elderly people should be cautious about exposure to colds, flu, or other infections.

2. The symptoms of cough, dyspnea on exertion, and breathlessness have been covered in the adult section (pp. 170 to 171).

3. Chest pain may be diminished in an older client.

Pleuritic pain may not be reported or sensed as intensely as it would be in a younger person. If chest pain does exist, be certain to examine the client for fractured ribs (sustained from a fall or from coughing) as well as arthritic changes in the rib cage.

4. It is a good idea to inquire about the effects of weather on the client. Some people have an increase in respiratory infections in cold, damp weather.

5. Ask about the incidence of colds, flu, and whether the number and/or severity of the episodes has been increasing.

6. The incidence of chronic respiratory disease is higher among the elderly population. Chronic bronchitis, emphysema, lung cancer, and tuberculosis are four of the major health problems. (Pulmonary edema associated with heart disease is covered in Chapter 9.) In addition to cough, dyspnea on exertion, chest pain, and breathlessness, chronic health problems can include:

   a. History of smoking (see *adult history* section for specific questions)

   b. Periodic bouts of low-grade fever

   c. Night sweats

   d. Remarkable weight change in the last 6 months or year

   e. New problems with fatigue

   f. Any sensations in the chest other than pain (e.g., feeling of heaviness)

   g. Family history of any respiratory problems

   h. Daily activities altered or decreased because of problems with fatigue, shortness of breath, or discomfort

7. Risk factors for respiratory disability with elderly individuals include:

   a. History of smoking

   b. History of frequent respiratory infections

   c. Immobilization or marked sedentary habits

   d. History of chronic exposure to environmental pollutants

   e. Difficulty swallowing

   f. Indication of weakened chest muscles (e.g., general physical disability, inability to cough or breathe deeply)

   g. Family history of respiratory disability

8. *Note:* It may be difficult for some clients to breathe deeply or to hold breath on command during the physical assessment.

Clinical variations associated with the geriatric client

Characteristic or area examined	Normal	Deviations from normal
1. Anterior and posterior chest		
a. Skin color and lips and nail beds	Pink, well oxygenated Dark-skinned clients' mucous membranes and nail beds appear pink and well oxygenated	Cyanosis, pallor Spider nevi
b. Nail configuration	160° angle at nail bed	Clubbing (angle disappears)
c. General appearance	Relaxed posture (Note elderly client's general condition of physical fitness: muscle weakness associated with general physical disability or sedentary life-style may affect client's ability to use respiratory muscles and to expand the chest.)	Apprehensive Tense, forward posture Restless Nostrils flaring Supraclavicular retractions Intercostal retractions Use of accessory muscles during breathing (*Note:* Pursed-lip breathing—chiefly expiration—is compensatory pattern associated with chronic obstructive pulmonary disease.)
d. Chest wall configuration	Symmetrical landmarks Downward and equal slope of ribs Bilaterally equal muscular development (may be slightly more muscle development on client's dominant side) Subcutaneous fat often decreased, and bony prominences more marked Costal angle less than 90° (*Note:* Kyphosis [Fig. 8-22] is a fairly common problem with elderly clients. Dorsal scoliosis may exist, accompanied by tracheal deviation. Loss of normal spinal curvature in the dorsal and lumbar regions may occur with arthritis.)	Asymmetry of landmarks Horizontal ribs Costal angle greater than 90° (*Note:* Chronic marked stooping or bending forward may affect lung expansion in localized areas.)

Characteristic or area examined	Normal	Deviations from normal

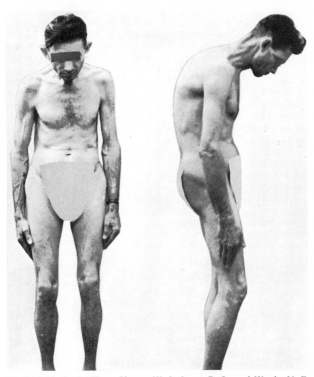

Fig. 8-22. Kyphosis. (From Phipps, W. J., Long, B. C., and Woods, N. F.: Medical-surgical nursing, St. Louis, 1979, The C. V. Mosby Co.)

Characteristic or area examined	Normal	Deviations from normal
e. Anteroposterior diameter of chest in relation to lateral diameter	1:2 to 5:7 ratio Kyphosis often accompanied by increased anteroposterior diameter	Barrel chest (Fig. 8-4)
2. Breathing pattern	Client able to close mouth and breathe through nose Diaphragmatic (male) Thoracic (female) Quiet, smooth, even breathing, relatively passive in nature During inspiration chest expands, costal angle increases, and diaphragm descends and flattens (*Note:* With elderly clients the vital capacity is reduced, and general chest expansion may be somewhat reduced. Calcification at rib articulation points may contribute to decreased chest expansion. These alterations may not be clinically evident.)	Mouth breathing Noisy breathing Breathing appears labored or painful; accompanied by grunting noises; inspiration interrupted by pain Irregular breathing patterns such as Cheyne-Stokes: periods of deep, rapid breaths alternating with periods of apnea Obstructive breathing pattern: expiration period prolonged and labored; may alternate with periods of shallow breathing
3. Rate of respiration	12 to 20 respirations per minute (*Note:* Anxiety or exertion will increase rate.)	Hyperpnea: increase in rate and depth Tachypnea: increased and relatively shallow respirations Bradypnea: decrease in rate Many heavy sighing respirations may exist in depressed or disturbed emotional states (*Note:* Some elderly clients with a chronic respiratory disturbance may present a general discoordinated breathing pattern: varying in rate, depth, and chest expansion. The exertion of moving from chair to

Continued.

Clinical variations associated with the geriatric client—cont'd

Characteristic or area examined	Normal	Deviations from normal
		examining table, of undressing, or sitting up from a lying position may disrupt a breathing pattern. Monitor the client's response to mild exertion.)
4. Posterior chest palpation		
a. General surface characteristics	Skin feels warm, smooth (*Note:* Elderly clients chill easily in a cool environment.)	Excessively dry or moist skin Poor skin turgor Cold or hot skin Crepitation
b. C_7 and T_1 spinal processes	May be quite prominent Kyphosis may be present Spine straight, nontender	Curved spine, tender on palpation
c. Scapulae and surrounding musculature	Symmetrical location	Asymmetry Asymmetrical muscle atrophy
d. General chest wall	Stable ribs, nontender	Tenderness Masses Crepitation
5. Respiratory excursion	Bilaterally equal expansion of ribs during inspiration (thumbs move equally away from the spine) (*Note:* Elderly client may have some difficulty breathing as deeply as a younger individual.)	Unequal excursion
6. Vocal fremitus response	Response varies among individuals due to intensity and pitch of voice Bilaterally equal mild vibratory sensation Most intense vibrations at upper posterior chest wall medial to scapulae	Increased fremitus: increased vibratory sense accompanies consolidaton of lung or portion of lung Decreased fremitus: occurs with decreased production of sound (air blockage) or increase in air space or muscle/tissue space between client's lung and examiner's hands (e.g., emphysema)
7. Entire posterior chest percussion	Resonance throughout lung fields	Hyperresonance found over emphysematous lung
a. Intensity	Moderately loud	Very loud
b. Pitch	Low	Very low pitch
c. Duration	Long	Longer
d. Quality	Hollow (*Note:* Some elderly clients manifest an increased distensibility of lungs and may respond with normal hyperresonance on percussion. However, all beginning examiners should refer hyperresonant responses to a physician.)	Booming Dullness over lung: occurs when fluid or solid tissue replaces normal lung tissue; or fluid in the pleural space
8. Diaphragmatic excursion percussion	Diaphragmatic dullness to percussion usually occurs at about tenth rib; level may be slightly higher on right Downward excursion (bilateral) should measure approximately 3 to 5 cm (1 to 2 inches), depending on size, age, and general physical condition of client	Asymmetrical response Diaphragm lower than usual in severe emphysema Diaphragm higher than usual if there is increase (of any form) of intraabdominal pressure Severe limited excursion of diaphragm
9. Posterior chest auscultation (*Note:* Elderly client may have difficulty breathing deeply and holding breath on command.)	Vesicular breath sounds heard over almost all of posterior lung fields Bronchovesicular breath sounds over right upper posterior lung field	Bronchial breath sounds over peripheral lung Bronchovesicular breath sounds over peripheral lung Adventitious sounds, including: Rales: discrete noncontinuous sounds produced by secretions in tracheobronchial tree, usually heard in inspiration Fine rales: high-pitched crackling noise heard toward end of inspiration; sound originates in alveoli Medium: lower, more moist sound, occurring earlier in inspiration and originating in

Characteristic or area examined	Normal	Deviations from normal
		bronchioles and small bronchi
		Coarse: loud, bubbling sound occurring in larger air passages, can sometimes be cleared with cough
		Rhonchi (wheezes): continuous sounds produced in narrowed air passages may be more prominent on expiration
		Sibilant: high-pitched musical sound occurring on inspiration or expiration, originating in smaller air passages
		Sonorous: low, loud, coarse sound originating in trachea or large bronchi; coughing may alter sound
		Pleural friction rub: dry, rubbing or grating sound usually due to inflammation of pleural surfaces
10. Vocal resonance bronchophony: client instructed to say "ninety-nine"	Auscultation sounds muffled: "nin-nin"	Sound increased in loudness and clarity: "ninety-nine"
11. Anterior chest palpation:		

a. Skin texture and temperature, manubrium, suprasternal notch, sternal angle, second rib, body of sternum, costochondral junctions, costal angle, ribs, and chest wall stability	Smooth, warm skin
	Stable, nontender chest wall and landmarks
	Symmetrical musculature
	Decreased subcutaneous fat
		Dry or moist skin
		Poor skin turgor
		Cold or hot skin
		Crepitation
		Thorax deformities:
		  Pectus excavatum (funnel chest): characterized by depression deformity of lower sternum; may impair breathing or cause compression of heart
		  Pectus carinatum (pigeon chest): characterized by outward deformity of sternum; increase in AP diameter
		Unequal muscle development, unstable chest wall, masses
		Tenderness on palpation (fairly common with arthritic clients at rib articulation points)

b. Tracheal position	Midline (position may be altered in scoliosis)	Lateral tracheal deviation
12. Vocal fremitus response	Varies from person to person due to intensity and pitch of voice Bilaterally equal mild vibratory sensation Most intense area of vibratory sensation upper medial chest area, lateral to sternum	Increased fremitus Decreased fremitus Unequal fremitus
13. Anterior chest percussion	Resonance throughout lung fields Flat sounds over sternum or heavy breast tissue Dull sounds over heart or liver Tympany over stomach	Hyperresonance Dullness over lung field
14. Anterior chest auscultation	Vesicular breath sounds over anterior peripheral lung fields Bronchial breath sounds over trachea Bronchovesicular breath sounds over large bronchioles	Bronchial breath sounds over peripheral lung fields Bronchovesicular breath sounds over peripheral lung fields Adventitious sounds such as rales (fine, medium, coarse), rhonchi (sonorous, sibilant), and pleural friction rub
15. Anterior chest vocal resonance		
a. Bronchophony	Muffled response: "nin-nin"	Sound increased in loudness and clarity: "ninety-nine"
16. Lateral thorax percussion	Resonance over lung area Dull sound as percussion reaches liver (on right) and spleen (on left)	Hyperresonance or dullness over lung fields
17. Lateral thorax auscultation	Vesicular breath sounds	Bronchovesicular breath sounds No breath sounds

Vocabulary

1. Adventitious sounds

2. Angle of Louis

3. Asthma

4. Biot breathing

   shallow breathing ⇄ apnea

5. Bradypnea

6. Bronchial breathing

7. Bronchitis

8. Bronchovesicular breathing

9. Consolidation

10. Costal angle

11. Cyanosis

12. Dyspnea

13. Egophony

14. Emphysema

15. Excursion

16. Fremitus

17. Friction rub

18. Hemoptysis

19. Hyperpnea

20. Hyperresonance

    emphysema

21. Increased fremitus

    consolidation

22. Kussmaul respirations

    deep & rapid

23. Kyphosis - *hunchback*
    ↑ convexity of thoracic spine

24. Manubrium

25. Orthopnea

26. Pectus carinatum

27. Pectus excavatum

28. Pleximeter

29. Rale

30. Rhonchi

31. Scoliosis
    lateral curve of spine

32. Singultus
    hiccup

33. Sternal angle

34. Stridor
    shrill, harsh - laryngeal obstruction

35. Tactile fremitus

36. Tympany

37. Vesicular breathing

38. Whispered pectoriloquy

Cognitive self-assessment

Mark each statement "T" or "F."

1. __F__ The right lung comprises two lobes, and the left lung comprises three lobes.
2. __T__ During inspiration the diaphragm descends and flattens.
3. __T__ Biot breathing may be seen in healthy persons.
4. __F__ The ratio of respiratory rate to pulse rate normally is 1:6. *1:4*
5. __F__ The nipple line is the common landmark for identifying the midclavicular line for all patients, with the exception of large-breasted women.
6. __F__ In palpating for rib identification, the initial rib felt below the clavicle is the first rib.
7. Complete the following table.

Comparison of duration
inspiration vs. expiration

Breath sounds	*(use < and >)*	*Sample location*
Vesicular	Inspiration __>__ expiration	lung fields
Bronchovesicular	Inspiration __=__ expiration	over branchus
Bronchial	Inspiration __<__ expiration	trachea

8. The trachea bifurcates at about the level of the:
   - ☐ a. cricoid cartilage
   - ☐ b. manubrium
   - ☐ c. costal angle
   - ☑ d. sternal angle
   - ☐ e. sternum

9. Tactile fremitus will be *decreased* with:
   - ☐ a. pneumonia (consolidation of lung)
   - ☑ b. chronic obstructive diseases
   - ☑ c. area of atelectasis
   - ☑ d. pneumothorax
   - ☑ e. large airway obstruction
   - ☐ f. all the above
   - ☐ g. all except e
   - ☐ h. a, c, and d
   - ☐ i. all except b
   - ☑ j. all except a

10. The best place to feel for tactile fremitus is:
    - ☐ a. the lower lateral chest wall
    - ☐ b. high in the axillary lateral chest wall
    - ☐ c. the posterior lower chest wall
    - ☐ d. over the scapulae—posterior chest wall
    - ☑ e. over the anterior chest, second or third ribs near the sternum

11. When percussing the posterior chest for inspiratory-expiratory excursion, one would expect to *normally* measure which of the following excursion distances?
    - ☐ a. Over 6 cm (2½ inches)
    - ☑ b. 4 to 6 cm (1½ to 2½ inches)
    - ☐ c. 3 to 5 cm (1 to 2 inches)
    - ☐ d. 2 to 4 cm (¾ inch to 1½ inches)
    - ☐ e. Below 3 cm (1 inch)

12. A client with increased density of the lung due to pneumonia would be expected to have which of the following lung percussion tones?
    - ☐ a. Resonance
    - ☑ b. Hyperresonance
    - ☐ c. Tympany
    - ☑ d. Dullness
    - ☐ e. Flatness

13. Bronchial breath sounds are normal when heard:
    - ☐ a. over the posterior lateral chest at the level of the scapulae
    - ☐ b. between the scapulae
    - ☑ c. over the trachea
    - ☐ d. in the anterior chest upper lateral areas
    - ☐ e. nowhere throughout the chest

14. A wheeze during expiration is most likely:
    - ☑ a. sibilant rhonchi
    - ☐ b. sonorous rhonchi
    - ☐ c. pleural friction rub

☐ d. fine rales

☐ e. medium rales

15. A high-pitched crackling noise heard toward the end of inspiration is most likely:

☐ a. sibilant rhonchi

☐ b. sonorous rhonchi

☐ c. pleural friction rub

☑ d. fine rales

☐ e. medium rales

PEDIATRIC QUESTIONS

16. The *normal* newborn may demonstrate which of the following breathing patterns?

☑ a. Cheyne-Stokes

☑ b. Biot

☐ c. Kussmaul respirations

☐ d. Stertorous respirations

☐ e. Tachypnea

☐ f. b and d

☑ g. a and b

☐ h. a, c, and d

☐ i. all except e

☐ j. all the above

17. When examining a 6-month-old child, the nurse must evaluate respiratory rate and depth as well as breath sound and percussion quality. Which of the following would indicate a *normal* response?

	Respiration rate	Expiratory distance	Breath sound	Percussion tone
☐ a.	52	3 inches	Vesicular	Hyperresonant
☐ b.	18	2 inches	Bronchovesicular	Resonant
☐ c.	22	5 inches	Vesicular	Hyperresonant
☑ d.	32	4 inches	Bronchovesicular	Hyperresonant
☐ e.	36	6 inches	Bronchovesicular	Resonant

18. When evaluating the vocal fremitus in a small child, which of the following client participation sounds would be most helpful?

☑ a. Crying

☐ b. No noise

☐ c. Babbling

☐ d. Whispering

19. *One* of the following examples demonstrates an abnormal finding requiring physician referral. Identify the child needing referral.

☐ a. Twelve-year-old boy, respiration rate 18/min, vesicular breath sounds over periphery of lungs, resonant percussion tones over lung fields

☐ b. Nine-year-old girl, thoracic breathing, respiration rate 18/min, vesicular breath sounds over periphery of lungs, resonant percussion tones over lung fields

☐ c. Six-month-old girl, abdominal breathing, respiration rate 36/min, bronchovesicular breath sounds, hyperresonant percussion tone

☐ d. One-year-old boy, abdominal breathing, respiration rate 20/min, bronchovesicular breath sounds throughout lung fields, resonant percussion tones

☑ e. Two-year-old girl, abdominal breathing, respiration rate 44/min, bronchovesicular breath sounds through lung fields, hyperresonant percussion tones

GERIATRIC QUESTIONS

20. The aging process of the lungs usually involves:
    - ☐ a. decreased residual volume
    - ☑ b. decreased vital capacity
    - ☑ c. decreased chest wall compliance
    - ☑ d. decreased force of elastic recoil of the lungs
    - ☐ e. decreased anteroposterior chest diameter
    - ☐ f. all the above
    - ☐ g. a, c, and e
    - ☐ h. a and d
    - ☑ i. b, c, and d
    - ☐ j. none of the above

21. Some of the risk factors for respiratory disability in elderly people include:
    - ☑ a. smoking
    - ☐ b. difficulty swallowing
    - ☑ c. history of frequent respiratory infections
    - ☑ d. immobility
    - ☑ e. decreased physical fitness
    - ☑ f. all the above
    - ☐ g. all except b
    - ☐ h. a, c, and e
    - ☐ i. a and d

22. An 80-year-old individual gets _____ as much oxygen into his cardiovascular system as a 20-year-old.
    - ☐ a. twice
    - ☐ b. half
    - ☑ c. one third
    - ☐ d. just

SUGGESTED READINGS
General

Barber, Janet M., Stokes, Lillian G., and Billings, Diane M.: Adult and child care: a client approach to nursing, ed. 2, St. Louis, 1977, The C. V. Mosby Co., pp. 765-774.

Bates, Barbara: A guide to physical examination, ed. 2, Philadelphia, 1979, J. B. Lippincott Co., pp. 112-138.

DeGowin, Elmer, and DeGowin, Richard: Bedside diagnostic examination, ed. 3, New York, 1976, Macmillan Publishing Co., pp. 259-322.

Judge, Richard D., and Zuidema, George, editors: Methods of clinical examination: a physiologic approach, Boston, 1974, Little, Brown and Co., pp. 105-140.

Littman, David: Stethoscopes and auscultation, Am. J. Nurs. **72**(7): 1238-1241, (July, 1972).

Malasanos, Lois, Barkauskas, Violet, Moss, Muriel, and Stoltenberg-Allen, Kathryn: Health assessment, St. Louis, 1977, The C. V. Mosby Co., pp. 195-215.

Nordmark, Madelyn T., and Rohweder, Ann W.: Scientific foundations of nursing, ed. 3, Philadelphia, 1975, J. B. Lippincott Co., pp. 53-77.

Patient assessment: examination of the chest and lungs, Am. J. Nurs. **76**(9):1-23, Nov., 1976.

Traver, Gayle: Assessment of thorax and lungs, Am. J. Nurs. **73**(3): 466-471, March, 1973.

Pediatric

Alexander, Mary, and Brown, Marie Scott: Physical examination. Part 12. Chest and lungs, Nursing' 75 **5**(1): 44-48, 1975.

Barness, Lewis A.: Manual of pediatric physical diagnosis, ed. 4, Chicago, 1974. Year Book Medical Publishers, Inc.

Johnson, Thomas, Moore, William, and Jeffries, James, editors: Children are different: developmental physiology, ed. 2, Montreal, 1978. Ross Laboratories, pp. 127-133.

Lowery, G. H.: Growth and development of children, ed. 6, Chicago, 1973, Year Book Medical Publishers, Inc., p. 186.

Prior, John A., and Silberstein, Jack S.: Physical diagnosis: the history and examination of the patient, ed. 5, St. Louis, 1977, The C. V. Mosby Co., pp. 462-464.

Geriatric

Burnside, Irene Mortenson, editor: Nursing and the aged, New York, 1976, McGraw-Hill Book Co., pp. 297-315, 404-405.

Caird, F. I., and Judge, T. G.: Assessment of the elderly patient, London, 1977, Pitman Medical Publishing Co. Ltd., pp. 26-30.

Campbell, Edward J., and LeFrak, Stephen: How aging affects the structure and function of the respiratory system, Geriatrics, **33**(6): 68-74, June, 1978.

Chinn, Austin B., editor: Clinical aspects of aging, Working with older people: a guide to practice, vol. 4, Rockville, Md., 1971, U.S. Department of Health, Education, and Welfare, Public Health Service, pp. 113-123.

CHAPTER 9

Assessment of the cardiovascular system

Cognitive objectives

At the end of this unit the learner will demonstrate knowledge of assessment of the cardiovascular system by the ability to do the following:

1. Identify the characteristics and phases of Korotkoff sounds.
2. Record a blood pressure, identifying the variables of auscultatory gap, first and second diastolic pressures, and pulse pressure.
3. Identify common variables that alter blood pressure in healthy individuals.
4. Identify the characteristics of arterial pulse that an examiner notes with inspection and palpation.
5. Identify causes attributed to selected variations of arterial pulse characteristics.
6. Identify major differences between observable signs of chronic venous insufficiency and chronic arterial insufficiency.
7. Identify major differences between carotid and jugular pulsation.
8. Identify some major characteristics of the normal jugular veins and jugular venous pressure.
9. Identify major characteristics and causes of leg varicosities.
10. Identify and locate the anatomical positions of the heart, the major components of the heart, and adjacent great vessels.
11. Identify some major characteristics of normal signs elicited during inspection and palpation of the precordium.
12. Identify the appropriate purpose and use of the bell and diaphragm of the stethoscope.
13. Identify the origin of the first and second heart sounds.
14. Identify the major auscultatory characteristics of the first and second heart sounds in terms of:
    a. Location
    b. Intensity

c. Frequency
d. Timing
e. Splitting

15. Identify the origin and major characteristics of the third and fourth heart sounds.
16. Recognize the following precordial auscultatory areas and identify selected auscultatory events in each area:
    a. Aortic area
    b. Pulmonary area
    c. Erb's point
    d. Tricuspid area
    e. Apical area
17. Identify the following six characteristics of cardiac murmurs that must be described during their assessment:
    a. Timing: systole, diastole, continuous
    b. Location: using precordial landmarks and/or distance in centimeters from a landmark
    c. Radiation: described in centimeters, landmarks
    d. Intensity: grades I through VI, or loud, medium, soft
    e. Pitch: high, medium, low
    f. Quality: blowing, harsh, rumbling, crescendo, decrescendo
18. Identify the origin and selected major characteristics of systolic and diastolic murmurs.
19. Identify selected major characteristics of "innocent" murmurs.
20. Identify selected common cardiovascular variations in pediatric and geriatric clients.
21. Define the terms in the vocabulary section.

Clinical objectives

At the end of this unit the learner will perform a systematic assessment of the cardiovascular system, demonstrating the ability to do the following:

1. Obtain a pertinent health history from a client.

2. Palpate and auscultate arterial blood pressure.
3. Assess carotid, radial, femoral, popliteal, dorsalis pedis, and posterior tibial pulses through inspection and palpation for:
   a. Rate
   b. Rhythm
   c. Amplitude
   d. Variations in amplitude
   e. Contour
   f. Symmetry
4. Conduct a predesignated maneuver to test for arterial sufficiency in extremities.
5. Evaluate and describe jugular venous pressure.
6. Inspect and describe jugular pulsation quality.
7. Inspect, palpate, and describe appearance of superficial veins and surface characteristics of the legs.
8. Maneuver the foot and describe results of an assessment for calf pains.
9. Inspect and palpate extremities for arterial and venous sufficiency.
10. Observe and describe the client's general condition (at rest) in terms of:
    a. Positioning and comfort
    b. Ease of respirations (in supine or 30° to 45° position)
    c. General skin color
11. Inspect and palpate the anterior chest precordium, sternoclavicular, aortic, pulmonary, right ventricular, apical, epigastric, and ectopic areas for:
    a. Contour
    b. General movement
    c. Pulsations
    d. Heaves or lifts
12. Palpate and describe the results of assessment of the apical impulse for:
    a. Amplitude
    b. Duration
    c. Location
    d. Diameter
13. Locate and auscultate the following sites with a stethoscope bell and diaphragm:
    a. Aortic area
    b. Pulmonary area
    c. Erb's point
    d. Tricuspid area
    e. Apical area
14. Describe the results of cardiac auscultation in terms of:
    a. Rate
    b. Rhythm
    c. S_1: location, intensity, frequency, timing, and splitting

d. S_2: location, intensity, frequency, timing, and splitting
   e. Systole: relative duration
   f. Diastole: relative duration
15. Identify additional systolic or diastolic sounds in terms of:
    a. Timing
    b. Location
    c. Radiation
    d. Intensity
    e. Pitch
    f. Quality
16. Auscultate and describe cardiac sounds while client is supine, turned to left decubitus position, and sitting up.
17. Summarize results with a written description of findings.

Health history related to the cardiovascular system additional to screening history

1. If the client complains of leg pains (cramps), inquire about specific situations or activities that worsen or relieve the problem.
   a. *Arterial insufficiency* results in pain that worsens with activity, particularly prolonged exercise (e.g., walking). The pain is usually quickly (within 2 minutes) relieved with cessation of movement (standing). Pain may occasionally occur when limbs are elevated and be relieved with dangling of feet. Claudication distance should be specified. Determine how many average city blocks (or yards, number of stairs, etc.) a client walks before pain occurs. Remember that variables such as a hilly terrain, walking in start-stop heavy traffic areas, environmental temperature, and pace of walking affect exertion intensity. Signs and symptoms indicating a severe problem are:
      (1) Sudden decrease in claudication distance
      (2) Diminished or absent pulses or cold, mottled, or bluish extremities
      (3) Cutaneous changes, such as reddened pressure areas, ulcers, taut shiny skin
      (4) Pain not relieved by rest
      Pain is most commonly located in the calf but may be in the lower leg or dorsum of the foot. Hip, buttock, or thigh pain may be present. The client should provide a clear description of the pain (e.g., numbness, feeling of cold, burning, tingling, sharp cramp, aching). Risk factors include family history of diabetes, vascular disease, or heart disease, hyperlipidemia, hypertension, and smoking.
   b. *Venous insufficiency* pain intensifies with pro-

longed standing or sitting in one position. Relief often occurs by elevating the leg, lying down, or exercise (walking). Edema often accompanies the problem. Varicosities may be present. Discomfort may be increased at the end of the day. Pain is commonly located in the calf and lower leg. It may be described as an aching, tiredness, or feeling of fullness. Risk factors include occupation involving prolonged sitting or standing, family or client history of varicosities, overweight, constrictive clothing (e.g., garters, girdles), pregnancy, history of thrombophlebitis, chronic systemic disease (e.g., heart disease, cirrhosis, hypertension).

c. Neurologically caused pain exhibits fewer predictable patterns. The pain often occurs at night and awakens the client. The pain may be associated with exercise or movement, but nothing in particular relieves it. There is usually no edema, cyanosis, cold extremities, or marked cutaneous changes associated with it. The pain may locate in the calf. A family or client history of diabetes mellitus should always be inquired about.

d. There may be other causes for leg pain, such as the following:

    (1) New type of shoe (e.g., very high heels, "negative heel" shoes)

    (2) Foot problems (with inadequate shoe support)

    (3) Participation in new type of exercise or increased exercise

    (4) Problems with back and pain radiating to legs (more information in Chapter 14)

    (5) Recent injury

e. Clients who complain of leg pain at night should

Exertion/exercise profile (sample form)

	Sleeping	Lying down	Sitting	Light exercise*	Moderate exercise†	Moderately heavy exercise‡	Other§
Hr/day	8	3 to 4	4	3	2 to 3		Twenty-eight stairs (climbs b.i.d.)
Hr/wk					5 to 6 (short walks to shopping center)	5 to 6 (heavy housework; occasional long walks)	
Hr/mo							
Symptoms and problems	None	Feels tired if unable to take AM and PM naps	None	None	None (however, carries out daily routines at a slow pace)	Occasional SOB and must rest after heavy housework	Feels "winded" midway at landing; rests for 2 minutes

*Walking from one room to another, fixing small meals, etc.
†Light housework, making bed, sweeping floor, dusting, office work, short walks (flat surface), etc.
‡Scrubbing floors, sexual intercourse, long walks (specify amount), stair climbing (specify flights), lifting, construction work, etc.
§Long periods of standing, exercise programs, jogging, stair climbing (may be recorded as unusual activity if many flights are climbed frequently).

clarify what specifically relieves it (e.g., rubbing leg, walking, dangling) and the duration of pain.

   f. All leg pain complaints should be treated with a full symptom analysis. The aforementioned descriptions may help the examiner to categorize a profile.

2. The following questions concern heart disease and hypertension:

   a. Have you experienced any visual changes? Loss of consciousness? Headaches? Marked weakness or fatigue?

   b. Are there any new or marked stress factors in your life (home, work, family, friends)?

   c. Have you noticed a weight change in the last 6 months?

   d. Do you feel dizzy? Does your body position affect the dizziness? (Postural hypotension might affect the client's safety in the home.) Have you ever fallen down?

   e. If orthopnea and paroxysmal nocturnal dyspnea are present, inquire about sleep habits.

   f. If edema is present, inquire about the times of day when it is most apparent (e.g., first thing in the morning vs. late afternoon or evening).

   g. Inquire closely about medications being consumed. (If nitroglycerin or other "prn" preparations are being taken, determine how often per day.) Review over-the-counter medications carefully. Some antacid medications contain large amounts of sodium. Many cold preparations (antitussives, decongestants), nose drops, nasal sprays, and weight control preparations contain sympathomimetic amines.

   h. Inquire closely about dietary habits. Consider calorie, cholesterol, and salt intakes.

   i. For clients with a history of heart disease, severe hypertension, or vascular disease, it may be helpful to establish an exertion/exercise profile. Definitions of light, moderate, or heavy exercise can be established in advance by the examiner or agency or can be defined for individual clients. The profile can be renewed periodically to follow client's progress. (See sample form on p. 201.)

   j. Chronic pain, shortness of breath, fatigue, or other symptoms must be related to reduction or change in functions of daily living. For example, dyspnea increases with stair climbing, and a client might live four flights up in an apartment building. Many people have to walk to the grocery store every day. Interference with sleep, work environment, physical demands, and family relationships should be explored.

3. Chest pain profile. Table 4 is not intended to be a complete guide to differential diagnosis. Gastrointestinal and musculoskeletal problems can mimic angina. It will, however, provide some ideas about specific questions to pose.

4. Risk factors for cardiovascular disease:

   a. Family history of diabetes mellitus, heart dis-

Table 4. Chest pain profile*

	Angina pectoris	Esophagitis	Musculoskeletal problems
Precipitated by	Effort (usually emotion, exercise, eating)	Eating Nervousness	Motion, especially neck movement Hyperventilation Coughing
Duration	10 to 15 min	Variable (up to several hours)	Variable
Alleviated by	Stopping activity or rest (often in 2 to 3 min) Nitroglycerin	Eructation Sitting upright Eating Antacids	Heat Analgesic Change of position
Worsening of pain	Soon after rising (AM) After heavy meal	Any time (especially at night)	Bedtime or after day of exertion
Onset	Often remembers date (pain seldom continues over 5 years without developing abnormal exercise ECG)	Uncertain	Uncertain
Disease	Myocardial infarction, diabetes, hypertension, rheumatic heart disease, obesity, indigestion	Indigestion	Trauma

*Data from Warner-Chilcott Laboratory, AEGIS Production: Differential diagnosis of chest pain, New York, 1967, American Heart Association. Wasson, J.. Walsh, B. T., Tompkins, R., and Sox, H.: The common symptom guide, New York, 1975, McGraw-Hill Book Co.

ease (especially under age 60), hypertension, or vascular disease
  b. Client history of hyperlipoproteinemia, diabetes, hypertension, obesity, heavy cigarette smoking,

lack of physical exercise, stressful life-style ("stressful" must be carefully defined by client)
  c. Age (increasing incidence over 30 years)

Clinical guidelines

The student will:	To identify:	
	Normal	**Deviations from normal**
1. Assemble equipment: **a.** Stethoscope **b.** Sphygmomanometer		
2. Palpate, then auscultate the brachial artery to determine arterial blood pressure in both arms (See *clinical strategies* for description of procedure for measuring blood pressure.)	Varies with sex, body weight, time of day Other variables that can be somewhat controlled by examiner listed in clinical strategies	
	Upper limits (adult): 140 mm Hg systolic 90 mm Hg diastolic 30 to 40 mm Hg pulse pressure	Elevated systolic (↑ 140)* Elevated diastolic (↑ 90)* Widened pulse pressure Narrow pulse pressure Low systolic (↓ 90) Low diastolic (↓ 60)
	Pressure in both arms same or does not vary more than 5 to 10 mm Hg systolic	Significant (↑ 5 to 10 mm Hg) discrepancy in pressure readings between upper extremities
3. Measure blood pressure while client is standing (as well as lying) if client offers history or complaint of syncope or dizziness or is taking antihypertensive medications	On standing, client may manifest drop of maximum of 10 to 15 mm Hg (systolic) and 5 mm Hg (diastolic)	Significant decrease of systolic (more than 15 mm Hg) or diastolic (more than 5 mm Hg) and/or symptoms of dizziness
4. Measure blood pressure in both legs if pedal, popliteal, and femoral pulses are weak or absent (See clinical strategies for technique.)	Popliteal artery auscultation reveals systolic pressure 5 to 15 mm Hg higher than brachial artery measurement; diastolic reading same or slightly lower	Systolic pressure lower in leg(s) then in arms
5. Palpate both carotid arteries **a.** Use flat surface of first three finger pads **b.** Place fingers between trachea and sternocleidomastoid muscle under mandible **c.** Client should flex neck and rotate head slightly toward side being examined (Fig. 9-1)		

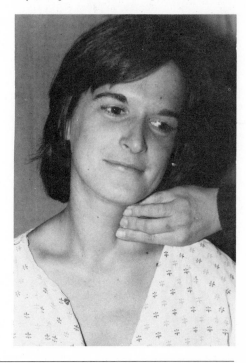

Fig. 9-1. Palpating for carotid pulse.

---

*If pressure is elevated, especially if accompanied by rapid pulse, repeat in 30 minutes.

Continued.

Clinical guidelines–cont'd

The student will:	To identify:	
	Normal	Deviations from normal
d. Palpate one artery at a time for:		
1. Rate	60 to 90 beats/min (conditioned athletes may be as low as 50/min)	↑ 90/min (tachycardia) (*Note:* Recent exertion, smoking, or anxiety will elevate pulse.) ↓ 60/min (bradycardia)
2. Rhythm	Regular (*Note:* Slight transient increase in rate during inspiration, especially in clients under 40 years.)	Irregular, without any pattern (e.g., atrial fibrillation) Regularity with occasional pauses or extra beats (e.g., premature contractions) Coupled beats (e.g., bigeminal pulse)*
3. Pulse amplitude and contour	Upstroke smooth, rounded, prompt	Upstroke exaggerated or bounding Pulse weak, small, or thready; peak prolonged
4. Amplitude pattern†	Series of pulse strokes unvaried in amplitude or contour	Upstrokes vary (e.g., strong and weaker beats alternate [pulsus alternans]) Force of beat reduced during inspiration (paradoxical pulse)
5. Symmetry	Symmetrical response (i.e., both carotid pulses manifest same rate, rhythm, amplitude, and contour)	Asymmetrical response
6. Arterial wall contour and consistency	Soft and pliable	Increased resistance to compression; beaded or tortuous

6. Using finger pads of first three fingers, palpate:

a. Both radial pulses at medial aspect of wrist (Fig. 9-2)

b. Both femoral pulses, immediately inferior to inguinal ligament, midway between anterior superior iliac spine and pubic tubercle (*Note:* Firmer compression may be necessary for accurate palpation of obese clients.) (Fig. 9-3)

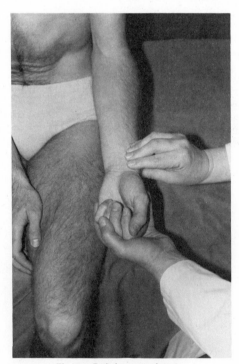

Fig. 9-2. Radial artery palpation.

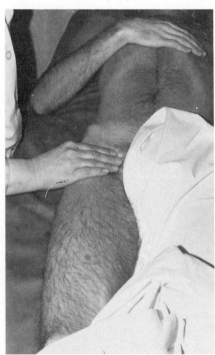

Fig. 9-3. Femoral artery palpation.

---

*An irregular, rapid, or slow pulse should be palpated simultaneously with auscultation of the apical pulse. Any difference between apical and peripheral pulse rate should be noted. If pulse irregularity is patterned (occurs in repeated sequences), note whether irregularity occurs during (1) inspiration or expiration and (2) systole or diastole.

†Pulse *amplitude* can be varied or uneven, and pulse *rate* can remain regular or may be irregular.

The student will:	To identify:	
	Normal	Deviations from normal

c. Both popliteal pulses: press fingers firmly into popliteal fossae (Fig. 9-4)

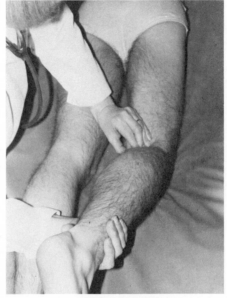

Fig. 9-4. Popliteal artery palpation.

d. Both dorsalis pedis pulses: press lightly over dorsum of foot; foot should be moderately dorsiflexed (Fig. 9-5)

(*Note:* Dorsalis pedis pulses may be difficult to find or absent in some normal individuals.)

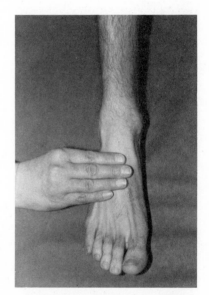

Fig. 9-5. Dorsalis pedis artery palpation.

e. Both posterior tibial pulses: curve fingers behind and slightly inferior to medial maleolus of ankle (Fig. 9-6)

(*Note:* Posterior tibial pulses may also be absent in some normal individuals.)

Fig. 9-6. Posterior tibial artery palpation.

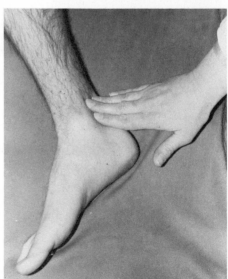

Continued.

Clinical guidelines–cont'd

The student will:	To identify:	
	Normal	Deviations from normal
7. Palpate all pulses for: **a.** Symmetrical response	All pulses should be full, strong, and symmetrical	Any asymmetry in force or pulse contour
b. Arterial wall contour and consistency	Soft and pliable	Increased resistance to compression; beaded or tortuous
8. Conduct the following maneuver if arterial insufficiency is suspected:		
a. With client lying down, elevate client's legs 30 cm (12 inches) above heart level		
b. Ask client to move feet up and down at ankles for 60 seconds	Extremities (feet) exhibit mild pallor	Marked pallor of one or both feet
c. Have client sit up and dangle legs	Original color returns in about 10 seconds Veins in feet fill in about 15 seconds	Delayed color return or mottled appearance (Fig. 9-7) Delayed venous filling Marked redness of dependent feet
(This maneuver can also be conducted with arms and hands.)		

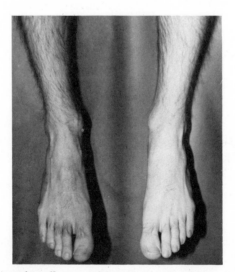

Fig. 9-7. Arterial insufficiency with contrasting pallor of foot in dependent position. Note increased venous filling on normal foot.

9. Evaluate venous pressure by inspecting both sides of client's neck as he lies at 30° to 45° angle; elevate chin slightly and tilt away from side being examined		

The student will:	To identify:	
	Normal	Deviations from normal
10. Identify highest point at which jugular vein blood level or pulsations can be seen, using sternal angle as reference point for "zero" level; estimate jugular venous pressure (JVP) in centimeters	JVP should not rise more than 3 cm (1 inch) above level of sternal angle* (Fig. 9-8)	JVP exceeds 3 cm above level of manubrium† (Fig. 9-9) Note if other veins in neck, shoulder, and upper chest distended

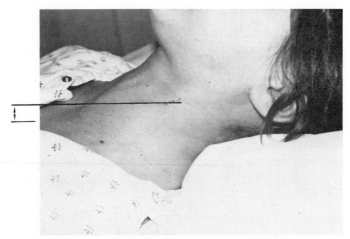

Fig. 9-8. Normal jugular venous pressure in external jugular vein. Blood level is less than 3 cm above the sternal angle.

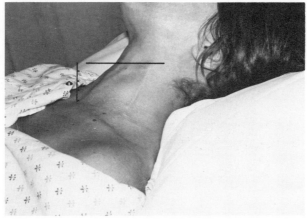

Fig. 9-9. Distended external jugular vein.

11. Inspect jugular pulsations for quality	Regular Soft and undulating Level of pulsation decreases with inspiration Pulsation increases in recumbent position	Fluttering or oscillating Irregular rhythm Unusually prominent waves

*If jugular vein is difficult to locate, ask client to lie flat for a few moments. Neck vein (particularly the external jugular) should distend with client in this position.

†If venous pressure is elevated (vein is distended up to neck), raise client's head until highest jugular pulsation can be detected. Record distance in centimeters above sternal angle *and* angle at which client is reclining.

Continued.

Clinical guidelines–cont'd

The student will:	To identify:	
	Normal	**Deviations from normal**
12. Inspect and palpate legs for presence and/or appearance of superficial veins	Distention in dependent position Venous valves may appear as nodular bulges Veins collapse with elevation of limbs	Distended veins in anteromedial aspect of thigh and lower leg or on posterolateral aspect of calf from knee to ankle (Fig. 9-10)

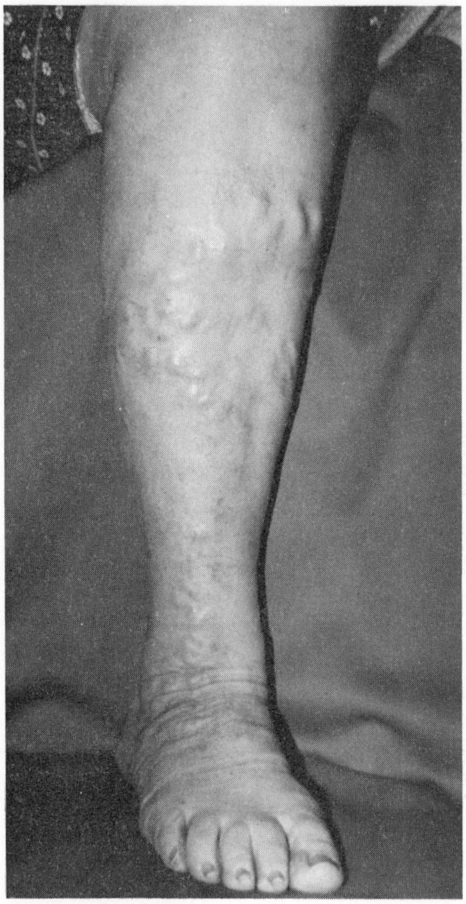

Fig. 9-10. Distended veins on lower leg with nodular bulges.

The student will:	Normal	Deviations from normal
13. Inspect and palpate thigh and calf for surface characteristics	Legs symmetrical Nontender No excess warmth	Swelling (or one leg, especially calf, appears larger than other)* Tenderness on palpation Warmth Redness
14. Sharply dorsiflex client's foot (with knee slightly flexed) to assess calf pain response	No pain	Pain (Homans sign)
15. Inspect and palpate extremities for evidence of adequate arterial supply	Absence of hair over digits or dorsum of hands and feet may be normal Skin pink and warm, nonedematous	Reduced or absent peripheral hair (over digits and dorsum of hands and feet) Thin, shiny, taut skin Cold extremities (in warm environment) Mild edema Marked pallor or mottling when extremity elevated Digit tips ulcerated Stocking anesthesia Tenderness on palpation

*If swelling is suspected, both thighs and calves should be measured with a tape to ensure accuracy.

	To identify:	
The student will:	**Normal**	**Deviations from normal**
16. Inspect and palpate extremities for evidence of venous sufficiency		Peripheral cyanosis Edema (pits on pressure), bilateral or unilateral* Pigmentation around ankles (See Fig. 3-2.) Thickening skin Ulceration (especially around ankles)
17. Observe client's general condition while lying supine or at elevation of 30° to 45°		
a. Positioning, comfort	Relaxed posture, without discomfort	Pain, coughing, or choking; "smothering" feeling; inability to lie flat for extended period
b. Respirations	Even and deep	Respirations uneven, shallow, gasping; inadequate exchange
c. Skin color	Pink/brown	Cyanosis, grayish pallor Mottling Note color around lips, neck, upper chest
d. Nail color and configuration	Pink 160° angle at nail bed	Cyanotic Clubbing (angle disappears)

*Edema should be measured against a bony prominence (over ankle or tibia). Record the following:

1. Type
   a. Pitting (Fig. 9-11)
   b. Nonpitting
2. Extent and location
   a. Ankle and foot
   b. Ankle only
   c. Foot to knee, etc.
   d. Hands and fingers
3. Degree of pitting
   a. 0 to 0.6 cm (0 to ¼ inch)—mild
   b. 0.6 to 1.3 cm (¼ to ½ inch)—moderate
   c. 1.3 to 2.5 cm (½ to 1 inch)—severe
4. Symmetrical or unilateral response

Continued.

Fig. 9-11. Moderate pitting edema at midcalf.

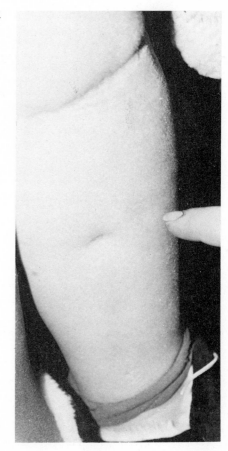

Clinical guidelines–cont'd

The student will:	To identify:	
	Normal	**Deviations from normal**
18. Inspect and palpate anterior chest		
a. Precordium		
1. Contour	Rounded, symmetrical	Kyphosis Sternal depression Any asymmetry
2. General movement: use the palmar surface of the hand and the finger pads (Fig. 9-12)	Even respiratory movements (precordium may lift slightly in thin people)	Entire chest heaving or lifting with heartbeat

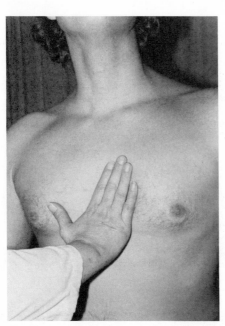

Fig. 9-12. Palpation over precordium. Note use of palmar surface of hand and finger pads.

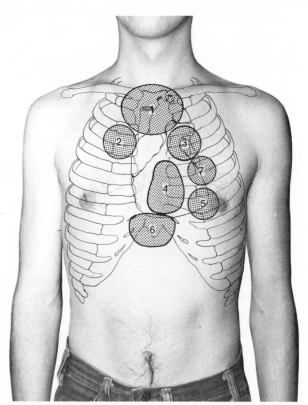

Fig. 9-13. Palpation areas for cardiac examination: *1,* sternoclavicular; *2,* aortic; *3,* pulmonary; *4,* anterior pericardium (right ventricular); *5,* apical; *6,* epigastric; *7,* ectopic.

19. Inspect and palpate the following specific areas (Fig. 9-13):		
a. Sternoclavicular area for pulsations	Slight or absent	Bounding
b. Aortic area (right second intercostal space adjacent to sternum) for pulsations	None	Pulsation, thrill (*Note:* Low-frequency vibrations can often be more easily felt than heard.)
c. Pulmonary area (left second intercostal space adjacent to sternum) for pulsations	None	Pulsation, thrill
d. Right ventricular area (left and right fifth intercostal space close to sternum) for heave or lift	May be present in hyperkinetic, thin, or pregnant adults	Diffuse lift or heave, pulsations

	To identify:	
The student will:	**Normal**	**Deviations from normal**
e. Apical area (fifth intercostal space, 5 to 7 cm [2 to 3 inches] from midsternal line) (Fig. 9-14) for:		
1. Pulsation	May be present	
2. Amplitude	Tapping	Thrusting
3. Duration	First third to half systole	Sustained throughout systole
4. Location	Fourth or fifth intercostal space, 5 to 7 cm from midclavicular line*	Displaced left lateral or down
5. Diameter	1 to 2 cm (⅓ to ½ inch)	Over 2 cm (½ inch)

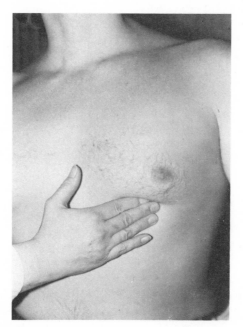

Fig. 9-14. Palpation for pulse at apical area. Finger pads are more sensitive to light pulsations.

f. Epigastric area for pulsations: slide fingers up under rib cage	Aortic pulsation with forward thrust Right ventricular pulsation with downward thrust	Bounding pulsation
g. Ectopic area (midway between pulmonary and apical areas) for pulsations	None	Outward pulsation

Note: Apical pulse location may displace slightly laterally if client turns to the left side.

Continued.

Clinical guidelines–cont'd

	To identify:	
The student will:	**Normal**	**Deviations from normal**

20. Auscultate the following specific areas (Fig. 9-15) (*Note:* Even though auscultation areas are pictured as separate locations, examiner should "inch" from one area to next.); use both diaphragm and bell to listen to all areas

  a. Aortic area (second right interspace)

  b. Pulmonary area (second left interspace)

  c. Erb's point (third left interspace)

  d. Tricuspid area (fifth left interspace near sternum)

  e. Apical area (fifth left interspace medial to midclavicular line)

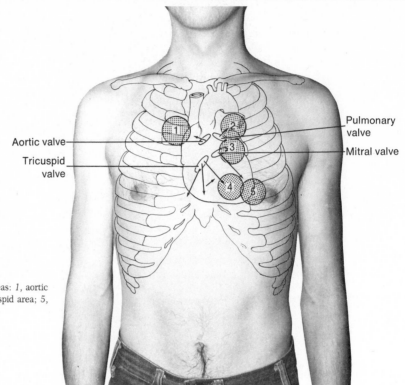

Fig. 9-15. Anatomical and auscultatory valve areas: *1,* aortic area; *2,* pulmonary area; *3,* Erb's point; *4,* tricuspid area; *5,* mitral area.

1. Rate	60 to 90 beats/min (conditioned athletes or "seasoned" joggers may have normally slower rate)	Over 90 Under 60
2. Rhythm	Regular	Irregular (without any pattern) Sporadic extra beats or pauses
3. S₁ sound		
a. Location	Usually heard at all sites	
b. Intensity	Often louder at apex (muscle, fat tissue, and air will diminish sound; rapid rate will accentuate sound)	Accented Diminished (muffled) Varying intensity with different beats (e.g., complete heart block)
c. Frequency	Usually lower in pitch than S₂	Frequency (pitch) becomes higher with accented intensity
d. Timing	Almost synchronous with carotid impulse Slightly longer in duration than S₂	
e. Splitting	May be heard occasionally in tricuspid area Normal S₁ splitting sound usually varies from beat to beat: occasionally single sound, occasionally narrow split	S₄ sound sometimes mistaken for S₁ splitting
4. S₂ sound		
a. Location	Usually heard at all sites	
b. Intensity	Often louder at base (intensity diminished with fat, muscle, or air)	Increased intensity, usually in aortic (e.g., arterial hypertension) or pulmonary area (e.g., pulmonary hypertension) Decreased intensity
c. Frequency	Usually higher in pitch than S₁	
d. Timing	Sound shorter in duration than S₁	

The student will:	To identify:	
	Normal	**Deviations from normal**
e. Splitting	Commonly heard in pulmonary area (on inspiration) in young adults	Wide splitting (e.g., right bundle branch block) Fixed splitting Paradoxical splitting (e.g., left bundle branch block)
5. Systole		
a. Duration	Shorter than diastole at normal heart rate (60 to 90 beats/min)	

b. Sounds	S_1 sound duration brief; silent interval	Early systolic ejection click:
		   Aortic—heard at base and apex
		   Pulmonary—heard in pulmonary area
		Middle and late systolic clicks (e.g., mitral valve deformity) heard at left sternal border
		Clicks high pitched and sharp in sound

6. Diastole		
a. Duration	Longer than systole at normal rate (60 to 100 beats/min) Shortens in duration as rate increases	
b. Sounds	S_2 duration brief Silent interval	
(1) S_3	*Young adults*	*Older adults*
(a) Location	Apex	Apex (may signify heart failure)
(b) Intensity	Dull, low pitched	Dull, low pitched
(c) Timing	Early in diastole (normal S_3 often disappear when client sits up)	Early in diastole
(2) S_4		
(a) Location		Medial to apex
(b) Intensity	Rarely heard in normal client	Higher pitch
(c) Timing		Late diastole (may be confused with split S_1)
(3) Other sounds		*Opening snap* At apex Higher pitch Very early in diastole
7. Murmurs	("Innocent" murmurs in children and young adults)	
a. Timing	Usually early systolic, but characteristics hard to differentiate from pathological sounds	Systolic: early, middle, late; continuous Diastolic: early, middle, late; continuous
b. Location	Usually at pulmonary area, apex or medial to apex	Area where sound heard may be small and confined or may cover most of precordium Describe in terms of precordial landmarks and centimeters distance from landmarks
c. Radiation		Describe in relation to landmarks and centimeters distance
d. Intensity	Soft, usually below grade III Varies with position and respiration	Grade I to VI, or loud, medium, soft Stable, or varies with respiration and position
e. Pitch		High, medium, low
f. Quality		Blowing, harsh, rumbling Crescendo Decrescendo
8. Other sounds		Pericardial friction rub (to-and-fro rubbing sound, usually heard during systole and diastole; sound usually increased when client sits up and leans forward)

21. Repeat palpation and auscultation maneuvers with client
  a. Lying in left decubitus position
  b. Sitting

Clinical strategies

1. Procedure for measuring arterial blood pressure (arm):
   a. The client should be comfortably seated, in a partially raised position or lying down.
   b. The arm should be stabilized at heart level with the elbow slightly flexed.
   c. The arm should be uncovered; shirt sleeves should be removed, not rolled up, if they are at all constrictive.
   d. The cuff:
      (1) Should be 20% wider than arm diameter, covering two thirds of the upper arm.
      (2) Bladder should be centered over the artery.
      (3) Lower edge should be placed 2 to 5 cm (1 to 2 inches) above the antecubital space.
      (4) Should be completely deflated when applied.
      (5) Should be snugly and smoothly wrapped around the arm.
      (6) Tubing will rest at the medial aspect of the arm (Fig. 9-16).
   e. The examiner should be positioned comfortably so that:
      (1) The aneroid or mercury gauge can be viewed at close range (closer than 90 cm [3 feet]).
      (2) The aneroid gauge can be viewed straight on (avoiding an oblique view) (Fig. 9-17).

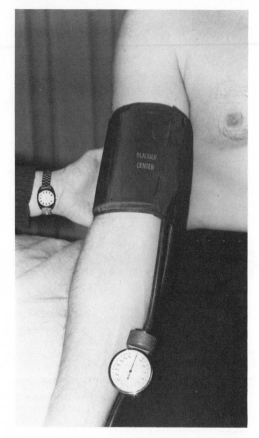

Fig. 9-16. Arterial blood pressure measurement. Note the following: (1) bladder is centered over the artery; (2) lower edge of cuff is 3 cm above antecubital space; (3) deflated cuff is wrapped snugly and smoothly around arm; (4) tubing rests at medial aspect of arm.

Fig. 9-17. Blood pressure measurement. Examiner views gauge "straight on" within a 90-cm range. Examiner palpates brachial artery before auscultation maneuver.

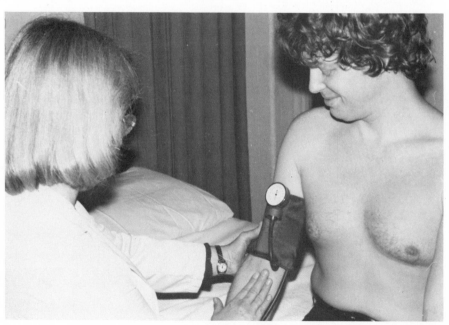

(3) The mercury column top is viewed at eye level.

f. If a mercury manometer is used, it should be placed on a flat surface.

g. The examiner should palpate the brachial or radial artery and inflate the cuff 30 mm Hg above the point where the pulse is no longer palpated (Fig. 9-17).

h. Deflate the cuff slowly (2 to 3 mm Hg per heartbeat) and note onset of pulse.

i. Apply the stethoscope bell to the previously palpated brachial artery. The bell should be applied as lightly as possible but with no space between the skin and stethoscope. The stethoscope should not be in contact with the cuff or clothing.

j. Inflate the cuff 30 mm Hg above the point where the previously palpated pulse was obliterated. Deflate slowly (2 to 3 mm Hg per heartbeat).

k. Note (1) onset of first sound, (2) muffling (or change in character) of sound, and (3) disappearance of sound.

l. If the blood pressure procedure must be repeated to clarify results, wait a minimum of 60 seconds to repeat. (Deflate cuff completely.)

m. Note variables that can alter client's blood pressure: exercise, anxiety, a cold environment, eating, drinking, or smoking within 30 minutes before measurement is taken, pain or discomfort, exertion, bladder distention.

2. Procedure for measuring arterial blood pressure (thigh):

a. Client should be lying prone.

b. The leg should be stabilized and uncovered (no restrictive clothing bunched or rolled at upper thigh).

c. The cuff:

(1) Should be wider and longer than that used for client's arm (e.g., an 18- to 20-cm bag).

(2) Should be applied over midthigh so that the bladder is centered over the posterior aspect.

d. The examiner must be positioned so that the aneroid or mercury gauge can be viewed at close distance. The mercury column should be at eye level.

e. The examiner should palpate the popliteal fossa and locate the pulsation.

f. Place the stethoscope over the artery and proceed as with brachial pressure maneuvers.

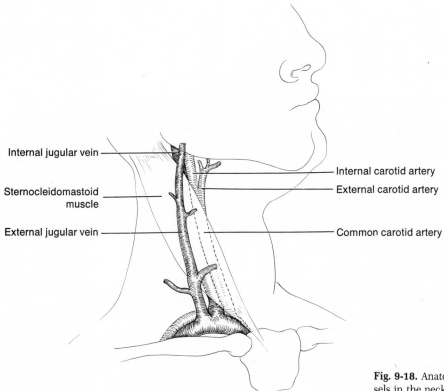

Internal jugular vein

Sternocleidomastoid muscle

External jugular vein

Internal carotid artery

External carotid artery

Common carotid artery

Fig. 9-18. Anatomical placement of carotid and jugular vessels in the neck.

g. *Note:* The examiner can anticipte that the popliteal systolic arterial pressure will register higher (5 to 15 mm Hg) than the brachial systolic pressure.

h. The diastolic pressure is usually the same or slightly lower.

3. If jugular pulsations are difficult to find, have the client lie flat for maximum venous distention. It is recommended that the internal jugular vein be viewed for registering venous pressure. However, it is often difficult to locate because of its anatomical placement (Fig. 9-18). Note the location of the carotid artery in relation to the jugular veins. Be certain not to confuse the arterial with the venous pulsations. Venous pulsations (a) are less vigorous (of an undulating quality), (b) can be eliminated by pressing over the clavicle, (c) increase in intensity when client is recumbent, and (d) are rarely palpable.

4. Inspect and palpate the extremities carefully. Foot pulses (dorsalis pedis) are sometimes difficult or impossible to find. *Note:* A cold environment may alter the appearance and temperature of extremities.

5. It is important to inspect the client carefully before proceeding with palpation and auscultation. Stand back and view the entire person. Establish a general picture of posture, comfort, character of respiration, tension, and general skin color.

6. Inspect the precordium *carefully.* Beginners sometimes tend to miss the obvious because they are anxious to auscultate. View the entire anterior chest. It is possible that the whole chest could be heaving. Then let your eyes focus on each inspection site described in the guidelines.

7. Good lighting is necessary for good inspection.

8. It is vital that the examiner develop a system for cardiac palpation and auscultation. There are a number of choices: moving from base to apex, apex to base, alternating diaphragm and bell, having the client sit first or lie down first, etc. Establish the mechanics, then develop a listening and concentration system. The characteristics of rate, rhythm, S_1, S_2, systole, diastole, and extra sounds are described in the guidelines. Each entity must be evaluated separately. It is impossible to hear everything at once.

9. When auscultating, avoid "jumping" from one site to another. "Inch" the endpiece along the route. This maneuver helps you avoid missing important sounds.

10. Stabilize the endpiece on the chest by letting your fourth and fifth fingers, or your wrist, rest on the adjacent chest wall. This will prevent sliding and extraneous noise. Use light pressure with the bell and a firmer pressure with the diaphragm.

11. Often heart sounds are better heard if the client breathes out and holds the expiration. Asking the client to breathe out and to lean forward while in a sitting position is helpful.

12. For women with large breasts, displace the breast upward with one hand and palpate or auscultate with the other. Some clients can assist in displacement.

13. It is sometimes helpful to place a hand on the client's shoulder to steady him while he is sitting.

Sample recording

Pulses, pressures: Carotid, radial, femoral, dorsalis pedis, and posterior tibial pulses symmetrical, strong, and regular. No bruits. Jugular venous pressure at the level of the sternal angle while client elevated at 30°.

Extremities: Warm, without pallor, cyanosis, edema. No varicosities or calf tenderness. Homans sign negative.

Precordium/heart: No thrills, heaves, or pulsations other than PMI barely palpable at fifth left ICS, 8 cm from midsternal line. AP = RP. S_1 and S_2 are brief and clear. No extra sounds or murmurs.

History and clinical strategies associated with the pediatric client

1. There are basically two types of cardiovascular disease in children. The first is a congenital problem with the heart itself or its pumping mechanisms. The second type, called acquired, occurs as the result of a systemic disease, such as rheumatic fever.

2. The examiner must use every sense available to evaluate the child's cardiovascular system. The obvious decompensating characteristics such as cyanosis, peripheral edema, and dyspnea will be recognized early and easily. But it is the subtle, early signs and symptoms that the examiner must be continuously watchful for. Early warning symptoms of a *potential* cardiovascular problem *may be:*

a. An infant that becomes tired of sucking and must rest periodically before able to finish

b. An infant who has tachycardia and tachypnea while eating

c. A child who is reported to tire frequently during playing (In this case it is important to clarify how much and what kinds of activities cause fatigue: an hour of playing tag vs. a short walk.)

d. A child who is reported to "turn blue" with prolonged crying episodes

e. A child who requires several rest/sleep periods during the day beyond what is normal for the age

f. A child who repeatedly complains that he does not want to go out and play because he cannot keep up with the others or because he becomes short of breath or tired when he plays

g. A child who assumes a knee-chest position during sleeping; or squats instead of sits when playing or watching television

h. A child who complains of leg pains with running (inquire as to how much running causes pains and what pains actually feel like)

i. Excessively labored breathing in an infant during defecation

j. A child who is falling behind the normal growth and development schedule

k. A child with a history of frequent headaches or nosebleeds accompanying a rise in blood pressure and/or leg cramping

Although any single symptom just listed may not be due to a cardiovascular dysfunction, it warrants full investigation of additional subjective and objective data.

3. Cardiovascular evaluation of the child extends far beyond examination of the heart. The evaluation should begin as the examiner first sees the child. The overall health, nutritional state, color, ease of respirations, and general overt qualities of the child should communicate information about the child's cardiovascular function.

4. The blood pressure of children under the age of 1 year may be difficult to obtain because of improper cuff size or excessive baby fat or simply because the child is extremely wiggly. The examiner can be assured that if the infant is screaming and pink, the blood pressure is substantial. It is the lethargic or ill-appearing infant who demands a blood pressure recording. If the examiner has difficulty obtaining an audible blood pressure, the "flush technique" may be used. Following are the steps:

a. Elevate the child's arm to drain its blood.

b. Wrap a 2-inch elastic bandage from the fingertips to the elbow.

c. Apply a blood pressure cuff (no more than two thirds or less than half the length of the upper arm).

d. Pump the cuffing to about 120 mm Hg.

e. Lower the infant's arm and remove the bandage.

f. Slowly deflate the cuff.

g. The point where there is a "flush" of the arm from white to pink is taken as the reading. This is generally considered to be the median reading between systolic and diastolic.

5. Following are general guidelines for obtaining blood pressure readings in children:

a. Every child 18 months and older should be screened for hypertension. This means that the child's blood pressure should be evaluated during every well-child examination.

b. Equipment for obtaining pediatric blood pressures is the same as for the adult. The cuff should not be larger than two thirds or smaller than half the length of the child's arm between the elbow and shoulder. Proper size cuffs are mandatory for the adequate evaluation of children. Pediatric cuffs are available in 2½ and 5-inch sizes.

c. The American Heart Association states that the muffling of the blood pressure tone in children should actually be considered the diastolic reading.

d. Crying or sudden jerking may alter the child's blood pressure between 5 and 10 mm Hg. The child should be evaluated during a quiet period.

e. Every child should have at least one or two thigh screening blood pressure measurements during early childhood to rule out a vast difference between upper and lower extremity pressure (a sign of coarctation of the aorta).

6. Fever in a child will normally increase the child's pulse. For every degree of fever, the pulse may increase 8 to 10 beats/min.

7. When physically examining the child's cardiovascular system, the techniques of inspection, palpation, and auscultation are normally used. Percussion may be used by the experienced examiner with the older child, but generally, small patients poorly tolerate the procedure.

8. All techniques require that the child be undressed to the underwear and sitting on the table (infants may be held). It is helpful for cooperative children to recline to a 45° angle during examination. If that is impossible, a supine position is preferable to an upright position because more cardiovascular "sounds" are generally heard with the child lying down.

9. Auscultating the hearts of infants and toddlers is a true feat. The child must be quiet during the

examination. Crying, talking, or pulling at the stethoscope tubing will defeat the process. The examiner is encouraged to examine the cardiovascular system early during the examination before the child becomes frightened, bored, or cold.

10. As will be discussed in subsequent clinical guidelines, a child's chest should be auscultated in the same spots as an adult's heart. Because of the rapidity of a child's heart rate, the examiner may need to listen to each selected area for a fairly long time to feel comfortable in describing the findings. Some parents may become concerned because of the long listening time, therefore it is suggested that the examiner explain to the parent that a long listening time is not a cause for concern.

11. If the examiner identifies any unusual findings, suggestive history, extra noises, or murmurs, it is recommended that the child be referred to a physician for further verification. The beginning examiner should *not* attempt to define a murmur as "functional" or an extra odd heart sound as insignificant. It is the examiner's duty at this time to identify normal findings and to recognize and refer abnormal or suggestive findings. The cardiovascular health of a young child is too valuable to provide an experimental opportunity for the examiner.

Clinical variations associated with the pediatric client

ASSESSMENT OF PRESSURES, PULSES, AND THE PERIPHERAL VASCULAR SYSTEM

Characteristic or area examined	Normal			Deviations from normal	
1. Blood pressure: technique described under clinical strategies		*Mean systolic** ($\pm$ 2 S.D.)	*Mean diastolic** ($\pm$ 2 S.D.)	Elevated blood pressures are those which exceed the following readings†	
				3 to 6 yr‡	>110/70
a. Sitting or lying, depending on age	Newborn	80 $\pm$ 16	46 $\pm$ 16	6 to 9 yr‡	>120/75
	2 mo to 1 yr	89 $\pm$ 29	60 $\pm$ 10	10 to 13 yr‡	>130/80
	1 yr	96 $\pm$ 30	66 $\pm$ 25	14 yr‡	
	2 yr	99 $\pm$ 25	64 $\pm$ 25	M	>133/82
	3 yr	100 $\pm$ 25	67 $\pm$ 23	F	>128/84
	4 yr	99 $\pm$ 20	65 $\pm$ 20	15 yr§	
	5 to 6 yr	94 $\pm$ 14	55 $\pm$ 9	M	>137/85
	6 to 7 yr	100 $\pm$ 15	56 $\pm$ 8	F	>128/84
	7 to 8 yr	102 $\pm$ 15	56 $\pm$ 8	16 to 19 yr§	
	8 to 9 yr	105 $\pm$ 16	57 $\pm$ 9	M	>140/85
	9 to 10 yr	107 $\pm$ 16	57 $\pm$ 9	F	>128/84
	10 to 11 yr	111 $\pm$ 17	58 $\pm$ 10		
	11 to 12 yr	113 $\pm$ 18	59 $\pm$ 10		
	12 to 13 yr	115 $\pm$ 19	59 $\pm$ 10		
	13 to 14 yr	118 $\pm$ 19	60 $\pm$ 10		
	Pressure in both arms same or does not vary more than 5 to 10 mm Hg			Significant (>5 to 10 mm Hg) discrepancy in pressure readings between upper extremities	
b. Standing	(Not routinely done with children. If problem is suspected, have child stand up. Follow adult guidelines.)				
	Pulse pressure between 20 and 50 mm Hg throughout childhood			Narrowing of pulse pressure seen with aortic stenosis	
				Widening of pulse pressure may be seen in children with patent ductus arteriosus or aortic regurgitation	
c. Thigh measurement: technique same as adult	In child less than 1 year systolic pressure in thigh should equal that of arm			Systolic pressure in thigh measurement *lower* than systolic arm measurement (sign of coarctation of aorta)	
	In child over 1 year systolic pressure in thigh greater than that in arm by 10 to 40 mm Hg; diastolic pressure in thigh equals that in arm				

*Data from Haggerty, R. J., Maroney, M. W., and Nadas, A. S.: Am. J. Dis. Child. **92**:536, 1956, Copyright 1973, American Medical Association.

†Data from Londe, S., and Goldring, D.: Am. J. Cardiol. **37**:650, 1976.

‡Supine reading.

§Seated reading.

Characteristic or area examined	Normal	Deviations from normal
2. Carotid artery palpation		
a. Rate	*Age** *Rate/min**	Any findings beyond limits stated
	Newborn 120 to 170	Increases may be due to factors such as toxic-
	12 mo 80 to 160	ity, fever, excitement, and respiratory
	2 yr 80 to 130	distress
	3 yr 80 to 120	Decreases may be due to heart block, digitalis
	4 yr 80 to 120	poisoning, sepsis, *Salmonella* infection
	6 yr 75 to 115	
	Beyond 6 yr 70 to 110	
b. Rhythm	Regular	Irregular pulse unrelated to breathing†
	Sinus arrhythmia: pulse rate will speed up with inspiration and slow down with expiration; makes pulse seem irregular in rhythm; to further evaluate, instruct child to hold breath while you continue to feel pulse; rate should become regular	
	Carefully watch respirations in infant to evaluate if pulse rhythm fluctuates with breathing	
	Common in children over age 3 years	
	Especially prominent at puberty	
	Extrasystoles or premature ventricular contractions (PVC) *may* be normal in healthy child; will feel like skipped beat; emotional factors may trigger; exercise will usually cause disappearance	Extrasystoles or PVCs heard for first time in ill child; child with known cardiac disease; or child with suggestive or questionable history
c. Pulse amplitude	Pulse upstroke smooth, rounded, and prompt	Upstroke exaggerated, bounding, weak, thready
d. Amplitude pattern	Series of pulse strokes unvaried in amplitude or contour	Upstrokes vary, for example, strong and weaker beats alternate (pulsus alternans)
e. Symmetry	Symmetrical response (i.e., both carotid pulses manifest same rate, rhythm, amplitude, and contour)	Asymmetrical response
f. Arterial wall contour	Soft and pliable	Increased resistance to compression, beaded or tortuous
3. Radial artery palpation	(Pulses in nos. 4 to 6 may or may not be evaluated, depending on the age and overall health of the child. Any child with known cardiovascular disease or suggestive symptomatology should receive a thorough evaluation. Other children are normally screened by evaluating carotid, femoral, radial, and apical pulses. Criteria for evaluation has been listed previously.)	Significant difference between radial and femoral pulses
4. Popliteal pulse palpation		
5. Dorsalis pedis pulse palpation		Weak or absent femoral pulses may indicate coarctation of aorta
6. Posterior tibial pulse palpation		
7. Femoral pulse palpation		
8. Evaluation of venous pressures (Not routinely done in well children.)	Jugular veins may be visible but should not pulsate or appear engorged	Noted pulsations of neck or engorgement
9. Evidence of adequate arterial supply	Warm, pink, nonedematous extremities	Thin, shiny, taut skin
	Mottling (if infant in cool environment and has been uncovered for some time)	Cold or mottled extremities in warm environment

*Data from Barness, L.: Manual of pediatric physical diagnosis, ed. 4. Copyright © 1972 by Year Book Medical Publishers, Inc., Chicago. Used by permission; Haggerty, R. J., Maroney, M. W., and Nadas, A. S.: Am. J. Dis. Child. **92**:536, 1956.
†An irregular (rapid or slow) pulse should be palpated simultaneously with auscultation of the apical pulse. Any difference between apical and peripheral pulse rate should be noted. If pulse irregularity is patterned (occurs in repeated sequences), note whether irregularity occurs during (1) inspiration or expiration and (2) systole or diastole.   *Continued.*

ASSESSMENT OF PRESSURES, PULSES, AND THE PERIPHERAL VASCULAR SYSTEM—cont'd

Characteristic or area examined	Normal	Deviations from normal
10. Evidence of adequate venous sufficiency		Edema* Marked pallor Tenderness of skin Peripheral cyanosis Edema* Thickening of skin

*Often one associates heart failure with peripheral edema. In children, however, the signs of heart failure are quite different. Signs may include a rapid respiratory rate in the supine position followed by slight dyspnea, liver enlargement, venous engorgement, orthopnea, pulsus alternans, and a gallop rhythm. Only very late in its course are signs of pulmonary or peripheral edema noticeable (Barness, 1972).

ASSESSMENT OF THE HEART AND PRECORDIUM

Characteristic or area examined	Normal	Deviations from normal
1. General appearance		
a. Positioning, comfort	Playing Relaxed posture, without discomfort	Client experiencing pain, coughing or choking, "smothering" feeling (unable to lie flat for extended period)
b. Respirations	Even and deep	Respirations uneven, shallow, gasping Inadequate exchange
c. Skin color	Pink/brown	Cyanosis, grayish pallor Mottling Note color around lips, neck, upper chest
d. Nail color and configuration	Pink 160° angle at nail bed	Cyanotic Clubbing (angle disappears)
2. Anterior chest precordium		
a. Contour	Rounded, symmetrical	Kyphosis Sternal depression Any asymmetry
b. General movement	Even respiratory movements (precordium may lift slightly in thin people)	Areas of bulging, or entire chest heaving or lifting with heartbeat Appearance of thrill across chest wall
3. Inspection and palpation (Child should be sitting and leaning forward.)		
a. Sternoclavicular area pulsations	Slight or absent	Bounding
b. Aortic area (second right intercostal space beside sternum) pulsations	None	Pulsation, thrill (*Note:* Low-frequency vibrations can often be more easily felt than heard.)
c. Pulmonary area (second and third left intercostal spaces near sternum) pulsations	May feel some slight pulsations following physical activity	Thrill or strong pulsations that continue even when patient at rest
d. Right ventricular area (third, fourth, and fifth intercostal spaces to right and left over sternum); note difference from adult	Very thin children may feel slight palpations	Systolic thrill, strong pulsations Heaves
e. Apical area (PMI) (infants and small children: fourth intercostal space to left of midclavicular line; after age 7 years, fifth intercostal space to right of the midclavicular line)		
1. Pulsation	May be present May be difficult to palpate in children under 2 years	
2. Amplitude	Tapping	Thrusting
3. Duration	First third to half systole	Sustained throughout systole

Characteristic or area examined	Normal	Deviations from normal
4. Location	As described	Displaced lateral left or down
5. Diameter	1 to 1.5 cm (⅓ inch)	Over 2 cm (¾ inch)
f. Epigastric area (at sternal angle) pulsations	Aortic pulsation with forward thrust Right ventricular pulsation with downward thrust	Bounding pulsation
g. Ectopic area (space between pulmonary and aortic area) pulsations	None	Outward pulsations
4. Auscultation (child sitting)		
a. Aortic area (location as discussed)		
b. Pulmonary area (location as discussed)		
c. Erb's point (third left intercostal space)		
d. Tricuspid area (fifth interspace near sternum to right in young children; to left in older children)		
e. Apical area (location as discussed)		
1. Rate	As previously discussed	As previously discussed
2. Rhythm	Described under pulses	Described under pulses
3. Pitch	Higher pitch/shorter duration than in adult	
4. S_1 sound		
a. Location	Usually heard at all sites	
b. Intensity	Often louder at apex (Muscle, fat tissue, and air will diminish sound; rapid rate will accentuate sound.)	Accented Diminished (muffled) Varying intensity with different beats (e.g., complete heart block)
c. Frequency	Usually lower in pitch than S_2	Frequency (pitch) becomes higher with accented intensity
d. Timing	Almost synchronous with carotid impulse Slightly longer in duration than S_2	
e. Splitting	May be heard occasionally in tricuspid area Normal S_1 splitting sound usually varies from beat to beat, occasionally a single sound, occasionally a narrow split	S_4 sometimes mistaken for S_1 splitting
5. S_2 sound		
a. Location	Usually heard at all sites May be loudest in pulmonary area	
b. Intensity	Often louder at base Intensity diminished with fat, muscle, or air	Increased intensity, usually in aortic area (e.g., arterial hypertension) or pulmonary area (e.g., pulmonary hypertension) Decreased intensity
c. Frequency	Usually higher in pitch than S_1	
d. Timing	Sound shorter in duration than S_1	
e. Splitting	Commonly heard in pulmonary area (on inspiration) in child Equal quality and intensity of sound	Wide splitting (e.g., right bundle branch block) Fixed splitting Paradoxical splitting (e.g., left bundle branch block) Area of apex
6. Systole		
a. Duration	Shorter than diastole at normal heart rate	
b. Sounds	S_1 sound duration brief; silent interval	Early systolic ejection click: aortic—heard at base and apex pulmonary—heard in pulmonary area Middle and late systolic clicks (e.g., mitral valve deformity) heard at left sternal border Clicks high pitched and sharp in sound

Continued.

ASSESSMENT OF THE HEART AND PRECORDIUM–cont'd

Characteristic or area examined	Normal	Deviations from normal
7. Diastole		
a. Duration	Longer than systole at normal rate	
	Shortens in duration as rate increases	
b. Sounds	S_2 duration brief	
	Silent interval	
8. S_3 sound	May be normal in children (may occur in as many as 30% of all children)	
a. Location	Apex	
b. Intensity	Different intensity from second sound, dull, low in pitch	
c. Timing	Early in diastole	
9. S_4 sound	Never normal	
a. Location		Medial to apex
b. Intensity		Higher pitch
c. Timing		Late diastole (may be confused with split S_1)
		Opening snap: at apex; higher pitch; very early in diastole
10. Other sounds		Pericardial friction rub: scratchy, high pitched, grating sound, unaffected by change in respirations
f. Murmurs	"Innocent" murmurs	"Organic" murmurs
1. Timing	Usually early systolic	Systolic or diastolic at any point during or continuous
2. Location	Second or third intercostal space along left sternal border	
3. Position in which heard	Usually supine	Heard in all positions
4. Duration	Short	Longer
5. Quality	Soft and musical	Louder, blowing, harsh, rumbling
6. Intensity	Soft (grades I, II)	Loud (grades III, IV, V)
7. Affected by exercise	Yes	Constant
5. Repeat palpation and auscultation with child lying and in left decubitus position		

History and clinical strategies associated with the geriatric client

The incidence of cardiovascular disease is higher in elderly individuals than in younger adults. However, the examiner should not assume that all elderly people are suffering from hypertension, cardiac or coronary artery disease, or vascular impairment.

The heart size of an older client who is not hypertensive or manifesting a heart disease often becomes smaller. Cardiac enlargement is usually associated with hypertension or other disease within the heart or vessels.

Cardiac output, at rest, decreases by 30% to 40% by 65 to 70 years of age. However, general organ atrophy and reduced exertion decrease the need for blood flow. Several authors have stated that the aging heart functions well under *normal* conditions but may not be able to respond efficiently to increased circulatory needs associated with extreme stress, blood loss, tachycardia, unusual exertion, or fever.

Although the process of arteriosclerosis advances with age, the amount of circulatory inadequacy at any given age is not predictable. This process may not cause symptoms or signs in many individuals.

Signs or symptoms associated with cardiovascular disease in the elderly are often the same as those manifested in younger adults (Refer to the history portion of the adult cardiovascular section for related questions.)

Following are special needs, concerns, and responses of older adults in relation to cardiovascular problems.

1. Angina pectoris. In some instances, the elderly individual may not experience chest pain to the extent that a younger person does. Dyspnea or palpitation on exertion may be reported as an initial symptom. Chest pain radiation may be reported as a "tightness" in the chest, neck, or shoulder. The pain radiation pattern is usually the same as with younger adults.
2. Confusion or slowed mental function may be an early sign of low cardiac output. Note that confu-

sion (even in mild form) alters the client's ability to provide an accurate account of symptoms.

3. Other early symptoms of cardiac distress are fatigue, light-headedness, or weakness.

4. Explore complaints such as "fatigue," "out of breath," and "tired" carefully. They are sometimes used interchangeably to indicate dyspnea. The precise amount of exertion that precedes the symptom should be described. Note that shortness of breath may indicate many problems other than heart disease. Sedentary elderly people with limited cardiac reserve may complain of breathlessness. Clarify whether shortness of breath interferes with sleep. If insomnia or wakefulness coexists with the dyspnea, clarify the number of times the client awakens each night and exactly what is done to deal with the symptom.

5. Coughing and wheezing may be indicative of heart disease, particularly if the onset is sudden or recent.

6. Dizziness, syncope, palpitations, or transient ischemia attacks may be associated with arrhythmias. Chest pain may accompany these symptoms.

7. Transient ischemial attacks are usually of limited duration (15 to 20 minutes) and are indicated by a variety of symptoms or signs. Dizziness, confusion, unilateral weakness or numbness, and aphasia are some of the complaints. These episodes often leave little or no aftereffects and frequently precede a stroke. Carotid arterial atherosclerosis can contribute to these "attacks." A history of "spells" or "attacks" should be a signal for immediate referral to a physician.

8. A complaint of hemoptysis may be associated with congestive heart failure or a pulmonary embolism.

9. Edema of both legs is often associated with heart disease. Clarify the pattern of swelling with the client in terms of frequency and time of day when it is most pronounced.

10. Weakness, bradycardia, hypotension, and confusion may indicate an excess of potassium, which sometimes occurs in conjunction with therapeutic measures for heart disease.

11. Weakness, fatigue, muscle cramps, and a variety of arrhythmias may be indicative of a low potassium level.

12. Digitalis toxicity may be indicated by anorexia, nausea, vomiting, diarrhea, headache, yellow vision, arrhythmias, or mental confusion.

13. Hypertension. Some authors state that the systolic pressure may normally rise gradually as an individual ages. Other authorities feel that the average systolic pressure is not altered by age. Most authors agree that the diastolic pressure does not change markedly with aging. The Joint National Committee on Detection, Evaluation, and Treatment of High Blood Pressure recommended in 1976 that blood pressures of individuals over 50 years of age in the range of 140/90 to 160/95 be rechecked in 6 to 9 months. The final diagnosis of hypertension is usually based on a number of blood pressure readings taken over a period of weeks or months. An elderly individual's blood pressure may fluctuate widely from one assessment to another (particularly the systolic pressure).

Most of the time, hypertension is asymptomatic. Severe hypertension may produce symptoms of headache (dull, in the morning), memory impairment, visual changes, epistaxis, angina pectoris, and dyspnea on exertion.

One of the major problems associated with hypertension is maintaining client compliancy with prescribed therapy. The following questions might be helpful in assessing the hypertensive client:

a. How much of a problem is hypertension for you in terms of:
  (1) Symptoms
  (2) Interference with activities of daily living
  (3) Taking medications

b. Do you feel the prescribed therapy is effective?

c. Do you have any difficulty with the therapy (e.g., fear of addiction ot drugs, side effects of drugs, false hope that drugs will "cure" the problem, only wishing to take medication when hypertensive symptoms occur)?

d. Have you had any experience with other family members (or close friends) who had hypertension?

14. If the examiner is assessing a client who offers a history of chronic heart or vascular disease, the effects of disability or symptoms, the client's coping skills and state of "chronicity" should be explored. (Review questions in Chapter 1 under activities of daily living assessment and psychological history.) The overall concerns to be covered are:

a. The client's understanding of his health state

b. The client's comprehension of his therapy

c. The client's overall *feelings* about his state of health and the success of the therapy

d. Interference with activities of daily living

e. The client's self-assessment of his and his family's coping ability

15. Risk factors (indicating more rigorous monitoring

or treatment) for borderline hypertensive clients include:

a. Left ventricular hypertrophy
b. Other target organ damage (e.g., kidney, eyes, brain)
c. High serum cholesterol
d. Diabetes mellitus
e. Smoking
f. Family history of hypertension with complications
g. Being a male

16. Risk factors for diagnosed coronary atherosclerosis clients include:

a. Hypertension
b. Obesity (an excess of 30% over ideal weight)
c. Smoking
d. Diabetes mellitus

e. Marked stress factors in life-style
f. Cardiotoxic drugs (e.g., antidepressants, phenothiazines)
g. Inactivity
h. Erratic strenuous exercise

17. *Note:* Some elderly clients have difficulty complying with examiner requests for body positioning or breathing patterns during the physical assessment. It may be impossible for an individual to lie flat for any extended period. It may be difficult to fully exhale and to hold the exhalation for the required period of examiner listening time. The examination may have to proceed more slowly, and the practitioner should be aware of variables contributing to and indicators of client discomfort (e.g., arthritis, emphysema, pulmonary congestion, kyphosis).

Clinical variations associated with the geriatric client

ASSESSMENT OF PRESSURES, PULSES, AND THE PERIPHERAL VASCULAR SYSTEM

Characteristic or area examined	Normal	Deviations from normal
1. Blood pressure (*Note:* For an initial examination the examiner should record blood pressure.)	Normal (adult) upper limits: Systolic—140 mm Hg Diastolic—90 mm Hg Pulse pressure—30 to 40 mm Hg	Low systolic ($\downarrow$ 90) Systolic pressure over 160 mm Hg
a. In both arms while client is lying down **b.** Client standing up during measurement	Some authorities state that maximum systolic pressure of 160 mm Hg may be within normal limits if: 1. It remains stable over period of time 2. Client has no symptoms or evidence of end organ damage 3. Client is checked regularly (every 6 to 9 months)*	Systolic pressure between 140 and 160 mm Hg with accompanying risk factors: 1. Left ventricular hypertrophy 2. Evidence of other end organ damage (e.g., kidneys, eyes, brain) 3. High serum cholesterol 4. Diabetes mellitus 5. Smoking 6. Family history of hypertension with complications 7. Male sex
	Most authorities agree that maximum diastolic pressure level is 90 to 95 mm Hg†	Diastolic pressure exeeding 90 mm Hg Low diastolic ($\downarrow$ 60) Widened pulse pressure (*Note:* Widened pulse pressure is fairly common due to decreased elasticity of aorta.) Narrow pulse pressure
	Pressures in both arms same or do not vary more than 5 to 10 mm Hg systolic	Significant ($\uparrow$ 5 to 10 MM Hg) discrepancy in pressure readings between upper extremities
	On standing, client may manifest drop of maximum of 10 to 15 mm Hg systolic and 5 mm Hg diastolic	Significant decrease of systolic (more than 15 mm Hg) or diastolic (more than 5 mm Hg) and/or symptoms of dizziness
c. Measurement of blood pressure in both legs if pedal, popliteal, and femoral pulses weak or absent	Popliteal artery auscultation reveals systolic pressure 5 to 15 mm Hg higher than brachial artery measurement Diastolic reading same or slightly lower	Systolic pressure lower in leg(s) than in arms

*If pressure is elevated (especially if accompanied by rapid pulse), repeat in 30 minutes.

†A nurse, physician, or agency protocol should be established to determine systolic and diastolic pressures warranting referral. *Note:* Systolic pressure may show a wide variation at different times. Several measurements should be taken (over a period of weeks) to determine accuracy.

Characteristic or area examined	Normal	Deviations from normal
2. Palpation of carotid, radial, femoral, popliteal, dorsalis pedis, and posterior tibial pulses for:		
a. Rate	60 to 90 beats/min (*Note:* The heart normally slows in rate with aging due to increase in vagal tone. Some individuals may normally manifest a rate of 50 beats/min; however, patients with slow heart rates should be referred for further evaluation.)	↑ 90 minute (tachycardia) (*Note:* Recent exertion, smoking, anxiety will elevate pulse.) ↓ 60 minute (bradycardia) (*Note:* Bradycardia and atrial fibrillation two of most common irregularities encountered; associated with "sick sinus syndrome." Often dizziness, syncope, or transient ischemia attacks accompany above signs.)
b. Rhythm	Regular (*Note:* Infrequent ectopic beats fairly common. However, all patients with irregularities should be referred for further evaluation.)	Irregular (without any pattern, e.g., atrial fibrillation) Regularity with occasional pauses or extra beats (e.g., premature contractions) Coupled beats (e.g., bigeminal pulse)*
c. Amplitude and contour	Pulse upstroke often more rapid in older adults Should be smooth and rounded	Upstroke exaggerated or bounding Pulse weak, small, or thready; peak prolonged
d. Amplitude pattern	Series of pulse strokes unvaried in amplitude or contour	
e. Symmetry	All pulses symmetrical (i.e., manifest same rate, rhythm, amplitude, and contour)	Asymmetrical response
(*Note:* If client has a history of hypertension, palpate femoral and brachial arteries at the same time.)	Femoral and brachial pulses occur at approximately same time with equal amplitude	Delayed, diminished femoral pulse (in comparison with brachial pulse)
3. Arterial wall contour and consistency	Arterial wall thickens; loses elasticity with aging, resulting in some increased resistance to compression (*Note:* Dorsalis pedis pulses may be difficult to find or absent in some normal individuals.) (*Note:* Posterior tibial pulses may also be absent or decreased in some normal individuals.)	
a. Conduct following maneuver if arterial insufficiency suspected: 1. With client lying down, elevate legs 30 cm (12 inches) above his heart level 2. Ask client to move feet up and down at ankles for 60 seconds	Extremities (feet) exhibit mild pallor	Marked pallor of (one or both) feet
3. Have client sit up and dangle legs (This maneuver can also be conducted with arms and hands.)	Original color returns in about 10 seconds Veins in feet fill in about 15 seconds	Delayed color return or mottled appearance Delayed venous filling Marked redness of dependent feet
4. Jugular venous pressure (JVP) (client sitting at 30° to 45° angle)	JVP should not rise more than 3 cm above level of sternal angle	JVP exceeds 3 cm above level of manubrium† Note whether other veins in neck, shoulder, and upper chest distended
a. Inspection of jugular pulsations for quality	Regular Soft and undulating Level of pulsation decreases with inspiration Pulsation increases in recumbent position	Fluttering or oscillating Irregular rhythm Unusually prominent waves
5. Inspection and palpation of arms	Distention in dependent position	Distended veins in anteromedial aspect of

*An irregular (rapid or slow) pulse should be palpated simultaneously with auscultation of the apical pulse. Any difference between apical and peripheral pulse rate should be noted. If pulse irregularity is patterned (occurs in repeated sequences), note whether irregularity occurs during (1) inspiration or expiration or (2) systole or diastole.

†If venous pressure is elevated (vein is distended up to neck), raise client's head until highest jugular pulsation can be detected. Record distance in centimeters above sternal angle and angle at which client is reclining.

Continued.

ASSESSMENT OF PRESSURES, PULSES, AND THE PERIPHERAL VASCULAR SYSTEM—cont'd

Characteristic or area examined	Normal	Deviations from normal
and legs for presence and/or appearance of superficial veins	Venous valves may appear as nodular bulges Veins collapse with elevation of limbs (*Note:* Vessels may appear tortuous or distended in elderly clients.)	thigh and lower leg or on posterolateral aspect of calf from knee to ankle
6. Inspection and palpation of thigh and calf for surface characteristics	Legs symmetrical Nontender No excess warmth	Swelling (or one leg, especially calf, appears larger than other) Tenderness on palpation Warmth Redness (*Note:* If swelling is suspected, both thighs and calves should be measured with tape for accuracy.)
a. Sharp dorsiflexion of client's foot (with client's knee slightly flexed) to assess calf pain response	No pain	Pain elicited (Homans sign)
7. Inspection and palpation of extremities for evidence of adequate arterial supply	Absence of hair over digits or dorsum of hands and feet may be normal Skin pink and warm, nonedematous (*Note:* Extremities may feel cool to touch in a cool environment. Loss of subcutaneous fat contributes to increased response to cool environment.)	Reduced or absent peripheral hair (over digits and dorsum of hands and feet) Thin, shiny, taut skin Cold extremities (in warm environment) Mild edema Marked pallor or mottling on elevating extremity Digit tips ulcerated Stocking anesthesia Tenderness on palpation
8. Inspection and palpation of extremities for evidence of venous sufficiency		Peripheral cyanosis Edema (pits on pressure), bilateral or unilateral* Pigmentation around ankles (see Fig. 3-2) Thickening skin Ulceration (especially around ankles)

*Edema should be measured against a bony prominence (over ankle or tibia). Record the following:
1. Type
   a. Pitting
   b. Nonpitting
2. Extent and location
   a. Ankle and foot
   b. Ankle only
   c. Foot to knee, etc.
   d. Hands, fingers
3. Degree of pitting
   a. 0 to 0.6 cm (0 to ¼ inch)—mild
   b. 0.6 to 1.3 cm (¼ to ½ inch)—moderate
   c. 1.3 to 2.5 cm (½ to 1 inch)—severe

ASSESSMENT OF THE HEART AND PRECORDIUM

Characteristic or area examined	Normal	Deviations from normal
1. Observation of general condition while client lying supine or at elevation of 30° to 45°		
a. Positioning, comfort	Relaxed posture, without discomfort	Client experiencing pain, coughing or choking, "smothering" feeling (unable to lie flat for extended period)
b. Respirations	Even and deep	Respirations uneven, shallow, gasping Inadequate exchange
c. Skin color	Pink/brown	Cyanosis, grayish pallor

Characteristic or area examined	Normal	Deviations from normal
		Mottling
		Note color around lips, neck, upper chest
d. Nail Color and configuration	Pink	Cyanotic
	160° angle at nail bed	Clubbing (angle disappears)
2. Inspection and palpation of anterior chest		
a. Precordium		
1. Contour	Kyphosis and scoliosis fairly common in elderly people; may distort normal rounded symmetrical contour and contribute to heart displacement	All asymmetry should be noted in summary
2. General movement	Even respiratory movements (precordium may lift slightly in thin people)	Entire chest heaving or lifting with heartbeat
3. Inspection and palpation of following areas:		
a. Sternoclavicular area pulsations	Slight or absent	Bounding
b. Aortic area (right second intercostal space adjacent to sternum) pulsations	None	Pulsation, thrill (*Note:* Low-frequency vibrations can often be more easily felt than heard.)
c. Pulmonary area (left second intercostal space adjacent to sternum) pulsations	None	Pulsation, thrill
d. Right ventricular area (left and right fifth intercostal space close to sternum) heave or lift	May be present in hyperkinetic, thin adults	Diffuse lift or heave, pulsations
e. Apical area (left fifth intercostal space 5 to 7 cm [2 to 2¾ inches] from midsternal line) for:		
1. Pulsation	May be present	
2. Amplitude	Tapping	Thrusting
3. Duration	First third to half systole	Sustained throughout systole
4. Location	Fourth or fifth intercostal space, 5 to 7 cm from midclavicular line*	Displaced left lateral or down
5. Diameter	1 to 2 cm	Over 2 cm
f. Epigastric area (slide fingers up under rib cage) pulsations	Aortic pulsation with forward thrust	Bounding pulsation
	Right ventricular pulsation with downward thrust	
g. Ectopic area (midway between pulmonary and apical areas) pulsations	None	Outward pulsation
4. Auscultation of following specific areas:		
a. Aortic area (second right interspace)		
b. Pulmonary area (second left interspace)		
c. Erb's point (third left interspace)		
d. Tricuspid area (fifth left interspace near sternum)		
e. Apical area (fifth left interspace medial to midclavicular line) for:		
1. Rate	60 to 90 beats/min (*Note:* The heart normally slows in rate with aging due to increase in vagal tone.) Some individuals may normally manifest rate of 50 beats/min; however, patients with	Over 90 Under 60

Note: Apical pulse location may displace slightly laterally if client turns to left side.

Continued.

ASSESSMENT OF THE HEART AND PRECORDIUM–cont'd

Characteristic or area examined	Normal	Deviations from normal
	slow heart rates should be referred for further evaluation	
2. Rhythm	Regular (*Note:* Infrequent ecoptic beats are fairly common with aging. However, all patients with irregularities should be referred.)	Irregular (without any pattern) Sporadic extra beats or pauses
3. S_1 sound a. Location	Usually heard at all sites	
b. Intensity	Often louder at apex (muscle, fat tissue, and air will diminish sound; rapid rate will accentuate sound)	Accented Diminished (muffled) Varying intensity with different beats (e.g., complete heart block)
c. Frequency	Usually lower in pitch than S_2	Frequency (pitch) becomes higher with accented intensity
d. Timing	Almost synchronous with carotid impulse Slightly longer in duration than S_2	
e. Splitting	May be heard in tricuspid area (normal S, splitting sound usually varies from beat to beat: occasionally single sound, occasionally narrow split)	S_4 sometimes mistaken for S_1 splitting
4. S_2 sound a. Location	Usually heard at all sites	
b. Intensity	Often louder at base (intensity diminished with fat, muscle, or air)	Increased intensity, usually in aortic area (e.g., arterial hypertension) or pulmonary area (e.g., pulmonary hypertension) Decreased intensity
c. Frequency	Usually higher in pitch than S_1	
d. Timing	Sound shorter in duration than S_1	
e. Splitting	Occasionally heard in pulmonary area (on inspiration)	Wide splitting (e.g., right bundle branch block) Fixed splitting Paradoxical splitting (e.g., left bundle branch block)
5. Systole a. Duration	Shorter than diastole at normal heart rate (60 to 90 beats/min)	

b. Sounds	S_1 sound duration brief, silent interval	Early systolic ejection click:
		  aortic—heard at base and apex
		  pulmonary—heard in pulmonary area
		Middle and late systolic clicks (e.g., mitral valve deformity) heard at left sternal border
		Clicks high pitched and sharp in sound

6. Diastole a. Duration	Longer than systole at normal rate (60 to 90) Shortens in duration as rate increases	
b. Sounds	S_2 duration brief Silent interval	
(1) S_3	Absent	May signify heart failure
(2) Location		At apex
(3) Intensity		Dull, low pitched
(4) Timing		Early in diastole (best heard when client in left lateral decubitus position, with bell of stethoscope)
(5) S_4	Absent (*Note:* Some authorities state that S_4 sounds are fairly common in the elderly and may just indicate decreased left ventricular compliance. However, all patients with extra sounds should be referred for evaluation.)	May indicate left ventricular hypertrophy or myocardial ischemia
(6) Location		Usually at apex or medial to apex

Characteristic or area examined	Normal	Deviations from normal
(7) Intensity		Slightly higher in pitch than S$_3$
(8) Timing		Late diastole (may be confused with split S$_1$)
		Best heard when client in left lateral decubitus position, with bell
c. Other sounds	None	Opening snap: At apex or left sternal border; higher pitch; very early in diastole
7. Murmurs		
a. Systolic	Most authorities agree that soft, early systolic murmurs may be "functional" in elderly client; commonly found, and due to aortic lengthening, tortuosity, and sclerotic changes	Loud aortic (ejection) murmurs that radiate into the neck may indicte obstructive aortic disease
	Best heard in aortic area or at base of heart; however, all patients with murmurs should be referred for further evaluation	Systolic murmurs heard at apex may indicate mitral calcification
b. Diastolic	Diastolic murmurs always abnormal	
c. Timing		Systolic—early, middle, late, continuous
		Diastolic—early, middle, late, continuous
d. Location		Area where sound heard may be small and confined or may cover most of precordium (Describe in terms of precordial landmarks and distance in centimeters from landmarks.)
e. Radiation of sound		(Describe in terms of landmarks and distance in centimeters.)
f. Intensity		Loud, medium, soft or grades I through VI
		Stable, or varies with respiration or position
g. Pitch		High, medium, low
h. Quality		Blowing, harsh, rumbling
		Crescendo
		Decrescendo
8. Other sounds		Pericardial friction rub: to-and-fro rubbing sound, usually heard during systole and diastole; sound usually increased when client sits up and leans forward

5. Repeat palpation and auscultation maneuvers with client (a) lying in left decubitus position and (b) sitting

Vocabulary

1. Anacrotic

2. Angina pectoris

3. Atherosclerosis

4. Apex

5. Arteriosclerosis

6. Atrial fibrillation

7. Atrial flutter

8. Auscultatory gap

9. Base (cardiac)

10. Bradycardia

11. Bruit

12. Circadian

13. Claudication

14. Coarctation

15. Depolarization

16. Diastolic

17. Dicrotic

18. Ectopic

19. Embolism

20. Heave (lift)

21. Holosystolic (pansystolic)

22. Homans sign

23. Hyperkinetic

24. Hypovolemic

25. Ischemia

26. Isovolumic (contraction)

27. "Inching"

28. Korotkoff sounds

29. Mediastinum

30. Palpitation

31. Pericardium

32. Point of maximum impulse (PMI)

33. Precordium

34. Protodiastolic

35. Pulse pressure

36. Pulsus alternans

37. Pulsus bigeminus

38. Pulsus paradoxus

39. Repolarization

40. Systole

41. Tachycardia

42. Thrombophlebitis

43. Thrombosis

44. Thrill

45. Valsalva maneuver

Cognitive self-assessment

1. Which of the following statements are true about Korotkoff sounds?
   - ☐ a. At phase one the arterial intraluminal pressure is the same as the cuff pressure.
   - ☐ b. At phase two the sounds are replaced by a bruit.
   - ☐ c. Systolic pressure is recorded at the beginning of phase two.
   - ☐ d. Muffling of the sounds (phase four) is thought by many authorities to be the most accurate indicator of diastolic pressure.
   - ☐ e. The second diastolic pressure is recorded when Korotkoff sounds are no longer heard.
   - ☐ f. c, d, and e
   - ☐ g. All the above
   - ☑ h. All except c
   - ☐ i. All except b
   - ☐ j. b and d

2. Which of the following statements are true about arterial blood pressure?
   - ☐ a. A difference of 5 to 10 mm Hg systolic pressure between arms is within normal limits.
   - ☐ b. The systolic pressure in the upper extremities is usually about 10 mm Hg higher than in the lower extremities.
   - ☐ c. A narrow cuff on an obese arm will yield a false low value.
   - ☐ d. Standing might lower the systolic pressure by 10 to 15 mm Hg in a healthy individual.
   - ☐ e. A wide cuff on a very small arm will yield a false low value.
   - ☐ f. a, b, and e
   - ☐ g. a, c, and d
   - ☐ h. All except c
   - ☑ i. a, d, and e
   - ☐ j. a, b, and c

3. Identify the variables that might alter a healthy client's blood pressure.
   - ☐ a. Age, sex, and weight
   - ☐ b. Circadian rhythm
   - ☐ c. Stress or anxiety
   - ☐ d. Food intake
   - ☐ e. Cuff/arm ratio
   - ☐ f. a, c, and e
   - ☑ g. All the above
   - ☐ h. All except b
   - ☐ i. All except d

4. You are auscultating Mrs. Jones' arterial blood pressure and hear a tapping sound at 210 mm Hg that continues until the mercury reaches 195. Then there is silence until the mercury reaches 185, at which time the tapping resumes and gradually intensifies. At 140, the loud, sharp sounds become muffled. At 110, the sounds disappear. How would you record this pressure?
   - ☐ a. 210/140
   - ☐ b. 210/110
   - ☐ c. 210/185/140
   - ☐ d. 195/185/110
   - ☑ e. 210/140/110

5. Which statement(s) is/are true about Mrs. Jones' blood pressure?
   - ☑ a. She has a wide pulse pressure.
   - ☐ b. She has a narrow pulse pressure.
   - ☑ c. She manifests an auscultatory gap.

    ☑ d. At 140 mm Hg the cuff pressure first fell below the arterial intraluminal pressure.

    ☐ e. At 110 mm Hg the cuff pressure first fell below the arterial intraluminal pressure.

    ☑ f. a, c, and d

    ☐ g. b, c, and d

    ☐ h. a, c, and e

    ☐ i. b and e

6. Identify the *true* statements about the following types of arterial pulses.

    ☐ a. Anxiety can create a bounding pulse.

    ☐ b. Aortic rigidity and atherosclerosis can create a bounding pulse.

    ☐ c. Obstructive lung disease can cause a paradoxical pulse.

    ☐ d. Pulsus alternans is evidence of left-sided heart failure.

    ☐ e. The normal pulse contour is smooth and rounded.

    ☐ f. a and d

    ☐ g. a, c, and e

    ☐ h. b and c

    ☑ i. All the above

    ☐ j. a, b, and e

7. Bates describes the differences between carotid and jugular pulsations. Which of the following statements are true about carotid pulsations?

    ☐ a. They are rarely palpable.

    ☐ b. Pulsation is not affected by inspiration.

    ☐ c. Pulsation is not affected by position.

    ☐ d. Pulsation usually increases in a recumbent position.

    ☐ e. Soft, undulating quality with two or three outward thrust components.

    ☐ f. b, d, and e

    ☑ g. b and c

    ☐ h. b and d

    ☐ i. a and d

    ☐ j. All except d

8. Which statement(s) is/are true about the jugular veins and jugular venous pressure?

    ☐ a. The internal jugular vein connects, without valves, to the right atrium.

    ☐ b. Jugular pulsation can usually be obliterated by moderate pressure at the scapular base of the neck.

    ☐ c. Neck veins frequently distend when a healthy client is in a supine position.

    ☐ d. The sternal angle is the common reference point for measuring jugular venous pressure.

    ☐ e. Pregnancy usually increases jugular venous pressure.

    ☑ f. All the above

    ☐ g. All except e

    ☐ h. b and d

    ☐ i. a, b, and c

9. Mr. Jones' feet are cool to touch. You have asked him to elevate both legs about 30 cm (12 inches) above his body for approximately 60 seconds. Both feet manifest a mild pallor. Then you ask him to sit up and dangle his legs. His normal (pink) skin color returns to his toes in about 15 seconds. Which statement(s) is/are true about what you have observed?

    ☐ a. Venous insufficiency should be suspected.

    ☐ b. Arterial insufficiency should be suspected.

- ☑ c. The results are within normal limits.
- ☑ d. The leg-raising drained the feet of most of the venous blood.
- ☐ e. The leg-raising drained the feet of most of the arterial blood.
- ☑ f. c and d
- ☐ g. a and d
- ☐ h. b and d
- ☐ i. c and e
- ☐ j. None of the above

10. Which statement(s) is/are true about varicosities in the legs?
    - ☐ a. Varicose means "dilated, swollen."
    - ☐ b. Varicosities can result from proximal obstruction in the pelvic vein.
    - ☐ c. Varicosities can result from inherent weakness in the saphenous vessel wall.
    - ☐ d. The great and small saphenous veins may both be involved.
    - ☐ e. The valves in the communicating veins between superficial and deep veins may be incompetent.
    - ☐ f. a, b, and d
    - ☐ g. c and e
    - ☐ h. a and c
    - ☑ i. All the above
    - ☐ j. All except d

11. Which of the following statements is/are true about the heart?
    - ☐ a. The heart lies within the mediastinum.
    - ☐ b. The base of the heart is normally found in the fifth intercostal space.
    - ☐ c. Most of the anterior cardiac surface consists of the right ventricle.
    - ☐ d. The left ventricle makes up a small portion of the anterior cardiac surface.
    - ☐ e. In a normal, average individual two thirds of the heart lies to the left of the midsternal line.
    - ☐ f. All the above
    - ☑ g. All except b
    - ☐ h. All except c
    - ☐ i. a, c, and d

12. Which of the following statement(s) is/are true?
    - ☐ a. Low-frequency vibration sounds might be palpated more easily than they can be auscultated.
    - ☐ b. A fever could create a palpable right ventricular impulse.
    - ☐ c. When the client rolls to the left side, the apical impulse is laterally displaced.
    - ☐ d. The normal apical impulse is palpated in an area 3 to 4 cm in diameter.
    - ☐ e. The normal apical impulse is sustained during the first third to half of systole.
    - ☐ f. a, c, and e
    - ☐ g. c, d, and e
    - ☐ h. All except e
    - ☐ i. b and c
    - ☑ j. All except d

13. Which of the following conditions would *not* produce right ventricular heave?
    - ☐ a. Anxiety

☐ b. Pulmonary stenosis
☐ c. Pregnancy
☒ d. Aortic stenosis
☐ e. Anemia

14. Which of the following statement(s) is/are true?
    ☐ a. When auscultating the heart, most low-pitched sounds are diastolic filling sounds or murmurs.
    ☐ b. Low-pitched sounds are often best heard when the client is supine.
    ☐ c. Auscultation should be performed using both the bell and the diaphragm.
    ☐ d. Loudness, quality and pitch of a sound may vary with the age and build of a client.
    ☐ e. Auscultation is performed only when the client is lying down.
    ☒ f. All except e
    ☐ g. All the above
    ☐ h. All except b
    ☐ i. All except a
    ☐ j. c and d

15. Which of the following statement(s) is/are true?
    ☐ a. Heart murmurs are of longer duration than heart sounds.
    ☐ b. Heart murmurs originate within the heart itself.
    ☐ c. Heart murmurs originate within the great vessels.
    ☐ d. Most "innocent" murmurs are faint or under grade 3 intensity.
    ☐ e. "Innocent" murmurs are usually soft ejection murmurs.
    ☐ f. a, b, and d
    ☐ g. All except e
    ☒ h. All the above
    ☐ i. a, c, and d

16. Which of the following statement(s) is/are true?
    ☐ a. Aortic regurgitation causes a diastolic murmur.
    ☐ b. Pulmonic regurgitation causes a diastolic murmur.
    ☐ c. Mitral stenosis causes a diastolic murmur.
    ☐ d. Tricuspid stenosis causes a diastolic murmur.
    ☐ e. a and b
    ☐ f. None of the above
    ☒ g. All the above
    ☐ h. c and d

17. A systolic ejection murmur occurs:
    ☐ a. at the mitral or tricuspid valves
    ☒ b. at the pulmonary or aortic valves

18. A systolic regurgitant murmur occurs:
    ☒ a. at the mitral or tricuspid valves
    ☐ b. at the pulmonary or aortic valves

Identify the characteristics of an arterial pulse that an examiner notes when palpating (as identified in the course clinical guidelines), beginning with:

Rate
Rhythm
19. _amplitude + contour_
20. _amplitude pattern_
21. _symmetry_
22. _wall contour/consistency_

23. Label the cardiac chambers, valves, and vessels as shown in the accompanying illustration.

a. _sup vena cava_
b. _if.   "   "_
c. _® atrium_
d. _tricuspid_
e. _R V_
f. _pulmonic_
g. _pulmonic veins artery_

h. _pulmonic veins_
i. _aorta_
j. _L A_
k. _mitral aortic_
l. _tr mitral_
m. _LV_

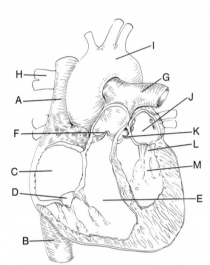

24. The first heart sound is due to closure of _mitral_ and _tricuspid_ valves. It occurs at the beginning of: Systole? Diastole?

25. The second sound results from _aorta_ and _pulmonic_ valve closure. It occurs at the beginning of: Systole? Diastole?

Each statement describes a sign related to chronic venous insufficiency (CVI) or chronic arterial insufficiency (CAI). Fill in the blanks with either CVI or CAI.

26. _A_ Extremity pulse diminished or absent
27. _A_ Extremity cool
28. _V_ Pigmentation and/or ulceration around ankles
29. _A_ Loss of hair over foot and toes
30. _V_ Marked pedal edema (with pitting)
31. _A_ Extremity turns "dusky red" in dangling (dependent) position
32. _A_ Thin, shiny, taut skin (over extremity)

The following statements describe characteristics of the first heart sound (S_1) or the second heart sound (S_2). Assign a (S_1) or b (S_2) to each statement.

33. _a_ Usually sounds louder at the apex of the heart.
34. _b_ Splitting heard near the pulmonary area.
35. _b_ Slightly higher frequency than the other sound.
36. _a_ Almost synchronous with carotid impulse.
37. _b_ Splitting heard in the tricuspid area.
38. _a_ Exercise shortens the P-R interval and results in a louder sound.
39. _b_ A right bundle branch block causes delay of pulmonary valve closure and results in splitting.

The following statements describe characteristics of the third heart sound (S_3) or the fourth heart sound (S_4). Assign a (S_3) or b (S_4) to each statement.

40. __a__ The sound originates in early diastolic rapid ventricular filling and wall vibration.
41. __b__ The sound originates in late diastole rapid ventricular filling.
42. __b__ Known as a presystolic gallop.
43. __a__ Known as a protodiastolic gallop.
44. __a__ Very commonly heard in normal children and young adults.
45. __a__ Often signifies myocardial failure in older adults.

Match the sounds in column B with the locations in column A (as shown on the accompanying illustration) where they can best be heard.

Column A	*Column B*
46. __d__ Aortic area	a. S^1—mitral valve closure
47. __c__ Pulmonary area	b. Aortic and pulmonary murmurs
48. __b__ Erb's point (or third left intercostal space)	c. S^2 splitting
49. __e__ Tricuspid area	d. Aortic stenosis—sound of hypertension
50. __a__ Apical area	e. Split S^1, ventricular septal defect

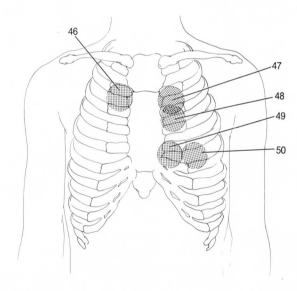

PEDIATRIC QUESTIONS

51. When examining 5-year-old John M., the examiner identifies the following findings:

    History: healthy child
    Pulse: 88 regular
    BP: 102/52
    Peripheral circulation good
    Heart sounds S_1, S_2 regular
    Extra sound consistently heard just following S_2 sound (split? S_3?)

    Murmur identified in systole; child was sitting; had soft short sound; remained audible following 30-second jumping exercise

    The examiner should:

    ☐ a. record the finding as a probable functional murmur and recheck the child in 8 weeks

   ☐ b. consider the cardiovascular examination normal; reevaluate child at next regularly scheduled well-child visit

   ☐ c. send the child *immediately* to the physician for further evaluation

   ☐ d. schedule the child for an ECG and stress test

   ☑ e. send the child for physician evaluation fairly soon, at a time convenient for both parties

52. Steven is a 7-year-old black boy. During his examination the nurse evaluates his pulse and blood pressure, which were normal. Which of the following readings would it have been?

   ☐ a. BP 94/40; pulse 88

   ☐ b. BP 128/72; pulse 84

   ☐ c. BP 112/78; pulse 74

   ☑ d. BP 102/48; pulse 102

   ☐ e. BP 120/62; pulse 94

53. At which of the following ages should routine blood pressure screening be initiated?

   ☑ a. 18 months

   ☐ b. 3 years

   ☐ c. 5 years

   ☐ d. 6 years

   ☐ e. 10 years

54. When auscultating the chest of a 4-year-old healthy child, all the following signs may be considered *normal* except one. Identify the abnormal finding.

   ☐ a. Sinus arrhythmia

   ☐ b. Single PVC

   ☐ c. S_1 split

   ☐ d. S_3 sound

   ☑ e. S_4 sound

GERIATRIC QUESTIONS

55. In elderly people, cardiac output:

   ☐ a. decreases by 30% to 40% over a 40- to 50-year span

   ☐ b. is the same as in younger adults unless there is disease present

   ☐ c. may not respond adequately during severe stress

   ☐ d. may not respond adequately to tachycardia

   ☐ e. increases due to normal left ventricular enlargement and increasing peripheral resistance

   ☐ f. none of the above

   ☐ g. d and e

   ☑ h. a, c, and d

56. Pulses in geriatric clients:

   ☑ a. may normally be slower than the average pulse of adults

   ☐ b. are normally irregular and rapid

   ☐ c. are normally irregular and slow

   ☐ d. are less symmetrical in timing and amplitude than younger adult pulses

57. The systolic pressure in an older individual:

   ☐ a. may be slightly higher because elderly people are often more excitable

   ☑ b. may be slightly higher than the young adult because of elasticity changes in the large arteries

   ☐ c. may be slightly lower than in the young adult because of loss of subcutaneous fat

☐ d. is within 5 to 10 mm Hg of 120 range unless the client is hypertensive

SUGGESTED READINGS
General

Bates, Barbara: A guide to physical examination, ed. 2, Philadelphia, 1979, J. B. Lippincott Co., pp. 139-185, 257-271.

Judge, Richard D., and Zuidema, George, editors: Methods of clinical examination: a physiologic approach, Boston, 1974, Little, Brown & Co., pp. 141-199.

Malasanos, Lois, Barkauskas, Violet, Moss, Muriel, and Stoltenberg-Allen, Kathryn: Health assessment, St. Louis, 1977, The C. V. Mosby Co., pp. 216-237.

Nordmark, Madelyn T., and Rohweder, Ann W.: Scientific foundations of nursing, ed. 3, Philadelphia, 1975, J. B. Lippincott Co., pp. 15-52.

Prior, John A., and Silberstein, Jack S.: Physical diagnosis: the history and examination of the patient, ed. 5, St. Louis, 1977, The C. V. Mosby Co., pp. 239-297.

Walker, H. Kenneth, Hall, W. Dallas, and Hurst, J. Willis: Clinical methods: the history, physical and laboratory examinations, Boston, 1976, Butterworth, Inc., pp. 154-196.

American Journal of Nursing: Programmed Instruction, Correcting common errors in blood pressure measurement, **65**:10, 1965.

American Journal of Nursing: Programmed Instruction, Patient assessment: examination of the heart and great vessels. Part I, **76**:11, 1976.

American Journal of Nursing: Programmed Instruction, Patient Assessment: auscultation of the heart. Part II, **77**:2, 1977.

American Journal of Nursing: Programmed Instruction, Patient assessment: Abnormalities of the heartbeat, **77**:4, 1977.

American Journal of Nursing: Programmed Instruction, Patient assessment: pulses, **79**:1, 1979.

Kirkendall, W. M., Burton, A. C., Epstein, F. H., and Fries, E. D.: Recommendations for human blood pressure determination by sphygniomanometers, New York, 1967, American Heart Association.

Audiovisual materials

Blue Hill Educational Systems, Inc. (videotape cassettes), New York, 1976.
Tape 12A. Cardiovascular system: Peripheral circulation (1 hr)
Tape 12B. Cardiovascular system: The heart (1 hr)
Tape 12C. Cardiovascular system: The heart (1 hr)
Tape 12D. Cardiovascular system: The heart (½ hr)
Concept Media Filmstrips: Physical assessment: heart and lungs, Costa Mesa, Calif., 1976.
Tape 5: Initial assessment of the heart
Tape 6: Auscultation of heart sounds
Warner-Chilcott Laboratory, AEGIS Production: Differential diagnosis of chest pain, New York, 1967, American Heart Association.

Pediatric

Alexander, Mary, and Brown, Marie: Pediatric physical diagnosis for nurses, New York, 1974, McGraw-Hill Book Co., pp. 131-148.

Barness, Lewis: Manual of pediatric physical diagnosis, ed. 4, Chicago, 1972, Year Book Medical Publishers, Inc., pp. 110-123.

Brown, Marie Scott, and Alexander, Mary: Physical examination. Part II. Examining the heart, Nursing '74 **4**(12):41-47, 1974.

Haggerty, R. J., Maroney, M. W., and Nadas, A. S.: Essential hypertension in infancy and childhood, Am. J. Dis. Child. **92**:536, 1956.

Johnson, T. R., Moore, W. M., and Jeffries, J. E., editors: Children are different: developmental physiology, ed. 2, Columbus, Ohio, 1978, Ross Laboratories, pp. 136-141.

Malasanos, Lois, Barkauskas, Violet, Moss, Muriel, and Stoltenberg-Allen, Kathryn: Health assessment, St. Louis, 1977, The C. V. Mosby Co., pp. 429-431.

Pillitteri, Adele: Nursing care of the growing family, Boston, 1977, Little, Brown and Co., pp. 551-556.

Prior, John A., and Silberstein, Jack S.: Physical diagnosis: the history and examination of the patient, ed. 5, St. Louis, 1977, The C. V. Mosby Co., pp. 464-466.

Geriatric

Babu, Thota N., Nazir, Farooq, Rao, Dodda, and Luisada, Aldo A.: What is "normal" blood pressure in the aged? Geriatrics **32**(1):73-76, Jan., 1977.

Caird, F. I., and Judge, T. G.: Assessment of the elderly patient, London, 1977, Pitman Medical Publishing Co. Ltd., pp. 31-39.

Chinn, Austin B., editor: Clinical aspects of aging, Working with older people: a guide to practice, vol. 4, Rockville, Md., 1971, U.S. Department of Health, Education, and Welfare, Public Health Service, pp. 81-112.

Foster, Sue, and Kousch, Deborah C.: Controlling high blood pressure: promoting patient adherence, Am. J. Nurs. **78**(5):829-832, May, 1978.

Harris, Raymond: Cardiopathy of aging: are the changes related to congestive heart failure? Geriatrics **32**(2):42-46, Feb., 1977.

Luisada, Aldo A.: Using noninvasive methods to study the aging heart, Geriatrics **32**(2):58-61, Feb., 1977.

Malasanos, Lois, Barkauskas, Violet, Moss, Muriel, and Stoltenberg-Allen, Kathryn: Health assessment, St. Louis, 1977, The C. V. Mosby Co., pp. 440-441.

Mead, William F.: The aging heart, Am. Fam. Phys. **18**(2):73-80, Aug., 1978.

Steinberg, Franz U., editor: Cowdry's the care of the geriatric patient, St. Louis, 1976, The C. V. Mosby Co., pp. 66-78.

Ward, Graham W., Bandy, Patricia, and Fink, Janis W.: Controlling high blood pressure: treating and counseling the hypertensive patient, Am. J. Nurs. **78**(5):824-828, May, 1978.

CHAPTER **10**

Assessment of the breasts

Cognitive objectives

At the end of this unit the learner will demonstrate knowledge of assessment of the breasts by the ability to do the following:

1. Identify the lymphatic system associated with the breasts and discuss lymphatic drainage patterns.
2. List inspection criteria associated with the examination of the breasts.
3. List palpation criteria associated with the examination of the breasts.
4. Identify client positions for examination of the breasts.
5. Describe selected signs and/or symptoms that would warrant physician referral or further investigation.
6. List instruction techniques associated with breast self-examination.
7. Identify the appropriate times of the month for women to perform breast self-examination.
8. Identify maturational variations associated with the breasts and their assessment.
9. Identify selected variations for pediatric and geriatric clients.
10. Define the terms in the vocabulary section.

Clinical objectives

At the end of this unit the learner will perform a systematic assessment of the breasts, demonstrating the ability to do the following:

1. Obtain a pertinent health history from the client.
2. Demonstrate and record results of inspection of the breasts while the client is seated and lying down. This assessment should include:
   a. General breast assessment
      (1) Size
      (2) Symmetry
      (3) Contour
      (4) Appearance of skin (color, texture, venous patterns)
      (5) Moles or nevi
   b. Areolar area
      (1) Size
      (2) Shape
      (3) Surface characteristics
   c. Nipples
      (1) Direction
      (2) Size and shape
      (3) Color
      (4) Surface characteristics
      (5) Discharge
3. Demonstrate and record results of palpation of the breasts while the client is seated and lying down, including:
   a. General breast assessment
      (1) Firmness
      (2) Tissue qualities
   b. Nipples
      (1) Elasticity
      (2) Tissue qualities
      (3) Discharge
   c. Lymphatic assessment
      (1) Supraclavicular and infraclavicular nodes
      (2) Central and lateral axillary nodes
      (3) Pectoral, scapular, and subscapular nodes
      (4) Brachial, intermediate, and internal mammary nodal chains
4. Demonstrate and record appropriate inspection and palpation of the male breasts.
5. Demonstrate instructional techniques and rationale in teaching self-examination of the breasts.

Health history related to assessment of the breasts additional to screening history

1. By synthesizing historical data, genetic factors, and information about exposure to carcinogenic agents, compile a risk profile for the client. Table 5 shows the assessment criteria that will help to develop a breast cancer risk profile for women living in the United States. Use these data to

Table 5. Assessment criteria for development of a breast cancer risk profile*

Questions for client	High-risk criteria	Low-risk criteria
Age	Women over 40 years of age	Women under 25 years of age
Race	White: affluent black	Low-income whites; low-income blacks
Ethnic ancestry	Northern European, Jewish	Latin or Mediterranean ancestry; American Indians, Orientals
Income (high, medium, low)	High and middle income	Lower incomes
Home location past 10 years (city, town, rural community)	Large cities, industrial cities, especially in Northeast	Medium cities, small towns, rural
Breast cancer in family that occurred prior to menopause (inquire about mother, sisters, maternal grandmother, maternal aunts, maternal first cousins)	Positive response to any of these if they occurred prior to menopause	Negative response to any of these; positive response if it occurred after menopause
Menarche and menopause history: early, late	Early menstruation, late menopause	Late menstruation, early menopause
History of breast abnormalities (may include fibrocystic diseases, adenomas, mastitis, breast abscesses, or breast injury)	Positive response to any items listed or other abnormalities	Negative response to any items listed
Diet history: whether it is high in animal proteins and fats or high in vegetable consumption and low in animal proteins and fats; caffeine	Diets high in animal proteins and/or animal fats. High consumption of caffeine	Diets mostly vegetarian or low in animal proteins and/or animal fats (e.g., Seventh Day Adventists). Low consumption of caffeine
Reproductive and sexual histories	Late beginning of sexual activity. No history of sexual activity	Early beginning of sexual activity
Children	No children	Has had children
Breast-fed children	No breast-feeding	Has breast-fed children
Age when children were born	Delivered first child after age 35 years	Delivered first child before age 20 years

*Adapted from Kushner, R.: Breast cancer risks for U.S. women. In Martin, L. L.: Health care of women, Philadelphia, 1978, J. B. Lippincott Co., p. 331.

develop a profile for *every* female client assessed. If the examiner determines that the client has a basically high-risk profile, then thorough examination, breast self-examination instruction techniques, and regular reevaluation periods become vitally important.

2. If the client has a symptomatic complaint of the breasts such as pain, tenderness, a lump, nipple discharge, skin rashes, or changes in the size or shape of the breasts, a thorough investigation must be made. In addition to the steps stated in the symptom analysis section, the following questions should be asked:
   a. How long has the lump or thickening been present?
   b. Have there been recent changes in the breasts' characteristics, such as pain, tenderness, size, shape, overlying skin characteristics? Describe.
   c. If there is pain, is it described as stinging, pulling, burning, or drawing?
   d. Is the pain unilateral or bilateral?
   e. Is the pain or discomfort localized or does it spread?

   f. Does the lump or discomfort change in size or character with menses?
   g. Has the client been involved in any strenuous activity that could contribute to the breast discomfort?
   h. Does client complain of nipple discharge? If so, inquire about:
      (1) Duration of problem
      (2) Drainage characteristics, including color, consistency, odor, amount
      (3) Times of presence (always, prior to menses, other)
      (4) Drug therapy such as oral contraceptives, phenothiazines, digitalis, diuretics, or steroids
   i. Continued questioning should include items from the risk profile assessment criteria in Table 5.

3. Does the client examine her own breasts regularly? Has she been taught the breast self-examination? At what part of the month does she examine her breasts? Have client explain the technique she uses.

Clinical guidelines

ASSESSMENT OF THE FEMALE BREASTS

The student will:	To identify:	
	Normal	Deviations from normal

1. Instruct client to *sit* comfortably and erect on side of cart; *arms should be at side;* gown should be around waist so that the breasts may be fully evaluated (Fig. 10-1)

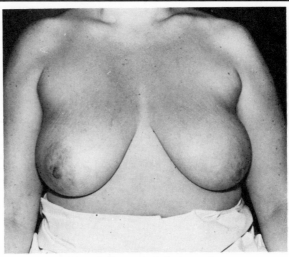

Fig. 10-1. Breasts ready for inspection.

2. Inspect and bilaterally compare:		
a. Breasts		
1. Size	Varies	
2. Symmetry	Bilaterally equal Slight asymmetry (Fig. 10-2)	Recent unilateral increase in size, marked asymmetry

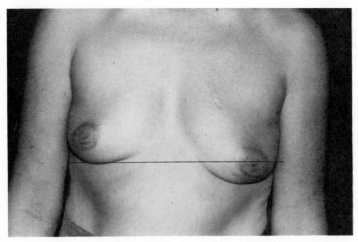

Fig. 10-2. Breast asymmetry.

3. Contour	Smooth, convex, even pattern	Dimpling, retraction Interruption of convex pattern Fixation
4. Skin color	Even throughout	Hyperpigmentation Erythema

The student will:	To identify:	
	Normal	**Deviations from normal**
5. Skin texture	Smooth, elastic, movable, striae	Thickened, rough Lesions or thickening Edema (peau d'orange) (Fig. 10-3)

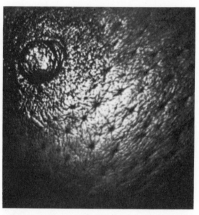

Fig. 10-3. Peau d'orange. (From Gallagher, S. G., Leis, H. P., Jr., Snyderman, R. K., and Urban, J. A., editors: The breast, St. Louis, 1978, The C. V. Mosby Co.)

6. Venous patterns	Bilaterally similar	Localized, unilateral increase in vascular pattern
7. Moles, nevi	Long history of presence Nonchanging Nontender	Newly developed or changed Tender
b. Areolar area		
1. Size	Bilaterally equal	Unequal
2. Shape	Round or oval	Other than round or oval
3. Surface characteristics	Smooth, bilaterally similar, Montgomery tubercles (Fig. 10-4)	Masses, lesions Color pigment changes Unilateral pigment change

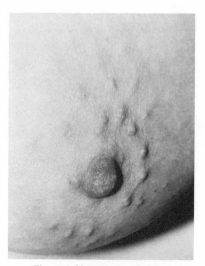

Fig. 10-4. Montgomery tubercles.

Continued.

Clinical guidelines—cont'd

ASSESSMENT OF THE FEMALE BREASTS—cont'd

The student will:	To identify:	
	Normal	**Deviations from normal**
c. Nipples 1. Direction	Bilaterally equal in pointing direction (Fig. 10-5, *A*) Supernumerary nipples	Asymmetrical deviations (Fig. 10-5, *B*)

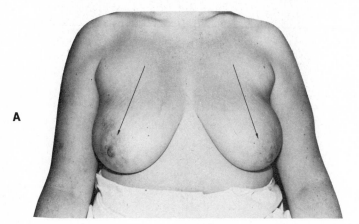
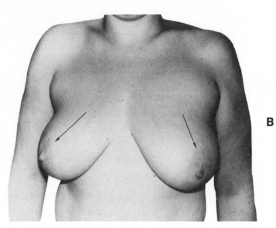

Fig. 10-5. A, Symmetrical breasts (note nipple position). **B,** Lateral deviation of right breast (note nipple position).

2. Size, shape	Bilaterally equal Long-standing inversion (unilateral or bilateral) (Fig. 10-6, *A*)	Asymmetrical Recent inversion or retraction (unilateral or bilateral) (Fig. 10-6, *B*)

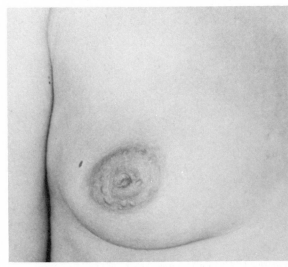
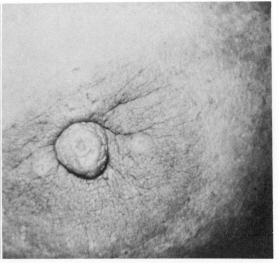

Fig. 10-6. A, Inverted nipple. **B,** Nipple retraction. (**B** from Gallagher, S. G., Leis, H. P., Jr., Snyderman, R. K., and Urban, J. A., editors: The breast, St. Louis, 1978, The C. V. Mosby Co.)

The student will:	To identify:	
	Normal	**Deviations from normal**
3. Color	Homogeneous	Edema, redness Bilaterally unequal Pigment changes
4. Surface characteristics	Smooth, may be slightly wrinkled Skin intact	Ulceration, crusting Erosion, scaling Wrinkled, dry, cracking, with lesions
5. Discharge (if present, describe odor, color, amount, consistency)	Absent	Serous, bloody, odorous, purulent discharges (Fig. 10-7)

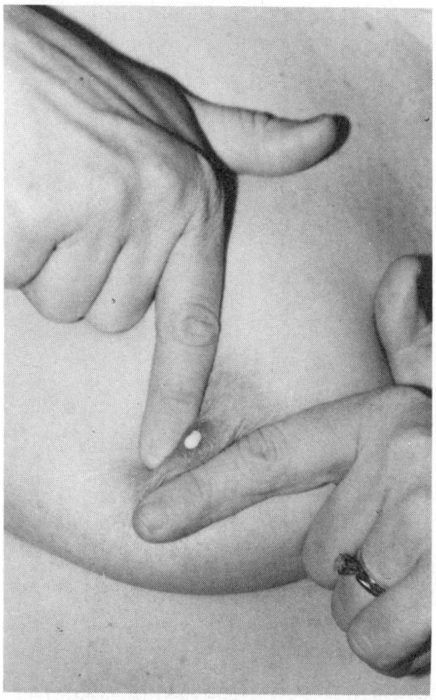

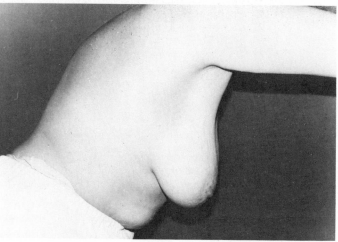

Fig. 10-7. Nipple discharge.

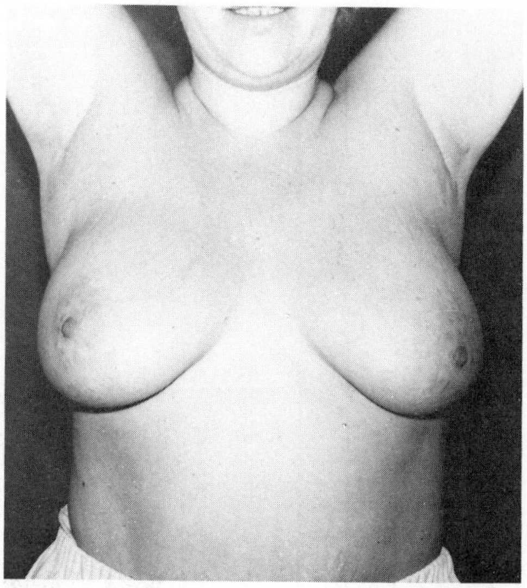

Fig. 10-8. Inspect breasts with arms extended overhead.

3. Inspect breasts while client is *seated with arms abducted overhead* (Fig. 10-8) to observe and bilaterally compare all items previously listed, as well as:
   a. Bilateral pull on suspensory ligaments

Equal; breasts bilaterally symmetrical

Asymmetry
Shortening or appearance of attachment of either breast (fixation)

4. Inspect breasts while client is *seated and leaning over,* to observe (Fig. 10-9) and bilaterally compare:

Fig. 10-9. Inspect breasts with client leaning forward.

Continued.

Clinical guidelines–cont'd

ASSESSMENT OF THE FEMALE BREASTS—cont'd

	To identify:	
The student will:	**Normal**	**Deviations from normal**
a. Symmetry	Breasts hang equally Smooth skin contour Equal; breasts bilaterally symmetrical	Asymmetry Bulging retraction
b. Bilateral pull on suspensory ligaments		Asymmetry Shortening or appearance of attachment of either breast (fixation)

5. Inspect breasts while client is *seated and pushing hands onto her hips or pushing palms together* (Fig. 10-10) and contracting pectoral muscles, to observe and bilaterally compare all items as previously listed

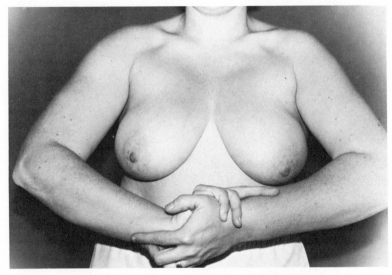

Fig. 10-10. Inspect breasts while client flexes pectoral muscles.

6. Palpate each breast in a systematic clockwise direction; client is seated with arms at sides (Fig. 10-11)

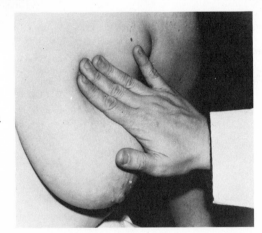

Fig. 10-11. Examiner using finger pads to examine breasts.

7. Palpate and bilaterally compare:
  a. Four quadrants, tail of the breast, and areolar area for:
    1. Firmness

    2. Tissue qualities (see clinical strategies for further description)

Bilaterally equal With aging or poor bra support, sagging of breast tissue may occur	Asymmetry
Smooth, diffuse tissue bilaterally Nodular, bilateral granular consistency Premenstrual engorgement Elastic, nontender Firm mammary ridge found along each breast at approximately 4 to 8 o'clock position	Tenderness unrelated to menstrual cycle Unilateral pain or tenderness, unilateral mass Heat of tissue

The student will:	To identify:	
	Normal	**Deviations from normal**
b. Nipple		
1. Elasticity and tissue characteristics	Bilaterally equal, nontender Smooth, skin intact	Tender, friable tissue, cracks, bleeding Lesions, dryness, crusting, erosion
2. Discharge (note color, odor, consistency, amount)	Absent	Present; serous, bloody, purulent, odorous
c. Lymph nodes associated with the lymphatic drainage system (Fig. 10-12); location and characteristics of lymph nodes, including supraclavicular and infraclavicular, central and lateral axillary, pectoral, subscapular, scapular, brachial, intermediate, and internal mammary chains (Fig. 10-13)	Nonpalpable	Palpable Note: 1. Location 2. Size 3. Contour 4. Consistency 5. Discreteness 6. Mobility 7. Tenderness

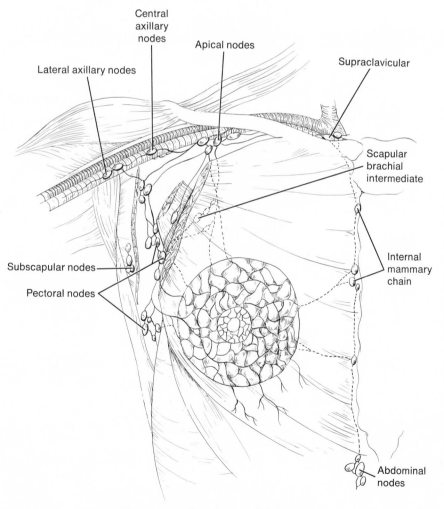

Fig. 10-12. Lymphatic drainage of the breast.

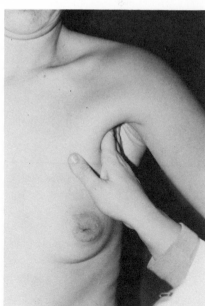

Fig. 10-13. Palpating axillary lymph nodes.

Continued.

Clinical guidelines–cont'd

ASSESSMENT OF THE FEMALE BREASTS—cont'd

	To identify:	
The student will:	**Normal**	**Deviations from normal**

8. Instruct client to remain *sitting* and *raise both arms over head;* may be most comfortable for client to grasp hands and rest on top of head; repeat and compare bilaterally the palpation of:
  a. Four quadrants of each breast
  b. Tail of each breast
  c. Areolar area
  d. Nipple
  e. Lymph nodes
	Criteria as previously described	Criteria as previously described

9. Instruct client to lie supine with the arm of the breast to be examined resting over her head (Fig. 10-14); place small towel under shoulder and back of breast to be examined; this displaces breast tissue more diffusely over the chest wall		

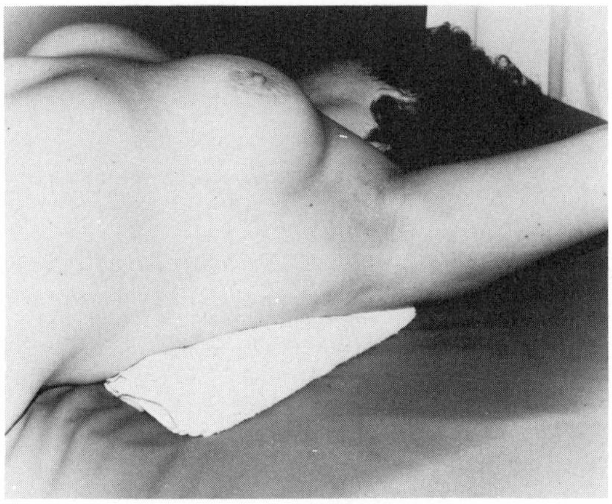

Fig. 10-14. Positioning for breast examination. Note placement of towel.

10. Inspect the
  a. Breasts, noting:
    1. Symmetry
    2. Contour
    3. Skin color
    4. Skin texture
    5. Venous patterns
    6. Moles, nevi
  b. Areolar area surface characteristics
  c. Nipple characteristics
	Criteria as previously described	Criteria as previously described

11. Palpate each breast in systematic clockwise direction; carefully evaluate:
  a. Four quadrants of each breast
  b. Tail of each breast
  c. Areolar area
  d. Nipple
  e. Lymph nodes
	Criteria as previously described	Criteria as previously described

Clinical guidelines

ASSESSMENT OF THE MALE BREASTS

The student will:	To identify:	
	Normal	**Deviations from normal**
1. Inspect the male client's breasts while he is seated, arms resting at sides.		
2. Inspect nipple and areolar area; compare bilaterally	Intact, smooth Bilaterally equal color Flat tissue	Ulcerated Masses, swelling Discolorations
3. Palpate client's breast and areolar area while he is seated, arms resting at sides; note skin texture, tissue consistency; compare bilaterally	Smooth, nontender Skin intact, nontender	Tenderness Unilateral or unequal swelling or masses
4. Palpate lymphatic system associated with the breast (similar to female breast assessment)		

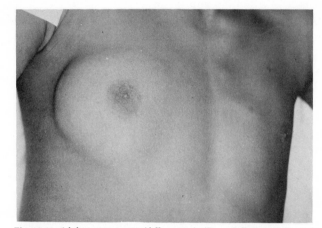

Fig. 10-15. Adult gynecomastia (diffuse type). (From Gallagher, S. G., Leis, H. P., Jr., Snyderman, R. K., and Urban, J. A., editors: The breast, St. Louis, 1978, The C. V. Mosby Co.)

Clinical strategies

1. Complete breast examination requires that the breast be evaluated in numerous positions. This facilitates pull on the suspensory ligaments that will most likely demonstrate retraction or dimpling of an affected breast. To summarize the previous clinical strategies, the evaluation positions include:
   a. Inspection: client sitting, arms at side; sitting, arms above head; sitting or standing, leaning over; sitting, hands pressed onto hips
   b. Palpation: client sitting, arms at side; sitting, arms above head
   c. Palpation: client lying, arm above head
   The total time required to completely evaluate the breasts should be between 5 and 10 minutes.
2. Symmetry is a key consideration in the assessment of the breasts. There should be a comparison of one side with the other throughout the assessment process.

3. For proper breast assessment, the client must be undressed to the waist. She must be encouraged to uncover both breasts at once so that they may be viewed together and compared. The examiner is not doing the client a favor by allowing her to uncover only one breast at a time.
4. Room lighting, for examination of the breast, is very important. The illumination should be overhead and adequate to shed an even light over all breast surfaces. Recognizing subtle coloring or surface characteristic changes of the breasts may depend on the lighting of the examination room.
5. The male client must be evaluated with the same sensitivity as the female client. Male breast cancer accounts for about 1% of all cancer of the breast. Beyond that, there are numerous other disease or inflammatory processes that can cause gynecomastia or areolar inflammation (Fig. 10-15).
6. When palpating the breast, the examiner must

learn to use the sensitive finger pads of the palmar surface of the hand (Fig. 10-11). The examiner must inch along the breast surface using a rotating exploratory manner. Try *not to lift* the fingers off the breast when moving from one point to the next. The examination technique should smoothly and continually move forward.

7. It is most beneficial to first palpate completely with a light palpation and then repeat the procedure using a deeper, heavier palpation. Most authorities state that the light exploratory palpation will yield more information than the deeper palpation.

8. For women with very large breasts, the palpation component of the seated examination is best performed when the examiner immobilizes the breast underneath with one hand while examining the above surface with the other hand. This bimanual palpation technique may assist in the detection of small mobile masses not picked up by other techniques.

9. If the examination takes place right before her menstrual period and the client has tender, engorged breasts, make arrangements for her to return following the end of her period for a thorough breast assessment.

10. During the examination of the nipples, the examiner should gently express the nipple using the index fingers of both hands and slowly strip the nipple between the fingers as they slide from the areola to the tip of the nipple. Palpation of the nipple should also include an exploration for small masses or duct thickening. If a nipple discharge is present, note if it is coming from a single or multiple duct openings.

11. Although it is relatively simple to palpate the areas where the lymph nodes are located, it is another issue to relate the lymph nodes with their drainage significance. Following is an outline of the patterns for breast lymphatic drainage. (See Fig. 10-12.)

    a. Lymphatic drainage of superficial breast tissue
       1. Mammary chain (located along medial and superior borders of breast tissue; drainage occurs toward opposite breast)
       2. Scapular ⎤ All located in upper outer
       3. Brachial ⎬ quadrant of breast; drainage
       4. Intermediate⎦ occurs toward axillary nodes

    b. Lymphatic drainage of deep breast tissue
       1. Supraclavicular
       2. Apical nodes or subclavicular or infraclavicular
       3. Central axillary
       4. Lateral axillary
       5. Pectoral (anterior)
       6. Subscapular (posterior)

       All these lymph nodes drain the breast. The most common drainage patterns are toward the *lateral axillary* (drains arm), *subscapular,* and *supraclavicular chains*. The medial and inferior deep breast tissue may also drain into the abdominal region.

    c. Areolar lymphatic drainage (areolar and nipple areas)
       1. Central axillary
       2. Apical nodes or subclavicular or infraclavicular
       3. Superior mammary chain

       Drainage of the areolar area involves an up-

Table 6. Physical findings helpful in the differential diagnosis of a breast lump*

Physical findings	Favors malignancy	Favors benignancy
Hard, dominant lump	Single, definite	Multiple, indistinct
Firm, palpable, radiating ducts	No help	Indicates cystic disease
Venous engorgement	Unilateral	Bilateral
Nipple deviation	Unilateral	Bilateral, symmetrical
Nipple excoriation	Unilateral	Bilateral
Skin dimpling	Present	Absent
Chest wall fixation	Present	Absent
Peau d'orange	Present	Absent
Bloody discharge	Present	Absent
Axillary or supraclavicular nodes	Present	Absent
Freely movable mass	No help	Typical of fibroadenoma
Tenderness	No help	May indicate cystic mass
Inflammation, heat	Ominous in nonlactating or nonpostpartum breast	Abscess in lactating or postpartum breast

*From Nance, F.: Clin. Obstet. Gynecol. **18**(2):188, 1975.

ward movement, toward the subclavicular and supraclavicular regions.

12. When dealing with a symptomatic breast problem, the examiner should start the evaluation procedure with the unaffected breast.

13. If the examiner identifies a lump or mass in the breast, it should be evaluated according to the following criteria:
    a. Location according to clock orientation and distance from the nipple
    b. Size
    c. Contour and shape—margin regularity vs. irregularity
    d. Consistency (soft, firm, rough)
    e. Discreteness (difficulty determining borders)
    f. Mobility
    g. Tenderness (marked or absent)
    h. Erythema of overlying skin
    i. Tissue characteristics over mass (bulging, dimpling)

14. In compiling the data associated with a breast mass or breast problem, the examiner must determine the urgency of the client's problem. Table 6 presents the physical findings related to benign and malignant breast masses and thus will help the examiner evaluate the data collected during physical assessment.

15. Work hard to develop a systematic assessment method. As in the assessment of all body systems, a patterned assessment process reduces the likelihood of missing a significant finding.

Techniques and strategies for teaching breast self-examination

One in every thirteen women in the United States will develop breast cancer. In 1980 alone, over 90,000 new cases will be discovered. Although it is impossible to prevent cancer of the breast, every health care provider must assume the position that it is possible to detect a breast mass early and to initiate prompt treatment. Each examiner must incorporate teaching breast self-examination techniques into the examination procedures because most breast masses will be detected by the women themselves. The American Cancer Society states that 85% of all women who are treated promptly for early breast cancer recover.

The examiner can facilitate client education and health maintenance by (1) developing a risk profile for the client and sharing the data collected and by (2) teaching breast self-examination techniques.

The teaching program should include both an informal and a structured presentation. The informal component will take place as the examiner is actually checking the client's breasts. Each step should be explained as it is being done. Involve the client in the process. If the client understands what is done and why, compliance is likely to increase.

The formal component involves scheduling 10 to 15 minutes with the client to systematically discuss anatomy of the breast, the sequence of the examination techniques, the anticipated findings, the appropriate times of the month to examine the breasts, and what the client should do about abnormal or questionable findings.

The following sequence of information provides the examiner with an instructional overview of breast self-examination*:

1. Breast cancer facts
   a. Over 90,000 women in the United States acquire breast cancer.
   b. Over 33,000 women die each year of breast cancer.
   c. Up to 85% of women who receive prompt treatment for breast cancer recover.
   d. Breast cancer is the leading cause of death from cancer in women.
   e. Breast cancer is the leading cause of death from all causes among women from 40 to 44 years of age.
   f. Breast cancer usually begins as a lump or thickening in the breast.
   g. About 90% of all breast lumps are found by the women themselves.
   h. About 80% of all breast lumps are benign.

2. Age of women who should examine breasts: *all* women from menarche through old age.

3. Best time of month to examine breasts
   a. Menstruating women: sixth to seventh day of menstrual period; at this time the breasts are least engorged or tender.
   b. Pregnant women: pick single day of each month; the birthdate is generally used.
   c. Postmenopausal women: pick a single day of each month; again, the birthdate is usually a convenient number to remember.

4. Breast anatomy the client must know
   a. Lymph nodes and locations associated with breast self-examination
   b. The four quadrants, the tail, the mammary ridge
   c. Areolar area
   d. Nipple
   e. Tissue characteristics: tenderness, nodular

5. Steps in teaching breast self-examination (Fig. 10-16); instructions for client

---

*Data from American Cancer Society: Teaching breast self-examination, Instructional material no. 77-1R-50M-6/77; 2015-LE.

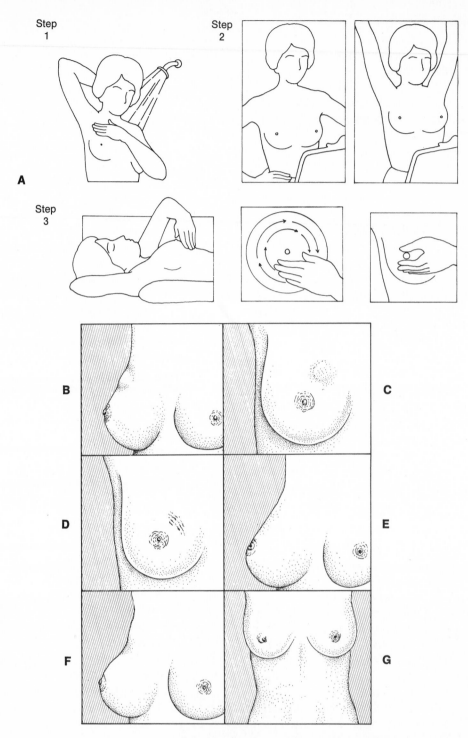

Fig. 10-16. A, Steps in breast self-examination. Inspect and palpate breasts *(1)* in the shower, *(2)* before a mirror, and *(3)* lying down. In all positions use the palmar surface of the examining fingers to inch along the breast tissue. Examine each breast using a circular movement until you are confident that the tail of the breast and all four quadrants have been evaluated. Gently express each nipple. Observe for discharge and bleeding. During inspection and palpation look for the following: swelling or elevated area **(B),** redness or inflammation **(C),** puckering or dimpling **(D),** nipple pulled inward **(E),** depression or sunken area **(F),** and nipple pulled askew compared with the other nipple **(G).** (Courtesy American Cancer Society: Teaching breast self-examination, Instructional Material no. 77-1R-50M, no. 2015-LE, June, 1977.)

Table 7. Maturational sequence in girls*

Stage	Breast development	Development description
1		Preadolescent
2		Breast and papilla elevated as small mound; areolar diameter increased
3		Breast and areola enlarged; no contour separation
4		Areola and papilla form secondary mound
5		Mature; nipple projects areolar part of general breast contour

*From Tanner, J. M.: Growth at adolescence, ed. 2, Oxford, England, 1962, Blackwell Scientific Publications.

6. What to do if lump or abnormality is identified
   a. Note time of month in relation to menses.
   b. Make appointment with physician for further evaluation.

Sample recording

Breasts moderate size.

Left slightly larger than right.

Firm, smooth texture bilaterally, without masses, retractions, bulges, or skin lesions.

Silver striae noted bilaterally.

Nipples erect, no discharge.

Areolar area intact and smooth bilaterally; pigmentation bilaterally equal.

No nodes palpated: axillary, supraclavicular, or infraclavicular.

Instructed on breast self-examination: return demonstration completed.

History and clinical strategies associated with the pediatric client

Although the breasts should be inspected during each well-child visit as part of the chest examination, there are basically two time periods when the examiner systematically evaluates the breasts: (1) following the birth of the child and during the newborn period; and (2) as a girl reaches puberty and her breasts begin to develop. Because the clinical guidelines for inspection and palpation remain the same for both the child and the adult, this section of the chapter has been developed to provide information about breast development and clinical strategies when approaching the pediatric client.

Often the neonate's breasts may be enlarged for 1 to 2 months. This is a simple hypertrophic breast, which is normal. Characteristics include flat nipple, small areola, and a small amount of milky discharge. Deviations requiring referral include hypertrophy extending beyond 3 months, redness, heat, or firmness around the nipple, and increased pigmentation around the areola.

Boys who are stocky or heavy may experience some hypertrophy of breast tissue. This may be a normal finding but many times is of great concern to the boy. He should be assured that, as he grows and thins, the hypertrophy will disappear. The examiner should assess the breasts to rule out actual breast development, tenderness, masses, redness, or inflammation. At puberty, true gynecomastia is normal for some boys, but for others it may be a symptom of a systemic disease process. Refer these boys for further evaluation.

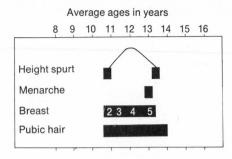

Fig. 10-17. Summary of maturational development of girls. For explanation of numbers 2 through 5, see Table 7.

As breast tissue in girls begins to develop, there will usually be protrusion of the nipple first. Breasts in girls normally develop between the ages 10 years 8 months and 13 years 6 months. Menarche occurs in most girls at about 12 years 3 months (Fig. 10-17). Table 7 summarizes the physical development of girls. If there is no evidence of breast or other puberty development by age 13 years, the girl should be referred to a physician. Once menarche has begun, the examiner should employ the same breast examination techniques as for the adult client. The young client will need much reassurance and assistance to feel comfortable during the breast examination.

Following are educational factors that may help the client feel more comfortable during examination of the breasts:

1. Breasts may develop at different ages; this is based on hereditary and hormonal characteristics and has nothing to do with the client's femininity.
2. The right and left breasts may not develop at the same rate.
3. Assess the client's understanding of breast development and menarche.
4. Begin educational instruction regarding care of the breasts, qualities of a supportive bra, and breast self-examination techniques.

History and clinical strategies associated with the geriatric client

The elderly client is subject to the same risk factors and physical change parameters as the younger client. The incidence of breast cancer (among women) rises steadily after the age of 40 and continues throughout the aging process. Breast self-examination remains an important consideration for older women.

The physical changes in the breasts that accompany aging follow:

1. Adipose tissue often increases (even if subcutaneous fat decreases over extremities).

2. In some women subcutaneous fat may decrease in the breasts.
3. Breast glandular tissue atrophies.
4. The suspensory ligaments relax and the breasts appear elongated or pendulous.
5. Chronic cystic disease diminishes after menopause.

In summary, breast palpation is often easier to accomplish because the nodular, glandular palpatory sensation associated with the breast glandular tissue in younger women is diminished. Breast lumps become even more significant in older clients. Refer to the adult section in this chapter for assessment guidelines.

Vocabulary

1. Areolar

2. Cooper's ligaments

3. Gynecomastia

4. Inversion

5. Mastitis

6. Peau d'orange

7. Pectoralis muscle

8. Piaget's disease

9. Retraction

10. Sebaceous gland

11. Striae

12. Supernumerary nipple

13. Tail of Spence

14. Tubercles of Montgomery

Cognitive self-assessment

1. The lymphatic system of the breasts drains to *two* major sites. These are:
   - ☑ a. axillary
   - ☐ b. internal mammary
   - ☑ c. supraclavicular
   - ☐ d. abdominal
   - ☐ e. pectoral

- ☑ f. a and c
- ☐ g. c and e
- ☐ h. b and e
- ☐ i. a and b
- ☐ j. b and d

2. All the following inspection findings are *normal except one*. Identify the *abnormal* findings.
   - ☐ a. Slight breast asymmetry
   - ☑ b. Deviated nipple
   - ☐ c. Venous pattern seen on both breasts
   - ☐ d. Inverted nipples (bilateral)
   - ☐ e. Montgomery tubercles

3. All the following palpation criteria are *normal except one*. Identify the *abnormal* finding:
   - ☐ a. Diffusely nodular
   - ☐ b. Mammary ridge
   - ☑ c. Palpable supraclavicular lymph node
   - ☐ d. Bilateral tenderness
   - ☐ e. Soft tissue bilaterally

4. Which of the following women should be referred to a physician for further evaluation?
   - ☐ a. A 26-year-old with multiple nodules palpated in each breast.
   - ☑ b. A 48-year-old who has a 6-month history of reddened and sore left nipple and areolar area.
   - ☐ c. A 35-year-old with asymmetrical breasts and inversion of nipples since birth of second child 8 years ago.
   - ☐ d. A 15-year-old with minimal breast development.
   - ☑ e. A 64-year-old with very slight ulcerated area tip of right nipple; no masses, tenderness, or lymph nodes palpated.
   - ☐ f. All except c
   - ☐ g. a, c, and d
   - ☑ h. b, d, and e
   - ☐ i. a and c
   - ☑ j. b and e

5. When palpating lymph nodes associated with drainage of the breasts, the examiner must palpate:
   - ☐ a. along the sternum
   - ☑ b. supraclavicular and subclavicular area
   - ☑ c. pectoral area
   - ☑ d. axillary area
   - ☐ e. lower thoracic area under breast
   - ☐ f. all the above
   - ☐ g. all except a
   - ☐ h. all except c and e
   - ☐ i. all except c
   - ☑ j. all except a and e

Mark each statement "T" or "F."

6. __F__ It is not necessary to examine a nonsymptomatic 20-year-old woman in both sitting and lying positions.

7. __T__ Nipples normally point slightly down and laterally.

8. __F__ Engorgement and an orange peel appearance of the breast tissue is a normal premenstrual finding.

9. __F__ A supernumerary nipple is considered a precancerous state, and the client should be referred to a physician.

10. __F__ Because of the vastness of breast tissue, large-breasted women should only receive breast palpation in a supine position.
11. __F__ Nipple inversion is always considered a cancerous sign.
12. __F__ As the breasts become engorged premenstrually, dimpling of breast tissue may normally occur.
13. __T__ It is just as important for a 25-year-old woman to perform breast self-examination as it is for a 75-year-old woman.
14. __T__ Breast tissue of an older woman that is found to be nodular and stringy is considered normal.
15. __T__ About 90% of all breast lumps were first detected by women themselves.
16. __F__ The presence of nipple discharge is usually indicative of an underlying malignancy.

PEDIATRIC QUESTIONS

17. Of the following children, *one* presents with an abnormal finding during the breast examination and should be referred. Identify the child with the abnormal finding.
    - ☐ a. John is a 9-day-old boy who presents with bilateral hypertrophy of the breast. A slight amount of milky-colored nipple discharge is observed.
    - ☐ b. Bonnie is a 1-month-old girl who has bilateral hypertrophy of the breast. There is no nipple discharge.
    - ☐ c. Amy is a 3-month-old female who has bilateral hypertrophy of the breast. There is no nipple discharge.
    - ☐ d. Michael is a 12-year-old husky boy who has recently developed bilateral hypertrophy of the breast. There is no nipple discharge.
    - ☐ e. Marilyn is a 13-year-old girl who is concerned because unlike all of her friends, she has had no breast development.
18. Which of the following 15-year-old girls should receive breast self-examination instructions?
    - ☐ a. Nancy: well developed, negative family history for breast cancer
    - ☐ b. Cindy: just beginning breast development, negative family history for breast cancer
    - ☐ c. Judy: has small breasts, both her aunt and grandmother have had breast cancer
    - ☐ d. Lynn: average breast development appropriate for age, has just started menstruating; mother has fibrocystic disease
    - ☐ e. Karen: very large breasted, started menstruating age 12 years; negative family history for breast cancer
    - ☐ f. a, b, and e
    - ☐ g. all except d
    - ☐ h. b, c, and e
    - ☐ i. all the above
    - ☐ j. none of the above

SUGGESTED READINGS
General

The American Cancer Society: Teaching breast self examination, Instructional pamphlet no. 77-1R-50M-6/77; no. 2015-LE.

Bates, Barbara: A guide to physical examination, ed. 2, Philadelphia, 1979, J. B. Lippincott Co., pp. 186-199.

DeGowin, Elmer, and DeGowin, Richard: Bedside diagnostic examination, ed. 3, New York, 1976, Macmillan Publishing Co., Inc., pp. 248-259.

Judge, Richard D., and Zuidema, George, editors: Methods of clinical examination: a physiologic approach, Boston, 1974, Little, Brown & Co., pp. 261-269.

Malasanos, Lois, Barkauskas, Violet, Moss, Muriel, and Stoltenberg-Allen, Kathryn: Health assessment, St. Louis, 1977, The C. V. Mosby Co., pp. 174-176, 182-194.

Martin, Leonide L.: Health care of women, Philadelphia, 1978, J. B. Lippincott Co., pp. 302-333.

Prior, John A., and Silberstein, Jack S.: Physical diagnosis: the history and examination of the patient, ed. 5, St. Louis, 1977, The C. V. Mosby Co., pp. 225-238.

Pediatric

Barness, Lewis: Manual of pediatric physical diagnosis, ed. 4, Chicago, 1972, Year Book Medical Publishers, Inc., p. 100.

Daniel, William A., Jr.: Adolescents in health and disease, St. Louis, 1977, The C. V. Mosby Co., pp. 29-38.

Pilliteri, Adele: Nursing care of the growing family, Boston, 1977, Little, Brown & Co., pp. 218, 310.

Tanner, J. M.: Growth at adolescence, ed. 2, Oxford, England, 1962, Blackwell Scientific Publications.

Geriatric

Malasanos, Lois, Barkauskas, Violet, Moss, Muriel, and Stoltenberg-Allen, Kathryn: Health assessment, St. Louis, 1977, The C. V. Mosby Co., p. 440.

Martin, Leonide L.: Health care of women, Philadelphia, 1978, J. B. Lippincott Co., pp. 209, 331.

CHAPTER 11

Assessment of the gastrointestinal system, the abdomen, and the rectal/anal region

Cognitive objectives

At the end of this unit the learner will demonstrate knowledge of assessment of the gastrointestinal system and abdomen by the ability to do the following:

1. Describe five activities or conditions that contribute to client comfort and relaxation in preparation for an abdominal examination.
2. Describe the location of the major abdominal organs in terms of abdominal quadrants.
3. Identify major abdominal organs in terms of location, relative size, and relationship to adjacent structures by completing an illustration.
4. Recognize normal findings associated with inspection of the abdominal surface, configuration, and pulsations.
5. Identify the rationale for performing auscultation of the abdomen before performing percussion and palpation.
6. Recognize normal findings associated with auscultation of the abdomen.
7. Recognize normal findings associated with percussion of the abdomen.
8. Recognize the major characteristics of a normal liver span and location.
9. Recognize the major characteristics of a normal spleen location and accessibility through percussion and palpation.
10. Describe the method for effective percussion and palpation of liver and spleen borders.
11. Describe three reasons for performing light palpation of the abdomen.
12. Describe three reasons for performing deep palpation of the abdomen.
13. Recognize major palpable characteristics of liver, kidney, small bowel, and pancreatic masses.
14. Identify abdominal areas that might be normally tender on deep palpation.
15. Recognize normal drainage patterns of the superficial inguinal nodes.
16. Identify specific examiner behaviors that will minimize client discomfort and enhance efficiency of the rectal examination.
17. Identify major characteristics of structures within the anal and rectal canals.
18. Identify selected common variations for pediatric and geriatric clients.
19. Define the terms in the vocabulary section.

Clinical objectives

At the end of this unit the learner will perform a systematic assessment of the abdomen and the inguinal area, demonstrating the ability to do the following:

1. Obtain a pertinent health history from a client.
2. Inspect the abdominal surface for:
    a. Skin color
    b. Surface characteristics
    c. Presence of scars
    d. Venous network pattern
    e. Umbilicus contour, placement, and surface characteristics
    f. Abdominal contour and symmetry
    g. Surface motion: peristalsis and pulsations
    h. General movement with respirations
3. Auscultate all four quadrants and the epigastrium for:
    a. Presence and timing of bowel sounds
    b. Presence and creation of vascular sounds
4. Percuss all four quadrants of the abdomen and describe tone(s) elicited in specific areas.

5. Percuss the upper and lower liver borders and estimate the midclavicular liver span and descent on inspiration.
6. Percuss in the left midaxillary line for splenic dullness or absence of dullness.
7. Percuss the gastric bubble and estimate its size.
8. Lightly palpate all four quadrants for:
   a. Tenderness
   b. Guarding
   c. Surface characteristics
   d. Masses
9. Deeply palpate all four quadrants for normal and abnormal tenderness and masses.
10. Deeply palpate at the right costal margin for:
    a. Liver border
    b. Contour
    c. Tenderness
11. Deeply palpate at the left costal margin for the splenic border.
12. Deeply palpate the abdomen for the right and left kidneys.
13. Deeply palpate the midline epigastric area for aortic pulsation.
14. Lightly palpate the inguinal regions for the presence of:
    a. Horizontal and vertical lymph nodes
    b. Contour
    c. Consistency
    d. Delimitation
    e. Tenderness
    f. Redness
    g. Size
15. Inspect and palpate the sacrococcygeal and perianal areas for surface characteristics and tenderness.
16. Inspect and palpate the anus for:
    a. Sphincter tone
    b. Tenderness
    c. Surface characteristics
17. Palpate the distal rectal walls for surface characteristics.
18. Summarize results with a written description of findings.

Health history related to gastrointestinal assessment additional to data base

1. Nutritional assessment. The screening questions, outlined in the original data base, provide the examiner with basic information about the client's food intake (through the use of a 24-hour recall chart), the client's weight measurement and stability, and major variables that might alter intake pattern. These data can be analyzed to assure the client and examiner that daily nutritional needs are being met in terms of the basic four food groups.

If food consumption or weight problems exist, further assessment is warranted.
a. The 24-hour recall intake record can be extended to cover a week's intake (to give an overview of day-to-day variations).
b. The final data can be analyzed in terms of recommended daily dietary allowances for calories, proteins, fats, carbohydrates, vitamins, and minerals.
c. Further variables that might affect food intake should be explored:
   (1) A survey of food preferences and dislikes
   (2) Family routines and values (e.g., food portions, eating times, control of food purchase and service, insistence on having a "clean plate," family values regarding ideal weight or appearance)
   (3) Cultural and religious values (e.g., forbidden foods, foods that are served frequently)
   (4) Psychological variables (e.g., depression, anxiety, compulsive eating habits)
   (5) Physical status (e.g., ill health, allergies or food idiosyncracies, mouth or dental problems, alterations in physical activity)
   (6) Access to food (e.g., transportation, type and availability of grocery store)
   (7) Personal habits or life-style (e.g., use of convenience foods due to limited time or interest in cooking, frequent dining out, night occupation and unusual eating schedule, dormitory or rooming house controls, disorganized life-style with no regular eating or shopping patterns, constant use of "fast food" restaurants for lunch or dinner, frequent entertaining or feasting on weekends and holidays, sedentary life-style with frequent snacks)
   (8) Eating behaviors (e.g., rapid eating, nibbling food all day, skipping meals, late night snacks)
   (9) Self-imposed dietary additions or restrictions (e.g., vitamin/mineral supplements, food supplements, vegetarian diet, low-calorie diet, low-carbohydrate diet, other diet forms)
   (10) Body image profile (self-assessment of satisfaction with present weight, weight distribution, recall of peer reaction to client's appearance)

(11) General knowledge of basic four food requirements, shopping within a budget, and content of fat, sugar, and proteins in basic foods

2. Abdominal pain may be reported as "indigestion," "heartburn," "stomachache," or other vague descriptions that need clarification and a full symptom analysis by the examiner. The client may experience pain that is diffuse and may be unable to specifically locate the discomfort. The pain may be precisely located and/or it may radiate to adjacent or remote areas. The discomfort may feel superficial or very deep. Referred pain often occurs as the pain intensifies. The following referral patterns may be helpful in eliciting information from the client (Fig. 11-1).

3. Indigestion. Various interpretations might include a feeling of fullness, heartburn, mild diffuse discomfort, excessive belching, flatulence, nausea, a bad taste, loss of appetite, or severe pain. The client must clarify the following:

a. Location of feeling or pain (if possible); radiation of pain (to arms, shoulders)
b. Symptoms associated with food intake (e.g., immediately before? immediately after? delayed response?)
c. Amount and type of food associated with discomfort
d. Associated symptoms (e.g., vomiting, headache, diarrhea)
e. Associated problems (e.g., anxiety, sleeplessness)
f. Time of day or night that symptom most often occurs
g. Does body position or activity cause or relieve pain?

4. Nausea. Might be described as an upset stomach, queasy stomach, a need to vomit, a fullness or tightness in the throat. Associated symptoms such as dizziness, increased salivation, headache, and weakness need to be explored. Again, onset, duration, and patterns should be clarified. Are

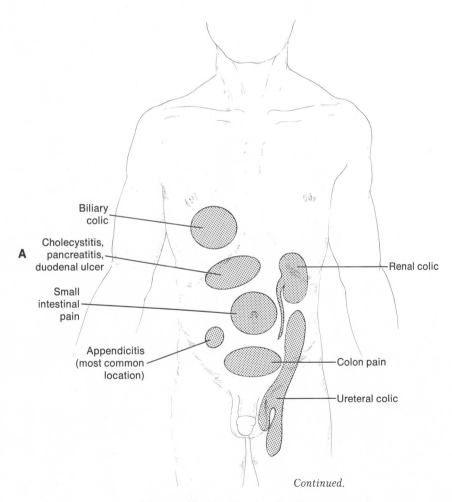

Continued.

Fig. 11-1. A, Anterior pain referral patterns.

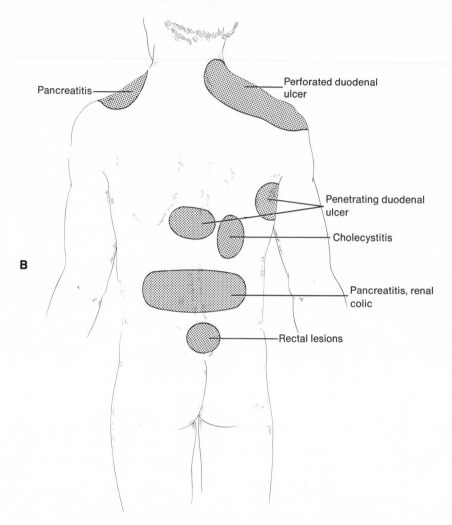

Fig. 11-1, cont'd. B, Posterior pain referral patterns. (Adapted from A. H. Robins Co.: GI series, Richmond, Va., 1974.)

there any notable stimuli (e.g., particular foods, odors, times of day, activity)? Does it occur with a certain meal? Before or after food intake? Is it associated with vomiting? If so, how?

5. Vomiting. To what extent is it associated with abdominal pain, nausea, retching? Are there other associated symptoms (e.g., fever, headache, diarrhea)? Clarify the timing between food intake and a vomiting episode. Once the symptom has been fully analyzed, the estimated quantity, color, consistency, odor, and taste should be established. If vomiting has occurred repeatedly, find out if the appearance of the vomitus has changed. Ask if there has been a weight loss. Determine whether fluid intake has been maintained, increased, or decreased. Specify which solids or liquids can be retained.

6. Heartburn. The location is usually substernal.

Ask if pain radiates to other areas (e.g., chest, neck, shoulders, back, or arms). Ask if body movement or position change alters the pain (e.g., bending over, sitting up, or lying down). Ask about specific food irritants (e.g., spices, coffee, alcohol). Establish the time of day or night when discomfort is most noticeable.

7. Appetite changes. A loss or gain of appetite should be explored in terms of particular foods that have been eliminated or added as well as an estimate of the quantity of food that has been changed. Careful inquiry about average weight and recent (last 3 to 9 months) loss or gain is important. Inquire about associated symptoms or situations that might interfere with appetite (e.g., increased stress, abdominal pain, bowel habit changes, other illnesses, or deliberate attempts to reduce caloric intake). Comparing a sample of a previous

"normal" of 24-hour intake with a present 24-hour intake might be helpful. (*Note:* Recent oral or dental problems can affect appetite.)

8. Diarrhea. The number of stools per day (24-hour period) or week should be established. Clarify whether this present pattern represents a change in bowel habits. If so, note the onset. Associated symptoms such as fever, nausea, vomiting, abdominal pain, abdominal distention, flatus, intermittent cramping, marked peristalsis, explosive diarrhea, or urgency to evacuate should be explored. The consistency, color, quantity, and odor of each stool should be noted. Does the client notice accompanying mucus, blood, or food particles with the stool? Is there nocturnal diarrhea? Has the client been taking antibiotics? Has there been a weight loss? Has the diarrhea interfered with activities of daily living?

9. Constipation: Usually defined as decreased number of stools, marked difficulty or pain with passage of stools, and/or excessive dryness or hardness of stools. Again the number of stools per day or week must be established. The date and time of the most recent stool should be noted. Establish whether this is a *change* of bowel habit. If so, was the onset sudden or gradual? Have the stools changed in size (smaller, thinner, larger)? Does the client feel that there is stool remaining in the rectum? Have there been any food intake changes recently (quantity or type of foods)? Has fluid intake been altered? Other associated abdominal or general symptoms should be inquired about. Has the client been depressed?

10. Anal discomfort. May be described in terms of itching, pain on defecation, a painful lump, or a stinging or burning sensation. Clarify whether body position (e.g., lying down or standing erect) alters the pain. Ask about the color, form, size, and consistency of stools. Ask if the client has noticed mucus or blood (streaks over stool, droplets on toilet paper, discoloration of water in the toilet bowl) at the time of bowel movement. Itching often interferes with sleep. Clarification of duration and daily patterns of itching is important.

11. General considerations for gastrointestinal symptom analysis:

    a. It is very important to list all medications that the client is taking in addition to careful exploration of medicines, enemas, or any self-help treatments that the client has been using.

    b. Severity of the symptom is often best determined by the client's account of symptom interference with activities of daily living (e.g., loss of sleep, marked eating habit change, loss of time at work, or alteration of daily tasks).

    c. The final accuracy of the description of the severity, duration, rhythmicity, and patterns of the pain depend greatly on the client's ability to articulate subjective sensations and a personal pain threshold and the examiner's ability to maintain a balance between nondirective and selective probing approaches.

Clinical guidelines

The student will:	To identify:	
	Normal	**Deviations from normal**

Abdomen

1. Assemble necessary equipment:
   a. Stethoscope
   b. Small ruler
   c. Marking pencil
2. Position client comfortably, making sure:
   a. Client's bladder recently emptied
   b. Arms on chest or at sides
   c. Small pillow under head
   d. Client's knees slightly flexed, supported by small pillow
   e. Client draped over breasts and at pubis
3. Take additional measures to ensure client comfort:
   a. Make sure room is warm

Continued.

Clinical guidelines–cont'd

The student will:	To identify:	
	Normal	Deviations from normal
b. Have warm hands, short fingernails, warm stethoscope		
c. Instruct client to breathe slowly through mouth if he appears anxious		
d. Offer explanations of examiner activity as assessment progresses		
4. Observe general behavior of client	Appears relaxed Facial muscles relaxed Lying quietly Respirations even and slow	Marked restlessness Marked immobility or rigid posture Knees drawn up Facial grimacing Respirations rapid, uneven, or grunting
5. Inspect the abdominal surface for:		
a. Skin color	May be paler than other parts due to lack of exposure	Jaundice Redness (inflammation) Lesions, bruises, discoloration, cyanosis (localized at umbilicus or generalized)
b. Surface characteristics	Smooth, soft Silver-white striae (usually lower abdomen) (See Fig. 3-7.)	Rashes, lesions Glistening, taut appearance Pink, red striae Purplish striae
c. Scars (configuration, location, length)		
d. Venous network	Very faint fine network may be visible	Prominent venous pattern Engorgement of veins around umbilicus
e. Umbilicus		
1. Placement	Centrally located	Displaced upward, downward, or laterally
2. Contour	Usually sunken, may protrude slightly	Visible hernia around or slightly above umbilicus
3. Surface characteristics	Smooth, noninflamed	Inflamed
f. Contour	Flat Rounded (Fig. 11-2) Scaphoid (concave profile) (Fig. 11-3)	Distention Marked concavity associated with general wasting signs or anterior-posterior rib expansion (Fig. 11-4)

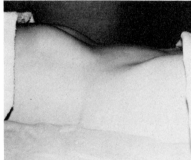

Fig. 11-2. Rounded abdominal contour.

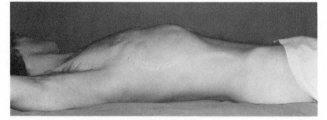
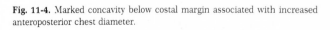

Fig. 11-3. Scaphoid abdominal contour.

Fig. 11-4. Marked concavity below costal margin associated with increased anteroposterior chest diameter.

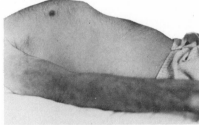

The student will:	To identify:	
	Normal	Deviations from normal
g. Symmetry (*Note:* Examiner must view abdomen at eye level from the side, as well as from behind client's head.)	Evenly rounded with maximum height of convexity at umbilicus	Distention of upper or lower half Visible masses or bulges in any area of abdominal surface
h. Surface motion		
1. Peristalsis	Usually not visible	Visible
2. Pulsation	Upper midline pulsation may be visible in thin people	Marked pulsation
i. General movement with respirations	Smooth, even movements Female exhibits chiefly costal movement Male exhibits chiefly abdominal movement	Grunting, labored Respirations accompanied by restricted abdominal movement
6. Instruct client to take a deep breath and hold it	Contour remains smooth and symmetrical	Bulges or masses appear
7. Instruct client to raise the head without using arms for support	Rectus abdominis muscles prominent Midline bulge may appear (Fig. 11-5)	Appearance of bulges through muscle layer
8. Auscultate all four abdominal quadrants and the epigastrium, using the diaphragm of the stethoscope and pressing lightly		

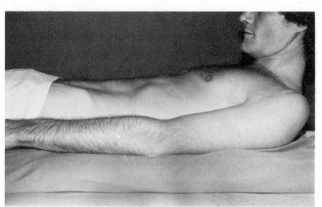

Fig. 11-5. Rectus abdominis muscles become prominent when head and neck are raised. Note that superficial masses will rise with muscles.

a. Presence and timing of bowel sounds	Usually 5 to 34/min Irregular in timing	Absence of sound established after 5 minutes of listening Note sounds that are infrequent
b. Quality of sounds	Gurgles, clicks Quality of sound varies greatly	High-pitched, tinkling noises
c. Arterial vascular sounds concentrated in epigastric area, in area surrounding umbilicus, over the liver, and at the posterior flank		Bruits (usually high pitched, soft "swishing" sound, and systolic in timing) (*Note:* Bruit will continue as client is moved into various positions.)
d. Bell of the stethoscope will pick up lower (venous) sounds		Venous hum (lower in pitch, softer, and continuous sound)
e. Friction rub		Infrequently heard sound, associated with respirations (soft, and may be confused with normal breath sounds) Rubs most often heard over spleen or liver

Continued.

Clinical guidelines–cont'd

	To identify:	
The student will:	**Normal**	**Deviations from normal**
9. Percuss lightly in all four quadrants (*Note:* Develop a system or route for percussion process.) (Fig. 11-6); note tone	General distribution of tympany (depending on amount of air and solid material in bowel) Suprapubic dullness heard over distended bladder	Marked dullness in local area

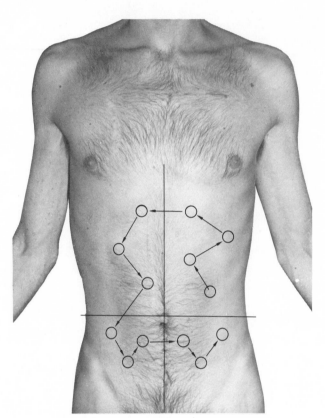

Fig. 11-6. Suggested percussion route for the abdomen.

a. Liver percussion 1. Percuss upward at right midclavicular line, beginning below level of umbilicus; continue percussing over tympanic area until dull percussion rate indicates liver border; note location of lower liver border with marker	Lower border of liver usually at costal margin or slightly below	Lower border of liver exceeds 2 to 3 cm (¾ to 1 inch) below costal margin

The student will:	To identify:	
	Normal	**Deviations from normal**
2. Percuss downward at right midclavicular line, beginning from area of lung resonance, and continue until dull percussion rate indicates upper liver border; note location of upper liver border with marker (Fig. 11-7)	Upper border of liver usually begins in fifth to seventh intercostal space	Upper border lowered Dullness extending above fifth intercostal space

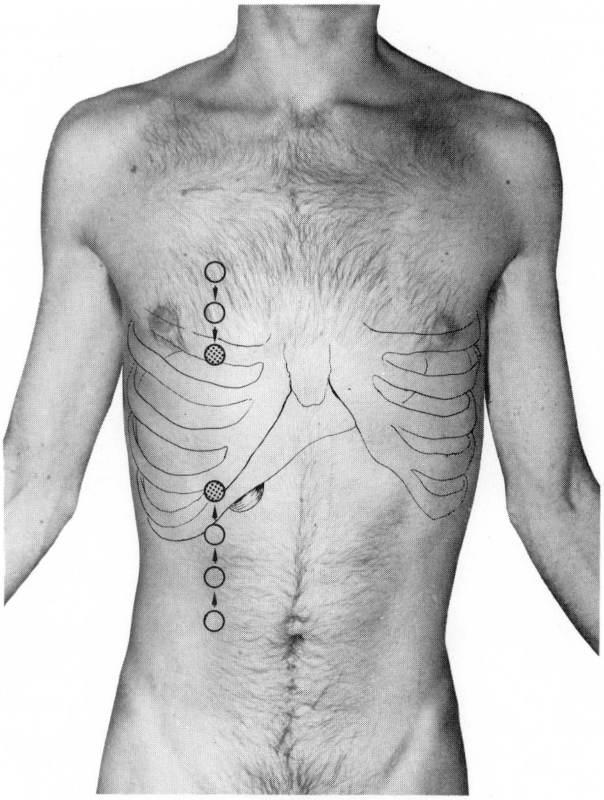

Fig. 11-7. Liver percussion route.

3. Estimate midclavicular liver span	6 to 12 cm (2½ to 4½ inches) Normal liver span usually greater in men than women and in taller individuals	Span exceeds 12 cm (4½ inches)
4. Additional liver percussion maneuvers		
a. Percuss upward then in downward direction over right midaxillary line	Liver dullness May be felt in fifth to seventh intercostal space	Dull percussion exceeds limits of fifth to seventh intercostal space
b. Percuss upward then in downward direction over midsternal line and estimate midsternal liver span	Normal midsternal liver span ranges from 4 to 8 cm (1½ to 3 inches)	Span exceeds 8 cm (3 inches)
c. Instruct client to take a deep breath and hold it; then percuss upward in right midclavicular line again; estimate liver descent	Lower border of liver should move inferiorly by 2 to 3 cm	Liver does not move with inspiration, or movement less than 2 cm

Continued.

Clinical guidelines–cont'd

	To identify:	
The student will:	**Normal**	**Deviations from normal**
b. Spleen percussion 1. Percuss down lower left thoracic wall in posterior midaxillary region beginning from an area of lung resonance to costal margin (Fig. 11-8)	Small area of splenic dullness may be heard at sixth to tenth rib, or tone may be tympanic (colonic)	Dullness extends above sixth rib or covers large area between sixth rib and costal margin

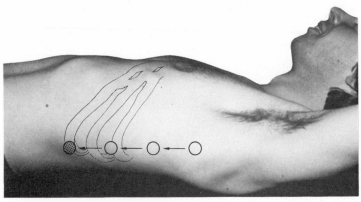

Fig. 11-8. Spleen percussion route.

2. Percuss lowest intercostal space in left anterior axillary line before and after client takes a deep breath (Fig. 11-9)	Area usually tympanic	Tympany changes to dullness on inspiration Enlarged spleen is brought forward on inspiration to produce dull percussion note

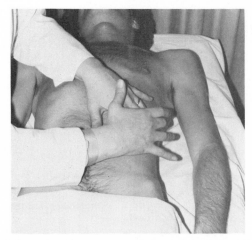

Fig. 11-9. Percussion at lowest intercostal space in left anterior axillary line before and after client takes a deep breath.

3. Percuss over left lower rib cage	Gastric "bubble" tympanic and varies in size	

The student will:	To identify:	
	Normal	**Deviations from normal**

10. Abdominal palpation

  a. Lightly palpate all four quadrants with pads of fingertips (Fig. 11-10, *A*)

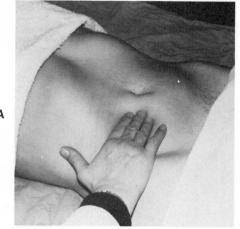

Fig. 11-10. A, Light palpation with distal pads of fingers.

1. Tenderness	Not present	Cutaneous (superficial areas of hypersensitivity)
2. Muscle tone	Abdomen relaxed Muscular resistance may be seen in anxious client	Involuntary resistance (muscles cannot be relaxed by voluntary effort)
3. Surface characteristics	Smooth; consistent tension felt by examiner	Masses (superficial) Localized areas of rigidity or increased tension

  b. Continue palpation of all four quadrants using moderate pressure with flat and sides of hand (Fig. 11-10, *B*)

(*Note:* This intermediate maneuver is performed as a method of gradually approaching deep palpation without alarming client and stimulating muscular resistance. If onset of resistance is noted, use a lighter touch and proceed again.)

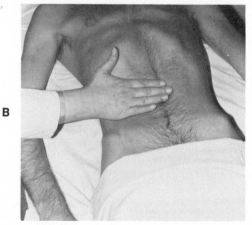

Fig. 11-10, cont'd. B, Palpation with moderate pressure, using flat and side of hand.

1. Tenderness	None	Present
2. Masses	None	Present
3. General tone and location of major structures	Abdomen surface feels smooth, and tension under palpating hand feels consistent throughout	Localized areas of rigidity or increased tension

Continued.

Clinical guidelines–cont'd

The student will:	To identify:	
	Normal	**Deviations from normal**

c. Deeply palpate all four quadrants; one of two methods may be used

   1. Distal flat portions of the fingers are pressed gradually and deeply into palpation areas (Fig. 11-10, *C*)

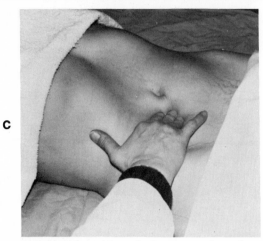

C

Fig. 11-10, cont'd. C, Deep abdominal palpation using flat surface of distal portion of fingers.

   2. Bimanual: lower hand rests lightly on the surface and upper hand exerts pressure for deep palpation (Fig. 11-10, *D*)

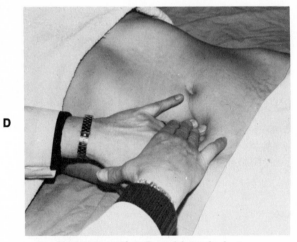

D

Fig. 11-10, cont'd. D, Deep abdominal palpation.

The student will:	Normal	Deviations from normal
a. Tenderness	Often present in midline near xiphoid process Often present over cecum May be present over sigmoid colon	Present in local or generalized areas Client response to pain may be muscle guarding and/or facial grimace, pulling away from examiner
b. Masses	Aorta often palpable at epigastrium and pulsates in forward direction Borders of rectus abdominis muscles Feces in ascending or descending colon Sacral promontory	Masses that descend on inspiration Pulsatile masses Laterally mobile masses Fixed masses

3. Palpate with fingertips around umbilicus for:
   a. Bulges
   b. Nodules
   c. Umbilical ring
	Umbilical ring round with no irregularities or bulges
	Umbilicus may be inverted or slightly everted
		Masses, bulges
		Umbilical ring may be incomplete or may feel soft in center

The student will:	To identify:	
	Normal	**Deviations from normal**

11. Specific organ identification
  a. Liver palpation
    1. Deeply palpate at right costal margin before and during deep inspiration; left hand is placed under eleventh and twelfth ribs; right hand is parallel to right costal margin (Fig. 11-11)

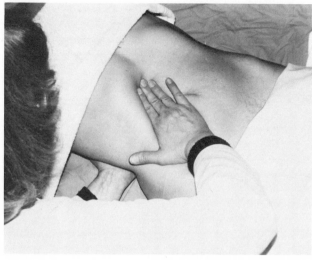

Fig. 11-11. Liver palpation with left hand under eleventh and twelfth ribs and right hand parallel to right costal margin.

a. Liver border and contour (*Note:* If border is felt, repeat palpation/inspiration maneuver at medial and lateral sites of costal border for better estimate of contour.)	Liver often not palpable Liver often "bumps" against fingers on inspiration (especially in thin clients)	(*Note:* Very enlarged liver may lie under examiner's hand as it extends downward into abdominal cavity.)
b. Liver border surface	Border feels smooth	Irregular surface or edge
c. Liver tenderness	None	Tenderness elicited (*Note:* Client's inspiration may be abruptly halted if pain exists.)

(*Note:* Both hands can be "hooked" over the right costal margin as the examiner faces the client's feet to palpate liver border on deep inspiration.)
  b. Spleen palpation
    1. Instruct client to turn to the right side; examiner stands to client's right and places left hand over client's left costovertebral angle; the right hand is pressed under the left anterior costal margin (Fig. 11-12)

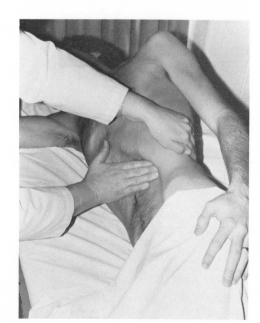

Fig. 11-12. Spleen palpation.

Continued.

Clinical guidelines–cont'd

The student will:	To identify:	
	Normal	**Deviations from normal**
2. Instruct the client to take a deep breath (*Note:* Both hands can be "hooked" over the left costal margin, as the examiner stands at the client's left side and faces the client's feet, to palpate the spleen border on inspiration.)	Spleen not normally palpable	Spleen palpated (as a firm mass)
c. Kidney palpation		
1. Left kidney		
a. The examiner stands to client's right; client returns to supine position		
b. The examiner's left hand is placed at the left posterior costal angle, and the right hand is placed at the client's left anterior costal margin		
c. The client is instructed to take a deep breath, and the examiner elevates the client's left flank with the left hand and palpates deeply with the right hand (Fig. 11-13)	Occasionally lower pole of the kidney can be felt in thin clients Contour smooth, and no tenderness on palpation	
2. Right kidney		
a. The same maneuver is repeated on the client's right side; the examiner remains at the client's right, elevates the posterior costal margin with the left hand, and palpates deeply at the anterior margin with the right hand	Lower pole of right kidney may be palpated (on inspiration) as smooth, firm, and nontender	

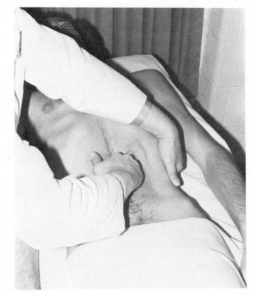

Fig. 11-13. Left kidney palpation.

The student will:	To identify:	
	Normal	Deviations from normal

d. Inguinal nodes
   1. Lightly palpate (with finger pads) the inguinal areas just below the inguinal ligament and the inner aspect of the upper thigh at the groin (Fig. 11-14) for horizontal and vertical inguinal nodes

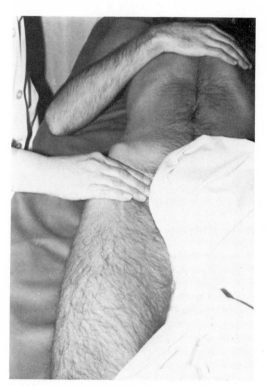

Fig. 11-14. Palpation of inguinal area; finger pads applied just below inguinal ligament.

    a. Presence   Small, mobile   Enlarged, tender
                    Nontender nodes often present
    b. Contour   Smooth or nonpalpable
    c. Consistency   Soft or nonpalpable   Hard
      (*Note:* Femoral pulses can also be palpated at this time. Techniques and palpable qualities are covered in Chapter 9.)
   2. Approach from behind as the client is seated; identify the right and left costovertebral angles

Continued.

Clinical guidelines–cont'd

The student will:	To identify:	
	Normal	**Deviations from normal**
3. Strike each angle with the ulnar surface of your right fist (Fig. 11-15)	Client perceives jar or thud	Tenderness elicited

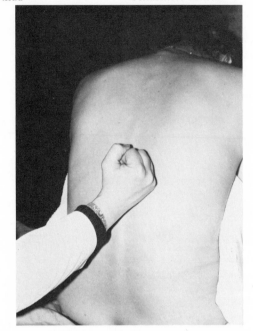

Fig. 11-15. First percussion over costovertebral angle.

Special maneuvers

1. If fluid within the abdomen is suspected:
   a. As the client remains in a supine position, fluid associated with ascites will pool in the lateral (flank) areas. Lines can be drawn on the abdomen to indicate the midline tympany percussion area in contrast to lateral dullness.
   b. If the client turns to the right side, the tympanic sound will shift toward the upper (left) side. As the fluid pools in the right side, the area of dullness will rise toward the midline.
   c. As the client turns to the left lateral position, the fluid will migrate to the left side and the left dullness will rise toward the midline.
2. Small amounts of free fluids can be identified if the client assumes an elbow-knee position. The fluid will pool in the periumbilical region, and the area of dullness can be identified through percussion.
3. If the client is experiencing pain, the examiner should test for rebound tenderness: Press firmly over an area of the abdomen that is remote from the area of discomfort. Release the hand suddenly. If the client experiences a sharp stabbing pain at the site of original discomfort, this can be interpreted as rebound tenderness.

Rectal/anal region

1. Evaluate anal and rectal region		
a. Inspect the sacrococcygeal and perianal areas while client is lying on the left side with the right hip and knee flexed		
1. Skin and surface characteristics	Surface smooth and clear	Lumps, rash, inflammation, scars, pilonidal dimpling, tuft of hair at pilonidal area
b. Palpate coccygeal area for tenderness	No tenderness	Tender
c. Spread buttocks with both hands; inspect anus for:		
1. Surface characteristics (penlight can be used)	Increased pigmentation Coarse skin	Inflammation Lesions Scars Skin tags Fissures Lumps Swelling Excoriation Hemorrhoids Mucosal bulging

The student will:	To identify:	
	Normal	**Deviations from normal**
d. Ask client to strain down; place gloved and lubricated finger at anal opening; as sphincter relaxes, slowly insert finger pointing toward client's umbilicus		
e. Ask client to tighten sphincter around finger to assess sphincter tone	Sphincter tightens evenly around finger with minimal discomfort to client	Hypotonic sphincter Hypertonic sphincter, with marked tenderness
f. Rotate finger to examine anal muscular ring for surface characteristics	Smooth, even pressure on finger	Nodules Irregularities
g. Insert finger farther to palpate all four rectal walls (*Note:* Prostate examination is covered in Chapter 12.)	Continuous, smooth surface with minimal discomfort to client	Nodules Masses (*Note:* The cervix is sometimes palpable on the anterior wall; do not mistake for a mass.) Tenderness
h. As finger is extracted, note characteristics of any stool 1. Color	Brown	Presence of blood, pus Black, tarry stool Pale or yellow Light tan or gray
2. Consistency	Soft	

Clinical strategies

1. Much has been said in textbooks about helping the client to feel comfortable before an abdominal examination. It is extremely difficult to complete an assessment if the abdominal muscles are not relaxed. The basic comfort measures described in the guidelines are essential; however, the examiner must be sensitive to the client's state of anxiety and should be prepared to be flexible with examination procedures if the client remains tense.
   a. If palpation stimulates muscle tension, it might be helpful to lighten the touch and to proceed more slowly.
   b. The abdominal examination can be delayed until later in the assessment when the client might feel more comfortable.
   c. Be certain that the client is draped as fully as possible.
   d. It is sometimes difficult to examine the abdomen while the client is talking; clients tend to lift and bob their heads as they converse. However, it is often soothing to have the examiner talking quietly, describing the procedures, perhaps reviewing the client's history.
2. This statement has appeared in other chapters, but it is worth repeating: *Look before you touch*. Once an individual begins using other senses, the impact of the visual sense diminishes. It is helpful to circle around the examining table and to view the abdomen carefully from all angles for surface and contour characteristics.
3. It is also helpful for the examiner to *visualize* organs or major structures within the abdominal cavity during inspection, auscultation, percussion, and palpation of the abdomen (Fig. 11-16). This mental picture heightens the tactile sense.
4. The examiner should inquire about a history of pain or discomfort *before* beginning palpation. If discomfort is described and located, begin the palpation in another region of the abdomen.
5. The beginning examiner must establish early and consistent routines for carrying out the mechanics of the assessment. Most individuals examine the abdomen from the client's right side. Making this decision early in the learning period is extremely helpful in expediting assessment skills.
6. If lesions, scars, masses, or fluid levels (lines) are identified, it is often easier and more clear to draw a picture of the finding and indicate dimensions and location rather than to attempt a description of it.

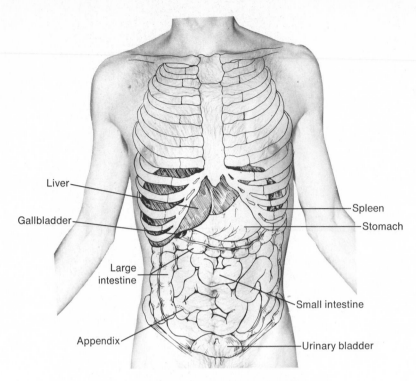

Fig. 11-16. Major structures of abdominal cavity.

Sample recording

Abdomen: Rounded and symmetrical with centrally placed umbilicus. No lesions, rashes, discolorations, scars, inflammation, or visible peristalsis. Normal bowel sounds and no bruits or venous hums. Tympanic on percussion. Abdomen relaxed and without tenderness or masses. Liver 10 cm in right midclavicular line. Spleen and kidneys not palpated. No CVA tenderness.

Rectal and anal region: Sacrococcygeal, perianal, and anal surfaces present no lesions, rash, inflammation, masses, or hemorrhoids. Good sphincter tone. Anal and distal rectal mucosa smooth and without masses.

History and clinical strategies associated with the pediatric client

1. Nutritional assessment. Entire textbooks have been written about the nutritional assessment of children. A basic list of nutritional questions has already been presented in Chapter 1. In addition to this, the examiner must be alert to common nutritional concerns associated with the child.
   a. Obesity is a common problem for children. Questions about a child's overweight situation should include those presented in the adult nutritional assessment section as well as those which follow:
      (1) Family history regarding obesity problems
      (2) Age of the child when overweight problems began
      (3) Whether the child is concerned about his overweight state
      (4) Whether the child understands the relationship between foods consumed and weight gained (For example, a story is told about one teenage girl who consumed three cases of liquid diet supplement every day to cancel the 1000 calories she consumed by eating three meals.)
   b. Toddler nutrition. Many parents of toddlers will express concern that their child's eating patterns have changed. The examiner must gather a food consumption profile from the past week as well as assess the child physically. If the child shows normal progression of height, weight, and maturational development, the examiner should try to decrease parental anxiety by sharing the growth and development progression facts as well as the normal developmental eating changes of the toddler.
   c. Adolescent nutrition. Studies have shown that less than 50% of all teenagers in the United States eat breakfast every day. This usually

arouses concern among parents who state that their teenager is not eating correctly. Likewise, studies done in the United States also show that most adolescents have adequate diets regardless of family income.

Although the examiner should develop a profile of the adolescent's nutritional style and food consumption, unless a problem arises such as overweight, underweight, anemia, fatigue, or systemic disease, there may be little the examiner can do to change the adolescent's style of food consumption.

It is important to assess the adolescent's knowledge of good nutrition and to supply educational facts where necessary.

d. Anorexia nervosa. This disease, referred to as a "socially acceptable" form of suicide, is becoming more common in the United States. Its assessment is included at this point because of the close correlation with adolescent nutrition. A hypothetical profile of a child affected by anorexia nervosa follows:

She is usually a female teenager from an upper middle class family. Her parents, who may be perfectionists, are successful and view themselves as being well adjusted and supportive. Both her mother and father have made many personal sacrifices for the child. The girl is popular and successful. Throughout her life she has conformed to the wishes of her parents. Hardly ever has she expressed her own wishes or translated her own desires into actions.

Anorexia nervosa is such a serious situation that the examiner must explore its potential with all really thin teenagers, especially those whose parents express a concern that the teenager has lost too much weight or will not eat. Although there is usually some significant event that triggers the situation, usually the first symptom to appear will be weight loss. As the anorexia nervosa cycle continues, the examiner will find the parent and the teenager in battle about eating, food, and weight loss. The more the parent harps, the more serious the situation becomes.

The examiner should use the following questions to gather data. Any teenager who appears at risk should be referred immediately.
(1) Is the client less than 25 years of age?
(2) Has there been a weight loss of more than 25% of the client's original weight?
(3) Does the client express an intractable or negative attitude about gaining weight or eating?

(4) Are there any other physical problems present?
(5) Are any of the following factors pertinent (a cluster of at least four is considered high risk)?
  (a) Distorted body image
  (b) Periods of amenorrhea
  (c) Periods of hyperactivity
  (d) History of being overweight
  (e) Denial of hunger
  (f) Denial of fatigue
  (g) History of self-induced vomiting to stay thin
  (h) Morbid fear of obesity
  (i) Preoccupation with food

2. Abdominal pain in the child is extremely difficult to assess. If the examiner asks the child if the palpation hurts or to point to the spot where it hurts, the child will usually comply and provide a response indicating discomfort or pain. More importantly, the examiner should rely on objective findings to assist in assessing the pain. Factors such as different pitch in a cry, a grimace or change in facial expression, or sudden protective movement by arms and legs are helpful indications.

3. A history of abdominal pain in the older child may have many causes. Some of the most common are anxiety, constipation, urinary tract infections, worms, or irritated bowel. The examiner should carefully question the child or parent about each of these.

4. Pinworms may be common in children, especially those who frequently have dirty hands and have their hands in their mouths. The child may complain of abdominal pain or nighttime rectal itching. The parent should be encouraged to observe the child's rectal area with a flashlight at night as the child sleeps. The worms are most likely to be seen at that time. If the parents suspect pinworms, they should attempt to collect a specimen for analysis. The best technique for this is to put cellophane tape, sticky side up, on the end of a tongue blade and gather the specimen as close to the anal opening as possible.

5. For crawling infants and toddlers the examiner should inquire about pica. Common items eaten are plaster, dirt, paint chips, grass, and blanket fuzz. Although it is normal for children to put nonfood items into their mouths, most learn by age 2 years what is and is not edible.

6. Constipation is a common problem during childhood, especially during the toilet training period. If this is a problem, the examiner should inquire about the following:

a. How long the problem has existed
b. Family history of similar problems or diseases affecting bowels
c. Whether toilet training has been associated with the problem
d. How many stools per day and week the child usually has (and within the past week)
e. Current family or home stresses (describe)
f. Food, juice, and water consumption last 48 hours
g. What parent has done about problem
h. How parent feels about problem

7. Symptoms such as indigestion, nausea, vomiting, and diarrhea should be explored as detailed in the adult history section.

8. The approach to the pediatric client is extremely important when attempting to assess the abdomen. The abdomen may be the place to start the entire physical examination of the child, but if the examiner moves in with both hands to palpate the abdomen of an 18-month-old, he or she is set to fail. The following approach may be helpful for assessing the young infant and child. By age 5 years the child should be ready to cooperate more fully.

a. Undress the infant or child to diaper and have child on the parent's lap. Do not attempt to examine the small child's abdomen by placing the child on the examination table. The child may tense, fight, or cry.
b. Observe the child's abdomen as he sits or lies on the parent's lap.
c. Instruct the parent to stand the child up for observation of the abdominal contour and "pot belly" appearance. This is also a time to observe for umbilical bulging or hernia.
d. For ausculation, percussion, and palpation, the child may be laid in the parent's lap with the child's legs extending onto the examiner's lap.
e. There is some disagreement as to the sequence of pediatric abdominal assessment elements. Should it be: (1) inspection, (2) ausculation, (3) percussion, and (4) palpation; or (1) inspection, (2) ausculation, (3) palpation, and (4) percussion? Some authorities suggest that percussion is a frightening procedure and should be done last. Try it both ways and then decide for yourself.
f. Even for a small infant the position that facilitates a soft abdomen is one in which both the knees and the neck are flexed. This is easy to achieve as the parent holds the child.
g. Because of the soft examination surface during palpation, it is helpful in both young and older children for the examiner to place the left hand under the child's back and palpate downward with the right hand directly over the same surface. This facilitates a ballottement approach to assessing the abdominal contents. Be gentle but firm during palpation.
h. An internal rectal examination is not routinely performed for the well child because of the invasiveness of the technique. If there is an obvious problem such as constipation requiring an internal rectal examination, the examiner should proceed with the same guidelines as for the adult. An ill child with an abdominal complaint should be referred for further evaluation.
i. It will be most helpful to undress the child and make some introductory attempts to touch the child during the history session. Another technique involves letting the child play with the examiner's stethoscope while the initial history and physical assessment is occurring.
j. If the examiner has a question about a finding but because of the parent's soft lap is unable to adequately assess, a last choice is to move both the parent and the examiner to the examination table. The child should be placed on the examination table, and the parent should assist in holding the child.
k. For the most part the abdomen is easy to assess early during the examination process, before the child becomes upset. If, however, the child is crying during the initial part of the examination, delay the assessment until later.
l. Crying tenses the abdominal muscles and interferes with accurate assessment.
m. Giving the infant a bottle during the abdominal examination is fine and will, in fact, assist in quieting the child and relaxing the abdominal muscle wall. Caution should be taken to avoid vigorous deep palpation in a child who has just consumed a large bottle of milk, juice, or formula.
n. Older children are generally eager to cooperate but may pose two new problems: ticklishness and firm abdominal muscles.
  (1) Ticklishness may be overcome by gentle continued contact with the child's skin. The sensation should decrease. If not, the examiner may place the child's hand under the examiner's hand.
  (2) A firm abdomen will be a problem in older children and especially in teenage boys. A pillow under the head and flexion of the knees may help to relax the abdominal muscles.
o. Tenseness of the abdominal wall in all children

may be a problem, especially if the child is afraid. The examiner should attempt to engage the child in small talk to take the child's mind off the examination. Although it is important for the examiner to observe the child's facial response during palpation of the abdomen, the examiner should try to avoid direct eye contact with the child continuously. This alone may increase tenseness of the child as well as the abdomen.

Clinical variations associated with the pediatric client

Characteristic or area examined	Normal	Deviations from normal
Abdomen		
1. Inspection		
a. Skin color	May be paler than other parts due to lack of exposure	Jaundice
		Redness (inflammation)
		Lesions, bruises, discoloration, cyanosis (localized at umbilicus or generalized)
b. Surface characteristics	Smooth, soft	Rashes, lesions
	Note scars, striae	Glistening, taut appearance
		Pink or red striae
		Purplish striae
c. Venous network	Very faint fine network may be visible, mostly during infancy	Prominent venous pattern
		Engorgement of veins around umbilicus
d. Umbilicus	Centrally located	Drainage from navel after cord falls off
	Newborn: should dry within 5 days; should drop off within 2 weeks with dry base remaining; cord should contain two arteries and one vein	Babies with cords containing one artery have high incidence of congenital anomalies
	Surface smooth, noninflamed	Inflamed, bluish, or nodular appearance
	Umbilical hernia common, especially in blacks	Umbilical hernia extending beyond 2 years of age in white children, beyond 7 years of age in black children
	Considered normal in white children until 2 years of age, black children until 7 years of age (by 1 month of age hernia should attain its maximum size)	
	Hernia may vary from few millimeters to 3 cm (1 inch)	Child with hernia over 2 cm (¾ inch) should be referred for further assessment
	Note if hernia present during crying only or also at quiet times; note how size changes	Hernia that continues to grow after 1 month of age requires referral
e. Contour	Infant, toddler: rounded "pot belly" both standing and lying (Fig. 11-17)	Scaphoid abdomen in infant or toddler
		Generalized distention

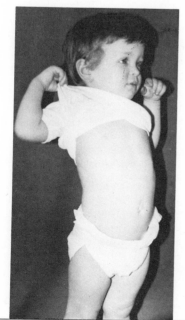

Fig. 11-17. Toddler displaying "pot belly" profile.

Continued.

Clinical variations associated with the pediatric client—cont'd

Characteristic or area examined	Normal	Deviations from normal

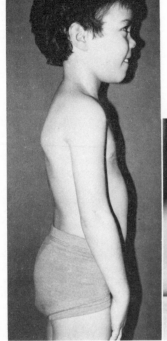 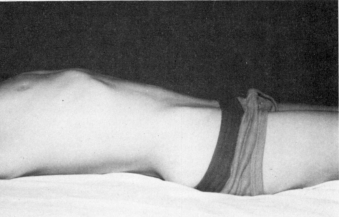

School age: may show some pot belly (lordotic stance) until age 13 years when standing; when child is lying, abdomen should appear scaphoid (Fig. 11-18)

Fig. 11-18. A, "Pot belly" stance of preschool-age child. **B,** Scaphoid contour of school-age child.

Characteristic or area examined	Normal	Deviations from normal
f. Symmetry	Evenly rounded with maximum height of convexity at umbilicus	Distention of upper or lower half Visible masses or bulges in any area of abdominal surface
g. Surface motion		
1. Peristalsis	Usually not visible	Marked peristalsis
2. Pulsations	Upper midline pulsation may be visible in thin children	Marked pulsation
h. Movement with respirations	Children, until approximate age 7 years, are abdominal breathers; after age 7 years boys exhibit chiefly abdominal movement, girls exhibit chiefly costal movement	Grunting, labored respirations accompanied by restricted abdominal movement
i. Tenseness of abdominal muscles	Diastasis recti abdominis condition in which two recti muscles do not approximate each other; common in black children; should disappear during preschool years May be 1 to 5 cm (½ to 2 inches) wide	Same condition with evidence of accompanying hernia Problem continues in 6-year-old
2. Auscultation		
a. Bowel sounds	Usually 5 to 34/min Irregular in timing	Absence of sound established after 5 minutes of listening; note sounds that are infrequent
1. Quality	Gurgles, clicks (quality of sound varies greatly)	High-pitched, tinkling noises May sound like metallic tinkling
b. Vascular sounds		Bruits (usually high-pitched, soft "swishing" sound, and systolic in timing) (*Note:* Bruit will continue as client is moved into various positions.) Murmur near umbilical area Venous hum (lower in pitch, softer, and a continuous sound)
c. Friction rub		Infrequently heard sound, associated with respirations (soft and may be confused with normal breath sounds) Rubs most often heard over spleen or liver

Characteristic or area examined	Normal	Deviations from normal
3. Percussion		
a. Tone	General distribution of tympany (depending on amount of air and solid material in bowel)	Marked dullness in local area
	Suprapubic dullness heard over distended bladder	
	Children's abdomens frequently sound louder in tympany tones than those of adults primarily because children often swallow more air during swallowing and eating	
b. Liver percussion	Upper liver border usually percussed at approximately sixth rib or interspace anteriorly and at ninth rib posteriorly	Upper border lower
		Dullness extending above fifth intercostal space
	Lower liver border usually percussed at approximately costal margin or 2 to 3 cm (¾ to 1 inch) lower	Lower border of liver exceeds 2 to 3 cm below costal margin
c. Liver span	Average: 5 years of age—7 cm (2¾ inches); 12 years of age—9 cm (3½ inches)	Span that exceeds these limits
d. Spleen percussion	May hear small area of dullness above ninth interspace along left midaxillary line	Dullness extends above sixth rib or covers large area between sixth rib and costal margin
	In young infants and children: may extend to 1 to 2 cm below costal margin	Spleen in any ill-appearing child that extends below costal margin
		Spleen in children over 1 year of age that extends below costal margin
4. Palpation		
a. Light and moderate palpation		
1. Tenderness	Not present	Cutaneous (superficial areas of hypersensitivity)
2. Muscle tone	Abdomen relaxed	Involuntary resistance (muscles cannot be relaxed by voluntary effort)
	Muscular resistance may accompany anxious child	
3. Surface characteristics	Smooth; consistent tension felt by examiner	Masses (superficial)
		Localized areas of rigidity or increased tension
4. Umbilical area	Note size of umbilical hernia if present	Tenderness
b. Deep palpation: (be gentle; use one hand)		
1. Tenderness	Often present in midline near xiphoid process	Present in local or generalized areas
	Often present over cecum	Client response to pain may be with muscle guarding and/or facial grimace, pulling away from examiner
	May be present over sigmoid colon	
2. Masses	Aorta often palpable at epigastrium and pulsates in forward direction	Masses that descend on inspiration
		Pulsatile masses
	Borders of rectus abdominis muscles	Laterally mobile masses
	Feces in ascending or descending colon	Fixed masses
		Wilms tumor located adjacent to vertebral column; does not extend across midline
3. Umbilical ring	Umbilicus may be inverted or slightly everted	Umbilical ring may be incomplete or may feel soft in center
	Umbilical ring round, with no irregularities or bulges	Masses, bulges
c. Organ identification		
1. Liver palpation		
a. Border location	0 to 6 months: palpable 0 to 3 cm below costal margin	Greater than 2 cm below right costal margin
	6 months to 4 years: palpable 1 to 2 cm below costal margin	
	Over 6 years: palpable 1 to 2 cm or not palpable below right costal margin	
b. Tenderness	None	Tenderness elicited
		(*Note:* Client's inspiration may be abruptly halted if pain exists.)

Continued.

Clinical variations associated with the pediatric client–cont'd

Characteristic or area examined	Normal	Deviations from normal
2. Spleen palpation	May feel at costal margin or slightly under ribs in small children Only tip (feeling like tongue) should be palpable	Able to palpate more than tip Palpable spleen in older child who also appears ill or has multiple other symptoms
3. Kidney palpation	Palpated periodically, not always Lies adjacent to vertebral column Descends slightly with inspiration Most likely able to palpate lower pole of right kidney; smooth contour	
4. Bladder	Frequently palpated as smooth mass extending midline, somewhere between pubis and umbilical area Ability to palpate should disappear following urination	Bladder distention following voiding
5. Inguinal nodes a. Presence	Small, mobile Nontender nodes often present	Enlarged, tender
b. Contour	Smooth or nonpalpable	
c. Consistency	Soft or nonpalpable	Hard
6. Costovertebral angle tenderness (kidney jarring)	Client perceives jar or thud No tenderness elicited	Tenderness elicited

Anal/rectal region

1. Evaluation of anal and rectal region **a.** Inspection 1. Skin surface characteristics	Surface smooth and clear	Lumps, rash, inflammation, scars, pilonidal dimpling, tuft of hair at pilonidal area
b. Palpation of coccygeal area for tenderness	No tenderness	Tender
c. Inspection of anus 1. Surface characteristics	Increased pigmentation Coarse skin	Inflammation Lesions Scars Skin tags Fissures Lumps Swelling Excoriation
d. Internal rectal examination not routinely done in children unless ill or specific problem exists; when performed, follow same guidelines as for adult client		

History and clinical strategies associated with the geriatric client

1. Nutritional assessment. Many authorities state that maintaining adequate nutritional intake is a major problem for the older adult. This problem is not confined to chronically ill individuals or to low-income persons. Following are risk factors for poor nutritional intake patterns:
   a. Individuals who live alone
   b. Physical disability (e.g., diminished vision, neurological deficits, decreased mobility, arthritic changes, diminished strength, general symptoms of fatigue, dyspnea, or pain)
   c. Depression; anxiety
   d. Mouth or dental problems
   e. Swallowing or choking problems
   f. Sedentary life-style (particularly if associated with boredom, depression, or obesity)
   g. Obesity (usually accompanied by long-standing overeating habits)
   h. Limited access to markets (especially if client is unable to drive, if stores are within walking

distance and require daily trips, or if client must rely on driving services of others)

   i. Limited cooking facilities or capability (often results in increased use of convenience foods, or "empty" calories)

   j. Limited income (this problem exists in all income ranges; fixed incomes do not reflect inflation trends)

   k. Numerous food idiosyncracies or general loss of senses of taste and smell

   l. Confusion (even mild, transient states of confusion will interrupt eating patterns)

  m. Misconceptions about nutritional requirements (e.g., the belief that fewer nutrients are required for the elderly)

   n. Special diets prescribed (especially if difficult to purchase or to prepare or if taste is less desirable)

   o. Medications (prescribed or over-the-counter drugs may cause gastrointestinal side effects such as dry mouth, anorexia, nausea, sedation, "heartburn") (*Note:* Aspirin is frequently the source of gastrointestinal symptoms.)

   p. Alcohol or drug abuse

The questions described in the original data base will help the examiner to elicit information related to the variables that alter food and fluid intake.

The actual *amounts* or *types* of food that are routinely consumed are sometimes difficult to assess because many older adults eat erratically (numerous meals are taken in small amounts scattered over a 24-hour period, or eating habits vary widely from day to day). A 24-hour recall may not reflect true eating patterns. A diary, covering a week or a month of food consumption, may be helpful if the client is sufficiently motivated to follow through with recording. Several appointments devoted to nutritional assessment may be necessary if the examiner suspects intake is inadequate.

2. Elimination assessment. Authorities state that elderly clients frequently express numerous problems associated with elimination and that individuals may be preoccupied with bowel movement regularity to the extent that it can alter daily living functions. Problems may be described as a "spastic" or "irritable" colon, colitis, "gas on the stomach," constipation, or diarrhea. Clarification of symptoms is necessary. Constipation and diarrhea are discussed in the adult history section of this chapter. If long-standing problems exist, inquire carefully about the client's effort to treat himself. Risk factors associated with bowel elimination problems follow:

   a. Hemorrhoids

   b. Individuals who take laxatives (clarify whether this is a long-standing or recent habit)

   c. Recent dietary changes: reduced intake; elimination of certain foods

   d. Dietary intake with insufficient bulk

   e. Limited fluid intake

   f. Depression (often associated with constipation)

   g. Anxiety

   h. Physical immobility

   i. Weakened abdominal muscles

   j. Medication side effects or abuse (prescribed or over the counter, e.g., iron, antibiotics, tranquilizers, antacids)

3. Major aging changes associated with gastrointestinal system include:

   a. Decrease in total volume of acid secretion

   b. Decreased hunger contractions

   c. Delayed gastric emptying

   d. Diminished tone of bowel wall

   e. Decreased peristalsis

   f. Decreased abdominal muscle strength

   g. Decreased anal sphincter tone

4. In many instances, the changes just listed do not produce any signs or symptoms that are significant to the client or the examiner. These changes take place at different rates with different individuals and are not predictable on a chronological basis. However, all symptoms should be explored carefully and not assumed to be a "functional" disorder by the examiner. Elderly clients may manifest less pain and less abdominal rigidity in acute or chronic conditions. Details related to the major symptoms are covered in the adult section of this chapter.

Clinical variations associated with the geriatric client

Characteristic or area examined	Normal	Deviations from normal
1. General behaviors of the client	Appears relaxed Facial muscles relaxed Lying quietly Respirations even and slow	Marked restlessness Marked immobility or rigid posture Knees drawn up Facial grimacing Respirations rapid, uneven, or "grunting"

Continued.

Clinical variations associated with the geriatric client–cont'd

Characteristic or area examined	Normal	Deviations from normal
Abdomen		
1. Inspection of abdominal surface		
a. Skin color	May be paler than other parts due to lack of exposure	Jaundice Redness (inflammation) Lesions, bruises, discoloration, cyanosis (localized at umbilicus or generalized)
b. Surface characteristics	Smooth, soft Silver-white striae (usually lower abdomen)	Rashes, lesions Glistening, taut appearance
c. Scars (configuration, location, length)		
d. Venous network	Faint fine network may be visible	Prominent venous pattern Engorgement of veins around umbilicus
e. Ubilicus		
1. Placement	Centrally located	Displaced upward or downward
2. Contour	Usually sunken, may protrude slightly	Visible hernia around or slightly above umbilicus
3. Surface	Smooth, noninflamed	Inflamed
f. Contour	Flat Rounded Scaphoid (concave profile) (*Note:* Elderly individuals may have increased fat deposits over abdominal area even though subcutaneous fat is decreased over extremities.)	Distention (common distress signal in elderly clients) Marked concavity associated with general wasting signs or associated with anterior-posterior rib expansion)
g. Symmetry	Evenly rounded with maximum height of convexity at umbilicus	Distention of upper or lower half Visible masses or bulges in any area of abdominal surface
h. Surface motion		
1. Peristalsis	Usually not visible	Visible
2. Pulsation	Upper midline pulsation may be visible in thin people	Marked pulsation
i. General movement with respirations	Smooth, even movements Women exhibit chiefly costal movement Men exhibit chiefly abdominal movement	Grunting, labored Respirations accompanied by restricted abdominal movement
2. Instruct client to take a deep breath and hold it	Contour remains smooth and symmetrical	Bulges or masses appear
3. Instruct client to raise the head without using arms for support	Rectus abdominis muscles prominent Midline bulge may appear	Appearance of bulges through muscle layer
4. Auscultatory bowel sounds	Usually 5 to 34/min Irregular in timing	Absence of sound established after 5 minutes of listening Note sounds that are infrequent
a. Quality	Gurgles, clicks Quality of sound varies greatly	High-pitched, tinkling noises
5. Vascular sounds		
a. Arterial: concentrate in epigastric area, in area surrounding umbilicus, over the liver, and at the posterior flank		Bruits (usually high-pitched, soft, swishing sound, and systolic in timing) (*Note:* Bruit will continue as client is moved into various positions.)
b. Venous		Venous hum (lower in pitch, softer, and continuous sound)
6. Friction rubs		Infrequently heard sound associated with respirations (soft, and may be confused with normal breath sounds) Rubs most often heard over spleen or liver
7. Percussion tones over entire abdomen	General distribution of tympany (depending on amount of air and solid material in bowel) Suprapubic dullness heard over distended bladder	Marked dullness in local area

Characteristic or area examined	Normal	Deviations from normal
8. Liver		
a. Lower border percussion	Lower border of liver usually at costal margin or slightly below; however, if elderly client has distended lungs, liver border will descend 1 to 2 cm into abdominal cavity	Lower border of liver exceeds 2 to 3 cm below costal margin
b. Upper border percussion	Upper border of liver usually begins in fifth to seventh intercostal space Upper border may descend 1 to 2 cm if liver has lowered with diaphragm, associated with distended lungs	Upper border lowered Dullness extending above fifth intercostal space
c. Midclavicular liver span	6 to 12 cm (2½ to 4½ inches) Normal liver span usually greater in men than women, and greater in taller individuals	Span exceeds 12 cm
d. Right midaxillary liver percussion	Liver dullness May be felt in fifth to seventh intercostal space	Dull percussion note exceeds limits of fifth to seventh intercostal space
e. Midsternal liver span	Ranges from 4 to 8 cm (1½ to 3 inches)	Span exceeds 8 cm
f. Liver descent with deep inspiration (*Note:* Deep inspiration may be difficult for elderly client.)	Lower border of liver should move inferiorly by 2 to 3 cm	Liver does not move with inspiration, or movement less than 2 cm
9. Spleen percussion		
a. At left posterior midaxillary line	Small area of splenic dullness may be heard at sixth to tenth rib, or tone may be tympanic (colonic)	Dullness extends above sixth rib or dullness covers large area between sixth rib and costal margin
b. At lowest left intercostal space in anterior axillary line (performed after client takes deep breath)	Area usually tympanic	Tympany changes to dullness on inspiration (An enlarged spleen is brought forward on inspiration to produce a dull percussion note.)
10. Percussion of gastric "bubble" in left lower rib cage	Tympanic and varies in size	
11. Palpation		
a. Muscle tone	(*Note:* Elderly clients often manifest a more lax abdominal tone.)	Involuntary resistance Elderly clients may not manifest rigidity response to extent that younger client does; rigidity may be replaced by distention
b. Tenderness	Not present on light or moderate palpation Deep palpation may cause discomfort in midline near xiphoid process Over cecum Over sigmoid colon	Cutaneous (superficial areas of hypersensitivity) or deep pain response in local or generalized area
c. Surface characteristics	Smooth	Induration Nodules Rough texture
d. General tone and location of major structures	Abdomen surface feels smooth, and tension under palpating hand feels consistent throughout	Localized areas of rigidity, distention, or increased tension
e. Masses	Aorta often palpable at epigastrium and pulsates in forward direction Borders of rectus abdominis muscles Feces in ascending or descending colon Sacral promontory	Masses that descend on inspiration Pulsatile masses Laterally mobile masses Fixed masses Aortic pulsations directed laterally
f. Umbilicus	Umbilical ring round, with no irregularities or bulges Umbilicus may be inverted or slightly everted	Masses, bulges Umbilical ring may be incomplete or may feel soft in center
12. Specific organ identification		
a. Liver palpation		
1. Border and contour	Liver often not palpable Liver often "bumps" against fingers on inspiration (especially with thin clients)	(*Note:* Greatly enlarged liver may lie under examiner's hand as it extends downward into abdominal cavity.)

Continued.

Clinical variations associated with the geriatric client—cont'd

Characteristic or area examined	Normal	Deviations from normal
	Liver commonly palpated 1 to 2 cm below costal margin in clients with distended lungs and lowered diaphragm	
2. Border surface	Smooth	Irregular, nodular surface or edge
3. Tenderness	None	Tenderness elicited (*Note:* Client's inspiration may be abruptly halted if pain exists.)
b. Spleen palpation	Spleen not normally palpable	Spleen palpated (as firm mass)
c. Kidney palpation	Kidneys rarely palpated in elderly clients Lower pole of right kidney may be felt in very thin clients; if palpated, contour smooth and no associated tenderness	
d. Inguinal nodes (horizontal and vertical)		
1. Presence	Small, mobile Nontender nodes often present	Tender, enlarged
2. Contour	Smooth or nonpalpable	
3. Consistency	Soft or nonpalpable	
(*Note:* Femoral pulses can also be palpated at this time. Techniques and palpable qualities are covered in Chapter 9.) *Note:* Special maneuvers for assessing fluid in the abdominal cavity and abdominal pain are conducted in the same manner as described in the adult section of this chapter (p. 274).		
Anal/rectal region		
1. Inspection of sacrococcygeal and perianal areas for:		
a. Skin and surface characteristics	Surface smooth and clear	Lumps Rash Inflammation Scars Pilonidal dimpling Tuft of hair at pilonidal area
2. Palpation of coccygeal area for tenderness	No tenderness	Tender
3. Inspection of anus for:		
a. Surface characteristics	Increased pigmentation Coarse skin	Inflammation Lesions Scars Skin tags Fissures Lumps Swelling Excoriation Hemorrhoids Mucosa (pinkish red in color) bulges through anal ring
4. Ask client to strain down to assess sphincter tone	Sphincter tightens evenly around examiner's finger with minimal discomfort to client	Client unable to tighten sphincter around finger or experiences discomfort with tightening
5. Palpation of anal muscular ring for:		
a. Surface characteristics	Smooth even pressure on finger	Nodules Irregularities

Characteristic or area examined	Normal	Deviations from normal
6. Palpation of all four rectal walls	Continuous smooth surface with minimal discomfort to client	Nodules Masses (*Note:* The cervix is sometimes palpable on the anterior wall. Do not mistake for a mass.) (*Note:* Elderly clients often have rectal polyps; however, they are soft and sometimes difficult to palpate.)
(*Note:* Prostate examination is covered in Chapter 12.) **7.** As finger is extracted, note characteristics of any stool **a.** Color	Brown	Presence of blood, pus Black, tarry stool Pale or yellow stool Mucus on stool surface
b. Consistency	Soft	

Vocabulary

1. Ascites

2. Ballottement

3. Borborygmi

4. Diastasis recti

5. Flank

6. Flatulence

7. Guarding

8. Linea alba

9. McBurney's point

10. Murphy's sign

11. Pilonidal (sinus)

12. Poupart's ligament

13. Pyrosis

14. Rebound tenderness

15. Riedel's lobe

16. Scaphoid

17. Shifting dullness

18. Striae

19. Tenesmus (rectal)

20. Tympanites

21. Verge (anal)

Cognitive self-assessment

1. Complete the illustration below, by drawing in the following organs:
   a. Liver
   b. Stomach
   c. Spleen
   d. Ascending colon
   e. Transverse colon
   f. Descending colon
   g. Bladder (distended)
   h. Aorta

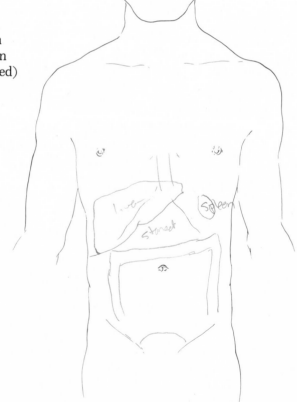

2. Describe five activities or conditions that contribute to client comfort and relaxation in preparation for an abdominal examination, beginning with:

a. Recently emptied bladder
b. _warm hands_
c. _warm stethoscope_
d. _mouth breathing_
e. _short nails_
f. _explanation_

Column A describes abdominal organs (or abdominal content). Column B names the four quadrants that serve as location landmarks for the abdominal contents. Assign a quadrant to each organ or abdominal structure.

Column A	*Column B*
3. _c_ Appendix	a. Right upper quadrant
4. _b_ Stomach	b. Left upper quadrant
5. _b_ Spleen	c. Right lower quadrant
6. _d_ Sigmoid colon	d. Left lower quadrant
7. _c_ Cecum	
8. _a_ Hepatic flexure of colon	
9. _a_ Pylorus	
10. _d_ Left ureter	

11. Which of the following statement(s) is/are true about findings associated with inspection of the abdomen?
    ☐ a. Silvery, white striae are often considered to be a finding within normal limits.
    ☐ b. A scaphoid abdominal contour may be a normal finding.
    ☐ c. A fine venous network may normally be visualized on the abdominal surface.
    ☐ d. A visible aortic pulsation may be a normal finding.
    ☐ e. A diastasis recti abdominis may be a normal finding.
    ☐ f. a, b, and d
    ☑ g. All the above
    ☐ h. All except e
    ☐ i. All except d
    ☐ j. c and e

12. Which of the following statement(s) is/are true?
    ☐ a. The normal liver span in the midclavicular line is 6 to 12 cm.
    ☐ b. The normal liver span in the midsternal line is 4 to 8 cm.
    ☐ c. The liver span is usually greater in tall people than in short people.
    ☐ d. Gas in the colon can obscure the liver border.
    ☐ e. On inspiration, the liver span will shift inferiorly 2 to 3 cm.
    ☐ f. All except c
    ☑ g. All the above
    ☐ h. All except e
    ☐ i. b, c, and d
    ☐ j. a, d, and e

13. Auscultation of the abdomen precedes percussion and palpation:
    ☐ a. only when one is examining an infant
    ☐ b. when the examiner suspects a pulsatile mass is present
    ☑ c. because the latter maneuvers may distort bowel sounds
    ☐ d. because palpation may displace organs and blood vessels

14. Which of the following statement(s) is/are true about findings associated with auscultation of the abdomen?
    ☑ a. The normal frequency for bowel sounds may range from 5 to 34 per minute.
    ☐ b. Peristaltic sounds are normally quite regular in frequency and duration.

☐ c. Gastroenteritis will often result in decreased bowel sounds.

☑ d. Surgical manipulation of the bowel will often result in decreased bowel sounds.

☑ e. Concluding that no bowel sounds are present can occur when the examiner fails to hear sounds after 5 minutes of listening.

☐ f. All the above

☐ g. All except b

☐ h. b, c, and d

☑ i. a, d, and e

☐ j. a, c, and e

15. Which of the following statement(s) is/are true about percussion findings associated with a normal abdomen?

☐ a. Tympany usually predominates as you percuss over the entire abdomen.

☐ b. Percussing a distended bladder will elicit a suprapubic resonance.

☐ c. Solid masses will percuss as dull.

☐ d. A gastric air bubble can usually be identified by percussing in the left upper quadrant.

☐ e. All the above

☐ f. All except d

☐ g. b and c

☑ h. All except b

☐ i. b and d

16. Which of the following statement(s) is/are true?

☐ a. The spleen is generally not palpable in the normal adult.

☐ b. Splenic dullness may be percussed from the ninth to the eleventh ribs in the left midclavicular line.

☐ c. Turning a supine client to the right brings the spleen closer to the abdominal wall.

☐ d. The spleen descends on inspiration.

☐ e. An enlarged spleen would lie anterior to the colon.

☐ f. All except a

☐ g. All except e

☑ h. All except b

☐ i. b, d, and e

17. Which of the following statement(s) is/are true?

☐ a. A liver mass would probably descend on inspiration when palpated.

☐ b. A kidney mass would probably be pulsatile.

☑ c. A small bowel mass would probably move from side to side when palpated.

☑ d. A pancreatic mass would probably be immobile when palpated.

☐ e. A splenic mass would probably be immobile when palpated.

☑ f. a, c, and d

☐ g. All the above

☐ h. All except d

☐ i. a, b, and c

☐ j. b and d

18. Deep palpation may normally elicit tenderness in which areas?

☐ a. over the liver

☑ b. over the cecum

☑ c. over the sigmoid colon

☐ d. just above the inguinal ligaments

☑ e. over the aorta (midline)

☐ f. all except e

    ☐ g. all except d
    ☑ h. b, c, and e
    ☐ i. a and d
    ☐ j. all the above

19. Which statement(s) is/are true about inguinal lymph nodes?
    ☐ a. Lymphatic drainage of the lower extremities consists of both superficial and deep systems.
    ☐ b. Only the superficial system of inguinal lymph nodes is accessible to physical examination.
    ☐ c. The vertical (or inferior) nodes receive drainage from the leg.
    ☐ d. The horizontal (or superior) nodes receive drainage from the skin of the lower abdominal wall.
    ☐ e. The horizontal (or superior) nodes receive drainage from the external genitalia.
    ☑ f. All the above
    ☐ g. a, b, and e
    ☐ h. All except d
    ☐ i. All except e
    ☐ j. a, c, and d

20. The anus:
    ☐ a. is approximately 2.5 to 4 cm in length
    ☐ b. is voluntarily closed by the external sphincter
    ☐ c. is contracted by the internal sphincter through sympathetic stimulation
    ☐ d. presents a surface of squamous epithelium that extends to the pectinate line
    ☐ e. forms a ring at the pectinate line called the valve of Houston
    ☐ f. all the above
    ☐ g. b and c
    ☐ h. a and b
    ☑ i. all except e
    ☐ j. all except d

21. The rectum:
    ☐ a. is lined with squamous epithelium
    ☐ b. is about 12 cm in length
    ☐ c. forms an ampulla at its distal end where it joins the anus
    ☐ d. is not accessible to manual palpation
    ☐ e. contains valves that, when well developed, are palpable
    ☑ f. b, c, and e
    ☐ g. a and d
    ☐ h. b and c
    ☐ i. a, b, and c
    ☐ j. all except d

PEDIATRIC QUESTIONS

22. The rectal examination in the child is routinely done in which of the following situations?
    ☐ a. Children at 1-year evaluation
    ☐ b. Children at preschool evaluation
    ☐ c. Children at time of puberty
    ☑ d. None of the above

23. Which of the following children should be referred for further evaluation?
    ☐ a. 2-month-old with 1 cm umbilical hernia
    ☐ b. 5-year-old black boy with 2 cm umbilical hernia

    ☐ c. 6-month-old whose liver is palpable 2 cm below the right costal margin

    ☐ d. 3-year-old with 1-inch gap in rectus abdominis muscles

    ☑ e. 18-month-old whose spleen is palpable 1 cm below the left costal margin

    ☐ f. None of the above

    ☐ g. a, b, and e

    ☐ h. b, c, and d

24. Which of the following organs may normally be palpated in a 9-month-old child?

    ☐ a. Kidney

    ☐ b. Bladder

    ☐ c. Liver

    ☐ d. Spleen

    ☐ e. Full descending colon

    ☑ f. All the above

    ☐ g. All except b

    ☐ h. All except d

    ☐ i. All except e

GERIATRIC QUESTIONS

25. Elderly individuals often describe constipation as a concern. Which of the following might be a contributing factor?

    ☐ a. Depression

    ☐ b. Decreased abdominal muscle tone

    ☐ c. Erratic eating habits

    ☐ d. Inactivity

    ☐ e. Insufficient bulk in diet

    ☐ f. b and e

    ☑ g. All the above

    ☐ h. All except a

    ☐ i. c, d, and e

26. When examining the abdomen of a healthy older individual, the examiner is likely to find:

    ☐ a. a liver span that is 1 to 2 cm longer than in a younger client

    ☐ b. moderate abdominal distention

    ☐ c. kidneys more readily palpable than in a younger client

    ☐ d. a palpable gallbladder

    ☑ e. tenderness (on deep palpation) over the epigastrium at the xiphoid process

SUGGESTED READINGS
General

Bates, Barbara: A guide to physical examination, ed. 2, Philadelphia, 1979, J. B. Lippincott Co., pp. 200-220, 249-256.

Diekelmann, Nancy: Primary health care of the well adult, New York, 1977, McGraw-Hill Book Co., pp. 37-50, 115-125, 227-232.

G.I. Series: Physical examination of the abdomen, Richmond, Va., 1974, A. H. Robins Co.

Malasanos, Lois, Barkauskas, Violet, Moss, Muriel, and Stoltenberg-Allen, Kathryn: Health assessment, St. Louis, 1977, The C. V. Mosby Co., pp. 238-270.

Prior, John A., and Silberstein, Jack S.: Physical diagnosis: the history and examination of the patient, ed. 5, St. Louis, 1977, The C. V. Mosby Co., pp. 298-322.

Walker, Kenneth, Hall, W. Dallas, and Hurst, J. Willis, editors: Clinical methods, vol. 1, Boston, 1976, Butterworths, Inc., pp. 69-129.

Pediatric

Alexander, Mary, and Brown, Marie Scott: Pediatric physical diagnosis for nurses, New York, 1974, McGraw-Hill Book Co., pp. 149-165.

Barness, Lewis: Manual of pediatric physical diagnosis, ed. 4,

Chicago, 1972, Year Book Medical Publishers, Inc., pp. 124-143.

Bates, Barbara: A guide to physical examination, ed. 2, Philadelphia, 1979, J. B. Lippincott Co. pp. 407-410.

Daniel, William: Adolescents in health and disease, St. Louis, 1977, The C. V. Mosby Co., pp. 234-247.

DeAngelis, Catherine: Basic pediatrics for the primary health care provider, Boston, 1975, Little, Brown & Co., pp. 197-210.

Feighner, J. P., et al.: Diagnostic criteria for use in psychiatric research, Arch Gen. Psychiatry **26:**57-63, 1972.

Johnson, Thomas: Developmental physiology. In Johnson, T. R., Moore, W. M., and Jeffries, J. E., editors: Children are different, Columbus, Ohio, 1978, Ross Laboratories, pp. 156, 157.

Prior, John A., and Silberstein, Jack S.: Physical diagnosis: the history and examination of the patient, ed. 5, St. Louis, 1977, The C. V. Mosby Co., pp. 466-469.

Geriatric

Burnside, Irene Mortenson, editor: Nursing and the aged, New York, 1976, McGraw-Hill Book Co., pp. 405-408, 414-416.

Caird, F. I., and Judge, T. G.: Assessment of the elderly patient, London, 1977, Pitman Medical Publishing Co., Ltd., pp. 40-43.

Chinn, Austin, editor: Working with older people: clinical aspects of aging, vol. IV, Rockville, Md., 1971, U.S. Department of Health, Education, and Welfare, Public Health Service, pp. 124-130, 267-278.

Diekelmann, Nancy: Primary care of the well adult, New York, 1977, McGraw-Hill Book Co., pp. 175-186.

Malasanos, Lois, Barkauskas, Violet, Moss, Muriel, and Stoltenberg-Allen, Kathryn: Health assessment, St. Louis, The C. V. Mosby Co., p. 441.

Steinberg, Franz U., editor: Cowdry's the care of the geriatric patient, St. Louis, 1976, The C. V. Mosby Co., pp. 93-114, 191-213.

CHAPTER **12**

Assessment of the male genitourinary system

Cognitive objectives

At the end of this unit the learner will demonstrate knowledge of assessment of the male genitourinary system by the ability to do the following:
1. Identify and locate the major internal and external structures of the male genitourinary system.
2. Identify observable and palpable characteristics of normal penis and scrotal contents.
3. Identify major inguinal and lower abdominal structures associated with assessment for hernias.
4. Locate, on a drawing, the three common pelvic area hernia sites.
5. Identify palpable characteristics of the normal prostate gland.
6. Identify common selected variations for pediatric and geriatric clients.
7. Define the terms in the vocabulary section.

Clinical objectives

At the end of this unit the learner will perform a systematic assessment of the male genitourinary system, demonstrating the ability to do the following:
1. Obtain a pertinent history from a client.
2. Inspect and palpate the pubic region for:
   a. Hair distribution
   b. Parasites
   c. Surface characteristics
3. Inspect and palpate the penis for:
   a. Surface characteristics
   b. Foreskin
   c. Meatus location
   d. Discharge
   e. Tenderness
4. Inspect and palpate the scrotum and scrotal contents for:
   a. Size and contour
   b. Testes
      (1) Size
      (2) Contour
      (3) Mobility
      (4) Tenderness
   c. Epididymides
   d. Vas deferens
   e. Additional scrotal contents
5. Transilluminate scrotal contents.
6. Evaluate inguinal region for hernias: palpate external inguinal ring and femoral area.
7. Inspect and palpate sacrococcygeal and perianal area for surface characteristics and tenderness.
8. Inspect and palpate the anus for:
   a. Sphincter tone
   b. Tenderness
   c. Surface characteristics
9. Palpate distal rectal walls for surface characteristics.
10. Palpate the prostate gland for:
    a. Size
    b. Contour
    c. Consistency
    d. Tenderness
11. Summarize results with a written description of findings.

Health history related to male genitourinary assessment additional to data base

1. Reproductive functions and sexuality. The examiner should screen all clients for sexual needs or problems by initially posing a broad, nondirective question. The question might be worded in this way: "Do you have any concerns regarding sexual practices or values that you would like to discuss?" This lets the client know that he can share his problems if he wishes to, and it does not direct

him toward any specific area of concern. Please note that anyone posing this question should be prepared to follow through with intervention skills in this area.

A more specific detailed assessment will help to clarify general concerns and can supplement the original data base.

  a. Present practices and values

    (1) Are you comfortable with your intimate relationships (with or without sexual activity)? Do you have difficulty meeting your needs for intimacy (or affection)?

    (2) Are you having a sexual relationship with anyone at present?

    (3) Do you feel satisfied with this relationship (e.g., do you and your partner share similar feelings about the methods and variety of sexual acts you perform; about the frequency of sex; about the kind and amount of affection displayed; about initiating sex? Do you talk about sexual feelings with your partner? Is there anything you would change about this relationship?)?

    (4) If you do not have a sexual partner, are your sexual needs being met?

    (5) Do you have more than one sexual partner? If so, is this a satisfactory arrangement?

    (6) How many partners have you had in the past year?

    (7) How do you feel about homosexuality (i.e., is it a personal issue with you)?

    (8) How do you feel about masturbation?

    (9) Have there been any recent changes in your sexual desire (arousal patterns), specific sexual acts or behaviors, frequency of sexual experiences, choice of sexual partners?

   (10) Do you and/or your partner(s) use contraception? What method do you use? Do you have questions or difficulty with this?

   (11) Do you have any questions about male sexuality, sexual function, female sexuality, sterility, venereal disease, other?

  b. Past history

    (1) Describe your personal experience with sex education (e.g., was sexuality discussed with family members? Was it discussed openly? Were there others outside the family who informed or influenced you sexually? Describe.).

    (2) Were your parents affectionate with each other?

    (3) What were your early experiences with masturbation; wet dreams; sex play with other children; adolescent relationships; dating (feeling comfortable with girls); petting?

    (4) How old were you when you first had sexual intercourse? How did you feel about it?

    (5) Have you ever had a homosexual experience? Describe.

    (6) How many sexual partners have you had?

  c. Genital health

    (1) Do you examine your penis and your scrotum (testicles)? How often? (*Note:* It is more helpful to allow the client to demonstrate how he examines himself during the physical assessment rather than to have him describe the procedure.)

    (2) Do you have any general concerns about your genitalia (e.g., size, shape, surface characteristics, texture)?

    (3) Are you able to pull back (and replace) the foreskin on your penis?

    (4) Have you ever noticed any sores, rashes, swelling, lumps, or discharge?

    (5) Have you felt any itching, burning, or stinging in your penis?

    (6) Are you able to have an erection? Do you have difficulty attaining or maintaining an erection?

    (7) Do you experience pain with an erection (either in your penis or scrotum)?

    (8) Do you ever have prolonged painful erections? If so, is it associated with sexual arousal?

    (9) When you have an erection, does your penis curve downward or to the side?

   (10) Do you have any difficulty with ejaculation (e.g., premature, inadequate, painful)?

   (11) Describe the fluid that discharges at the time of ejaculation (color, consistency, odor, amount).

   (12) Do you ever feel any irregularities, lumps, soreness, or heaviness in your testicles?

   (13) Have you ever been treated for (or ever been exposed to) any venereal diseases: gonorrhea, syphilis, herpes simplex, ve-

nereal warts? If so, describe symptoms, treatment, follow-up procedures.

(14) Do you take any precautions to prevent exposure to sexually transmitted diseases?

(15) Do you have specific questions or concerns about symptoms or disease transmission?

2. Genitourinary symptoms

a. Urinary frequency. How many times do you void (urinate) in a 24-hour period? Does this frequency involve sleeping hours as well as waking hours? Can you estimate the volume voided each time? Has the volume increased or decreased?

b. Nocturia. How many times do you have to urinate at night? Is this a *change* of habit for you? Has your daytime or nighttime fluid intake changed?

c. Urgency. Does urgency occur with every urination, occasionally, or rarely? Does urgency occur without voiding? Is it associated with other symptoms such as frequency, dysuria, or incontinence?

d. Hesitancy. Do you have to wait a while for your stream to start? Once you have started, can you pass 80% to 90% of your urine in a continuous stream? Do you have to strain to start or to maintain your stream?

e. Flow of urinary stream. Have you had any decrease in the size of your stream? Are you having to stand closer to the toilet to avoid urinating on the floor? (The examiner is concerned with the force as well as caliber of the stream.)

f. Urethral discharge. What color is it? Has the amount of discharge increased or decreased since it started? Is the discharge associated with pain? With urination? Is an unusual odor associated with discharge? Describe.

g. Hernia. If you feel a lump in your scrotum, are you able to push the lump back inside? Does the lump ever change size? How long has it been since you were able to push the lump back inside (a day; a week)? Do you have a heavy feeling or a dragging sensation in your scrotum?

Clinical guidelines

The student will:	To identify:	
	Normal	**Deviations from normal**
1. Assemble equipment		
a. Rectal glove		
b. Lubricant		
c. Penlight		
2. Inspect and palpate the general pubic region (Palpation of inguinal lymphatics is described in Chapter 11.)		
a. Hair distribution	Variable in adults	Patchy growth or loss
	Diamond-shaped pattern often extending to umbilicus	Absence of hair
		Female configuration: triangular, with base over pubis
b. Parasites	Absent	Nits, pubic lice
c. Skin surface characteristics	Smooth, clear	Scars
		Lower abdominal or inguinal lesions
		Rash (especially in folds)
3. Inspect the penis		
a. Skin color and surface characteristics	Usually dark	Reddened
	Hairless	Lesions
	Wrinkled; surface vascularity may be apparent	Swelling
		Nodules

The student will:	To identify:	
	Normal	**Deviations from normal**
b. Foreskin	Uncircumcised: prepuce present and folded over glans (Fig. 12-1) Circumcised: prepuce often absent, or small flap remains at corona (Fig. 12-2)	

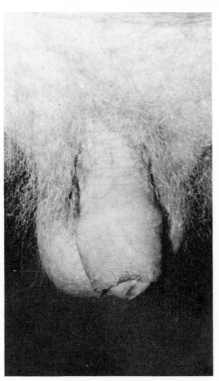

Fig. **12-1.** Uncircumcised penis.

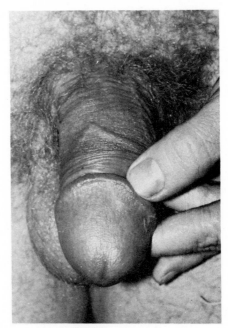

Fig. **12-2.** Circumcised penis.

| **4.** Ask client to retract foreskin if present (Fig. 12-3) | Foreskin retracts easily to expose glans and returns to original position with ease | Failure to retract; discomfort with retraction
Difficulty returning prepuce to original position |

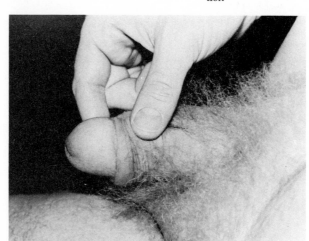

Fig. **12-3.** Client retracting foreskin.

Continued.

Clinical guidelines–cont'd

The student will:	To identify:	
	Normal	Deviations from normal
5. Inspect glans and under prepuce fold		Lesions Crusting under fold or around tip of glans Redness, swelling
6. Inspect urethral meatus for: **a.** Location	Central, at distal tip of glans	Dorsal location Ventral location
b. Discharge	Usually not present	Yellow-green discharge Milky-white discharge Discharge with foul odor
7. Ask client to compress the glans anteroposteriorly to open distal end of uretha (Fig. 12-4); inspect for surface characteristics	Pink, smooth No discharge	Reddened, swollen Discharge Crusting

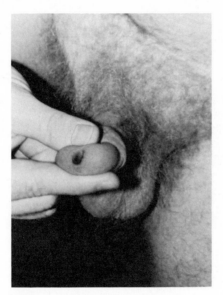

Fig. 12-4. Client compressing glans to open urethral meatus.

The student will:	Normal	Deviations from normal
8. Palpate entire penis between thumb and first two fingers for palpable characteristics; use glove if lesions or discharge is visualized	Nontender Smooth, semifirm consistency	Tenderness Swelling Nodules Induration
9. Ask the client to hold penis out of the way, inspect the scrotum for size and contour	Sac divided in half by septum Left scrotal sac may be longer than right Size varies: may appear pendulous Scrotal contents contracted when surface temperature cool	
10. Lift scrotum to examine underside surface characteristics (spread rugated surface for better view)	Deeply pigmented Hairless Rugous surface	Reddened Edematous Rugae not present Rash Lesions

The student will:	To identify:	
	Normal	Deviations from normal

(*Note:* While viewing surface of scrotum, visualize scrotal contents: placement, proximity, size; tactile maneuvers will be more efficient [Fig. 12-5].)

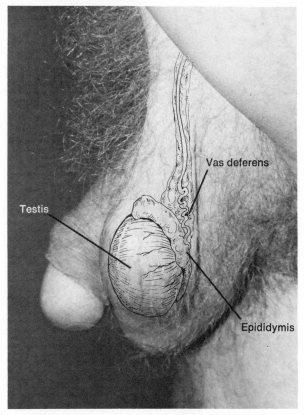

Vas deferens

Testis

Epididymis

Fig. 12-5. Palpable scrotal contents.

11. Palpate each half of the scrotum for surface characteristics

12. Palpate testes simultaneously between thumb and first two fingers (Fig. 12-6)

Nontender
Thin loose skin over muscular layer
No pitting

Marked tenderness
Swelling
Pitting

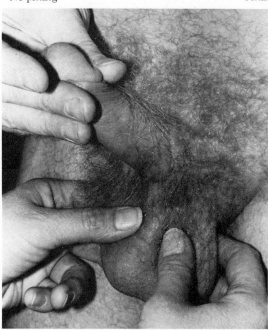

Fig. 12-6. Examiner palpating scrotum.

Continued.

Clinical guidelines–cont'd

The student will:	To identify:	
	Normal	Deviations from normal
a. Presence	Present in each sac	Not present
b. Size	Approximately 4 × 3 × 2 cm (1½ × 1 × ¾ inches)	Enlarged (unilateral/bilateral)
		Atrophied
	Equal in size	
c. Tenderness	Mildly sensitive to moderate compression	Markedly tender
d. Contour	Smooth, ovoid	Nodular
		Irregular
e. Mobility	Movable	Fixed
13. Palpate epididymides for palpable characteristics	Nontender	Tender
	Usually located on posterolateral surface of each testis	
	Discretely palpable	
	Comma shaped	Irregular
	Smooth	Enlarged
		Indurated
		Nodular
14. Palpate vas deferens for palpable characteristics (use thumb and forefinger)	Nontender	Tender
	Discretely palpable from epididymis to external inguinal ring	Tortuous
	Smooth and cordlike	Thickened; beaded
	Movable	Indurated
15. Palpate for additional scrotal contents	None	Mass distal or proximal to testis either tender or nontender
a. Transilluminate each scrotal sac if mass or irregularity is suspected	Testes and epididymides do not transilluminate	Hydrocele ⎱ Transilluminate Spermatocele ⎰
		Tumors ⎫ Hernias ⎬ Do not transilluminate Epididymitis ⎭
16. Evaluate inguinal region for hernia: if possible, the client should be standing and the examiner sitting		
17. Inspect inguinal region for bulges; then ask client to strain, and continue to inspect the area		Bulges at area of external ring, Hesselbach's triangle, femoral area
18. Palpate both right and left inguinal rings: use index finger or little finger of hand on client's corresponding side; client should be standing is possible, and examiner seated (Fig. 12-7); ask client to strain	Finger follows spermatic cord upward to triangular slitlike opening, which may or may not admit finger	Palpable mass touches examiner's fingertip or pushes against side of finger

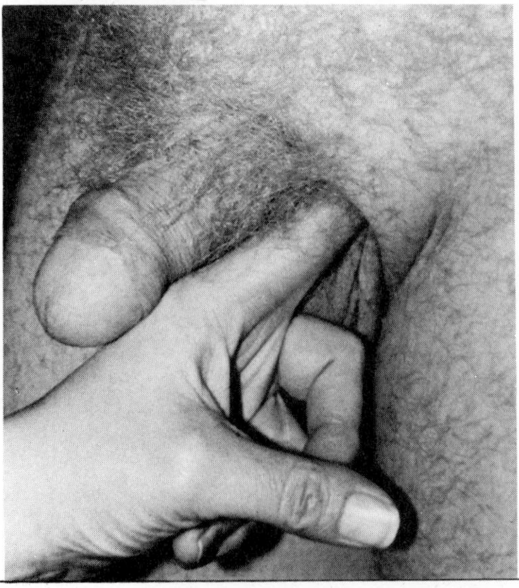

Fig. 12-7. Palpation for inguinal hernia.

The student will:	To identify:	
	Normal	Deviations from normal
19. Palpate each femoral area (fossa ovalis) for bulges; ask client to strain		Soft bulge emerges at fossa
20. Evaluate anal and rectal region (also described in Chapter 11)		
a. Inspect the sacrococcygeal and perianal areas (client lying on left side with right hip and knee flexed)		
1. Skin and surface characteristics	Surface smooth and clear	Lumps Rash Inflammation Scars Pilonidal dimpling Tuft of hair at pilonidal area
b. Palpate coccygeal area for tenderness	No tenderness	Tender
c. Spread buttocks with both hands and inspect anus for:		Inflammation Lesions Scars
1. Surface characteristics (penlight can be used)	Increased pigmentation Coarse skin	Skin tags Fissures Lumps Swelling Excoriation
d. Ask client to strain down; place gloved and lubricated finger at anal opening; as sphincter relaxes, slowly insert finger pointing toward client's umbilicus; ask client to tighten sphincter around finger to assess tone	Sphincter tightens evenly around finger with minimal discomfort to client	Hemorrhoids Mucosal bulging Hypotonic sphincter Hypertonic sphincter with marked tenderness
e. Rotate finger to examine anal muscular ring for surface characteristics	Smooth, even pressure on finger	Nodules Irregularities
f. Insert finger further to palpate all four rectal walls	Continuous, smooth surface with minimal discomfort to client	Nodules Masses Tenderness

Continued.

Clinical guidelines–cont'd

The student will:	To identify:	
	Normal	**Deviations from normal**
g. Palpate the entire prostate gland (Fig. 12-8) at the anterior surface for:		Tenderness

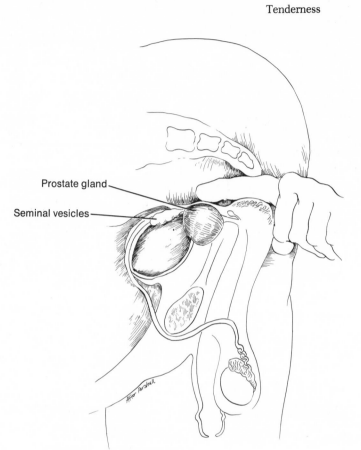

Fig. 12-8. Prostate palpation. (Modified from Malasanos, L., Barkauskas, V., Moss, M., and Stoltenberg-Allen, K.: Health assessment, St. Louis, 1977, The C. V. Mosby Co.)

1. Size	Approximately 4 cm (1½ inches) in diameter; projecting less than 1 cm into rectum	Enlarged
2. Contour	Symmetrical	Asymmetrical
	Bilobed with palpable sulcus	Median sulcus obliterated
3. Consistency	Firm, smooth	Boggy feeling
		Irregular
		Nodular
4. Tenderness	Nontender	Tender
h. Ask client to strain; palpate area above prostate if possible		Masses or bulges touch finger
i. Slowly withdraw finger and examine any fecal material adhering to glove	Stool brown, soft	Presence of blood, pus
		Black, tarry stool
		Pale or yellow stool
		Light tan or gray stool

Clinical strategies

1. Several authors discuss the female practitioner's possible emotional discomfort with examination of male genitalia. One way of avoiding discomfort is to be well prepared with the baseline cognitive data. Read carefully about surface, consistency, and contour characteristics of male genitalia. Have a clear mental picture of the size, location, contour,

and palpable characteristics of scrotal contents before engaging in physical assessment (Fig. 12-5). It is also helpful to observe a seasoned examiner during the process of examination.

2. One author indicates that male genitalia examinations are often deferred for some of the following reasons: ". . . patient refused . . . . will do later. . . . too cold in room. . . . no time. . . . patient too nervous. . . . VIP."* The male genital examination should be considered a routine part of any physical examination.

3. Testicular tumors are often asymptomatic. Educating a client to examine his own genitalia regularly is important. Self-examination on a weekly or a monthly basis is advisable. A regular time and place for self-assessment is helpful. Examination during the shower or bath might be convenient and simple. Many clients are not familiar with their scrotal contents and do not know what normal structures would feel like. The actual process of the examination is an excellent opportunity to explain the procedure and why it is being done. It is helpful to guide the client through the process of self-examination.

4. The examiner must have short fingernails!

Sample recording

Circumcised penis with no lesions, induration, or discharge. Scrotal contents palpated without tenderness or masses. External inguinal canals palpated without masses, bulges, or tenderness.

Sacrococcygeal, perianal, and anal surfaces present no lesions, rash, inflammation, masses, or hemorrhoids. Good anal sphincter tone. Anal and distal rectal mucosa are smooth with no masses. Bilobed prostate is firm, not enlarged, and nontender to palpation.

History and clinical strategies associated with the pediatric client

1. The examiner must assess two types of clients in this area. One will be the infant or little boy and the second the maturing, developing adolescent. Although the techniques of examination are similar, the observations and histories are unique.

2. The examiner must ask the parents of the male infant or little boy the following questions:
   a. Does the child have difficulty voiding?
   b. Is the stream straight?
   c. Does the child's urination stream seem ade-

quate? (That is, is there a very fine high pressure stream or a heavier easy flow?)
   d. Does the child cry and hold his genitalia as if something were hurting?
   e. Has the parent ever noticed any swelling, discoloration, or sores about the penis or scrotum?
   f. Has the child ever had a urinary tract infection?
   g. Does child have difficulty because of bed-wetting or wetting himself? How much of a problem is this? What has the parent done about it? Any tests for the problem? How does the child feel about the problem? Is there a family history of bed-wetting?
   h. To the parents' knowledge, are the child's testes descended?
   i. Has the child ever been told he has a hydrocele or hernia?
   j. Has the parent ever noticed that the child's scrotum appears to swell or change size with crying or coughing?
   k. Has child ever caused trauma to his genitalia either through an accident or during play?

3. For older boys, the examiner will fluctuate back and forth between asking significant subjective questions appropriate for the smaller boys and those appropriate for the adult male. Much will depend on the actual maturation, development, and interest of the client. For example, it would be appropriate to ask a mature 16-year-old who is known to be dating, "Do you have any concerns regarding sexual practices or values that you would like to discuss?" Other specific interview questions regarding sexuality are thoroughly discussed in the adult section of this chapter.

4. As boys mature, it should be anticipated that they will have many educational needs regarding what is happening to their own bodies, as well as how to sexually explore with others. The examiner should be alert to these needs and be prepared to develop a beginning profile of the boy's current knowledge and understanding. Not every boy will feel comfortable sharing this information with the examiner, but the examiner should be prepared for and alert to an adolescent asking for clarification and assistance. Profile questions should include items such as:
   a. Has he ever had education classes regarding the changes that boys' bodies go through? If so, is he able to describe the type of material presented?
   b. Were girls involved in the education classes?

---

*Warren, M. M.: Testicular tumors, Continuing Ed., March, 1975, p. 31.

Did they also study about the changes girls' bodies are making?

c. How does his family feel about discussing this information at home?

d. Within his family, who does he talk with about sexual changes and dating?

e. If he needs information clarified, who does he go to?

f. Has he ever had any classes or organized discussions about dating, petting, birth control?

g. What does he know about venereal disease?

5. Most adolescents are not intimidated by direct questioning, as long as it does not appear that someone is pointing a punitive finger toward them. Therefore the level of questioning may relate directly to *normal* activities that the young adolescent may be experiencing, may feel guilty about, or may have incorrect information about, such as homosexual desires, masturbation, sexual fantasies, nocturnal emissions, or erections. The examiner may ask questions such as: Many fellas your age are experiencing new and normal sensations, such as wanting to touch other boys or having wet dreams at night. Do you have any concerns that I could perhaps provide more information about?*

6. The examination strategies will vary with age.

a. Infants through age 2 years should present no problem; the assessment is usually done following the abdominal examination. The examiner simply moves from the abdomen to the genitalia and inguinal area.

b. Boys 3 to 8 years of age should be examined in their undershorts. After the abdominal examination, matter-of-factly tell the child what is going to happen and then slip down his pants to examine the genitalia and inguinal area. During and following the examination, the examiner should reassure the child that everything is perfectly normal and healthy.

c. For boys over age 8, provide them with a drape, just as you would for an adult. A reassurance of normal findings is also recommended.

7. Evaluation for undescended testes

a. History. If the parent reports that at one time the testes were found in the scrotum, the testes should not be considered undescended.

b. Rugae. If the scrotum shows well-formed rugae, it usually means that the testes have descended at some time.

c. Techniques to force testes into the scrotum

(palpation of scrotum should confirm presence)

(1) Have the child stand; slightly milk the inguinal canal region to pull the testes into the scrotum.

(2) Have the child sit on chair or the examination table, feet next to the buttocks, with the knees pulled tight to the chest.

(3) Have the child sit Indian style (cross-legged); this will relax the cremasteric reflex.

(4) Child may be placed into very warm water.

d. Palpate the inguinal canal. If the testis is located in the inguinal canal but cannot be pushed down or if no testis is felt, an undescended testis is very likely.

e. Boys whose testes have not descended by age 4 years should be referred to a physician.

8. If the testis is palpated momentarily in the scrotum but it quickly slips up into the inguinal canal prior to adequate assessment, the examiner may block the slippage by gently placing the index finger of the left hand over the inguinal canal and palpating the testis with the right hand.

9. Inguinal hernias are fairly common in children. Generally, the parent will describe a bulge in the child's inguinal region. The inguinal region of a larger boy may be palpated in the same manner as for the adult, but for the smaller boy it is better to try to produce the hernia or bulge by external techniques such as the following:

a. Instruct the child to stand; give him a balloon to blow up.

b. Have the infant or toddler in a standing position on the examination table. The examiner should place one hand behind the child's back and with the other hand pump in and out on the child's abdomen. The external abdominal pressure may produce the inguinal bulge.

c. Instruct the child to sit on the examination table and pull his knees to his chest. The examiner then tries to straighten the leg on the questionable side. Again, intra-abdominal pressure should fill the hernia sac and produce a bulge.

10. Hydroceles are a common finding in children under 2 years of age. Any child with what appears to be a large scrotum should be evaluated for a hydrocele. To do this, the examiner must darken the examination room and transilluminate the scrotum. A fluid-enlarged scrotum shows a pink, light shadow. With scrotal palpation the examiner is not able to reduce the fluid.

---

*Daniel (1977) provides an excellent discussion of the normal experimentation of adolescent males.

Clinical variations associated with the pediatric client

Characteristic or area examined	Normal	Deviations from normal
1. Pubic region		
a. Skin surface	Smooth, clear	Scars, rashes, lesions
b. Hair distribution	Variable as male develops (Table 8)	Patchy growth or loss
		Female configuration: triangular with base over pubis

Continued.

Table 8. Pubic hair development in males*

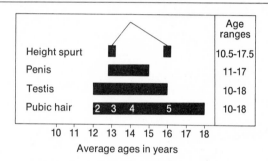

Development	Stage	Characteristics
	1	None; preadolescent
	2	Scant, long, slightly pigmented
	3	Darker, starting to curl, small amount
	4	Resembles adult, but less quantity; coarse, curly
	5	Adult distribution, spread to medial surface of thighs

*From Tanner, J. M.: Growth at adolescence, ed. 2, Oxford, England, 1962, Blackwell Scientific Publications.

Clinical variations associated with the pediatric client–cont'd

Characteristic or area examined	Normal	Deviations from normal
2. Penis **a.** Skin color and surface characteristics	Penis size in newborn 2 to 3 cm (3/4 to 1 1/4 inches) long Variable as male develops (Table 9)	Reddened Lesions Swelling Nodules

Table 9. Penis and testes/scrotum development in males*

Development	Stage	Characteristics
	1	Penis, testes, and scrotum preadolescent
	2	Enlargement of scrotum and testes, texture alteration; scrotal sac reddens; penis usually does not enlarge
	3	Further growth of testes and scrotum; penis enlarges and becomes longer
	4	Continued growth of testes and scrotum; scrotum becomes darker; penis becomes longer; glans and breadth increase in size
	5	Adult in size and shape

*From Tanner, J. M.: Growth at adolescence, ed. 2, Oxford, England, 1962, Blackwell Scientific Publications.

Characteristic or area examined	Normal	Deviations from normal
b. Foreskin	Uncircumsised: prepuce present and folded over glans (Fig. 12-9)	Continually retracted foreskin in uncircumcised male

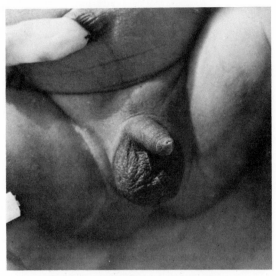

Fig. 12-9. Uncircumcised penis in newborn.

	Circumsised: prepuce often absent, or small flap remains at corona (Fig. 12-10)	

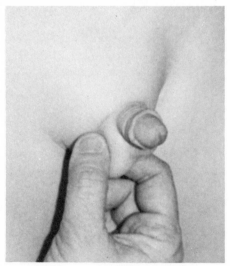

Fig. 12-10. Circumcised penis in small child.

1. Foreskin retraction	For uncircumcised males after age 3 or 4 months (be gentle; if tissue resists, do not force)	Unable to retract, or very tightly attached foreskin of child over 3 months of age
	Foreskin retracts easily to expose glans and returns to original position with ease	Failure to retract; discomfort with retraction
		Difficulty returning prepuce to original position
c. Glans and under prepuce fold		Lesions
		Crusting under fold or around tip of glans
		Redness, swelling
		Pinpoint opening

Continued.

Clinical variations associated with the pediatric client–cont'd

Characteristic or area examined	Normal	Deviations from normal
d. Urethral meatus		
1. Location	Central, at distal tip of glans	Pinpoint opening
		Dorsal location
		Ventral location
2. Discharge	Usually not present	Yellow-green discharge
		Milky white discharge
		Discharge with foul odor
e. Penis shaft palpation	Nontender	Tenderness
	Smooth, semifirm consistency	Swelling
		Nodules
		Induration
3. Scrotum		
a. Contour	Sac divided in half by septum	
	Left scrotal sac may be longer than right	
	Scrotal contents and scrotum may retract upward with cool temperature	
b. Size	Size varies; may appear pendulous	Fluctuates in size greatly with crying or coughing
		Hydrocele common in boys under 2 years of age; nontender mass
4. Scrotum and testes palpation	Testis present in each sac	Hydrocele, unable to reduce (see clinical strategies)
		Solid scrotal mass
		Testes not present in sac (see clinical strategies)
a. Size	Birth: 1 to 2 cm	Unilateral or bilateral testicle size
	11 to 18 years: 3.5 to 4.5 cm	
	Equal in size	
b. Tenderness	Mildly sensitive to slight compression	Markedly tender
c. Contour	Smooth, ovoid	Nodular
		Irregular
d. Mobility	Movable	Fixed
5. Epididymis	Nontender	Tender
	Usually located on posterolateral surface of each testis	Irregular shape
		Enlarged
	Discretely palpable	Indurated
	Comma shaped	Nodular
	Smooth	
6. Vas deferens	Nontender	Tender
	Discretely palpable from epididymides to external inguinal ring	Tortuous
		Thickened; beaded
	Smooth and cordlike	Indurated
	Movable	
7. Inguinal hernia inspection (see clinical strategies); older boys may palpate right and left inguinal rings *if hernia is suspected;* child should stand and bear down after finger is in place	Using little finger, follow spermatic cord upward to triangular slitlike opening; opening may or may not admit finger	Bulges appearing at area of external ring, Hesselbach's triangle, femoral area
		Palpable mass touches examiner's fingertip or pushes against side of finger

History and clinical strategies associated with the geriatric client

1. Sexual functions. Physiological changes occurring in the aging male result in sexual function alterations.
   a. Erections develop more slowly in response to stimulation. Erection time may be longer or may be delayed until shortly before ejaculation.
   b. The erection may feel less full or firm.
   c. Ejaculation is less intense, invoking fewer contractions.
   d. The volume of seminal fluid expelled is lessened. The production of spermatozoa diminishes.
   e. The refractory phase is longer, lasting for about 12 hours to several days.

Note that the changes described occur gradually and at different rates according to the individual. Despite testosterone level decreases, an elderly man is capable of sexual function indefinitely if he is generally healthy and is within a sexually stimulating environment.

The questions posed to the adult male regarding his sexual and reproductive functions are generally appropriate for the elderly client (pp. 294-296).

The questions about early childhood and adolescent experiences may not have as much bearing on present sexual concerns as they would with a younger client. An older man may be preoccupied with his present needs for intimacy and sexual activity. Some of the variables that could alter sexual function follow:

a. Feelings that he is too old or too frail to engage in sexual activity; election to withdraw from all sexual encounters or stimulation
b. Loss of spouse, isolation, unavailability of a sexual partner, or a sexually restrictive environment
c. Depression related to sexual or to other concerns
d. Physical illness resulting in fatigue, anxiety about health status, or pain (from arthritis, respiratory or cardiac problems, etc.)
e. Effects of certain diseases (neurogenic or vascular impairment, diabetes mellitus)
f. Side effects of medications (e.g., some antihypertensive drugs, sedatives, tranquilizers, alcohol)
g. Surgery for prostatism (may or may not affect erection status); retrograde ejaculation a possible concern
h. Inadequate nutrition
i. Diminished strength of muscles associated with the act of intercourse

Several authors have stated that the majority of men requesting help for impotence offer no organic basis for the problem. It is imperative that the examiner be well informed about sexual needs and behaviors of the geriatric client and prepared to follow through with a thorough assessment in this area.

2. Genitourinary symptoms. The symptoms of urinary frequency, nocturia, urgency, hesitancy, abnormal flow of urinary stream, urethral discharge, and scrotal masses are described in the adult section of this chapter. Additional concerns or questions follow:
   a. Nocturnal frequency is a common concern. Ask the client what amount and type of fluids he drinks in the evening. Also, ask if he is taking diuretics.
   b. Incontinence: Was the onset sudden or slow? Does the client feel (or sense) any warning that he has to urinate?
3. Prostatism. Early symptoms include the following:
   a. Hesitancy in initiating stream
   b. Diminished force of stream
   c. Urinary frequency
   d. Nocturia
   These symptoms may be subtle, ignored, or tolerated by the client. The later symptoms of hematuria or urinary tract infection alarm the client. *Note:* The size of the prostate gland (as estimated when palpated) may not be indicative of the degree of obstruction of the urethra. The number and intensity of symptoms offered by the client may not correlate with the estimated palpatory enlargement of the gland.
4. Cancer of the prostate gland is often asymptomatic.
5. Pain associated with genitourinary illness may be ill defined or vague, located in the groin, low back, perineum, abdomen or flank.

Clinical variations associated with the geriatric client

The assessment procedure and physical findings for the geriatric male are the same as for the younger client. The following alterations may be noted:
1. The genital examination should be preceded by an abdominal assessment to palpate and percuss the bladder for fullness (after the client has been asked to urinate), discomfort, or dullness.
2. The scrotal sac may appear elongated or pendulous. Elderly clients sometimes have the problem of sitting on the scrotum, resulting in trauma or excoriation of the surface.
3. The testes may feel slightly softer than in a younger man and may be slightly smaller.
4. The prostate gland may feel larger than in a younger client.

Vocabulary

1. Ampulla

2. Anuria

3. Chordee

4. Corona

5. Cryptorchism

6. Dysuria

7. Enuresis

8. Epididymis

9. Epispadias

10. Fossa ovalis

11. Glans (penis)

12. Hematuria

13. Hesselbach's triangle

14. Hydrocele

15. Hypospadias

16. Oliguria

17. Paraphimosis

18. Phimosis

19. Prepuce

20. Pyuria

21. Rugous

22. Spermatocele

23. Tenesmus (rectal)

24. Tunica vaginalis

25. Varicocele

Cognitive self-assessment

Match the lettered structures with the corresponding numbered label.

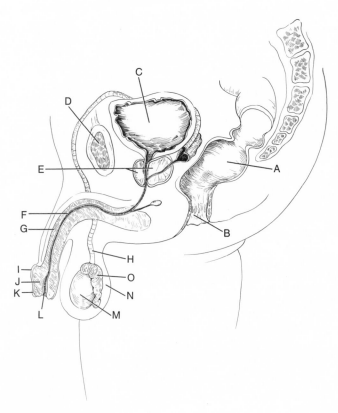

1. __N__ Scrotum
2. __G__ Shaft of penis
3. __O__ Epididymis
4. __B__ Anus
5. __H__ Vas deferens
6. __F__ Urethra
7. __C__ Bladder
8. __L__ Urethral meatus
9. __K__ Prepuce
10. __D__ Pubis
11. __J__ Glans
12. __I__ Corona
13. __M__ Testis
14. __A__ Rectum
15. The skin of the penis is usually:
    ☑ a. dark red
    ☐ b. moderately deep red
    ☐ c. pale red

16. Scrotal skin is:
    ☐ a. pale
    ☒ b. deeply pigmented
17. Scrotal skin is:
    ☐ a. thick
    ☒ b. thin
18. Testes are usually:
    ☒ a. firm
    ☐ b. soft
19. Testes are approximately _____ in length.
    ☒ a. 4 to 5 cm
    ☐ b. 1 to 2 cm
    ☐ c. 5 to 6 cm
20. Normal testes are _____ sensitive to mild compression.
    ☐ a. markedly
    ☐ b. never
    ☒ c. slightly
21. The epididymides are usually located _____ to the testes.
    ☒ a. posterolateral
    ☐ b. anteromedial
22. Which statement(s) is/are true about the normal epididymides?
    ☐ a. They are slightly tender to palpation.
    ☒ b. They are nontender to palpation.
    ☒ c. They are discretely palpable within the scrotum.
    ☒ d. They may visibly bulge in the posterior portion of scrotal sac.
    ☐ e. All except b
    ☒ f. All except a
    ☐ g. a and c
    ☐ h. b and d
23. The vas deferens is usually:
    ☐ a. taut or fixed to surrounding tissue
    ☒ b. movable
24. Which of the following structures, if present in the scrotum, would transilluminate?
    ☒ a. Hydrocele
    ☐ b. Testis
    ☐ c. Scrotal hernia
    ☒ d. Spermatocele
    ☐ e. Varicocele
    ☐ f. Epididymal nodule
    ☐ g. All the above
    ☐ h. None of the above
    ☒ i. a and d
    ☐ j. a, c, and e
25. Which of the following structures (or conditions), if present in the scrotum, would usually be described as painful by the client?
    ☐ a. Spermatocele
    ☒ b. Epididymitis
    ☐ c. Hydrocele
    ☐ d. Testicular tumor
    ☐ e. Anteverted epididymis
    ☐ f. All the above
    ☐ g. None of the above
    ☐ h. a and d
    ☐ i. b, c, and e

Match the lettered structures with the corresponding numbered label.

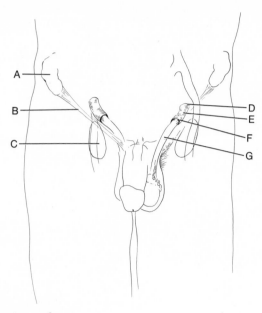

26. __G__ Spermatic cord
27. __D__ Internal inguinal ring
28. __F__ External inguinal ring
29. __E__ Inguinal canal
30. __A__ Anterosuperior iliac spine
31. __C__ Fossa ovalis
32. __B__ Poupart's ligament

PEDIATRIC QUESTIONS

33. The *average* age for the beginning development of pubic hair in males is:
    ☐ a. 9 years
    ☐ b. 10 years
    ☐ c. 11 years
    ☑ d. 12 years
    ☐ e. 13 years
34. When examining the uncircumcised male, the examiner should attempt to retract the foreskin after which of the following ages?
    ☐ a. 6 weeks
    ☐ b. 2 months
    ☑ c. 4 months
    ☐ d. 6 months
    ☐ e. never
35. Which of the following techniques should be used to attempt to force the testes back into the scrotum of a boy who is being evaluated for undescended testes?
    ☑ a. Child should stand; examiner attempts to milk testes into scrotum.
    ☑ b. Child is sitting on examination table, feet against buttocks, pulling knees tight to chest.
    ☑ c. Child sits cross-legged (Indian style) to relax cremasteric reflex.
    ☐ d. Child stands and examiner pushes on child's abdomen.
    ☑ e. Place child in warm tub of water.
    ☐ f. All the above
    ☐ g. a, c, and d
    ☐ h. All except c

☑ i. All except d
☐ j. b, d, and e

GERIATRIC QUESTIONS

36. In older men a palpable scrotal mass:
   ☐ a. is usually indicative of cancer
   ☐ b. is common because the testicle hypertrophies and becomes irregular in shape with aging
   ☑ c. may be a hydrocele
   ☐ d. none of the above

37. Early symptoms of prostatism:
   ☑ a. include hesitancy in initiating urine stream
   ☐ b. include hematuria
   ☐ c. include inability to maintain an erection
   ☐ d. none of the above

38. Physiological sexual function changes that normally occur with the aging male include:
   ☑ a. an extended erection period
   ☐ b. slow detumescence
   ☑ c. longer refractory phase
   ☑ d. decrease in volume of seminal fluid at time of ejaculation
   ☐ e. loss of ability to maintain erection
   ☐ f. a and b
   ☐ g. a and d
   ☐ h. c and e
   ☑ i. a, c, and d
   ☐ j. all except e

SUGGESTED READINGS
General

Bates, Barbara: A guide to physical examination, ed. 2, Philadelphia, 1979, J. B. Lippincott Co., pp. 179-187, 221-229, 249-256.

Conklin, Margaret, Klint, Karen, Marway, Ann, and Shepard, Roberta: Should health teaching include self examination of the testes? Am. J. Nurs. **78**(12):2073-2074, 1978.

Diekelmann, Nancy: Primary health care of the well adult, New York, 1977, McGraw-Hill Book Co., pp. 51-69, 127-137, 139-149, 217-223.

Malasanos, Lois, Barkauskas, Violet, Moss, Muriel, and Stoltenberg-Allen, Kathryn: Health assessment, St. Louis, 1977, The C. V. Mosby Co., pp. 262-270, 271-282, 442.

Murray, Barbara L. S., and Wilcox, Linda J.: Testicular self examination, Am. J. Nurs. **78**(12):2074-2075, 1978.

Prior, John A., and Silberstein, Jack S.: Physical diagnosis: the history and examination of the patient, ed. 5, St. Louis, 1977, The C. V. Mosby Co., pp. 315-319, 323-338.

Pediatric

Alexander, Mary, and Brown, Marie Scott: Pediatric physical diagnosis for nurses, New York, 1974, McGraw-Hill Book Co., pp. 166-178.

Barness, Lewis.: Manual of pediatric physical diagnosis, ed. 4, Chicago, 1972, Year Book Medical Publishers, Inc., pp. 134-139.

Bates, Barbara: A guide to physical examination, ed. 2, Philadelphia, 1979, J. B. Lippincott Co., pp. 410-412.

Daniel, William A.: Adolescents in health and disease, St. Louis, 1977, The C. V. Mosby Co., pp. 27-39, 65-71.

Prior, John A., and Silberstein, Jack S.: Physical diagnosis: the history and examination of the patient, ed. 5, St. Louis, 1977, The C. V. Mosby Co., pp. 469-470.

Rauh, Joseph, and Brookman, Richard: Children are different: developmental physiology. In Johnson, T. R., Moore, W. M., and Jeffries, J. E., editors, Columbus, Ohio, 1978, Ross Laboratories, pp. 26-29.

Geriatric

Caird, F. I., and Judge, R. D.: Assessment of the elderly patient, London, 1977, Pitman Medical Publishing Co. Ltd.

Chinn, Austin B., editor: Clinical aspects of aging, Working with older people: a guide to practice, vol. 4, Rockville, Md., 1971, U.S. Department of Health, Education, and Welfare, Public Health Service, Part VII, pp. 131-148.

Diekelmann, Nancy: Primary health care of the well adult, New York, 1977, McGraw-Hill Book Co., pp. 187-199.

Steinberg, Franz U., editor: Cowdry's the care of the geriatric patient, St. Louis, 1976, The C. V. Mosby Co., pp. 275-283, 393-400.

CHAPTER 13

Assessment of the female genitourinary system

Cognitive objectives

At the end of this unit the learner will demonstrate knowledge of assessment of the female genitourinary system and rectal/anal region by the ability to do the following:

1. Identify and locate the major internal and external structures of the female genitourinary system.
2. Identify observable and palpable characteristics of normal external genitalia and perineum.
3. Identify observable and palpable characteristics of normal internal structures:
   a. Vagina
   b. Cervix
   c. Fornices
4. Identify the major characteristics of normal vaginal discharge.
5. Identify the appropriate and effective procedures for using a vaginal speculum.
6. Identify specific examiner behaviors that will minimize client discomfort and enhance effectiveness of the pelvic examination.
7. Identify common normal palpable findings elicited during a bimanual examination.
8. Identify common normal deviations of findings related to pelvic examination associated with:
   a. Nulliparous clients
   b. Multiparous clients
   c. Early pregnant clients
9. Identify major palpable characteristics of the anteverted, retroverted, anteflexed, and retroflexed uterus.
10. Identify the reasons for performing a rectovaginal examination.
11. Identify common pediatric and geriatric variations of the female genitourinary system.
12. Define the terms in the vocabulary list.

Clinical objectives

At the end of this unit the learner will perform a systematic assessment of the female genitourinary system and rectal/anal region, demonstrating the ability to do the following:

1. Obtain a pertinent history from a client.
2. Inspect the pubic region and external genitalia for:
   a. Hair distribution
   b. Parasites
   c. Inguinal skin surface characteristics
   d. Labia majora surface
   e. Labia minora surface
      (1) Vestibule surface
      (2) Clitoris size and surface
      (3) Urethral meatus contour and surface
   f. Vaginal introitus contour and surface
   g. Perineum surface
   h. Anal surface
3. Palpate external genitalia for:
   a. Labia and vestibule consistency and tenderness
   b. Urethral duct tenderness and discharge
   c. Bartholin's gland tenderness, discharge, and swelling
   d. Perineum consistency and tenderness
4. Palpate vaginal introitus and test for bulging (or straining) and urinary incontinence.
5. Perform a vaginal examination and inspect for:
   a. Cervix
      (1) Color
      (2) Position
      (3) Size
      (4) Surface characteristics
      (5) Os configuration
      (6) Discharge color, odor, and texture
   b. Vagina

315

(1) Color
(2) Surface characteristics
(3) Consistency
(4) Secretions: color, odor, and texture
6. Obtain specimens for cervical cytological evaluation.
7. Perform a bimanual vaginal examination to identify:
    a. Vaginal wall surface characteristics and tenderness
    b. Cervix
        (1) Size
        (2) Contour
        (3) Consistency
        (4) Surface texture
        (5) Mobility
        (6) Location in vaginal tube
        (7) Os patency
    c. Uterus
        (1) Fundus location, contour, surface consistency, shape, size, mobility, and tenderness
        (2) Isthmus consistency
    d. Adnexa
        (1) Ovary location and surface characteristics
        (2) Masses
        (3) Pulsations
8. Perform a rectovaginal examination to identify:
    a. Rectovaginal septum and pouch characteristics
    b. Tenderness in pouch
    c. Rectal wall surface characteristics
    d. Anal sphincter surface and tone
    e. Tenderness
9. Summarize results with a written description of findings.

Health history related to female genitourinary assessment additional to data base

1. Sexual history. A screening question might be worded in the following manner: "Do you have any sexual difficulties or concerns that you would like to share with me?" or "Are you satisfied with your sexual habits and activities as they occur now?" This gives the client an opportunity to express concerns and does not direct her toward any particular issue. More specific questions might be posed if the client indicates that she wishes to discuss specific sexual matters.
    a. Are your needs for intimacy and affection being met?
    b. Are you sexually active at present?
    c. Are your sexual activities meeting your physical needs?
    d. Do you and your partner talk about sex? Do you generally agree on sexual needs, sexual expression, and modes of behavior?
    e. Do you have any problems with sexual arousal, arousing your partner, or completing a sexual experience satisfactorily?
    f. If particular problems exist, what do you feel is the cause?
    g. Have you attempted to solve the problem? If so, in what way? What was the outcome of these attempts?
    h. Do you have any questions about sexual behaviors or sexuality in general that you would like to pose (e.g., concerns about venereal disease, sexual anatomy, orgasm, masturbation, sexual fantasies)?
2. Abnormal bleeding
    a. If associated with menses, it might fall into one of the following categories:
        (1) Too many periods (menstrual interval is less than 19 to 21 days)
        (2) Infrequent menses (menstrual interval is over 37 days)
        (3) Amenorrhea
        (4) Extended menses (duration is over 7 days)
        (5) Intermenstrual bleeding
        (6) Flow pattern increased during menses
    b. Amount of flow (normal or abnormal) is difficult to determine. Inquire about the nature of the *change* in the amount of flow. Ask about the number of pads or tampons used during the heavy flow in a 24-hour period. Find out if the pad or tampon is soaked when it is changed. Do clots accompany the bleeding?
    c. Is there bleeding associated with intercourse? With douching?
3. Premenstrual tension should be defined by the client. Is it associated with headaches? Weight change? Edema? Breast tenderness? Marked (or difficult) mood swings? Does it occur before every period or just occasionally? Are premenstrual problems incapacitating (e.g., do they interfere with activities of daily living)?
4. Vaginal discharge. Discharge is normal with many women and often occurs in cycles with an increase at midcycle or just before menses. If vaginal discharge is a complaint, establish the *change* that has occurred in terms of estimated amount, color, odor, consistency, and times or intervals of increased discharge.
    a. Are you taking any medications for other problems (especially broad-spectrum antibiotics, metronidazole, or steroids)? Do you take birth control pills?
    b. Do you douche? If so, how often, what solution,

and what amount? Were you douching before or after the discharge?

c. Is the discharge associated with itching? (If itching is present, is there a family or client history of diabetes mellitus?)

d. Do you wear cotton or ventilated underwear or pantyhose?

e. Was the onset of the discharge sudden or gradual?

f. Does your sexual partner have any problem with discharge, itching, rash or lesions, pain?

5. Birth control. If any measure is used, establish the type used, length of time it has been used, and the client's assessment of its effectiveness, convenience, noninterference with sexual activity, and noninterference with the client's general physical and mental health. More specific questions include the following:

a. Birth control pills. Do you take them regularly? Do you have any symptoms or physical problems associated with taking the pill?

b. Diaphragm. Are you able to use it each time you have intercourse? Do you use cream (or jelly) every time you use the diaphragm? Do you have any problems inserting, removing, or retaining it? Do you examine your diaphragm periodically for thinning or weak spots, cracks, holes, or tears? How long before intercourse do you insert it? How long do you leave it in place following intercourse? How long ago were you fitted with your diaphragm?

c. IUD. Do you insert your finger in your vagina to feel for the string periodically? How often? Do you have any problem with bleeding or spotting between periods? Do you have any problem with menstrual cramps?

6. Menopause. If it has been established that the client is approaching, in the midst of, or completing the menopausal phase, a general question about any concerns should be posed. More specific questions include:

a. Do you recall your mother experiencing menopause? How old was she? Did she describe her experience to you?

b. Do you have any concerns or problems with menstrual irregularity, mood changes, tension, back pain, hot flashes, painful intercourse, changes in sexual desire or sexual behaviors, other physical changes?

c. What kind of birth control measures are you using? Describe.

d. What general feelings do you have about menopause?

7. Pelvic discomfort associated with the menstrual cycle is normal with some women. If the client complains of pain, establish the *change* that has occurred in terms of timing (with menstrual cycle) and location (e.g., vulvar or vaginal, localized in lower abdomen, or general pain). Is the pain associated with intercourse? If so, does it occur at the time of insertion, deep penetration throughout intercourse, and/or is there a residual pain following intercourse?

Clinical guidelines

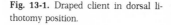

The student will:	To identify:	
	Normal	**Deviations from normal**

1. Assemble equipment:
   a. Gloves
   b. Speculum
   c. Sterile cotton swabs
   d. Glass slides
   e. Wooden spatula
   f. Lubricant
   g. Cytology fixative
   h. Examining lamp
   i. Culture plates for gonorrhea screening
2. Check with client to be certain that bladder has been recently emptied
3. Position draped client in lithotomy position (Fig. 13-1)
   (*Note:* Examiner may assist client in positioning her buttocks at the edge of the examining table

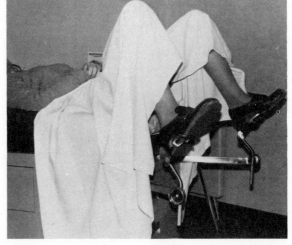

Fig. 13-1. Draped client in dorsal lithotomy position.

Continued.

Clinical guidelines–cont'd

The student will:	To identify:	
	Normal	**Deviations from normal**
after checking to see that client's feet are secure in stirrups.)		
4. See that equipment is within easy reach and arrange light for good visualization of external genitalia		
5. Wear gloves on both hands; warn the client that examiner is going to touch her to begin procedure		
6. Inspect the external genitalia		
a. Hair distribution	Variable in adults Usually inverse triangle with base over pubis; some hair may extend up midline toward umbilicus No parasites	Male hair distribution (diamond-shaped pattern) Patchy loss of hair Absence of hair in client over 16 years Nits, pubic lice
b. Inguinal and mons pubis skin surface characteristics	Smooth, clear	Scars Inguinal swelling, excoriation, lesions, rash
c. Labia majora surface characteristics	Darker pigmentation Shriveled or full Gaping or closed Usually symmetrical Skin surface smooth May appear dry or moist	Inflammation, ulceration Lesions Nodules Marked asymmetry
7. Spread labia to view:		
a. Inner surface of labia majora; labia minora and surface of vestibule (Fig. 13-2)	Dark pink pigmentation and moist Usually symmetrical	Inflammation Leukoplakia Lesions Nodules Varicosities Marked asymmetry Swelling Excoriation

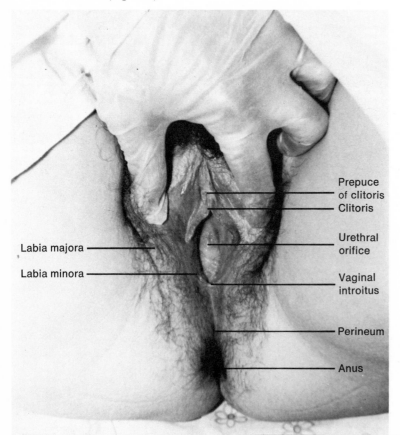

Labia majora

Labia minora

Prepuce of clitoris

Clitoris

Urethral orifice

Vaginal introitus

Perineum

Anus

Fig. 13-2. Labia spread with thumb and fingers to view external genitalia.

The student will:	To identify:	
	Normal	**Deviations from normal**
b. Clitoris		
1. Size	2 cm (¾ inch) length visible	Enlargement
	0.5 cm diameter	Atrophy
2. Surface	Medial aspect covered by prepuce	Inflamed
c. Urethral meatus and immediate surrounding tissue surface	Irregular opening or slit	Discharge from surrounding glands (Skene's) or urethral opening
	May be close to or slightly within vaginal introitus	Polyp
		Inflammation
	Usually located midline	Urethral caruncle
		Lateral position of meatus
d. Vaginal introitus and immediate surrounding tissue surface	Thin vertical slit or large orifice with irregular edges (hymenal caruncles)	Surrounding inflammation
		Profuse vaginal discharge
	Moist tissue	Swelling
		Lesions
e. Perineum surface	Smooth or evidence of episiotomy	Inflammation, fistula
	Scar (midline or mediolateral) may be visible	Lesions, mass
f. Anus surface	Increased pigmentation and coarse skin	Scars, skin tags
		Lesions, inflammation
		Fissures, lumps
		Excoriation
8. Palpate external genitalia		
a. Labia and vestibule (Fig. 13-3)		
1. Consistency	Soft, homogeneous	Irregular, nodular
2. Tenderness	Nontender	Tender

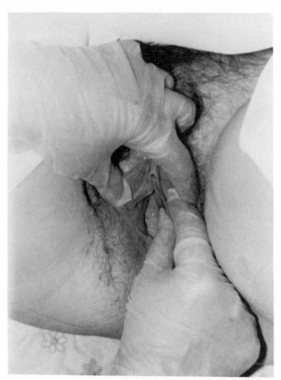

Fig. 13-3. Palpation of labia.

Clinical guidelines–cont'd

The student will:	To identify:	
	Normal	Deviations from normal
b. Insert index finger in vagina and milk urethral ducts (Fig. 13-4) to test for: 1. Tenderness 2. Discharge	Nontender No discharge	Tenderness Discharge*

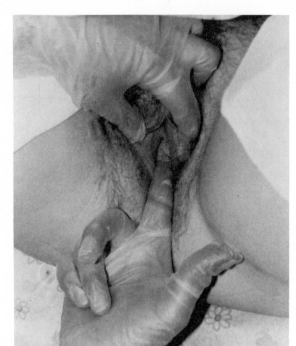

Fig. 13-4. Milking urethral duct.

c. Palpate lateral and posterior areas surrounding introitus (Fig. 13-5) to test for:

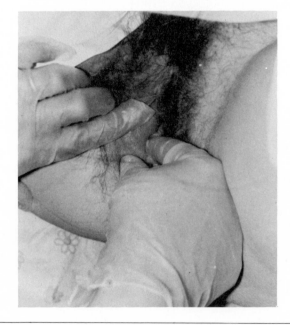

Fig. 13-5. Palpation of lateral and posterior areas surrounding vaginal introitus.

*Prepare a culture of any discharge.

The student will:	To identify:	
	Normal	Deviations from normal
1. Tenderness	Nontender	Tenderness
2. Discharge	No discharge	Discharge*
3. Surface characteristics	Homogeneous	Swelling
d. Palpate perineum between index finger and thumb (Fig. 13-6) for:		
1. Consistency	Nulliparous: thick, smooth Multiparous: thin, rigid Scarring	Paper thin
2. Tenderness	Nontender	Tender

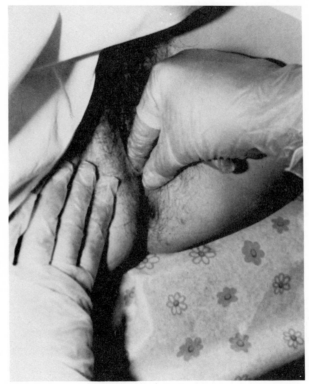

Fig. 13-6. Palpating perineum.

9. Ask client to squeeze vaginal orifice around examiner's finger; insert middle and index fingers into vagina; ask client to strain down or bear down to elicit:	Nulliparous client squeezes tightly Multiparous client demonstrates less tone	Client unable to constrict vaginal orifice around examiner's finger
a. Bulging	No bulging	Cystocele (anterior wall bulging) Enterocele Rectocele (posterior wall bulging) Uterine prolapse (cervix visible on straining, or uterus protrudes on straining)
b. Incontinence	No urinary incontinence	Urinary incontinence
10. Select speculum of appropriate size, and warm and lubricate with water (if necessary)		

*Prepare a culture of any discharge.

Continued.

Clinical guidelines–cont'd

The student will:	To identify:	
	Normal	Deviations from normal

11. Place two fingers just inside vaginal introitus and apply pressure over posterior wall (Fig. 13-7); wait for relaxation

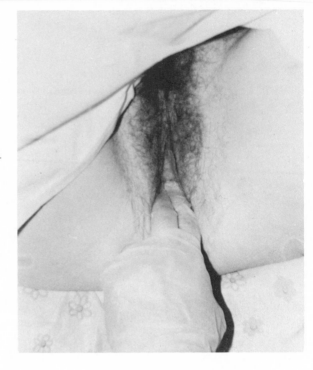

Fig. 13-7. Applying pressure in posterior vaginal orifice with two fingers.

12. Insert closed speculum (held at oblique angle) over fingers and direct at 45° angle downward; remove fingers; lock speculum in place (Fig. 13-8) to inspect cervix

a. Color	Pink color evenly distributed	Inflamed
	Bluish (in pregnancy)	Pale (associated with anemia)
		Cyanotic (other than pregnancy)
	Symmetrical, circumscribed erythema surrounding os may indicate normal condition of exposed columnar epithelium; however, beginning examiners should consider any reddened appearance a problem for consultation	Erythema, especially if patchy or if borders irregular or asymmetrical around os
b. Position	Midline	Cervix situated laterally
	Cervix and os may be pointed in anterior or posterior direction	
	May project into vaginal tube 1 to 3 cm (resulting in 1 to 3 cm fornices surrounding cervix)	Projection of over 3 cm (1 inch) into vaginal tube
c. Size	Usually 2.5 cm (1 inch) diameter	Over 4 cm (1½ inches) diameter
d. Surface	Smooth	Reddened granular area around os (especially asymmetrical)
	Occasional visible squamocolumnar junction (symmetrical reddened circle around os)	Friable tissue
	Nabothian cysts (smooth, round, small, yellowish raised areas)	Red patches, lesions
		Strawberry spots
		White patches
e. Os	Nulliparous: small, evenly round	
	Multiparous: slitlike, may be star shaped or irregular	
f. Cervical discharge	Mucous plug may be present at os	
	Odorless	Odor
	Creamy or clear	Colored (yellowish, greenish, gray)
	Thin, thick, or stringy	
	Discharge often heavier at midcycle or immediately before menstruation	

Continued.

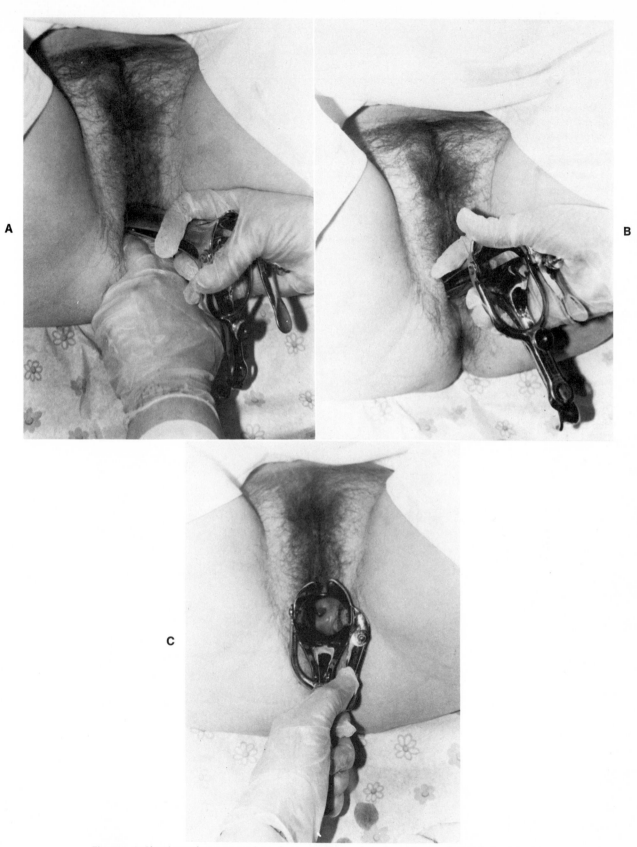

Fig. 13-8. A, Closed speculum is inserted over fingers. Insert speculum at an oblique angle if vaginal opening is not relaxed. **B,** Fingers removed; closed speculum is inserted in a downward (45° angle) direction. **C,** Speculum in place, locked, and stabilized. (Note cervix in full view.)

Clinical guidelines–cont'd

The student will:	To identify:	
	Normal	**Deviations from normal**

13. Obtain specimens for:
  a. Papanicolaou smear
  b. Gonorrheal culture (see clinical strategies if indicated)
14. Inspect vagina: as unlocked, partially opened speculum is rotated and slowly removed, it tends to close itself		

a. Color	Pink	Reddened Lesions Pallor (associated with anemia)
b. Surface	Transverse rugae (rugae diminish after vaginal deliveries) Moist, smooth	Leukoplakia Dried Lesions, cracks Bleeding
c. Consistency	Smooth, homogeneous	Nodular Swollen
d. Secretions	Thin Clear or cloudy Odorless	Thick, curdy, frothy Gray, greenish, yellowish Foul odor
e. Amount	Minimal to moderate	Profuse

15. Perform a bimanual vaginal examination
  a. Rise to standing position; remove glove from one hand, lubricate the other, and insert middle and index fingers into vaginal opening; compress posteriorly; wait for a moment and vaginal opening will relax; insert fingers gradually
  b. Palpate vaginal wall		

1. Surface	Smooth, homogeneous	Nodules
2. Tenderness	Nontender	Tender
16. Locate cervix with gloved hand; place palmar surface of other hand in abdominal midline, midway between umbilicus and pubis and press lightly toward intravaginal hand **17.** Palpate cervix and fornices with palmar surface of both fingers (Fig. 13-9)		

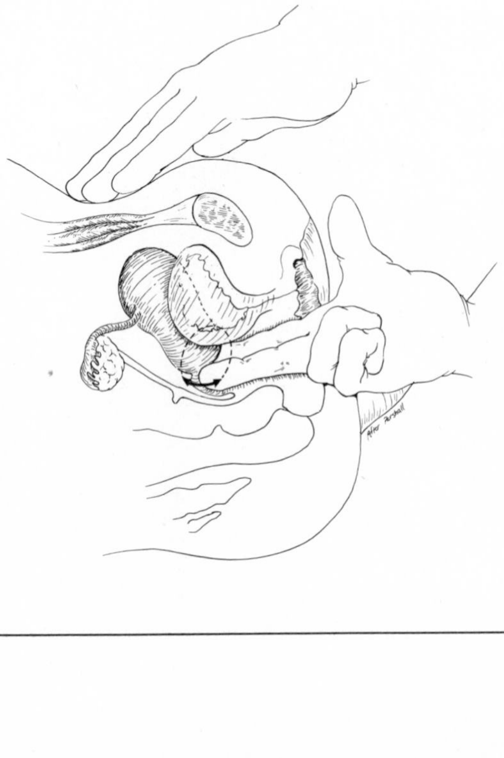

Fig. 13-9. Cervical palpation.

	To identify:	
The student will:	**Normal**	**Deviations from normal**
a. Cervical size	2.5 to 4 cm	Enlarged
b. Contour	Evenly rounded Slightly ovoid	Irregular
c. Consistency and surface	Firm (like tip of nose), smooth	Soft, nodular Hard
d. Mobility	Cervix moves 1 to 2 cm in each direction without discomfort	Immobile (fixed), or discomfort associated with movement
e. Location	Anterior or posterior midline	Laterally displaced
18. Insert one finger gently into cervical os to evaluate:		
a. Patency	Os admits fingertip 0.5 cm	Os stenosed
b. Fornices (pockets surrounding cervical protrusion)	Pliable and smooth Nontender	Hardened, nodular, or irregular surface Tender on palpation
19. Palpate uterus: place intravaginal fingers in anterior fornix; slowly slide abdominal hand toward pubis with flattened fingers pressing downward to evaluate:		
a. Location of fundus		
1. Anteverted (Fig. 13-10)	Fundus at level of pubis palpated between abdominal and gloved hand; cervix aimed posteriorly (*Note:* Most women have an anteverted uterus. The fundus should be palpated at the level of the pubis.)	

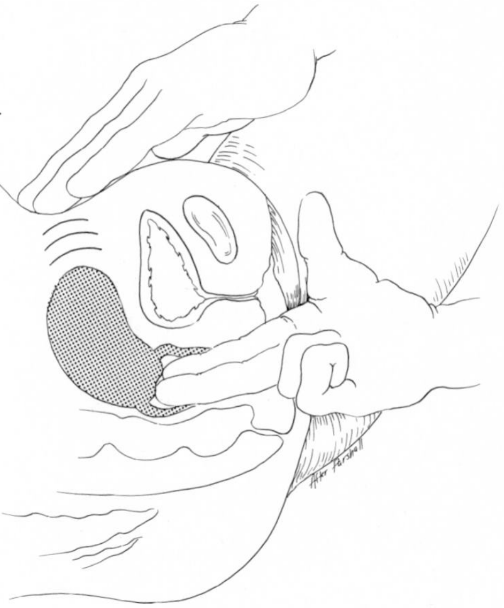

Fig. 13-10. Anteverted uterus.

2. Midposition (Fig. 13-11)	Fundus may not be palpable (depending on amount of abdominal adipose tissue and degree of abdominal muscle relaxation); cervix pointed along axis of vaginal canal	

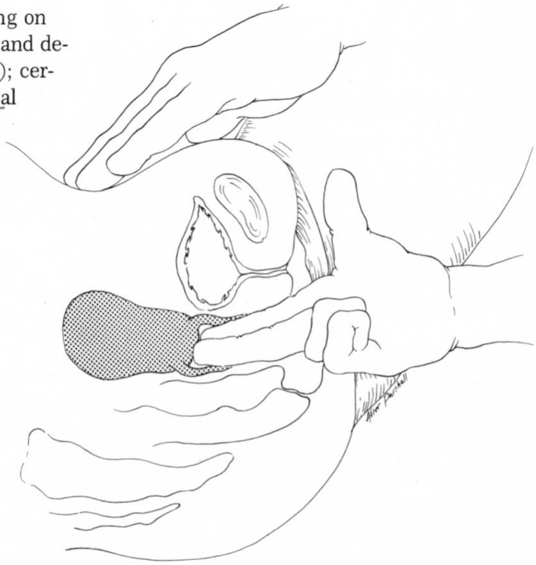

Fig. 13-11. Midposition uterus.

Continued.

Clinical guidelines—cont'd

The student will:	To identify:	
	Normal	**Deviations from normal**
3. Anteflexed (Fig. 13-12)	Fundus palpable at pubis between abdominal and gloved hand; cervix pointed along axis of vaginal canal *Post.*	

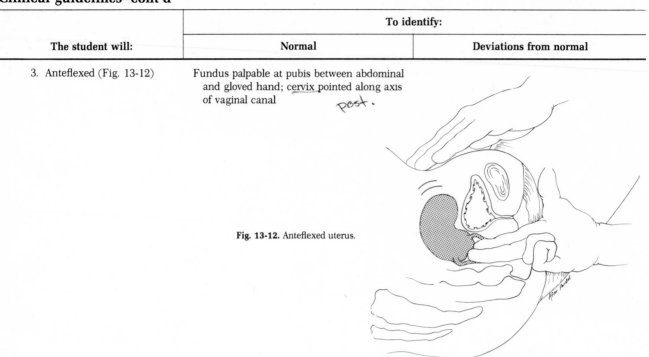

Fig. 13-12. Anteflexed uterus.

| 4. Retroflexed (Fig. 13-13) | Fundus not palpable; cervix directed along axis of vaginal canal | |

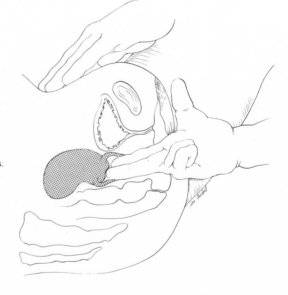

Fig. 13-13. Retroflexed uterus.

The student will:	To identify:	
	Normal	**Deviations from normal**
5. Retroverted (Fig. 13-14)	Fundus not palpable; cervix aimed anteriorly	Enlarged; fundus above level of pubis

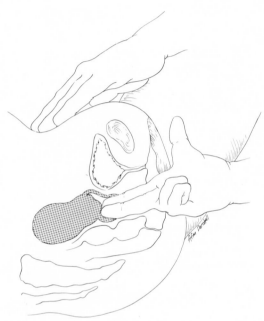

Fig. 13-14. Retroverted uterus.

b. Contour of fundus	Rounded	Irregular
c. Consistency and surface of uterine wall	Firm, smooth	Soft, nodular Masses
20. After the fundus is palpated, spread the fingers within the vagina and press into and upward within the posterior, anterior, and lateral fornices to palpate the lateral uterine wall		
a. Shape and size of uterine wall	Pear shaped, 5.5 to 8 cm long Somewhat enlarged in multiparous client	Nodular Enlarged Tender on palpation
b. Consistency	Smooth	Nodular
21. Gently "bounce" uterus between intravaginal and abdominally placed hands for:		
a. Mobility	Freely movable	Fixed
b. Tenderness	Nontender	Tender

Continued.

Clinical guidelines—cont'd

The student will:	To identify:	
	Normal	**Deviations from normal**
22. Place outside hand in right lower abdominal quadrant and intravaginal hand in right fornix; slide flat portion of fingers toward intravaginal hand (Fig. 13-15) to evaluate:		

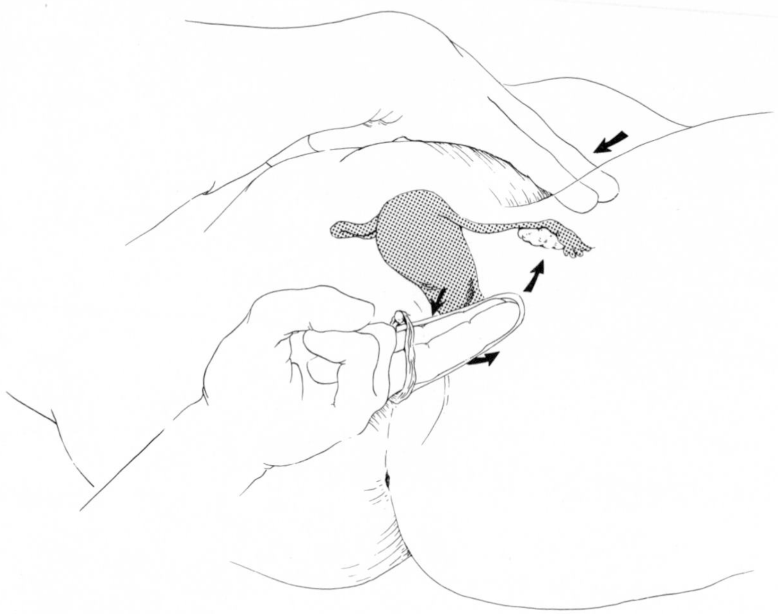

Fig. 13-15. Palpation of left adnexal area.

a. Right ovary	Slightly tender on palpation	Markedly tender
b. Palpable characteristics*	Not always palpable	
	Firm, smooth, ovoid	Nodular
	Walnut sized	Enlarged
	Approximately 4 cm	
	Mobile	Immobile mass felt
c. Other organs, masses, pulsations	Usually no other structures palpable except occasional round ligaments	Masses
		Nodularity
		Pulsations
		Fallopian tubes usually not palpable; if palpated, may indicate problem
23. Repeat procedure for left side		
24. Withdraw fingers from vagina; examine secretions on fingers for:		
a. Odor	None	Foul odor
b. Color	Clear or creamy	Gray, yellow, frothy
c. Amount	Minimal to moderate	Profuse
25. Perform a rectovaginal examination: withdraw fingers; change glove; lubricate and reinsert index finger into vagina and middle finger into anus; place other hand on abdomen		
26. Palpate anterior rectal wall for:		
a. Rectovaginal septum characteristics	Thin, smooth, pliable	Thickened, nodular
b. Rectovaginal pouch characteristics	Smooth	Nodular
	Uterine body (occasionally the fundus) may be felt	Tenderness
	Nontender	
27. Rotate finger in rectum to explore rectal wall for surface characteristics	Continuous smooth surface with minimal discomfort	Masses
		Nodules
		Induration
		Tenderness

*Remember, most palpation is done with the *intravaginal* hand, using the palmar surfaces of the fingers.

The student will:	To identify:	
	Normal	Deviations from normal
28. Withdraw fingers slowly, noting: **a.** Anal sphincter tone	Sphincter evenly tight around finger	Sphincter markedly relaxed Nodules, induration, masses
b. Tenderness	Nontender	Tenderness
29. Examine gloved finger for stool	If present, brown	Black Blood present

Clinical strategies

1. Procedure for obtaining Papanicolaou smears
   a. This procedure is performed after the cervix and surrounding tissue have been inspected and while the speculum is still in place in the vagina. The examiner should not apply lubricant to the speculum if the intent is to collect a Pap smear specimen.
   b. The bifid end of the wooden spatula is introduced into the vagina.
   c. The longer projection at the end of the spatula is inserted into the cervical os.
   d. The spatula is then rotated in a full circle, flush against the surrounding cervical tissue (light pressure is sufficient to keep the spatula in contact with the cervix).
   e. The spatula is then withdrawn, and the specimen is spread on a microscopic slide. A single light stroke with each side of the spatula enables the examiner to thin out the specimen over the slide surface. Avoid scraping the slide with back and forth motions.
   f. The slide is labeled and sprayed with a fixative solution or placed in a fixative solution container and labeled.
   g. The rounded end of the spatula is then introduced into the vagina and gently scraped over the posterior fornix area to collect a vaginal pool specimen.
   h. The spatula is withdrawn, and each side is lightly spread over another slide.
   i. This slide is labeled and sprayed or immersed in a fixative solution.
2. Procedure for obtaining a gonorrhea culture specimen
   a. Endocervical culture
      (1) The specimen for this culture can be collected immediately following the Pap smear procedure.
      (2) A sterile cotton applicator is introduced into the vagina and inserted into the cervical os.
      (3) The examiner holds the applicator in place for 10 to 30 seconds (there is no need to rotate the applicator).
      (4) The applicator is withdrawn and spread (and rotated) in a large **Z** pattern over the medium of a Thayer-Martin plate, or the applicator is placed in a Thayer-Martin culture tube.
      (5) The plate or tube is labeled.
      (6) The examiner must be familiar with agency routines for keeping the specimen warm, cross-streaking, and immediate transport to the laboratory.
   b. Anal culture
      (1) The specimen for this culture is collected after the vaginal speculum has been removed.
      (2) The sterile cotton-tipped applicator is inserted about 2.5 cm (1 inch) into the anal canal and rotated in a full circle. The applicator is also moved from side to side while inserted.
      (3) The examiner holds the applicator in place for 10 to 30 seconds.
      (4) The applicator is withdrawn and spread (and rotated) in a large **Z** pattern over the medium in a Thayer-Martin plate.
      (5) The plate is labeled. (*Note:* If the swab contains feces, it must be discarded and another specimen taken.)
      (6) The examiner must be familiar with agency routines for keeping the specimen warm, cross-streaking the medium, and transporting the specimen to the laboratory.
3. Mechanics of the pelvic examination
   a. The examiner must make a decision about which hand will insert and hold the speculum; then she must decide which will be the intravaginal hand during the bimanual examination. Once the decision is made, the examiner should maintain this routine. Often the dominant hand is more efficient with speculum insertion as well as serving as the internal hand for the bimanual assessment.
   b. The beginning examiner should become famil-

iar with the vaginal speculum before using it in a clinical setting. The metal speculum is very different from the plastic disposable speculum. The plastic speculum base widens as a portion of it moves in an adjacent groove. When the base is stabilized, it snaps into place with a resounding snap that often alarms both examiner and client! The metal speculum opens and stabilizes in position with the aid of twisting lever nuts and rods. It is most helpful to "play" with these instruments in advance until the examiner feels comfortable with them (Fig. 13-16).

4. Promoting client comfort
   a. Inquire about whether the client has had a pelvic examination before and ask if she has any concerns. Showing and explaining instruments, equipment, and the procedure will alleviate some anxiety.
   b. Assist the client in stabilizing her feet in the stirrups (she should wear her shoes). Help her to place her buttocks at the *edge* of the examining table.
   c. A client who is ill or weak may need assistance in maintaining her legs in position (an assistant may be necessary to support the client's legs).
   d. If the client is unable to assume the lithotomy position, an assessment can be accomplished while the client assumes the Sims position.
   e. Be certain that the room is warm and privacy is ensured.

   f. When draping the client, be certain to fully cover her knees with the drape.
   g. Posing questions during the examination is difficult, particularly if you are unable to establish eye contact. However, we have found it helpful to maintain a relaxed dialogue, describing our activities as we do them, so that the client feels included and informed.
   h. Some practitioners carry small hand mirrors and offer the client the opportunity to view her

---

Sample recording

External: Female hair distribution with no masses, lesions, scars, rash, or swelling in inguinal area. Labia, vestibule, urethral meatus are intact without inflammation, swelling, lesions, discharge, or tenderness. No bulging at vaginal orifice. Perineum intact with healed episiotomy scar.

Internal: Cervix multiparous, pink, firm, mobile, and midline without lesions.
Vaginal surface rugous and moist without inflammation. No discharge visualized. Nonodorous.
Uterine fundus anterior and firm under symphysis pubis, contour smooth, nontender.
Ovaries and tubes not palpable. No masses or tenderness on palpation.

Rectovaginal: Septum smooth and firm. Cul-de-sac and rectum without nodules, tenderness, or masses. Good anal sphincter tone.

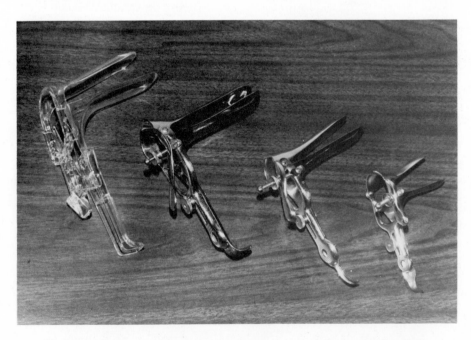

Fig. 13-16. Variety of metal specula in graduated sizes, and plastic speculum (left).

own genitalia with explanations and guidance from the examiner.

i. If the client becomes tense during the examination, stop the procedure but keep examining hands in place as you urge her to breathe slowly through her mouth and to concentrate on the breathing rhythm.

j. Be certain all equipment is close at hand before beginning the examination.

History and clinical strategies associated with the pediatric client

1. The extent of the gynecological examination of the child will depend on the child's age and presenting complaints. For the well child, during a screening examination, the extent of the examination includes only inspection and palpation of the external genitalia. The vaginoscopy examination is done for a young child only when a problem is anticipated or for a teenager who is sexually active and requests birth control information or who is experiencing abdominal, gynecological, or urinary problems.

2. Because of the complexity of the procedure, the vaginoscopy examination of the young child is beyond the scope of this text. Although it may at times become necessary to perform a speculum examination, it requires special equipment and a well-prepared and knowledgeable practitioner who frequently performs pediatric gynecological examinations.

3. Examining the external genitalia of any child should be anticipated as a stressful event for both the client and her parent, if present. The examiner must explain to the child and the parent exactly what will be done prior to the examination as well as continue to explain throughout the inspection and palpation of the external genitalia. It may be necessary to explain to the parent that thorough inspection of the child's external genitalia is part of every complete examination.

   The young infant and child will usually participate cooperatively if the examination is completed in a matter-of-fact manner.

   By the time the child reaches 4 to 6 years of age, the examiner will need to spend even more time reassuring the child that the procedure involves only looking at her gentialia and touching her on the outside. If necessary, the examiner should enlist the help of the child by taking the child's hand and having her first touch herself; then the examiner can palpate the genitalia.

   A school-age or young teenage child will not like the examination but will allow it to occur uneventfully. The child's mother may or may not be present during the examination. If the child appears fearful or anxious, the mother may be able to provide comfort. If the child is older, the examiner should be alert to the child's embarrassment because her mother is present. The examiner should confer with the child prior to the examination and, if appropriate, ask the mother to wait outside.

   As the child begins to mature she will become very interested in her own body and what she looks like. The examiner may use a mirror to allow the child to look at herself. Education could coincide with the examination.

   Older teenagers deserve to be examined without their mothers present if they desire or if the examiner wants to talk with the adolescent alone. As for the younger adolescent, a mirror may be used as an educational tool and to involve the teenager in the actual assessment process.

4. Positioning the child for the examination will depend on the child's age.

   a. Birth to 3 years of age. The child should be on the parent's lap with the child's back reclining at about a 45° angle against the parent's chest. The child should feel secure in this position, and the parent can help by holding the child's legs in a frog position up against her chest. This will allow the examiner full access to the external genitalia. The examiner should be sitting opposite the mother and have an adequate light source.

   b. Three to 5 years. Because of the child's size, she will need to be moved to the examination table. If possible, the head of the table should be up about 30°. The child should be resting back on the incline and her legs again held up by her parent in a frog position against her chest. The child does not need to be at the end of the examination table.

   c. Six to 15 years. The child should be on the examination table in a modified lithotomy position, lying flat or at an upward slight angle. Her legs must be flexed at the knee, and her heels should be close to her buttocks. The knees are then separated so that the genitalia may be viewed. If the mother is present, she should stand near the girl's head and assist in maintaining a spread-knee position. Depending on the child's age and the length of her legs, she may need to be toward the end of the table. If the examiner has difficulty visualizing the genitalia, a small pillow may be placed under the child's hips. Although the conventional gynecological stirrups are extremely convenient for the examiner, they are often frightening to the young adolescent and spaced too widely for comfort.

d. Over age 15 years. The adolescent will require the same lithotomy positioning as the adult. The success and adequacy of this positioning will depend on the examiner's approach to the client.

5. Frequently the examiner performs the first speculum examination for the teenage or young adult client. The first examination is perhaps the client's most important, since during that examination the client is developing perceptions that will remain with her for future examinations. Special preparations the examiner should make follow:

a. Discuss the procedure with the client while she is still dressed.

b. If possible, use illustrations or models to show exactly what will happen and what the examiner will be observing.

c. Prepare all necessary equipment so that once the procedure is started, there will be no interruptions.

d. Use an appropriate size speculum.

(1) There are pediatric and virginal specula that are approximately 1 to 1.5 cm wide. These can be carefully inserted with minimal discomfort.

(2) A small adult speculum may be used if the client is sexually active.

6. The history questioning about the genitourinary system of girls should focus on the following three areas:

a. Urinary functioning. Does the child have any difficulties with voiding, such as urinary incontinence, bed-wetting, inability to maintain a steady stream until the bladder is emptied, burning or urgency with urination? If any of these are present, explore in detail including family history of similar problems, use of bubble bath, and frequency of urinary tract problems.

b. Vaginal itching or discharge. These are both frequent problems that require in-depth investigation. Common causes of these include inconsistent or inadequate cleansing of the area; foreign bodies such as a toy, toilet tissue, crayons, or coins; sexual abuse or genital fondling. The parent and/or child must be questioned about these possibilities, and the examiner must be careful to consider them during the physical assessment.

c. Maturational changes. Girls over 9 years of age who are also showing breast and pubic hair development should be questioned about whether they have begun menstruation and whether they understand about the developmental changes their bodies are undergoing. Areas of specific investigation include:

(1) The girl's awareness and information about menstruation

(2) The girl's feelings about menstruation

(3) The girl's information regarding sexual activities and techniques to prevent pregnancy

Clinical variations associated with the pediatric client

Characteristic or area examined	Normal	Deviations from normal
1. Position child as previously discussed		
2. Careful examination of external genitalia of the infant to make sure it is unambiguous		Inability to identify the labia majora, labia minora, clitoris, urethera, vaginal introitus
3. Inguinal and mons pubis surface characteristics	Smooth, clear surface area Parasites absent	Poor perineal hygiene Scars, swellings, discolorations Excoriated surface Lesions, rash Lice
4. Hair distribution	See Table 10 for maturational development	Absence of pubic hair by child's thirteenth birthday
5. Labia majora surface characteristics	Pink, smooth surface Symmetrical, dry appearance Becomes prominent and hair covered during puberty	Swelling, redness Discoloration, excoriated or rash surface
6. Labia minora	Very prominent in infants (may normally protrude from labia majora)	Labia fused by adhesions
	By puberty labia minora recede to adult configuration	Inflammation, swelling, nodules, varicosities Marked asymmetry
	Light pink color in infants and small children, changing to dark pink by puberty Symmetrical	Tissue appearing white and thin

Characteristic or area examined	Normal	Deviations from normal
7. Clitoris size	From 3 mm to 1 cm (½ inch) in length, depending on age and maturational development	Enlargement, atrophy Ambiguous appearance
8. Uretheral meatus and surrounding tissue	Irregular opening or slit Usually located midline; may be close to or slightly within vaginal introitus	Redness, rashes, or lesions Lateral position of meatus Discharge from surrounding Skene's glands or urethral opening
9. Vaginal introitus and immediate surrounding tissue	Moist tissue, even pink color Hymen may or may not be across or partially across vaginal opening; by menarche, opening should be at least 1 cm wide Vaginal opening present	If hymen intact (imperforate hymen), bluish color or bulging behind the hymen may mean presence of blood; most commonly found in (1) newborn: will generally reabsorb on own; (2) adolescent: menstrual blood Any time imperforate hymen found, client should be referred Lesions, redness, rashes, swelling
10. Perineum surface	Smooth, pink	Inflammation, fistula, lesion, mass
11. Anus	Deeper pigmentation and coarse skin	Lesions, rash, skin tags, inflammation, lumps, excoriation, unclean surface Presence of pinworms

Continued.

Table 10. Pubic hair development in females*

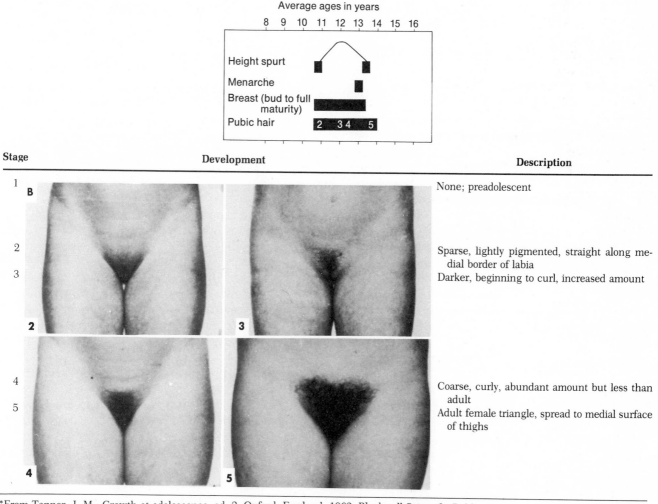

Stage	Development	Description
1		None; preadolescent
2		Sparse, lightly pigmented, straight along medial border of labia
3		Darker, beginning to curl, increased amount
4		Coarse, curly, abundant amount but less than adult
5		Adult female triangle, spread to medial surface of thighs

*From Tanner, J. M.: Growth at adolescence, ed. 2, Oxford, England, 1962, Blackwell Scientific Publications.

Clinical variations associated with the pediatric client–cont'd

Characteristic or area examined	Normal	Deviations from normal
12. External genitalia palpation		
a. Labia and vestibule	Soft, homogeneous, nontender	Nodular, tender
b. Skene's glands	Not visible or palpable	Tender or swollen glands; presence of discharge
c. Bartholin's glands	Not visible or palpable	Tender or swollen glands Unilateral swelling Presence of discharge
d. Vaginal discharge	Mucoid or sanguineous discharge in newborn Watery discharge present for 2 to 3 years prior to onset of menstruation Within 1 year following onset of menstruation, discharge as seen in adult	Thick or foul odorous discharge

Note: If speculum examination is required in a small child, she should be referred to a physician. If speculum examination is required in a menstruating adolescent, techniques previously described should be used; the findings are similar to those for the adult.

History and clinical strategies associated with the geriatric client

1. Sexual history. The elderly woman is capable of sexual functioning during her entire lifetime. Changes associated with aging do occur in the external and internal genitalia, but they occur slowly and at different rates according to the individual. A summary of the aging changes follows:
   a. The vaginal tube becomes shorter and narrower.
   b. Vaginal fluids lessen and may secrete at a slower rate to direct stimulation.
   c. The vaginal walls are thinner and more friable.
   d. Excitement phase: the time and extent of the expansion phase of the vagina is diminished.
   e. Plateau phase: uterine elevation is reduced; vasocongestion of the labia is diminished.
   f. Orgasmic phase: duration of orgasm is lessened, and the number of uterine contractures are fewer. Occasionally the uterine muscles will lapse into spasm, which can be painful.
   g. Resolution phase: this phase is more rapid than in younger women.
   Some of the changes mentioned accelerate if the woman experiences no sexual stimulation for an extended period of time (either with a sexual partner or through masturbation). Lack of a sexual partner can be a problem. Some older women, even though they have sexual needs and a desire for intimacy, are not comfortable with extramarital relationships, masturbation, or other life-style alterations if they have no sexual partner.

   All the intimacy and sex-related questions listed in the adult section of this chapter are appropriate for the elderly woman. Additional questions might be considered if the client indicates that she is interested in pursuing the topic of sexuality.
   a. If you have a male sexual partner, do you feel that he is comfortable with his sexual behaviors, responses, and capabilities?
   b. Do you ever experience pain in response to direct stimulation of the vagina? During orgasm?
   c. Do you have difficulty with urinary frequency or urgency during sexual stimulation?
   d. Do you have other physical problems that interfere with sexual behavior (e.g., painful joints, fatigue, dyspnea, fear of injuring yourself or causing illness)?
   e. Does your partner have any other physical problems that interfere with sexual behaviors?
   f. Are adequate privacy and time available for you to meet your sexual needs?
   g. Do you have any problems with family members objecting to your friendships or sexual habits?
   (*Note:* Some elderly women have consciously made the decision to discontinue sexual activity. An overly enthusiastic practitioner might create conflict and cause embarrassment. Other older females are quite creative and zealous in pursuing needs for sexual fulfillment. Homosexual encount-

ers, masturbation, extramarital experiences, and creative sexual methods with a partner may be part of their life-style. The practitioner should be well informed about elderly individuals' needs and capabilities before pursuing a detailed sexual history.)

2. Symptoms associated with the genitourinary system
   a. Vulvitis may occur with immobilization, poor hygiene practices, urinary incontinence, poor nutrition, and obesity. Associated symptoms are itching (which is worsened by scratching) and local discomfort or burning.
   b. Vaginitis may occur because of limited vaginal secretions, an increased alkaline condition (associated with diminished estrogen output), or pessary irritation. Symptoms are itching, pain during intercourse, general localized soreness, and perhaps a resulting increase in vaginal discharge that may be yellowish or brown and foul in odor.
   c. Uterine cancer is first suspected with postmenopausal bleeding. *Any bleeding episode* is cause for immediate referral to a physician.
   d. Genital prolapse may feel like pressure or heaviness in the genital area. Back pain, attacks of cystitis (urgency, frequency, burning on urination), urinary retention, urinary incontinence, and constipation may accompany this problem. (*Note:* The severity and number of complaints may not correlate with the severity of prolapse that the examiner observes.)
   e. Stress incontinence is common. Involuntary urination with coughing, sneezing, laughing, moving from sitting to standing position, or general movement may occur.
   f. The questions listed in the adult section of this chapter regarding vaginal discharge and pelvic pain are appropriate for the aging woman.
   g. The client should be asked if she has any concerns or information to share about her menopausal phase.
   h. If the client is undergoing estrogen therapy, inquire specifically about bleeding episodes, fluid retention, breast enlargement, or pain. Ask the client to evaluate the effects and side effects of the therapy.

3. Clinical strategies
   a. Many clients may assume the lithotomy position with help and support from the examiner. Another individual might be needed to support the client's legs, since they may tire easily when the hip joints remain in abduction for extended periods.
   b. Clients with orthopneic problems will have to have the head elevated during the examination.
   c. Disabled clients may assume the Sims position for a pelvic examination if they are unable to maintain the dorsolithotomy pose.
   d. Papanicolaou smears should be obtained for aging women with the same frequency as with younger women.
   e. Read the clinical strategy section in the adult section of this chapter for further suggestions regarding client comfort and examination procedures.

Clinical variations associated with the geriatric client

Characteristic or area examined	Normal	Deviations from normal
1. External genitalia inspection		
a. Hair distribution	Pubic hair thinned, perhaps sparse, often gray	Patchy loss of hair
		Total absence of hair
	Parasites absent	Nits, pubic lice
b. Inguinal, mons pubis, skin surface characteristics	Smooth, clear	Scars
		Inguinal swelling, excoriation, lesions, rash
c. Labia majora surface characteristics	Labial folds flattened or may disappear into surrounding skin	Shrinkage accompanied by inflammation
	Decrease in subcutaneous fat in folds usually corresponds to degree of loss of subcutaneous fat elsewhere on client's body	Thickening or induration of small areas
		Maceration, ulceration, lesions, nodules
	Symmetrical	Marked asymmetry
	Skin appears smooth, often shiny, and paler than in younger adult	
d. Inner surface of labia majora and labia minora	Shiny, usually dry, paler than in young adult	Inflammation
	Fewer folds	Maceration
	Usually symmetrical	Lesions, nodules
		Varicosities
		Swelling, thickening

Continued.

Clinical variations associated with the geriatric client–cont'd

Characteristic or area examined	Normal	Deviations from normal
e. Clitoris size	Slightly smaller than in younger adult	Induration Marked asymmetry Enlargement Marked atrophy
f. Clitoris surface	Medial aspect covered by prepuce Pink	Inflammation
g. Urethral meatus and immediate surrounding tissue	Irregular opening or slit (relaxed perineal musculature may result in meatus being situated more posteriorly; very near or within vaginal introitus) Midline location	Discharge from surrounding glands or urethral opening Polyp Inflammation Urethral caruncles fairly common, appearing as a bright red nodule near urethral meatus Lateral position of meatus
h. Vaginal introitus and immediate surrounding tissue	May be smaller (admit only one finger) than younger adult, or multiparous client may manifest gaping introitus with vaginal walls rolling toward opening	Surrounding inflammation Profuse vaginal discharge Swelling Lesions Large rectocele, cystocele, enterocele, or marked uterine prolapse will show mucosal tissue bulging through vaginal orifice
i. Perineum surface	Smooth, or episiotomy scar (midline or mediolateral) may be visible	Inflammation, fistula Lesions, mass
j. Anus surface	Increased pigmentation and coarse skin	Scars, skin tags Lesions, inflammation Fissures, lumps Excoriation Hemorrhoids
k. External genitalia palpation	Soft, homogeneous Nontender	Irregular, nodular Tender
1. Urethral duct	No discharge from urethral duct Nontender	Discharge* Tenderness
2. Bartholin's gland area	No tenderness, no swelling, homogeneous tissue No discharge	Tender, swelling nodules Discharge*
3. Perineum	Thin, rigid Lateral episiotomy scar may be visible Nontender	Paper thin Tender
(*Note:* At time of insertion of finger into vaginal orifice estimate opening and vaginal orifice tone)	Opening may be very narrow and admit one finger only Opening may be very relaxed; client has difficulty squeezing examiner's finger with voluntary vaginal constriction	
2. Insert middle finger and index finger (if possible) in vagina; press posteriorly with firm gradual motion; ask client to strain down or bear down to elicit: **a.** Bulging	Vaginal wall may roll slightly outward	Bulge appears from anterior wall Bulge appears from posterior wall Uterus emerges at opening (cervix may be visible at opening, or may protrude beyond opening) (*Note:* The cervix is often eroded and hypertrophied with marked uterine prolapse.)
b. Urinary incontinence (*Note:* A speculum with narrow blades may have to be used if client has small introitus.) **3.** Internal inspection **a.** Cervix	No incontinence	Incontinent

*Prepare a culture of any discharge.

Characteristic or area examined	Normal	Deviations from normal
1. Color	Paler than in younger woman; color evenly distributed Symmetrical, circumscribed erythema surrounding os may indicate normal condition of exposed columnar epithelium; however, beginning examiners should consider any reddened appearance a problem for consultation	Inflamed (red) in local areas or generally Markedly pale Cyanotic Erythema, especially if patchy or if borders irregular around os
2. Position	Midline Cervix and os may be pointed in anterior or posterior direction Cervix protrudes less into vaginal tube; may be flush against back of vaginal wall Surrounding fornices diminish or may disappear	Situated laterally Projection of over 3 cm (1¼ inches) into vaginal tube
3. Size	Cervix decreases in size with aging	Over 4 cm (1½ inches) in diameter
4. Surface	Smooth; may appear paler than in younger woman Occasional visible squamocolumnar junction (symmetrical reddened circle around os) Nabothian cysts common (smooth, round, yellowish raised areas)	Reddened granular area around os (especially asymmetrical), friable tissue Red patches, lesions Strawberry spots White patches
5. Os	Often very narrow or stenosed; in some instances may be obliterated	Absence of os should be reported as problem (*Note:* If secretions from uterus are trapped by nonfunctional os, the uterus may be enlarged and tender on palpation.)
6. Cervical discharge	Often scanty; if present, should be clear or slightly opaque and odorless	Odor foul Colored (yellowish, greenish, gray) Also note odor of stale urine Bloody discharge
b. Vagina	Length of tube shortens with aging	
1. Color	Appears paler than in younger women	Reddened Lesions Pallor (associated with anemia)
2. Surface	Less moisture Smooth (rugae diminish with aging) Shiny	Leukoplakia Dried Lesions, cracks, petechiae Bleeding
3. Consistency	Smooth, homogeneous	Nodular Swollen
4. Secretions	If present, should be clear or slightly opaque Odorless	Thick, curdy, frothy Gray, greenish, yellowish Foul odor
5. Amount of secretion	May be absent or sparse	Profuse
4. Bimanual examination		
a. Vaginal wall surface (*Note:* Examiner may be able to insert one finger only.)	Smooth, homogeneous Nontender	Nodular Tender
b. Cervix	Cervical protrusion into vaginal vault diminishes Cervix may be flush against back of vault In some instances examiner may not be able to palpate cervix	
1. Size	Diminished	Enlarged
2. Contour	Evenly rounded, may be slightly ovoid	Irregular in shape
3. Consistency and surface	Firm (like tip of nose) Smooth	Soft, nodular, or hard
4. Mobility	Cervix remains mobile, but mobility may be less noticeable if protrusion into vaginal vault greatly diminished	Immobile, fixed, or discomfort associated with movement

Continued.

Clinical variations associated with the geriatric client–cont'd

Characteristic or area examined	Normal	Deviations from normal
	Movement should not cause discomfort	
5. Location	Midline	Laterally displaced
6. Patency of os	Os may be smaller but should be palpable	Stenosis of os may be normal finding; however, beginning examiners should report this as problem
7. Fornices surrounding cervix	Diminish (may disappear) with aging; if palpable, should be pliable, smooth, and nontender	Irregular or nodular surface, tender on palpation
c. Uterus	Greatly diminishes in size; most often not palpable at all	Enlarged
		Nodular, irregular, hardened, or indurated areas; tender on palpation
	If body of uterus palpated with internal hand, should be smooth, firm, freely movable, and nontender	Fixed
d. Ovaries	Atrophy with age and rarely palpable in aging women	Marked tenderness in adnexal area
		Nodulation or mass palpated
	Fallopian tubes not palpable	Pulsations
		Ascites and pleural fluid accumulation sometimes associated with adnexal masses
5. Rectovaginal examination		
a. Palpable characteristics	Rectal wall should feel smooth and homogeneous	Nodular, thickened
		Tender
	Nontender	Pouching on anterior rectal wall
	Rectovaginal septum should feel thin, smooth, and pliable	Any palpated mass abnormal
		Uterus bulging into rectal wall
	Uterine body rarely palpated, and posterior fornix difficult to locate	Anal sphincter manifesting no tone
	Anal sphincter tone may be somewhat diminished but should be nontender	

Vocabulary

1. Adnexa

2. Amenorrhea

3. Bartholin's glands

    Secrete mucus vulvovaginal

4. Cystocele *herniation of bladder → vagina*

5. Douglas' cul-de-sac (pouch)

6. Dysmenorrhea *painful menstruation*

7. Dyspareunia

8. Enterocele *intestinal hernia*

9. Escutcheon

pattern of pubic hair distribution

10. Fornix

11. Fourchette

post. junction of labia minora

12. Gravida

pregnancies

13. Hymenal caruncles

14. Introitus

vaginal entrance

15. Leukorrhea

vaginal discharge white or yellow

16. Menarche

17. Menorrhagia

excessive menstruation

18. Metrorrhagia

uterine bleeding, irregular intervals

19. Mons pubis

20. Parous

viable offspring

21. Pudendum

external structures mons, labios

22. Retrocele

23. Rugae

24. Skene's glands

mucus secreting, inside urethral meatus

25. Vestibule

between labia minora

Cognitive self-assessment

Match the lettered structures with the corresponding numbered label.

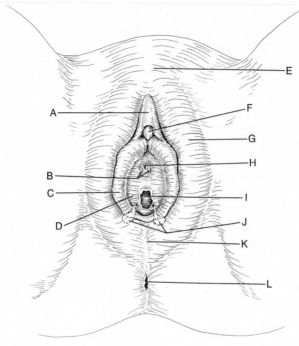

1. __L__ Anus
2. __F__ Clitoris
3. __C__ Labia minora
4. __K__ Perineum
5. __H__ Urethral meatus
6. __A__ Prepuce
7. __E__ Mons pubis
8. __I__ Vaginal introitus
9. __B__ Opening of Skene's gland
10. __G__ Labia majora
11. __D__ Vestibule
12. __J__ Bartholin's gland
13. Which of the following statements is/are true?
    - ☐ a. The labia majora extend from the mons pubis to the fourchette.
    - ☑ b. The labia minora are darker in color and thinner than the majora.
    - ☑ c. The visible part of the clitoris is normally no more than 2 cm long and 1 cm wide.
    - ☑ d. The perforated hymen can leave visible rounded fragments at the introital margins.
    - ☑ e. The perineum usually feels thicker and more flexible in a nulliparous woman.
    - ☐ f. All except c
    - ☐ g. b and e
    - ☑ h. All except a
    - ☐ i. a, c, and e
14. Which of the following statements is/are true?
    - ☑ a. Bartholin glands are lateral and slightly posterior to the vaginal orifice.
    - ☐ b. Bartholin glands are usually not visible but can be palpated.
    - ☑ c. Skene's ducts are located in the paraurethral area.

☐ d. When Skene's ducts are "milked," they usually exude a small amount of clear discharge.

☑ e. A visible discharge from Bartholin's glands should be considered abnormal.

☐ f. All except e

☑ g. a, c, and e

☐ h. All the above

☐ i. All except d

☐ j. b and d

15. Which of the following statements is/are true about preparation of the client for a pelvic examination?

☐ a. A vinegar douche administered the night before a scheduled pelvic examination is usually recommended.

☐ b. Demonstrating the instruments used for a pelvic examination prior to using them generally increases anxiety on the part of teenage clients.

☑ c. Covering the client's knees with the drape while she is in lithotomy position maintains the illusion that she is "decently" covered.

☑ d. If the client breathes deeply and slowly through her mouth and concentrates on the breathing rhythm, she is more likely to relax.

☑ e. If a disabled client cannot assume or maintain the lithotomy position, the Sims position can be used.

☐ f. a and d

☐ g. b, d, and e

☑ h. c, d, and e

☐ i. All except e

Match the lettered structures with the corresponding numbered label.

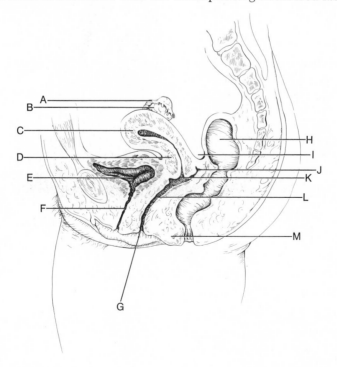

16. ___D___ Uterus (isthmus)
17. ___G___ Introitus
18. ___B___ Ovary

19. __H__ Rectum
20. __K__ Cervix
21. __C__ Uterus (fundus)
22. __M__ Perineum
23. __F__ Urethra
24. __A__ Fallopian tube
25. __L__ Vagina
26. __J__ Rectouterine pouch
27. __E__ Bladder
28. __S__ Fornix
29. Which of the following statements is/are true?
    ☑ a. The vagina inclines posteriorly at about a 45° angle with the vertical plane of the body.
    ☑ b. The anterior vaginal wall is more sensitive to pressure than the posterior wall.
    ☑ c. Vaginal discharge is normally odorless.
    ☐ d. A whitish, creamy vaginal discharge should be considered abnormal.
    ☑ e. The vaginal surface often appears thinner and paler in an elderly client.
    ☐ f. a, b, and c
    ☐ g. c, d, and e
    ☐ h. All except c
    ☐ i. All the above
    ☑ j. All except d
30. Which of the following statements is/are true about normal deviation of findings related to pelvic examination?
    ☐ a. The cervix softens in the fourth to sixth week of pregnancy.
    ☑ b. The cervix usually appears bluish or purplish in early pregnancy.
    ☑ c. The multiparous cervical os is slitlike in appearance.
    ☑ d. The uterus size is decreased in an elderly client.
    ☑ e. Vaginal mucosa may become increasingly friable with aging.
    ☑ f. All the above
    ☐ g. All except e
    ☐ h. a, c, and e
    ☐ i. b, c, and d
31. Retroversion of the uterus:
    ☐ a. rarely occurs
    ☑ b. is a tilting backward of the entire uterus
    ☐ c. occurs with aging
    ☑ d. when marked, may permit palpation of the fundus through the rectum
    ☑ e. results in the cervix facing more anteriorly in the vagina
    ☑ f. b, d, and e
    ☐ g. all except c
    ☐ h. all except a
    ☐ i. b, c, and d
32. Anteflexion of the uterus:
    ☐ a. results in the cervix facing more posteriorly in the vagina
    ☑ b. results in easy palpation of the fundus
    ☐ c. is a tilting forward of the entire uterus
    ☐ d. occurs with aging
    ☐ e. may permit palpation of the fundus through the rectum
    ☐ f. all except e
    ☑ g. a, b, and c

☐ h. c and d

☐ i. b and c

33. A normal cervix:

    ☑ a. is covered by a smooth, pink epithelium

    ☐ b. is a granular, vascular membrane

    ☑ c. has an os with a slitlike appearance after childbirth

    ☐ d. is immobile

    ☑ e. feels firm, like the tip of your nose

    ☐ f. all except a

    ☑ g. a, c, and e

    ☐ h. b, d, and e

    ☐ i. all except b

    ☐ j. a and d

34. When you use the vaginal speculum:

    ☑ a. it is usually warmed and lubricated with water

    ☐ b. a commercial lubricant should be used at all times

    ☐ c. on insertion, exert pressure against the anterior wall to avoid client discomfort

    ☐ d. the blades are vertical on initial insertion

    ☐ e. on insertion the blades are partially open to permit viewing of the vaginal wall

    ☐ f. all except e

    ☐ g. all except d

    ☐ h. a, c, and d

    ☐ i. b and e

35. During bimanual palpation, the normal uterus:

    ☐ a. is immobile

    ☐ b. feels spongy at the fundus

    ☑ c. is usually 5 to 8 cm long

    ☑ d. feels firm

    ☐ e. feels nodular

    ☐ f. all except b

    ☐ g. a and d

    ☐ h. a, b, and c

    ☑ i. c and d

36. Which of the following statements is/are true about normal palpable findings during a bimanual examination?

    ☑ a. The cervix is freely movable (1 to 2 cm in each direction) when manipulated by the examiner's fingers.

    ☐ b. The normal cervical os is closed and will not admit a fingertip.

    ☑ c. Approximately 85% of uteri are in an anteposition and can be palpated anteriorly.

    ☑ d. Normal ovaries are 4 to 6 cm, firm to touch, and movable.

    ☑ e. Round ligaments are sometimes palpated as cordlike structures.

    ☐ f. a, d, and e

    ☐ g. b and c

    ☑ h. All except b

    ☐ i. b, c, and d

37. The rectovaginal examination is performed:

    ☐ a. to confirm the uterine position

    ☐ b. to reassess adnexal areas

    ☑ c. to palpate the rectovaginal cul-de-sac and septum

    ☑ d. to palpate the rectal wall

    ☑ e. to assess anal sphincter tone

- [ ] f. all except c
- [x] g. all the above
- [ ] h. d and e
- [ ] i. a, c, and d
- [ ] j. all except b

Mark each statement "T" or "F."

38. __T__ The labia may appear somewhat shriveled in a normal multiparous woman.
39. __F__ Skene's ducts are often normally somewhat tender when palpated (or milked).
40. __F__ Bartholin's gland openings are usually visible.
X 41. __FF__ The perineum usually feels thinner and more rigid in a nulliparous woman.
42. __T__ The squamocolumnar junction may occasionally be visible on a normal cervix.
43. __T__ A normal cervix should extend (project) no more than 3 cm into the vaginal vault.

PEDIATRIC QUESTIONS

Mark each statement "T" or "F."

44. __T__ By age 13 years all girls should start to develop pubic hair.
45. __F__ All teens should have a speculum examination by age 16.
46. __T__ The hymen must be perforated for the adolescent to menstruate.
47. __T__ The best method to examine the external genitalia of a 2-year-old is to have the child on the parent's lap.
48. __T__ Perineal irritation in the preschool child is commonly due to the use of bubble bath.
49. __F__ The labia majora in the infant are more prominent than the labia minora.

GERIATRIC QUESTIONS

50. Common genital findings in the aging female are:
    - [ ] a. ✗ a flaccid boggy uterus that can usually be palpated in the anterior rectal wall
    - [x] b. diminished vaginal secretions
    - [ ] c. ✗ increased protrusion of cervix into the vaginal vault, resulting in deep fornices surrounding the cervix
    - [x] d. paler appearing vaginal walls
    - [x] e. flatter labia majora and diminished skinfolds
    - [ ] f. all the above
    - [x] g. b, d, and e
    - [ ] h. a, c, and e
    - [ ] i. all except b
    - [ ] j. none of the above
51. Sexual functioning of the elderly female:
    - [ ] a. usually ceases after age 65 years
    - [ ] b. is not usually advisable if the client has osteoarthritis or cardiac disease
    - [x] c. may be consciously relinquished by the individual
    - [ ] d. should be rigorously promoted by the practitioner
    - [ ] e. none of the above
52. Vulvitis may occur because of:
    - [ ] a. poor nutrition

☐ b. poor hygiene practices
☐ c. urinary incontinence
☐ d. excess vaginal secretions
☐ e. obesity
☐ f. all the above
☐ g. none of the above
☑ h. all except d
☐ i. b and c

SUGGESTED READINGS
General

American Journal of Nursing: Programmed Instruction, Patient assessment: examination of the female pelvis. Part I, **78**(10), 1978.

American Journal of Nursing: Programmed Instruction. Patient assessment: examination of the female pelvis. Part II, **78**(11), 1978.

Bates, Barbara: A guide to physical examination, ed. 2, Philadelphia, 1979, J. B. Lippincott Co., pp. 230–248, 249–256.

Malasanos, Lois, Barkauskas, Violet, Moss, Muriel, and Stoltenberg-Allen, Karthryn: Health assessment, St. Louis, 1977, The C. V. Mosby Co., pp. 283–304.

Martin, Leonide L.: Health care of women, Philadelphia, 1978, J. B. Lippincott Co., pp. 29–56, 201–218.

Prior, John A., and Silberstein, Jack S.: Physical diagnosis: the history and examination of the patient, ed. 5, St. Louis, 1977, The C. V. Mosby Co., pp. 338–356.

Walker, Kenneth, Hall, W. Dallas, and Hurst, J. Willis, editors: Clinical methods, vol. 1, Boston, 1976, Butterworths, Inc., pp. 223–263, 272–281.

Pediatric

Alexander, Mary and Brown, Marie Scott: Pediatric physical diagnosis for nurses, New York, 1974, McGraw-Hill Book Co., pp. 179–185.

Barness, Lewis: Manual of pediatric physical diagnosis, ed. 4, Chicago, 1972, Year Book Medical Publishers, Inc., pp. 134–136.

Daniel, William A., Jr.: Adolescents in health and disease, St. Louis, 1977, The C. V. Mosby Co., pp. 27–41, 132–150.

Huffman, John W.: Gynecologic examination of the premenarcheal child, Pediatric gynecology, Pediatric Annals, December, 1974, pp. 6–18.

Mager, Joni: The pelvic examination: a view from the other end of the table, Ann. Intern. Med. **83**:563–564, 1975.

Prior, John A., and Silberstein, Jack S.: Physical diagnosis: the history and examination of the patient, ed. 5, St. Louis, 1977, The C. V. Mosby Co., p. 470.

Rauh, Joseph, and Brookman, Richard R.: In Johnson, T. R., Moore, W. M., and Jefferies, J. E., editors: Children are different: developmental physiology, Columbus, Ohio, 1978, Ross Laboratories, pp. 28–29.

Geriatric

Burnside, Irene Mortenson: Nursing and the aged, New York, 1976, McGraw-Hill Book Co., pp. 99–111, 452–463.

Chinn, Austin B., editor: Clinical aspects of aging, Working with older people: a guide to practice, vol. 4, Rockville, Md., 1971, U.S. Department of Health, Education, and Welfare, Public Health Service, pp. 149–155.

Griggs, Winona: Sex and the elderly, Am. J. Nurs. **78**(8):1352–1354, Aug., 1978.

Steinberg, Franz U.: Cowdry's: the care of the geriatric patient, St. Louis, 1976, The C. V. Mosby Co., pp. 292–299, 393–400.

CHAPTER 14

Assessment of the musculoskeletal system

Overview

Assessment of the musculoskeletal system can be performed on many levels, from gross observations of function to the electrical evaluation of selected muscle fiber groups. For the purpose of this chapter, musculoskeletal evaluation is directed toward functional assessment and detection of the presence, location, and extent of dysfunction. Emphasis is placed on observation of gait, symmetry and function of joints, bones, and muscles, and range of motion as it relates to activities of daily living.

Cognitive objectives

At the end of this unit the learner will demonstrate knowledge of assessment of the musculoskeletal system by the ability to do the following:
1. State the anatomy and function of a joint.
2. Describe assessment criteria for evaluating joint function.
3. Describe selected methods by which to evaluate a symptomatic joint, including the drawer test, the McMurray test, and the Thomas test.
4. List the normal range of motion position of the joints to be assessed during a screening examination.
5. Describe a systematic method by which to evaluate the skeletal system.
6. Describe a systematic method by which to evaluate muscle function during a screening evaluation using the make/break technique.
7. Describe the normal gait sequence and assessment criteria by which to evaluate gait functioning.
8. Identify selected characteristics of the pediatric musculoskeletal examination.
9. Identify selected characteristics of the geriatric musculoskeletal examination.

Clinical objectives

At the end of this unit the learner will perform a systematic assessment of the musculoskeletal system, demonstrating the ability to do the following:
1. Obtain a health history appropriate to the screening evaluation of the musculoskeletal system. This should include demonstration of knowledge of the client's ability to perform the activities of daily living as well as in-depth investigation of symptoms such as musculoskeletal pain analysis and skeletal, muscle, or joint problems.
2. Demonstrate inspection of the client's musculoskeletal system, including body build, bone structure and contour, symmetry, posture, gait, strength, and coordination.
3. Demonstrate inspection of the client's range of motion of all joints. Communicate an interpretation of findings as related to normal.
4. Demonstrate palpation of the client's musculoskeletal system, noting the following:
   a. Bone structure and contour
   b. Joint stability and characteristics and any deviations from normal
   c. Muscle mass, including hypertrophy or atrophy
5. Demonstrate screening techniques to evaluate muscle strength of the fingers, hands, wrists, triceps, biceps, deltoids, feet, ankles, hips, hamstrings, gluteals, abductors, adductors, quadriceps, and trunk muscle groups.
6. Demonstrate ability to perform special evaluation techniques for the knee, hip, and lower back, including:
   a. Knee-fluid evaluation
   b. Drawer test
   c. McMurray's test

d. Thomas' test

e. Back pain evaluation techniques

7. Summarize results of the assessment with a written description of findings.

Health history related to musculoskeletal assessment additional to data base

1. Review the client's employment situation both past and present. What are the working conditions and risks regarding lifting or accident proneness for the musculoskeletal system?

2. To what extent does client walk or exercise each day?

3. Are there recent weight changes that could have stressed the musculoskeletal system?

4. Inquire regarding client's ability to perform activities of daily living. (The following questions are arranged according to function. If the interviewer receives a response indicating difficulty, that area should be further evaluated during the physical assessment.)

  a. Eating

    (1) Opening containers

    (2) Cutting meat

    (3) Chewing and swallowing

    (4) Preparing food

    (5) Getting food to mouth

    (6) Measuring and taking medications

  b. Bathing

    (1) Running water and testing temperature

    (2) Undressing self

    (3) Getting into and out of tub or shower

  c. Dressing

    (1) Getting clothes

    (2) Putting on prosthesis

    (3) Putting on clothes

    (4) Using zippers

    (5) Buckling

    (6) Tying

    (7) Buttoning

    (8) Putting on shoes (shoelaces)

  d. Grooming

    (1) Washing hair

    (2) Brushing hair

    (3) Brushing teeth

    (4) Shaving

    (5) Grooming nails

    (6) Applying makeup

    (7) Washing clothes

  e. Elimination

    (1) Bowel routine

    (2) Bladder routine

  f. Activity (consider safety factor)

    (1) Walking

    (2) Getting into and out of chair

    (3) Getting into and out of bed

    (4) Transferring

    (5) Turning

  g. Communication

    (1) Speech

    (2) Telephone

5. Often clients complain of musculoskeletal problems. The following outline details the symptom analysis profile for the complaint of *pain*. This profile may be slightly adapted to collect information about any client with a musculoskeletal complaint. Following the detailed pain analysis profile are numerous other musculoskeletal complaints. Accompanying each of the items listed are important evaluative components. These components may be added to or may replace certain components of the pain analysis profile.

  a. Pain

    (1) When was the client last well?

      (a) When did *this type* of pain start occurring?

      (b) How long has client been bothered with musculoskeletal pain in general?

    (2) Date of current problem onset

    (3) Character of specific complaint

      (a) Pressure sensation

      (b) Stiffness

      (c) Numb, tingling sensation

      (d) Single area, multiple areas

      (e) Sharp vs. dull or shooting pain

      (f) If radiation of pain occurs, note to where (hips, buttocks or legs, unilateral vs. bilateral)

    (4) Nature of onset

      (a) Slow over several weeks, days, hours

      (b) Abrupt over several minutes

    (5) Client's hunch of precipitating factors

      (a) Recent injury

      (b) Recent strenuous activity, exercise, lifting

      (c) Sudden movement

      (d) Stress

    (6) Course of problem

      (a) Comes and goes

      (b) Becoming progressively worse or better

      (c) Relieved by medication, rest, exercise, etc.

    (7) Location of problem

      (a) Anatomical location

      (b) Unilateral vs. bilateral

    (8) Relation to other entities

    (a) Clumsiness
    (b) Weakness
    (c) Paralysis
    (d) Anesthesia (hypoesthesia, hyperesthesia)
    (e) Gastroenterological complaints (ulcer disease, pancreatitis, bowel problems, biliary colic)
    (f) Gynecological complaints (e.g., endometriosis)
    (g) Urological complaints (calculi, prostatic disease)
    (h) Chills
    (i) Fever
    (j) General malaise
    (k) Stiffness
  (9) Patterns
    (a) Worse with movement or better with activity
    (b) Worse following coughing or defecation
    (c) Worse in AM or PM (gets better or worse as day progresses)
    (d) Worse following exercise or specific movements
    (e) Worse with riding in car
    (f) Episodes of problem getting closer together and worse
    (g) Episodes of problem getting closer together but not worse
  (10) Efforts to treat
    (a) Exercise program
    (b) Weight reduction program
    (c) Rest
    (d) Medications
    (e) Physician evaluation
  (11) How does pain interfere with client's activities of daily living?
  b. Gait difficulty
    (1) Clumsiness
    (2) Weakness
    (3) Client unaware of position in space
    (4) Pain
    (5) Stiffness
    (6) Systemic difficulty such as dizziness or vision problem
  c. Voluntary muscle complaints
    (1) Muscle weakness or fatigue
    (2) Stiffness
    (3) Pain
    (4) Wasting (atrophy)
    (5) Paralysis
    (6) Tremor
    (7) Tic

    (8) Cogwheel movement
    (9) Spasms
    (10) Aching muscles
    (11) Muscle hypertrophy
  d. Skeletal complaints
    (1) Recent fractures
    (2) Abnormalities in skeletal contour
    (3) Absence of or change of movement in a part
    (4) Crepitus
    (5) Pain with movement
    (6) Ecchymosis or hematoma of injured part
  e. Joint complaints
    (1) Recent injury (explore the event in detail, including the direction the joint was stressed)
    (2) Change in contour or size of joint
    (3) Limitations of joint motion
    (4) Swelling or redness of skin around joint
    (5) Local pain or ache that increases with muscle contraction

6. Any client complaining of vague or generalized musculoskeletal complaints should be questioned in detail regarding history of both self and family, social history, personal psychological history; a detailed review of systems should be carried out.

7. Any client with a musculoskeletal complaint should be questioned regarding activities of daily living and occupational history. Both areas should include questions about the type of work or activity (present and past), working conditions, accident proneness, and safety precautions.

8. As well as evaluating clients with complaints or injuries, the practitioner must develop a profile to identify clients at risk and intervene with preventive education techniques. Although the following is not an inclusive list, it represents the type of risk profile data that should be collected regarding the musculoskeletal system.
  a. Client who only exercises, jogs, plays tennis, etc. sporadically or less than twice a week
  b. Athlete playing contact sports without a structured conditioning program
  c. Participation in athletics without proper supportive or protective equipment
  d. Occupation requiring lifting of awkward or heavy items
  e. Occupation requiring operation of press machines or equipment such as farm machinery that could catch clothing or limbs, causing crushing or mutilating injury
  f. Client overweight for height and body build
  g. Family history of arthritis or musculoskeletal diseases

h. Pregnancy
i. Clients with poor eyesight or unsafe environment (such as throw rugs or darkened stairway)
j. Client with systemic complaint such as dizziness, light-headedness, or difficulty determining body position in space
k. Any client unable to perform activities of daily living

Clinical guidelines

Prior to the assessment of the musculoskeletal system, the practitioner must study and memorize several things: (1) the anatomy of the skeletal system and the name of the bones to be assessed, (2) the anatomy and normal range and degree of motion of the joints to be assessed, and (3) the major muscle groups to be evaluated and the anticipated normal response to each group. It is assumed that the student is knowledgeable in these areas.

Because of the vast complexity of the assessment of the musculoskeletal system, an integrated body-region approach will be used. During examination of each region, the bones, joints, and muscles will be evaluated. This should save the examiner time as well as provide a more integrated assessment of each region.

The student will:	To identify:	
	Normal	Deviations from normal
1. Have goniometer at hand (if ranges of motion are to be measured) (*Note:* For musculoskeletal assessment, client should be undressed to underpants alone or underpants and bra and a gown.)		
2. Observe client walking into room (Fig. 14-1)	Gait smooth, coordinated, rhythmic Walks with ease, arms extended to sides, standing erect; gaze straight forward	Walks with difficulty or with assistance Fasciculations, tremor

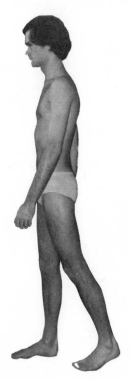

Fig. 14-1. Inspect client's gait.

Continued.

Clinical guidelines–cont'd

The student will:	To identify:	
	Normal	Deviations from normal
3. Measure client's height and weight	(See Tables 11 and 12.)	

Table 11. Desirable weights for men 25 years of age and over*†

Height with shoes on (1-inch heels)		Small frame	Medium frame	Large frame
Feet	Inches			
5	2	112-120	118-129	126-141
5	3	115-123	121-133	129-144
5	4	118-126	124-136	132-148
5	5	121-129	127-139	135-152
5	6	124-133	130-143	138-156
5	7	128-137	134-147	142-161
5	8	132-141	138-152	147-166
5	9	136-145	142-156	151-170
5	10	140-150	146-160	155-174
5	11	144-154	150-165	159-179
6	0	148-158	154-170	164-184
6	1	152-162	158-175	168-189
6	2	156-167	162-180	173-194
6	3	160-171	167-185	178-199
6	4	164-175	172-190	182-204

*Courtesy Metropolitan Life Insurance Co.: How to control your weight, New York, 1960 supplement. Based on 1959 Build and blood pressure study.
†Weight in pounds, according to frame (in indoor clothing).

Table 12. Desirable weights for women 25 years of age and over*†

Height with shoes on (2-inch heels)		Small frame	Medium frame	Large frame
Feet	Inches			
4	10	92-98	96-107	104-119
4	11	94-101	98-110	106-122
5	0	96-104	101-113	109-125
5	1	99-107	104-116	112-128
5	2	102-110	107-119	115-131
5	3	105-113	110-122	118-134
5	4	108-116	113-126	121-138
5	5	111-119	116-130	125-142
5	6	114-123	120-135	129-146
5	7	118-127	124-139	133-150
5	8	122-131	128-143	137-154
5	9	126-135	132-147	141-158
5	10	130-140	136-151	145-163
5	11	134-144	140-155	149-168
6	0	138-148	144-159	153-173

*Courtesy Metropolitan Life Insurance Co.: How to control you weight, New York, 1960 supplement. Based on 1959 Build and blood pressure study.
†Weight in pounds, according to frame (in indoor clothing).

The student will:	To identify:	
	Normal	Deviations from normal

Trunk

The student will:	Normal	Deviations from normal

1. Observe client standing erect (front, back, and side) (Fig. 14-2)	Stands erect
	Symmetry of body parts
	Straight spine
	Normal spine curvature:
	    cervical spine concave;
	    thoracic spine convex;
	    lumbar spine concave
	Knees in direct straight line between hips and ankles
	Feet flat on floor pointing directly forward
		Asymmetry
		Unable to maintain straight posture
		Lateral spine curvature
		Asymmetry in height of shoulders or iliac crest
		Lordosis or kyphosis, varus or valgus deformity
		Medial or lateral rotation of feet

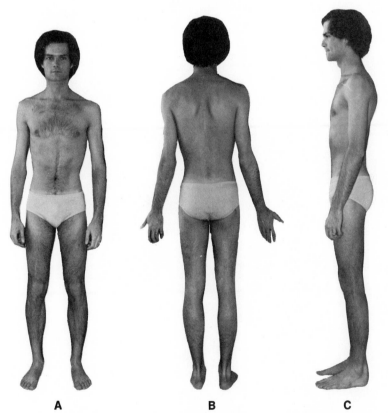

Fig. 14-2. A, Anterior inspection. **B,** Posterior inspection. **C,** Lateral inspection.

Continued.

Clinical guidelines–cont'd

	To identify:	
The student will:	**Normal**	**Deviations from normal**
2. With client standing observe spine from posterior as client bends from waist to touch toes; note range of motion and symmetry (Fig. 14-3)	Straight spine Iliac crests to equal height Shoulders of equal height Convexity of thoracic spine	Lateral deviation of spine Asymmetry of shoulder height ("razor back" deformity) (Fig. 14-4)

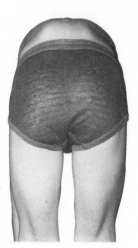

Fig. 14-3. Inspect shoulder and hip symmetry and spine straightness during forward bending.

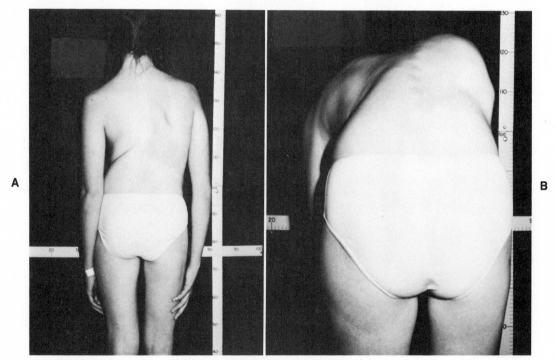

Fig. 14-4. A, Asymmetry of shoulder height. **B,** Same patient, bending forward. (From Prior, J. A., and Silberstein, J. S.: Physical diagnosis: the history and examination of the patient, ed. 5, St. Louis, 1977, The C. V. Mosby Co.)

The student will:	To identify:	
	Normal	Deviations from normal
3. Observe client hyperextending spine (Fig. 14-5)	30° hyperextension from neutral position	Unable to hyperextend without losing balance, or pain with hyperextension

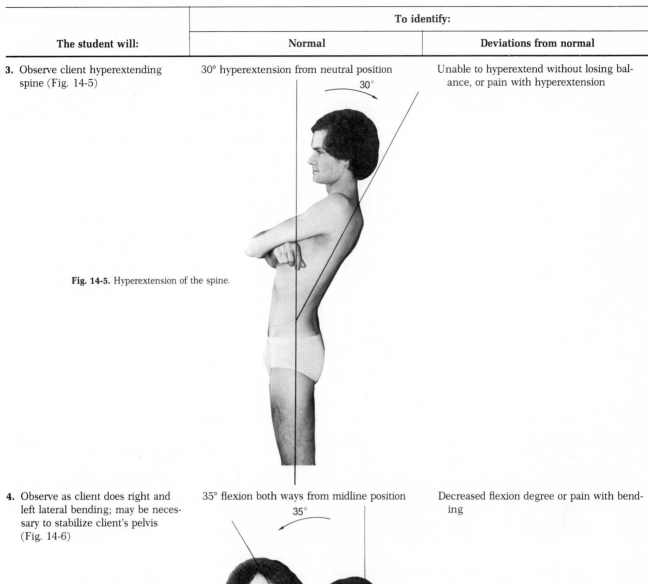

Fig. 14-5. Hyperextension of the spine.

The student will:	Normal	Deviations from normal
4. Observe as client does right and left lateral bending; may be necessary to stabilize client's pelvis (Fig. 14-6)	35° flexion both ways from midline position	Decreased flexion degree or pain with bending

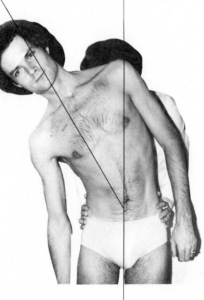

Fig. 14-6. Lateral bending of the spine.

Continued.

Clinical guidelines–cont'd

The student will:	To identify:	
	Normal	Deviations from normal
5. Observe as client rotates upper trunk (stabilize pelvis) to right and left (Fig. 14-7)	30° rotation in both directions from direct forward position	Decreased rotation capability Rotation with discomfort

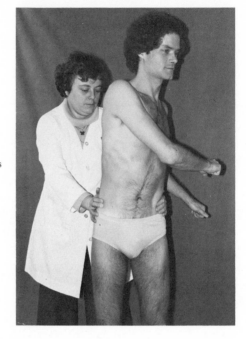

Fig. 14-7. Functional testing of trunk rotation; examiner stabilizes client's hips.

6. Palpate along spinal processes and paravertebral muscles; may be helpful to have client hunch shoulders forward and slightly flex (Fig. 14-8)	Straight spine Nontender	Curvature of spine Tenderness Spasm of paravertebral muscles

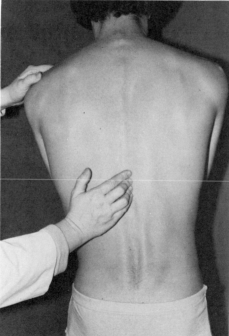

Fig. 14-8. Palpation of vertebral column.

The student will:	To identify:	
	Normal	**Deviations from normal**

Gait

1. Have client walk across room and back; observe for rhythm and smoothness
   a. Gait phase — Conformity; ability to follow gait sequencing of both stance and swing — Pain or discomfort with gait
   b. Cadence — Symmetry of gait / Regular smooth rhythm — Unsteady / Jerky
   c. Stride length — Symmetry in length of leg swing — Asymmetry or irregularity
   d. Trunk posture — Smooth swaying related to gait phase — Irregular or jerky
   e. Arm swing — Smooth, symmetrical — Jerky, asymmetrical, or unrelated to gait

Head and neck

1. With client sitting on examination table, observe musculature of face and neck — Symmetrical appearance — Asymmetry / Atrophy or hypertrophy of muscles
2. Palpate each temporomandibular joint just anterior to tragus of ear while client opens and closes mouth (Fig. 14-9) — Smooth movement of mandible — Pain, limited range of motion, or crepitus of temporomandibular joint

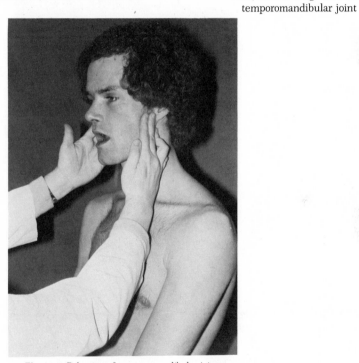

Fig. 14-9. Palpation of temporomandibular joint.

3. Inspect and palpate posterior neck, cervical spine, paravertebral, and trapezius muscles — Locate landmarks C_7 and T_1 / Nontender cervical spine — Tenderness / Nodules / Muscular spasm
4. Evaluate range of motion of neck by asking client to:
   a. Flex chin to chest — 45° from midline — Limited or painful range of motion
   b. Extend head — 55° from midline — Crepitus of cervical spine
   c. Laterally bend neck to right and left — 40° each way from midline
   d. Rotate chin to shoulders right and left — 70° from midline

Continued.

Clinical guidelines–cont'd

The student will:	To identify:	
	Normal	Deviations from normal
5. Evaluate neck muscle strength		
a. Have client flex chin to chest; instruct client to maintain position while examiner tries to manually force head upright (Fig. 14-10)	With reasonable strength, unable to force head upright	Able to break muscular flexion before anticipated point

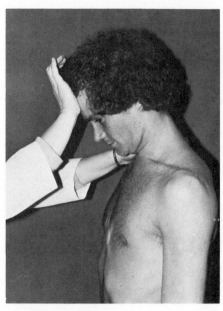

Fig. 14-10. Maintaining flexion of neck against resistance.

b. Have client hyperextend head; instruct client to maintain position while examiner tries to manually force head upright (Fig. 14-11)	With reasonable strength, unable to force head upright	Able to break muscular flexion before anticipated point

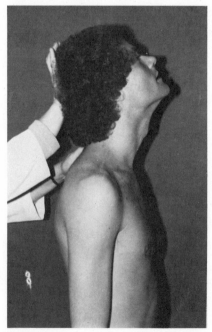

Fig. 14-11. Maintaining hyperextension of neck against resistance.

The student will:	To identify:	
	Normal	**Deviations from normal**

Hands and wrists

1. Observe and palpate hands and wrists, including joints

Smoothness; no swelling or deformities noted
Fingers able to maintain full extension

Irregular finger contour
Swelling
Deformities
Tenderness
Muscular atrophy
Heberden's nodes

2. Observe muscular function and range of motion of fingers and hands; instruct client to:
  a. Extend and spread fingers of both hands (Fig. 14-12, *A*)

Symmetrical response
Smooth movement without complaints of discomfort
Full flexion and extension

Asymmetrical response
Pain on movement

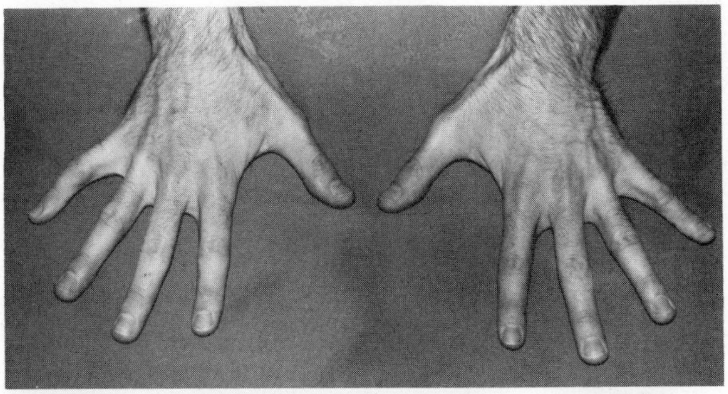

Fig. 14-12. Functional assessment of hands. **A,** Fingers extended and spread.

A

  b. Make fist with thumb across fingers (Fig. 14-12, *B*)

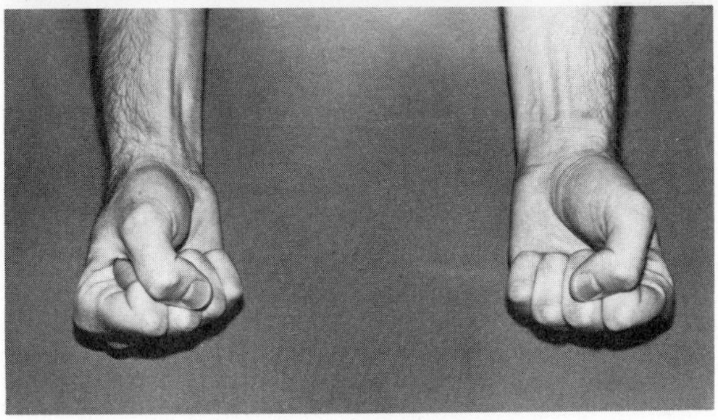

Fig. 14-12, cont'd. B, Fist formation.   **B**

  c. Grip examiner's first two fingers (Fig. 14-12, *C*)

Bilaterally equal response
Tight grip

Unequal response
Decreased response

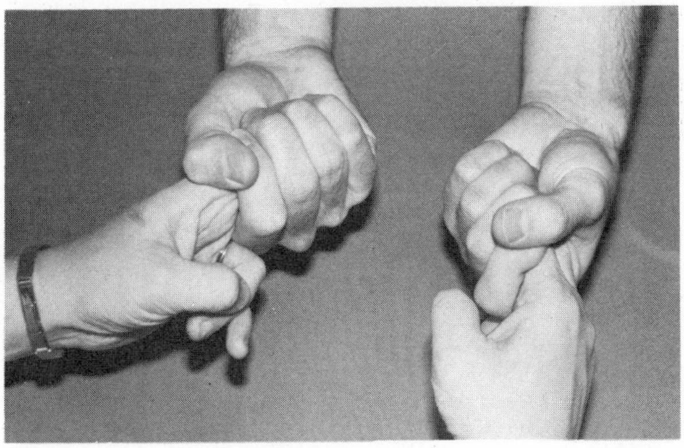

Fig. 14-12, cont'd. C, Hand grip.   **C**

Continued.

Clinical guidelines–cont'd

The student will:	To identify:	
	Normal	Deviations from normal
3. Observe range of motion of wrist (Fig. 14-13)		
a. Radial deviation (*A*)	20° movement from central position	Pain with movement Decreased movement
b. Ulnar deviation (*B*)	55° movement from central position	
c. Extension (*C*)	70° movement from central position	
d. Flexion (*D*)	90° movement from central position	

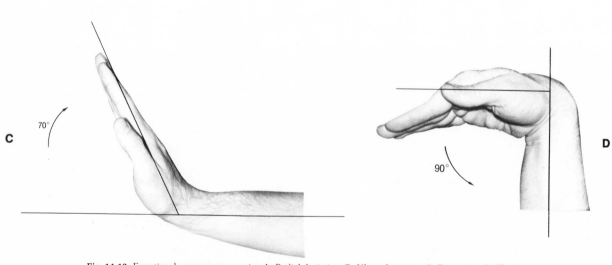

Fig. 14-13. Functional assessment of wrist. **A,** Radial deviation. **B,** Ulnar deviation. **C,** Extension. **D,** Flexion.

The student will:	To identify:	
	Normal	Deviations from normal
4. Evaluate wrist strength; instruct client to maintain position against examiner's force		
a. Client flexes wrists; examiner attempts to straighten	Bilaterally strong Unable to break position	Asymmetrical response Able to easily break position
b. Client extends wrists; examiner attempts to straighten (Fig. 14-14)	Bilaterally strong Unable to break position	Asymmetrical response Able to easily break position

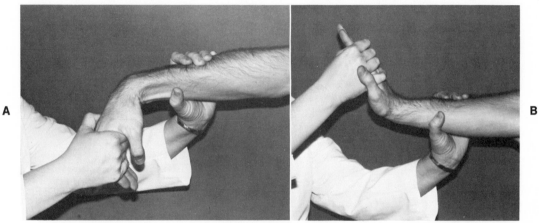

Fig. 14-14. A, Maintaining flexed position of wrist against resistance. **B,** Maintaining hyperextended position of wrist against resistance.

Elbows

The student will:	Normal	Deviations from normal
1. Flex client's arm and support; inspect and palpate elbow, including:		
a. Extensor surface of ulna	Skin intact	Swelling
b. Olecranon process	Smooth	Inflammation
c. Groove on either side of olecranon	Surface nontender without nodules or discomfort	General tenderness Subcutaneous nodules Point tenderness
d. Lateral epicondyle		
e. Epitrochlear nodes (palpate lateral groove between biceps and triceps muscle)	Lymph nodes not palpable	Lymph nodes palpated

Continued.

Clinical guidelines–cont'd

| | To identify: | |
The student will:	Normal	Deviations from normal
2. Evaluate range of motion **a.** Ask client to bend and extend elbow (Fig. 14-15)	160° full movement Bilaterally equal No discomfort	Limited range of motion Asymmetrical movement Pain at elbow

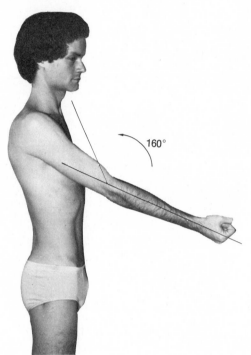

160°

Fig. 14-15. Functional assessment of elbow extension.

b. Bend client's forearm to 90° angle from shoulder; have client pronate and supinate forearm (Fig. 14-16)	90° each direction Bilaterally equal No discomfort	Limited range of motion Asymmetrical movement Pain at elbow

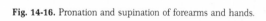

Fig. 14-16. Pronation and supination of forearms and hands.

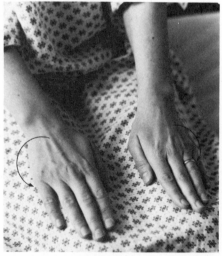

The student will:	To identify:	
	Normal	Deviations from normal

Shoulders

1. Inspect shoulders, including shoulder girdle and acromioclavicular junction
2. Palpate shoulders, including sternoclavicular joint, acromioclavicular joint, shoulder in general, humerus, and biceps groove
3. Evaluate range of motion of shoulders
   a. Extends arms straight up beside head (Fig. 14-17, A)

   b. Client hyperextends arm backward (Fig. 14-17, B)

	Normal	Deviations from normal
1.	Intact Smooth and regular Bilaterally symmetrical	Redness Swelling Nodules
2.	Nontender Smooth and regular Bilaterally symmetrical	Tender, painful Swelling
3a.	180° from resting neutral position Bilaterally equal No discomfort	Limited range of motion Pain with movement Crepitations with movement Asymmetry
3b.	50° Bilaterally equal No discomfort	Limited range of motion Pain with movement Crepitations with movement Asymmetry

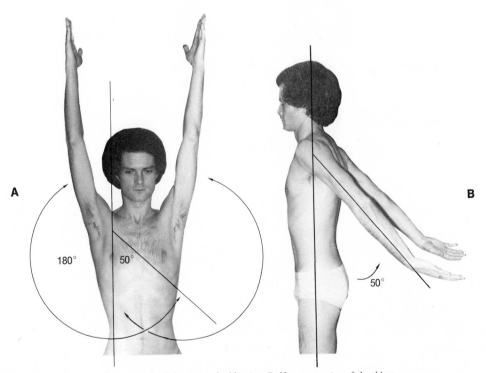

Fig. 14-17. A, Abduction and adduction. **B,** Hyperextension of shoulders.

Continued.

Clinical guidelines–cont'd

The student will:	To identify:	
	Normal	**Deviations from normal**
c. External rotation: client places hands behind head, elbows out (Fig. 14-17, *C*)	90° Bilaterally equal No discomfort	Limited range of motion Pain with movement Crepitations with movement Asymmetry
d. Internal rotation: client places hands behind small of back (Fig. 14-17, *D*)	90° Bilaterally equal No discomfort	Limited range of motion Pain with movement Crepitations with movement Asymmetry

90°

C

90°

D

Fig. 14-17, cont'd. C, External rotation. **D,** Internal rotation.

Arm muscles

(using make/break technique)

1. Deltoids: client holds arms up while examiner attempts to push them down (Fig. 14-18)	Bilaterally strong Unable to break position	Symmetrically unequal Weak response Pain during technique Muscular spasm

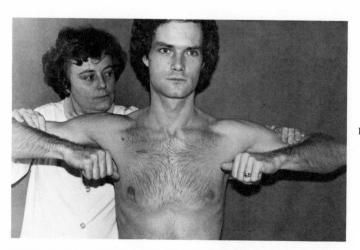

Fig. 14-18. Testing deltoid strength against resistance.

The student will:	To identify:	
	Normal	Deviations from normal
2. Biceps: client tries to flex arm into fighting position while examiner tries to extend forearm (Fig. 14-19)	Bilaterally strong Unable to break position	Symmetrically unequal Weak response Pain during technique Muscular spasm

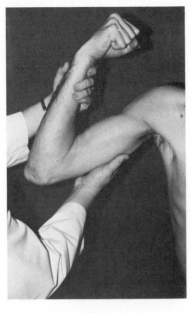

Fig. 14-19. Testing bicep strength against resistance.

3. Triceps: client tries to straighten forearm while examiner attempts to flex forearm (Fig. 14-20)	Bilaterally strong Unable to break position	Symmetrically unequal Weak response Pain during technique Muscular spasm

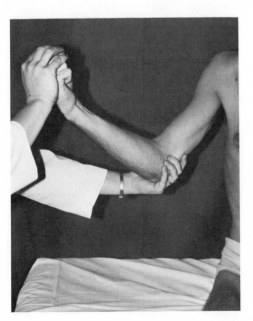

Fig. 14-20. Maintaining extended position of forearm against resistance.

Continued.

Clinical guidelines–cont'd

The student will:	To identify:	
	Normal	**Deviations from normal**

Feet and ankles

1. Inspect feet and ankles with client lying down

   Smoothness; no swelling or deformities noted
   Toes maintain extended and straight position
   Toenails intact and neatly trimmed
   Feet maintain straight position

   Inflammation
   Swelling over any joints
   Hallux valgus (Fig. 14-21, *A*)
   Medial deviation of toes
   Clawtoes (Fig. 14-21, *B*)
   Hammertoes
   Calluses

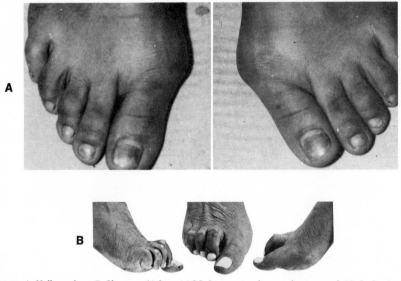

Fig. 14-21. A, Hallux valgus. **B,** Clawtoes. (**A** from AAOS: Instructional course lectures, vol. 22, St. Louis, 1973, The C. V. Mosby Co.; **B** from Mann, R. A.: DuVries' surgery of the foot, ed. 4, St. Louis, 1978, The C. V. Mosby Co.)

2. Palpate feet and ankles

   Smooth
   Nontender

   Tenderness
     (diffuse vs. pinpoint)
   Swelling
   Inflammation
   Ulcerations
   Nodules

The student will:	To identify:	
	Normal	**Deviations from normal**
3. Evaluate range of motion of feet and ankles		
a. Client dorsiflexes and plantar flexes foot (Fig. 14-22)	Dorsiflexion 20° from midline position Plantar flexion 45° from midline position Bilaterally equal No discomfort	Limited range of motion Pain with movement Crepitations Asymmetry
b. Inversion and eversion of foot (stabilize heel) (Fig. 14-23)	Inversion 30° from midline position Eversion 20° from midline position Bilaterally equal No discomfort	Limited range of motion Pain with movement Crepitations Asymmetry

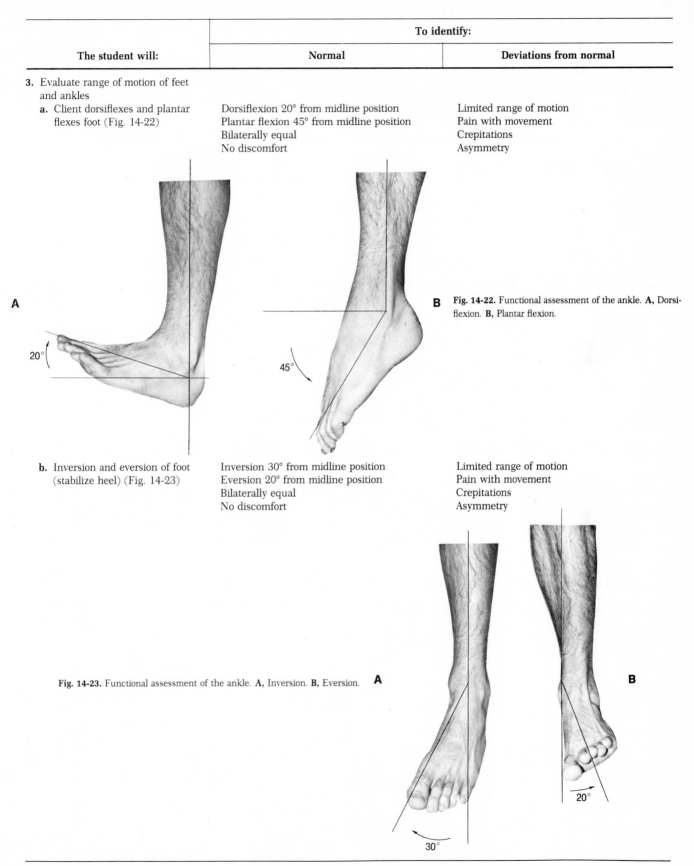

Fig. 14-22. Functional assessment of the ankle. **A,** Dorsiflexion. **B,** Plantar flexion.

Fig. 14-23. Functional assessment of the ankle. **A,** Inversion. **B,** Eversion.

Continued.

Clinical guidelines–cont'd

The student will:	To identify:	
	Normal	Deviations from normal
c. Flexion and extension of toes	Active movement without discomfort	Painful movement
4. Evaluate muscles of foot and ankle by make/break technique		
a. Client is instructed to flex foot upward and maintain position; examiner presses down on big toe (Fig. 14-24)	Bilaterally strong Unable to break position	Unequal Weak response Pain during technique

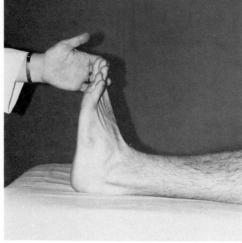

Fig. 14-24. Dorsiflexion of foot against resistance.

Knee

1. Inspect knees; note alignment and characteristics	Symmetrical Smooth Hollowness present adjacent to and above patella	Swelling Thickness Bogginess Inflammation
2. Palpate knees on:		
a. Each side of patella and over tibiofemoral joint space	Smooth, nontender	Bogginess Thickening Tenderness Painful
b. Popliteal space	Smooth, nontender	Tenderness, redness Nodules and swelling
3. Evaluate range of motion of knees by asking client to flex knees (Fig. 14-25) (May postpone until hip range of motion is evaluted.)	130° from straight extended position No discomfort or difficulty	Decreased range of motion Pain with movement Crepitations

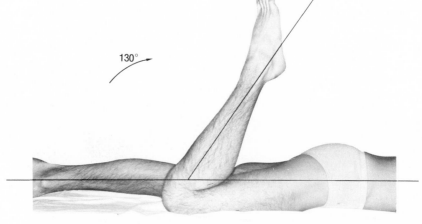

Fig. 14-25. Evaluating knee flexion.

130°

The student will:	To identify:	
	Normal	**Deviations from normal**

Hips and pelvis

1. With patient lying down, inspect and palpate hips for position and stability (Fig. 14-26)

Bilaterally symmetrical
Stable and painless with palpation

Painful hip area (diffuse vs. pinpoint tenderness)
Crepitations

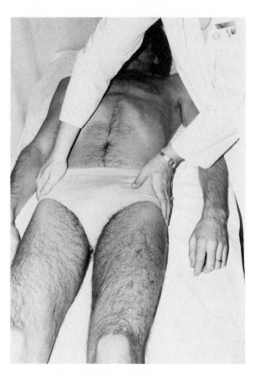

Fig. 14-26. Evaluating pelvic stability.

2. Evaluate range of motion of hip
  a. Instruct client to alternately pull each knee up to chest (Fig. 14-27)

120° from straight extended position

Limited range of motion
Pain or discomfort with movement
Flexion of opposite thigh
Crepitations

Fig. 14-27. Evaluating hip flexion.

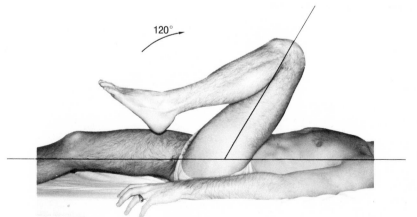

Continued.

Clinical guidelines–cont'd

The student will:	To identify:	
	Normal	Deviations from normal
b. Instruct client to flex hip as far as possible without bending knee (Fig. 14-28)	90° from straight extended position	Limited range of motion Pain or discomfort with movement Crepitations

90°

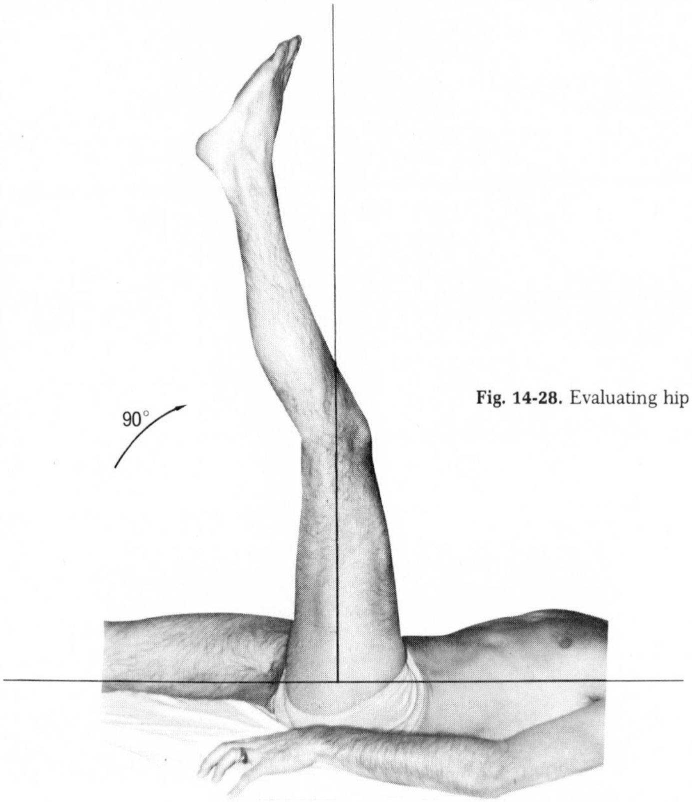

Fig. 14-28. Evaluating hip flexion with leg extended.

c. Instruct client to place foot on opposite patella; press knee down laterally (external hip rotation) (Patrick's test) (Fig. 14-29)	40° from straight midline position	Limited range of motion Pain or discomfort with movement Crepitations

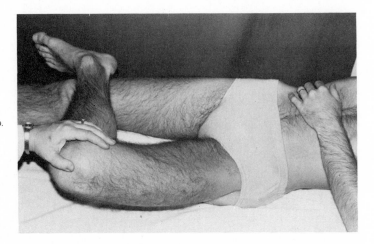

Fig. 14-29. Evaluating external rotation of hip.

	To identify:	
The student will:	**Normal**	**Deviations from normal**
d. Instruct client to flex knee and turn medially; examiner pulls heel laterally (internal hip rotation) (Fig. 14-30)	40° from straight midline position	Limited range of motion Pain or discomfort with movement Crepitations

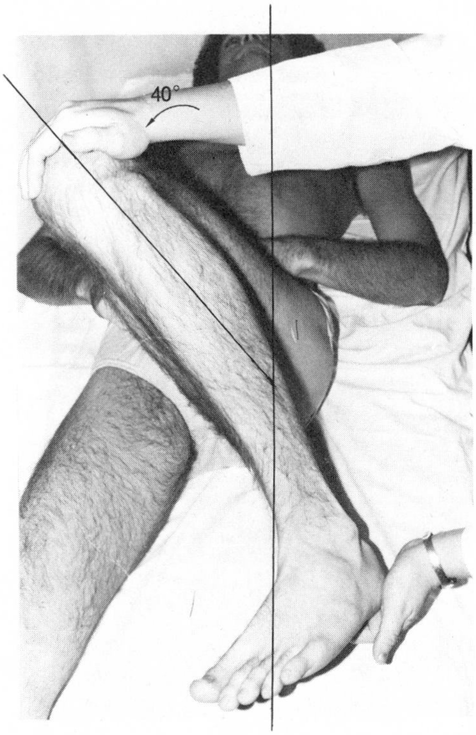

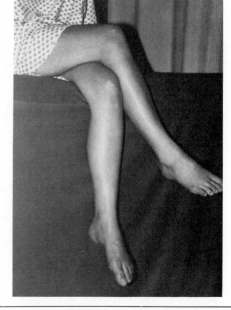

Fig. 14-30. Internal hip rotation.

Leg, hip, and pelvis muscles

(using make/break technique)

1. Hip strength: client in supine position attempts to raise legs while examiner tries to hold them down; evaluate one leg at a time	Bilaterally strong Unable to break position	Symmetrically unequal Weak response Pain during technique
2. Hamstrings, gluteals, abductors, and adductors: instruct client to sit and alternately cross legs (Fig. 14-31)	Able to perform Bilaterally equal and without difficulty	Unable to perform Performs with pain or great difficulty

Fig. 14-31. Assessment of adductors and hamstring.

Continued.

Clinical guidelines–cont'd

The student will:	To identify:	
	Normal	Deviations from normal
3. Quadriceps: client extends leg at knee; examiner attempts to flex knee (Fig. 14-32)	Bilaterally strong Unable to flex knee	Symmetrically unequal Weak response Pain during technique

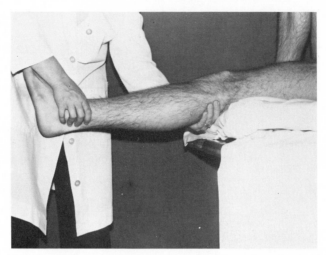

Fig. 14-32. Maintaining extended position of anterior thigh muscles against resistance.

4. Hamstrings: client tries to bend knee while examiner attempts to straighten knee (Fig. 14-33)	Bilaterally strong Unable to flex knee	Symmetrically unequal Weak response Pain during technique

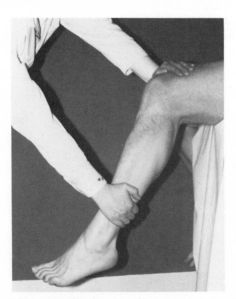

Fig. 14-33. Maintaining flexed position of hamstring against resistance.

The student will:	To identify:	
	Normal	**Deviations from normal**

Special techniques

1. Knee evaluation

   a. Fluid within knee joint

     1. Palpate the patella against the femur with the leg in full extension; tap on one side of joint

   b. Drawer test to evaluate intactness of the cruciate ligaments: client sitting with knees flexed to 90°

     1. Pull and push tibia, trying to displace its position from under the femur (Fig. 14-34)

	Normal	Deviations from normal
Palpate patella	No fluid waves or bulging on opposite side of joint	Fluid waves palpable on opposite side of joint
Drawer test	Unable to displace its position	Tibia can be pulled anteriorly from under femur (indicates injury to anterior cruciate ligament) Tibia can be pushed posteriorly from under femur (indicates injury to posterior cruciate ligament)

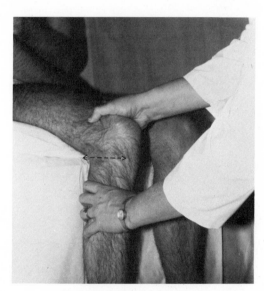

Fig. **14-34.** Performing drawer test.

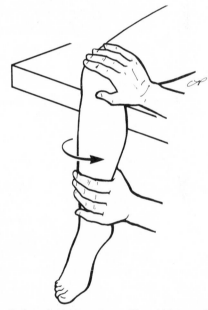

Fig. **14-35.** Performing McMurray's test. (From Malasanos, L., Barkauskas, V., Moss, M., and Stoltenberg-Allen, K.: Health assessment, St. Louis, 1977, The C. V. Mosby Co.)

   c. McMurray's test to evaluate presence of foreign body within knee or torn meniscus: client sitting, knee flexed

     1. Stabilize one hand on client's knee and with other hand grasp ankle and rotate lower leg internally and externally while gradually extending leg (Fig. 14-35)

	Normal	Deviations from normal
McMurray's test	Stable knee No discomfort	Positive findings: pain, clicking feeling, or inability to extend lower leg

Continued.

Clinical guidelines–cont'd

The student will:	To identify:	
	Normal	Deviations from normal

2. Hip evaluation
   a. Thomas' test to evaluate for flexion contractures of the hip: client supine
     1. Instruct client to pull one knee up toward chest as far as possible
	Easy flexion
	Opposite leg remains flat on table (Fig. 14-36, A)
		Opposite leg and hip flex in response to flexing leg
		Note degree of flexion (Fig. 14-36, B)

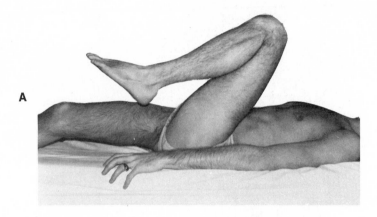

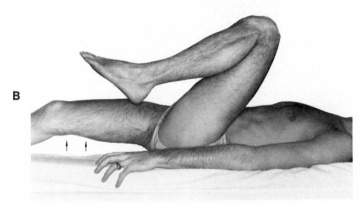

Fig. 14-36. Thomas test. **A,** Negative. **B,** Positive.

3. Low back pain evaluation
   a. Four specific areas of assessment
     1. Observe curvature of lumbar region
	Lumbar lordosis: concavity of lumbar region	Reversal or flattening of lumbar curvature

2. Observe trunk positioning	Upright trunk position	Slightly flexed back Slight lateral bending of trunk
3. Palpate erector spinae muscles	Muscle not in spasm Nontender muscles	Muscle spasms of erector spinae group Tender
4. Evaluate range of motion of lumbar spine	(See normal values for movement.)	Limited, difficult, or painful range of motion

The student will:	To identify:	
	Normal	**Deviations from normal**
b. Lasègue's sign, or sciatic stretch test to evaluate low back pain arising from nerve root irritation: client supine		
1. Perform single and alternating straight leg raising	Tightness may be felt, but should be no pain	Pain felt with elevation of leg; then flex knee: pain should be gone as leg further raised
c. Evaluation of lumbar disc injury		
1. Observe client supine and perform alternating straight leg raising	Tightness may be felt, but should be no pain	Pain felt with elevation of leg Dorsiflexion of foot causes feeling of pressure in lumbosacral area

Clinical strategies

1. Assessment of the musculoskeletal system should begin as the client enters the examination room. Use that time to observe ambulatory capabilities and body posturing.
2. Assessment of the musculoskeletal system involves an individual evaluation of bone stability, joint function, and muscle strength and function. The clinical guidelines describe in detail what the examiner must do, as well as the anticipated response. It is essential that the examiner *continuously* keep in mind *what* bones, muscles, or joints are being evaluated as well as the *normal* anticipated response.
3. Many clients complain of vague aches or muscular weakness. The examiner must thoroughly explore the complaint as well as perform a systematic evaluation. In addition, the examiner should watch how the client moves, postures, rises from a sitting position, takes off a coat, and so on.
4. A key consideration when evaluating the musculoskeletal system is symmetry.
5. The client must be undressed. This means shoes and socks, too.
6. It does not matter whether the examination sequence is from the top down or vice versa, but a method of client assessment must be developed and maintained every time a client is evaluated.
7. How much musculoskeletal assessment each client requires will be individually determined. A young athlete who comes to see the examiner for a college physical will require a basic screening evaluation, whereas a 67-year-old chronically ill woman will require a more thorough assessment. Many times the data collection and early inspection of the client's ability to ambulate, sit, and undress are the keys for determining the necessary extent of the assessment.
8. It should be remembered that the practitioner's purpose in collecting data about the musculoskeletal system is to assess the client's functional capabilities, including activities of daily living. If the examiner isolates areas of distress or injury, the client should be referred to the physician for differential diagnosis.
9. While performing extremity evaluation, the examiner should incorporate the assessment of the skin, peripheral vascular system, and neurological system.
10. If the examiner notes a difference in muscle size or arm or leg diameter or length, a measurement should be recorded. A circumference or length difference of more than 1 cm should be considered abnormal. The examiner *must* be careful to measure from the same spot bilaterally.
11. The technique for measuring the range of motion of a joint follows:
    a. Start with joint in fully extended position.
    b. When the joint is flexed as much as possible, the angle is measured. This is recorded as the angle of greatest flexion (AGF).
12. Although normal flexion angles of joints have been identified in this text, the examiner should realize that there are many deviations from these angles which are considered normal for various individuals of different ages. It is most important that the examiner compare one side of the client's body to the other when measuring angles and considering abnormal findings.
13. When measuring the client's muscle strength, there are many techniques to use, from actual number scoring to evaluation of minimal or severe weakness. We have used the make/break screening technique to grossly evaluate the client's ability to make and maintain a flexed muscle position while the examiner attempts to break the flex.

Although the results will be subjectively interpreted, the examiner will, with practice, determine what an abnormal response is for his or her own strength.

An absolute baseline of muscle testing involves the client's ability to move the limbs or trunk against gravity (e.g., lift the arm up in the air). Any client having difficulty moving the trunk or limbs against gravity should be referred for further evaluation.

Sample recording

Muscular development and skeletal structure bilaterally equal, normal for age. No joint deformities, tenderness, or crepitations. Full active range of motion without pain. Normal spinal curve without deformity. No CVA or spinal tenderness on palpation. Adequate muscle tone and strength bilaterally.

History and clinical strategies associated with the pediatric client

1. Assessment of the child's musculoskeletal system can range from a basic functional screening examination to an extensive joint by joint evaluation. The extent of the actual evaluation should be determined for each individual child, based on subjective data as well as gross objective assessment. An active and coordinated toddler who demonstrates basic gross and fine motor functioning appropriate for age will require a less extensive musculoskeletal assessment than a 7-year-old complaining of joint pains and generalized weakness.

2. To subjectively evaluate motor functioning appropriate for age, the examiner must be aware of normal values. Table 13 details the sequencing of motor development and approximate age of achievement. The practitioner should consider this

Table 13. Normal age and sequence of motor development in children*

Age	Fine motor	Gross motor
4 weeks (1 month)	Follows with eyes to midline	Turns head to side Keeps knees tucked under abdomen When pulled to sitting position, has gross head lag and rounded swayed back
8 weeks (2 months)	Follows objects well; may not follow past midline (major developmental milestone)	Holds head in same plane as rest of body Can raise head and maintain position; looks downward
12 weeks (3 months)	Follows past midline When in supine position puts hands together; will hold hands in front of face	Raises head to 45° angle Maintains posture; looks around with head May turn from prone to side position When pulled into sitting position, shows only slight head lag
16 weeks (4 months)	Grasps rattle Plays with hands together	Actively lifts head up and looks around Will roll from prone to supine position When pulled to sitting position, no longer has head lag When held in standing position, attempts to maintain some weight support
20 weeks (5 months)	Can reach and pick up object May play with toes	Able to push up from prone position and maintain weight on forearms Rolls from prone to supine and back to prone Maintains straight back when in sitting position
24 weeks (6 months)	Will hold spoon or rattle Will drop object and reach for second offered object	Begins to raise abdomen off table Sits, but posture still shaky May sit with legs apart and hands (arms straight) as prop between legs Supports almost full weight when pulled to standing position
28 weeks (7 months)	Can transfer object, one hand to another Grasps objects in each hand	Sits alone; still uses hands for support When held in standing position, bounces Pulls feet to mouth
32 weeks (8 months)	Beginning thumb-finger grasping	Sits securely without support (major developmental milestone)
36 weeks (9 months)	Continued development of finger-thumb grasp	Steady sitting; can lean forward and still maintain position

*Data from Frankenburg, W. K., and Dodds, J. B.: Denver Developmental Screening Test, Denver, 1969, University of Colorado Medical Center.

Age	Fine motor	Gross motor
	May bang objects together	Begins creeping (abdomen off floor)
		Can stand holding onto stabilizing object when placed in that position; still may not be able to pull self into standing position
40 weeks (10 months)	Practices picking up small objects	Can pull self into standing position; unable to let self down again
	Points with one finger	
	Will offer toys to people but unable to let go of object	
44 weeks (11 months)		Moves about room holding onto objects
		Preparing to walk independently, wide-base stance
		Stands securely, holding on with one hand
48 weeks (12 months)	May hold cup and spoon and feed self fairly well with practice	Able to twist and turn and maintain posture
		Able to sit from standing position
	Can offer toys and release them	May stand alone at least momentarily
15 months	Can put raisins into bottle	Walks alone well
	Will take off shoes and pull toys	Able to seat self in chair
18 months	Holds crayon	May walk up and down stairs holding a hand
	Scribbles spontaneously (major developmental milestone)	May show running ability
2 years	Able to turn doorknob	May walk up stairs by self, two feet on each step
	Able to take off shoes and socks	
	Able to build two-block tower	Able to walk backward
	Dumps raisin from bottle following demonstration	Able to kick ball
2½ years	Able to build four-block tower	Able to jump from object
	Scribbling techniques continue	Walking becomes more stable; wide-base gait decreases
	Feeding self with increased neatness	
	Dumps raisins from bottle spontaneously	Throws ball overhanded
3 years	Can unbutton front buttons	Walks upstairs, alternating feet on steps
	Copies vertical line within 30°	Walks downstairs, two feet on each step
	Copies "○"	Pedals tricycle
	Able to build eight-cube tower	Jumps in place
		Able to perform broad jump
4 years	Able to copy " + "	Walks downstairs, alternating feet on steps
	Picks longer line three out of three times	Able to button large front buttons
		Able to balance on one foot for approximately 5 seconds
5 years	Able to dress self with minimal assistance	Hops on one foot
	Able to draw three-part human figure	Catches ball bounced to child two out of three times
	Draws □ following demonstration	
	Colors within lines	Able to demonstrate heel-toe walking
6 years	Copies □	Jumps, tumbles, skips, hops
	Draws six-part human figure	Able to walk straight line
	Printing skills increase	Able to skip rope with practice
		Able to ride two-wheel bicycle
		Able to demonstrate heel-toe backward walking
7 years	Able to read small print	Able to play hopscotch and to skip well
	Able to print well	Running, climbing abilities becoming more coordinated
	Able to write in script with practice	
8 years	Handwriting skills show maturity	Movements become more graceful
9 years	Writing skills continue to show maturity and less awkwardness	Development of hand-eye coordination; assists with playing baseball, basketball, soccer
10 years		Girls taller than boys
		Continued sports and coordinated activities
11 years		Physically more active
		May appear awkward because of preadolescent growth spurt
		May do less well in sports
12 years		Growth spurt begins
		Coordination decreases
13 years		Continues to have coordination difficulty
		Poor posture may become problem

sequence when collecting data base information. Any child who lags behind in two or more areas at any given age should be carefully evaluated. Although it is unrealistic to believe that all children develop at the normal rate, nonmastery of these criteria should serve as red flags indicating necessity of a thorough physical evaluation. Conversely, an active, playful, and maturing child that is on or ahead of schedule will need a less detailed evaluation. Some of the values in Table 3 have been extracted from the Denver Developmental Screening Test (DDST).

Children who appear to be lagging behind in musculoskeletal development may be screened more closely through tests such as the DDST.

3. The approach used to examine the musculoskeletal system in the child will vary greatly, depending on the child's age.

   a. Up to 6 months (Fig 14-37). Assessment should occur with the child undressed to the diaper and supine on the examining table or the parent's lap. Although the examiner should observe the symmetry and overall kicking and wiggling movement of the child, the actual palpation and joint and muscle evaluation will occur with the child's passive participation. As the child becomes older, the examiner must position the child in a way that facilitates the evaluation. For example, place a 4-month-old in prone position to evaluate his ability to push up on hands and roll from prone to supine position; place in a standing position to evaluate muscle strength of the legs.

   b. Six months to 1 year (Fig. 14-38). Approach the child slowly. Start the evaluation by playing with his fingers and toes. As the child becomes accustomed to your touching, slowly move from distal limb evaluation to neck, hip, and spine evaluation. Much can be observed about the child's musculoskeletal and neurological systems by watching the child sitting and playing with hands and feet. If the examiner charges toward the child and frightens him, the child may stiffen up, cry, or decide not to cooperate. An inaccurate musculoskeletal evaluation will follow.

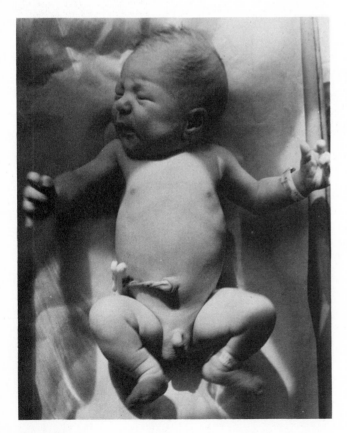

Fig. 14-37. Make a general observation of the musculoskeletal system of the neonate.

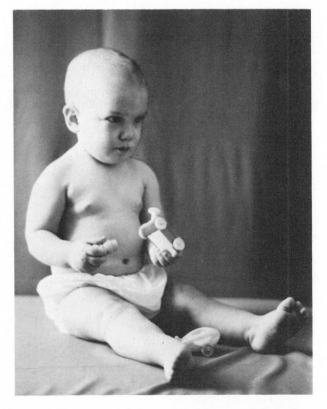

Fig. 14-38. Make a general observation of the musculoskeletal system of the infant.

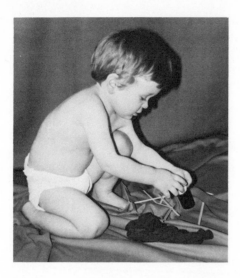

Fig. 14-39. Make a general observation of the musculoskeletal system of the toddler.

c. One to 3 years (Fig. 14-39). The examiner should let the toddler show off a little: watch him walk, play with blocks, and climb onto the examining table. Much can be learned about the development and functioning of the musculoskeletal system through observation.

Once the child is situated for the examination, the examiner should again start with the hands and feet. To evaluate the child's range of motion and ability to follow directions, a game of imitation might follow: instruct the child to "Do as I do"; if that does not work, games such as catching and kicking a ball, building a tower of blocks, and playing peek-a-boo may facilitate the examination.

Although much of the assessment can be done by playing and watching, techniques such as hip examination require specific manipulations that must be worked into the total physical evaluation.

d. Three to 6 years (Fig. 14-40). A slow, "let's play" approach is still helpful for the unsure preschooler. The examiner should watch the child undress and climb onto the examination table. The child should be ready to play hopping games and jumping, squatting, and bending exercises that will facilitate the physical evaluation. The challenge for the examiner with this age child is to invent techniques that will evoke cooperation from the child. Sometimes a game of "Simon Says" works. For example, "Simon says keep your arm as stiff as a tree and don't let me push it down."

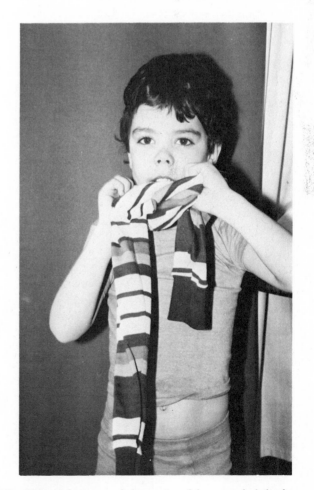

Fig. 14-40. Make a general observation of the musculoskeletal system of the preschooler.

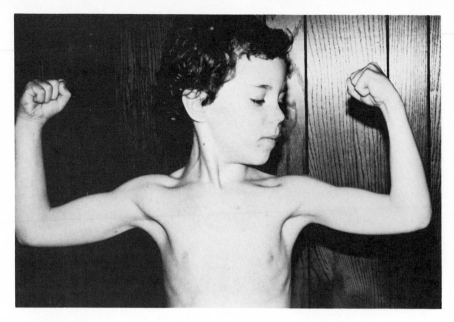

Fig. 14-41. Assessing the musculoskeletal system of a cooperative 7-year-old.

e. Over age 6 years (Fig. 14-41). These children should be ready to fully cooperate with the examiner. The degree of cooperation will usually depend on how the examiner approaches the child. The brisk examiner may get less cooperation and fewer data than will the examiner who takes a few minutes to play with the child, watch him write his name, and demonstrate how strong he is by allowing him to show off his muscles and squeeze the examiner's hand.

4. Many parents may express concern that their children have foot problems. Following are some principles of foot evaluation:

a. Examine the foot for complete range of motion.

b. Do not limit the evaluation to the foot only; also evaluate for stability, deformity, and range of motion of the knee, hip, and spine.

c. Palpate the underside of the foot to evaluate for deformities of the forefoot or the hindfoot.

d. Observe for tibial torsion or bowing.

e. Observe the older infant or child walking without shoes. (Note that a cold floor on bare feet may distort the child's gait.)

f. Observe for muscular weakness or asymmetry.

g. Inspect the child's shoes for evidence of abnormal wear. Normal heel-toe gait wears the shoes more on the outer border of the heel and the inner border of the toe. Walking babies will normally wear down the medial edge of the shoe first.

h. Inspect the child's shoes for size and general fit.

(1) High shoes that cover the ankle are necessary only if the child walks out of low-cut shoes. The ankles are not supported by high shoes, nor is the support necessary.

(2) Shoes should be long enough to allow the thumb to be pressed between the end of the big toe and the end of the shoe while the child maintains a weight-bearing position.

i. Evaluation for flat feet

(1) Before a child begins to walk, the foot does not actually have any arch.

(2) When a child first begins to stand, the feet normally pronate slightly inward (Fig. 14-42). The child assumes a wide-base stance, and the weight line normally falls toward the inner side of the foot.

(3) Between 12 and 30 months the arch strengthens, and the weight bearing falls more directly with the middle of the foot (Fig. 14-43).

(4) Any child older than 30 months whose feet maintain a pronated medial position where the medial border of the foot becomes prominent should be referred for further evaluation.

j. Evaluation for pigeon toes

(1) Many children may demonstrate inward bending of the foot (either of the ankle or toes), the tibia (tibial torsion), or the femur (femoral torsion).

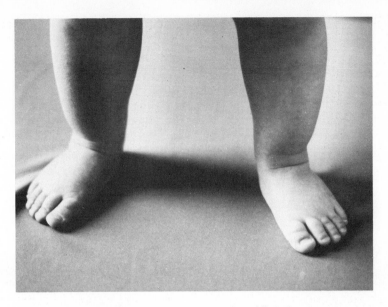

Fig. 14-42. Normal pronation of a toddler's foot.

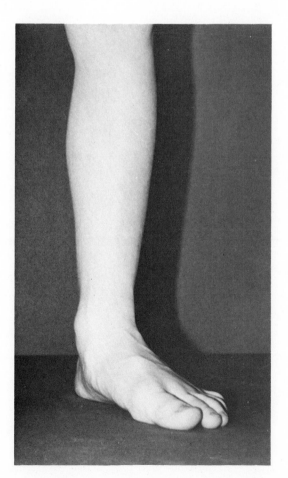

Fig. 14-43. Normal arch of a foot in an older child.

(2) If the examiner notes any inward bending of any of these areas, the child should be referred for further evaluation.

k. Evaluation of toe walking. Babies and older children may demonstrate toeing downward or toe-walking techniques. Toe walking may be normal, or it may be found in children with spastic diseases, congenital shortening of the Achilles, tendon, early muscular dystrophy, or infantile autism. The examiner should manually dorsiflex the child's foot to evaluate the stretchability of the Achilles tendon. Any child with a tight or shortened Achilles tendon (dorsiflexion less than 20°) should be referred. Likewise, any child demonstrating other musculoskeletal or neurological problems should be referred.

5. Children may complain of muscular aches and pains. Although a thorough history and physical evaluation are mandatory, the examiner must also be aware of normal "growing pains." Boys between 11 and 18 years and girls between 9 and 16 years experience rapid growth spurts. At times the skeletal system grows faster than the muscular system; therefore the children may feel discomfort in their limbs.

6. Curvature of the spine is a common finding in children, particularly during puberty. There are two types of scoliosis:

a. Functional: most frequent type found in young children. The spine is curved when the child stands, but if the child bends over to touch toes, the curvature disappears.

b. Idiopathic: the spine remains curved when the child is sitting as well as bending forward. There is pelvic tilt, and there may be a shortened leg. Even though all children must be evaluated for lateral spinal bending, teenagers are at high risk. Teenage girls (12 to 13 years old) are at highest risk to show development of scoliosis. Any child with noted spinal curvature should be referred for further evaluation. Most studies have shown that the approximate time of spinal curvature development is the same time that pubic hair develops. Each child deserves a care-

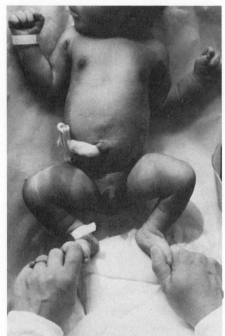

A

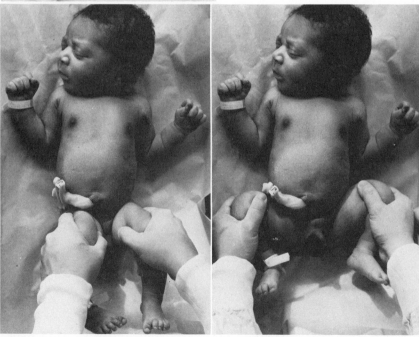

B　　　　　　　　C

Fig. 14-44. Ortolanis' test. **A,** Initial observation of symmetry. **B,** Hips flexed at 90° angle. **C,** Hips externally rotated.

ful inspection and palpation of the spine.
7. Hip evaluation for possible congenital hip dislocation (Ortolanis' test)
   a. Problem is found more in girls than boys.
   b. Parent may report difficulty diapering the child.
   c. Infant should be checked at every visit from newborn stage until about 2½ years of age.
   d. Technique (Fig. 14-44)
      (1) Baby supine, knees brought to 90° angle with back
      (2) Examiner's hands on knees, index finger along lateral thigh to feel click vibration if present
      (3) Knees brought up then flexed laterally; newborn knees should almost lie flat on bed (160° to 175°)
   e. Abnormal findings
      (1) Pop, click, or snap during manipulation technique
      (2) Bilaterally unequal response
      (3) Sudden cry of pain during procedure
8. Hip and knee evaluation for teenage boys, who are at risk for two specific types of skeletal problems:
   a. Slipped capital femoral epiphysis. Even though this is a hip injury, the boy will usually have pain in the knee or lateral distal thigh. Many times an injury precipitated by an activity such as jumping off an object will precede. Any boy with these complaints should be referred. Objective assessment data include the following:
      (1) Deep palpation to the hip causes pain and tenderness.
      (2) There is increased pain with abduction, internal or external rotation, or flexion of the hip.
      (3) In severe cases the examiner may see a shortening of the affected leg due to muscle spasm and upward displacement of the femoral head.
   b. Osgood-Schlatter disease. The boy will usually complain that his knee hurts. Although no specific injury may precede, an increase in running or jumping will aggravate the pain. Any teenage

boy with this complaint should be referred. Objective assessment data include the following:
   (1) Specific location of pain by one finger will not be at kneee itself but at a point inferior to the knee, on the head of the tibia.
   (2) Inspection of the area will reveal a slight elevation.
   (3) Tapping the area with the knuckles will cause pain.
Although Osgood-Schlatter disease has traditionally been referred to as the disease of the young athletic teenage male, many orthopedists believe that, as more girls become active in athletics, there will be a greater incidence of the disease among females.

Clinical variations associated with the pediatric client

The clinical guidelines for musculoskeletal system of children vary greatly depending on the age of the child, his cooperation, and his motor development. The examiner will spend a great deal of time developing routines for examining different ages. The guidelines and motor development sequence presented here represent normal findings for various aged children.

Special techniques for evaluation of feet and shoes, muscle aches and pains, scoliosis, and hips have been discussed under clinical strategies. These must be incorporated into the following guidelines.

To use the guidelines, the examiner must know the developmental norms for age of the child being examined and have the cleverness to collect these data during the examination. If the examiner does not have the cooperation of the child, an inaccurate evaluation will result.

By age 6 years a child should be able to fully cooperate with the examiner. Evaluation of a child less than 6 years of age will probably not require following the guidelines in order. Instead, the examiner must watch the child walk, climb, play patty-cake, jump and skip to gather the necessary data. Other more specific suggestions such as "kiss your knee" or "touch your toes" will aid specific joint and muscle evaluation.

Characteristic or area examined	Normal	Deviations from normal
1. Weighing and measuring child	(See Figs. 14-45 and 14-46.)	

Text continued on p. 386.

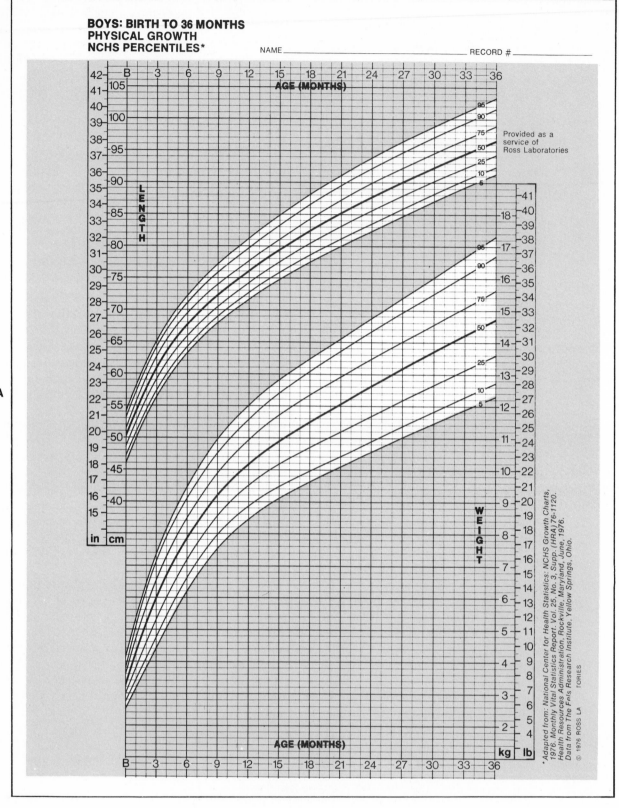

Fig. 14-45. A, Male physical growth chart, birth to 36 months.

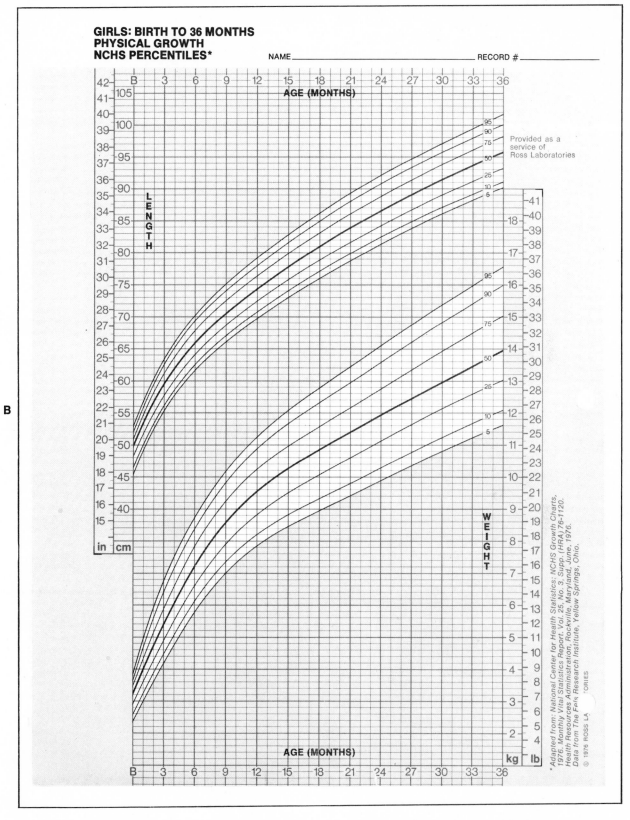

**GIRLS: BIRTH TO 36 MONTHS
PHYSICAL GROWTH
NCHS PERCENTILES***

NAME _____   RECORD # _____

Provided as a
service of
Ross Laboratories

* Adapted from: National Center for Health Statistics: NCHS Growth Charts, 1976. Monthly Vital Statistics Report. Vol. 25, No. 3, Supp. (HRA) 76-1120. Health Resources Administration. Rockville, Maryland, June, 1976. Data from The Fels Research Institute, Yellow Springs, Ohio.

© 1976 ROSS LABORATORIES

B

Fig. 14-45, cont'd. B, Female physical growth chart, birth to 36 months. (Courtesy Ross Laboratories, Columbus, Ohio, 1976.)

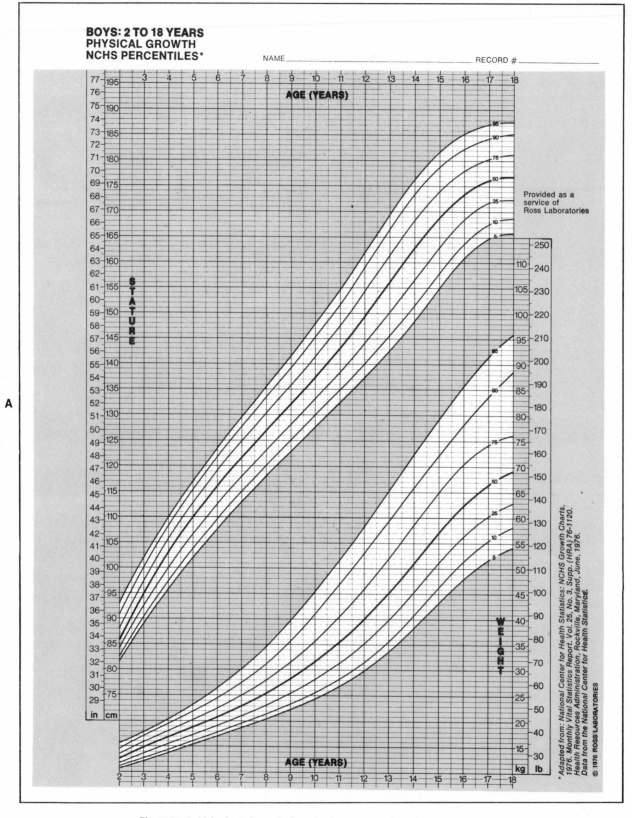

Fig. 14-46, A, Male physical growth chart showing stature and weight, 2 to 18 years.

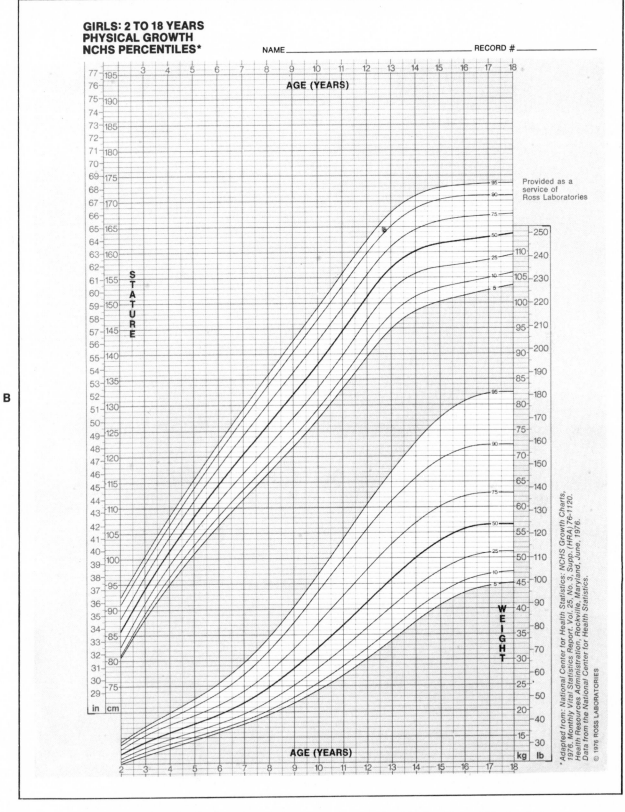

Fig. 14-46, cont'd. B, Female physical growth chart showing stature and weight, 2 to 18 years. (Courtesy Ross Laboratories, Columbus, Ohio, 1976.)

Clinical variations associated with the pediatric client–cont'd

Characteristic or area examined	Normal	Deviations from normal

2. Trunk (child lying or standing)
    a. Spine

Spine straight
Newborn: convex spine (Fig. 14-47)
3 to 4 months: cervical curve develops as child
    holds head up

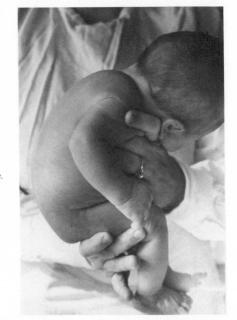

Fig. 14-47. Normal convex curvature of newborn's spine.

12 to 18 months: lumbar curve develops as
    child learns to walk (Fig. 14-48)
Lumbar lordosis in toddlers

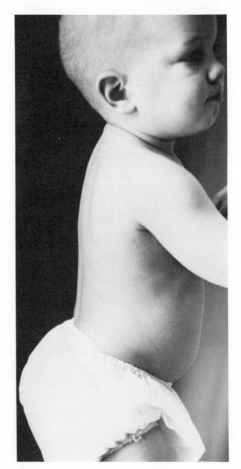

Fig. 14-48. Normal lumbar curvature of toddler's spine.

Characteristic or area examined	Normal	Deviations from normal
	Beyond 18 months: cervical spine concave; thoracic spine convex, but less than that of adult; lumbar spine concave, like that of adult (Fig. 14-49)	

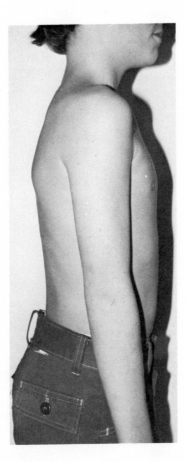

Fig. 14-49. Adult curvature in school-age child.

Characteristic or area examined	Normal	Deviations from normal
	No dimpling or bulges along spine	Dimpling or bulges along spine or thickening
	Black children may more frequently show lordosis	Lumbar lordosis in children over 6 years
		Curved spine either in standing or bent over position
1. Bending to touch toes	Straight spine, both in upright and bending position	Functional vs. idiopathic scoliosis (see clinical strategies)
	Iliac crests of equal height	Unequal iliac crests in either standing or bent over position
	Shoulders equal height	
	Convexity of thoracic spine	
2. Hyperextension	30° hyperextension from neutral position	Unable to hyperextend without losing balance, or pain with hyperextension
3. Lateral bending	35° flexion both ways from midline position	Decreased flexion degree or pain with bending
4. Lateral rotation	30° rotation in both directions from direct forward position	Decreased rotation capability
		Rotation with discomfort
5. Spinal process palpation	Straight spine	Curvature of spine
	Nontender	Tenderness
		Spasm of paravertebral muscles

Continued.

Clinical variations associated with the pediatric client–cont'd

Characteristic or area examined	Normal	Deviations from normal
3. Gait	Newly walking babies and toddlers have wide stance and wide waddle gait pattern; normal, and tends to disappear by approximately 2 to 2½ years (Fig. 14-50) Gait should become progressively stronger, steadier, and smoother as child matures; any deviation from this, or history of increasing falls or balance problems, should be considered abnormal (also evaluate shoes; see clinical strategies) Smooth regular gait with symmetrical arm swing	Unsteady or jerky Pain or discomfort Irregular or jerky trunk posturing Asymmetrical or jerky arm swing unrelated to gait

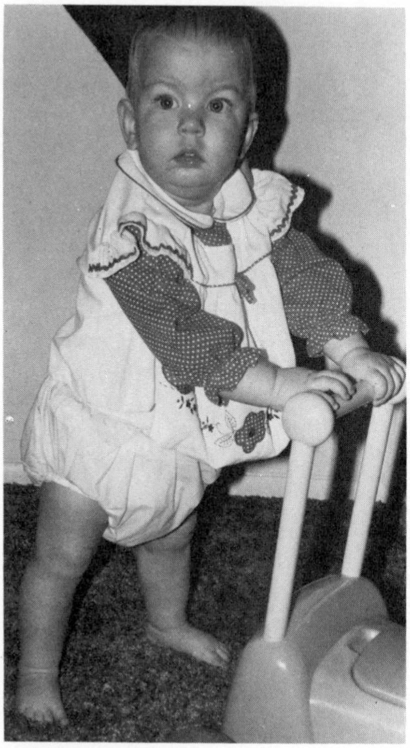

Fig. 14-50. Wide-base stance of toddler.

Characteristic or area examined	Normal	Deviations from normal
4. Head and neck		
a. Musculature	Symmetrical appearance	Asymmetry Atrophy or hypertrophy of muscles
b. Temporomandibular joint	Smooth movement of mandible	Pain, limited range of motion, or crepitus of temporomandibular joint
c. Posterior neck	Locating landmarks may be difficult in small child due to short neck and excess baby fat Locate C_7, T_1, nontender cervical spine	Tenderness, spasms Nodules
d. Range of motion of neck		
1. Chin flexion	45° from midline	Limited or painful range of motion
2. Head extension	55° from midline	Crepitus of cervical spine
3. Lateral bending	40° each way from midline	
4. Rotation of chin to shoulders	70° from midline	
e. Muscle strength of neck		
1. Chin flexion, position maintenance	With reasonable strength, unable to force head upright	Able to break muscular flexion before anticipated point
2. Head hyperextension, position maintenance	With reasonable strength, unable to force head upright	Able to break muscular flexion before anticipated point
5. Hands and wrists	Smoothness; no swelling or deformities noted Fingers able to maintain full extension position	Irregular finger contour Swelling Deformities Tenderness Muscular atrophy Heberden's nodes Long spider or short clubbed fingers

Characteristic or area examined	Normal	Deviations from normal
a. Range of motion of fingers and wrists		
1. Finger extension	Symmetrical response	Asymmetrical response
	Smooth movement without complaints of discomfort	Pain on movement
	Full flexion and extension	
2. Fist	Bilaterally equal response	Unequal response
		Decreased response
3. Grip	Tight grip	
4. Radial deviation	20°	Pain with movement
		Decreased movement
5. Ulnar deviation	55°	
6. Extension	70°	
7. Flexion	90°	
b. Wrist strength		
1. Wrist flexion, position maintenance	Bilaterally strong	Asymmetrical response
	Unable to break position*	Able to easily break position
2. Wrist extension, position maintenance	Bilaterally strong	Asymmetrical response
	Unable to break position	Able to easily break position
6. Elbows		
a. Palpation	Skin intact	Swelling
	Smooth	Inflammation
	Surface nontender, without nodules or discomfort	General tenderness
		Subcutaneous nodules
	Lymph nodes not palpable	Point tenderness
		Lymph nodes palpated
b. Range of motion		
1. Extension and flexion	160° full movement	Limited range of motion
	Bilaterally equal	Asymmetrical movement
	No discomfort	Pain at elbow
2. Pronation and supination	90° each direction	Limited range of motion
	Bilaterally equal	Asymmetrical movement
	No discomfort	Pain at elbow
7. Shoulders		
a. Inspection	Intactness	Redness
	Skin smooth and regular	Swelling
	Bilaterally symmetrical	Nodules
b. Palpation	Nontender	Tender, painful
	Smooth and regular	Swelling
	Bilaterally symmetrical	
c. Range of motion		
1. Extension	180° from resting neutral position	Limited range of motion
	Bilaterally equal	Pain with movement
	No discomfort	Crepitations with movement
		Asymmetry
2. Hyperextension	50°	Limited range of motion
	Bilaterally equal	Pain with movement
	No discomfort	Crepitations with movement
		Asymmetry
3. External rotation	90°	Limited range of motion
	Bilaterally equal	Pain with movement
	No discomfort	Crepitations with movement
		Asymmetry
4. Internal rotation	90°	Limited range of motion
	Bilaterally equal	Pain with movement
	No discomfort	Crepitations with movement
		Asymmetry
8. Arm muscles: use make/break technique		
a. Deltoids	Bilaterally strong	Symmetrically unequal

*Throughout pediatric guidelines, according to resistance appropriate for age.

Continued.

Clinical variations associated with the pediatric client—cont'd

Characteristic or area examined	Normal	Deviations from normal
	Unable to break position	Weak response
		Pain during technique
		Muscular spasm
b. Biceps	Bilaterally strong	Symmetrically unequal
	Unable to break position	Weak response
		Pain during technique
		Muscular spasm
c. Triceps	Bilaterally strong	Symmetrically unequal
	Unable to break position	Weak response
		Pain during technique
		Muscular spasm
9. Shoulder muscles: lift infant under arms	Infant able to maintain position on examiner's hands (Fig. 14-51)	If muscles weak, child will slip through examiner's hands

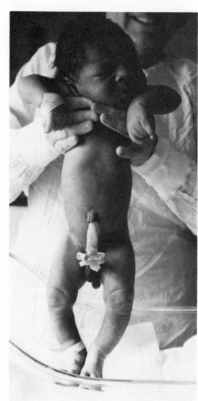

Fig. 14-51. Newborn shoulder muscle assessment.

10. Feet and ankles		
a. Inspection	Smoothness; no swelling or deformities noted	Inward or lateral deviation of feet or toes, tight Achilles tendons
	Toes maintain extended and straight position	Flat feet
	Toenails intact and neatly trimmed	
	Feet maintain straight position	
	(See clinical strategies for additional observation criteria.)	
b. Palpation	Smooth	Tenderness: diffuse vs. point
	Nontender	Swelling
		Inflammation
		Nodules
c. Range of motion		
1. Dorsiflexion and plantar flexion	Dorsiflexion 20° from midline position	Dorsiflexion less than 20° due to tight tendon
	Plantar flexion 45° from midline position	Limited range of motion
	Bilaterally equal	Pain with movement

Characteristic or area examined	Normal	Deviations from normal
(Instruct child to stand on toes.)	No discomfort	Crepitations Asymmetry
2. Inversion 3. Eversion	Inversion 30° from midline position Eversion 20° from midline position Bilaterally equal No discomfort	Inversion or eversion when foot at rest Limited range of motion Pain with movement Asymmetry
d. Muscular evaluation: maintain dorsiflexed position against opposite pull	Bilaterally strong Unable to break position	Unequal Weak response Pain during technique
11. Knee	Knees in direct straight line between hip, ankle, great toe	Deviation of line so that it maintains position of hip, knee, ankle, fourth or fifth toe Rotation of feet or lower legs (see clinical strategies)
	Valgum: medial malleolus > 2.5 cm (1 inch) apart with knees touching; normal for children 2 to 3½ years old (may be present and normal in some children up to 12 years) (Fig. 14-52) Varum: medial malleolus touching, knees > 2.5 cm (1 inch) apart; needs further evaluation for tibial torsion (may be normal until 18 months to 2 years of age)	May be seen with systemic diseases such as polio, rickets, syphilis
	Smooth, symmetrical	Swelling, thickness Inflammation Inflamed painful joints in black children may be sign of sickle cell anemia Enlargement of tibial tubercles in teenage boys may be sign of Osgood-Schlatter disease

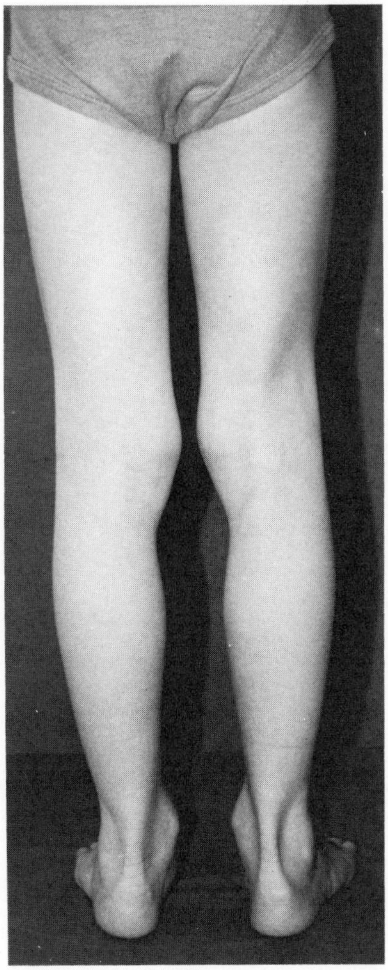

Fig. 14-52. School-age child: normal valgum position.

Characteristic or area examined	Normal	Deviations from normal
a. Palpation of knees and popliteal space	Smooth, nontender	Bogginess Thickening Tenderness, redness Painful Nodules and swelling
b. Range of motion evaluation	130° from straight extended position No discomfort or difficulty	Decreased range of motion Pain with movement Crepitations
12. Hips and pelvis **a.** Inspection and palpation		

Continued.

Clinical variations associated with the pediatric client—cont'd

Characteristic or area examined	Normal	Deviations from normal
1. Babies to 3 years	Gluteal folds bilaterally equal No click, snap, or dislocation felt Hip rotation of 160° to 175° bilaterally equal	Difference in height of gluteal folds Click, snap felt Unequal range of motion Sudden cry during procedure
2. Children over 3 years: use adult technique to evaluate		
a. Knee to chest	120° from straight extended position	Limited range of motion Pain or discomfort with movement Flexion of opposite thigh Crepitations
b. Hip flexion without bending knee	90° from straight extended position	Limited range of motion Pain or discomfort with movement Crepitations
c. External rotation	40° from straight midline position	Limited range of motion Pain or discomfort with movement Crepitations In teenage boys with slipped femoral epiphysis: much pain with external rotation or abduction of hip
d. Internal rotation	40° from straight midline position	Limited range of motion Pain or discomfort with movement Crepitations
b. Muscular evaluation		
1. Hips		
a. Flexion against examiner's pushing	Bilaterally strong Unable to break position	Symmetrically unequal Weak response Pain during technique
2. Hamstring		
a. Leg crossing	Able to perform Bilaterally equal and without difficulty	Unable to perform Performs with pain or great difficulty
b. Bending of knee against examiner's pushing	Bilaterally strong Unable to flex knee	Symmetrically unequal Weak response Pain during technique
3. Quadriceps		
a. Extension of lower leg against examiner's pushing	Bilaterally strong Unable to flex knee	Symmetrically unequal Weak response Pain during technique

History and clinical strategies associated with the geriatric client

1. The normal aging process is accompanied by numerous musculoskeletal changes:
   a. A decrease in bone mass, which results in increased vulnerability to stress in weight-bearing areas and predisposes to fractures
   b. Thinning (possibly collapse) of intervertebral discs
   c. Calcification within cartilage and ligaments
   d. Less elastic tendons
   e. A decrease in muscle mass, tone, and strength (however, at age 60 the decrease usually does not exceed a 10% to 20% loss)
      (1) Less ability to perform intense, sudden exercise
      (2) Decreased endurance with exercise (less ability to hold isometric contractions)
      (3) Decreased agility

2. Risk factors. As with all other aging changes, these alterations occur at different rates in different individuals. The changes are gradual and not often presented as a complaint. The rate of change is greatly affected by a number of variables or risk factors.
   a. General physical health of client
      (1) Decreased respiratory capacity and reserve
      (2) Diminished circulatory supply
      (3) Arthritic changes accompanied by symptoms
      (4) Neurogenic disorders affecting voluntary muscle response or sensory alterations
      (5) Other physical changes that are accompanied by symptoms which interfere with

body function or fitness: pain, diminished vision, fatigue, and weakness

b. Obesity
c. Immobility, either short term (2 to 3 weeks) related to injury or episodic illness, or long term
d. Sedentary life-style (a hypokinetic state can perpetuate itself)
e. Depression
f. Inadequate nutrition and/or fluid intake
g. Mind-altering drugs (e.g., tranquilizers, sedatives, alcohol)
h. Fear of falling
i. Confusion or altered mental state (inattentiveness)

All the variables mentioned contribute to reduced physical activity, which in turn promotes and hastens the changes associated with the aging musculoskeletal system.

3. Presenting symptoms related to musculoskeletal problems:
   a. The major symptoms to inquire about are listed in the geriatric data base in Chapter 2. These complaints relate to the following:
      (1) General feeling of well-being
      (2) Muscle function
      (3) Joint and bone function and appearance
      (4) Extremity function
      (5) Back and spine function
      (6) Gait
      (7) Sleeping patterns
   b. Further details about symptom analysis are offered in the adult section of this chapter:
      (1) Pain
      (2) Gait difficulty
      (3) Voluntary muscle function complaints
      (4) Skeletal complaints
      (5) Joint complaints
   c. Symptoms that should be explored in detail follow:
      (1) Weakness
         (a) Onset sudden or slow?
         (b) Isolated to a specific body part or generalized (e.g., difficulty swallowing, lid drooping, unilateral weakness, or weakness in feet, ankles, hands)?
         (c) Associated with any particular activity (e.g., stair climbing [how many], rising from a chair, walking on level ground)?
         (d) Does weakness occur at onset of activity or after activity has been sustained (how long or how much)?
         (e) Associated symptoms (e.g., dizziness, "black-outs," numbness or tingling,

pain, tics or fasciculations, tremors, shortness of breath)
         (f) Associated stiffness of joints, spasms, or muscle tension (do these symptoms occur at night?)
         (g) Associated weight gain or loss
         (h) Associated mood or mental changes
         (i) Medications being taken
      (2) "Restless" legs (usually at night)
         (a) Associated symptoms of back pain, muscle cramps in legs, numbness or coldness of extremities?
         (b) How is this relieved?
      (3) History of injuries, falls (inquire specifically about all accidents, minor "spills," or injuries that are recent; client may not be aware that a pattern of increased stumbling, falls, or limited agility is emerging if injuries are not obvious or incapacitating)
      (4) Decrease in height (ask client to estimate number of inches over last few years; last year)

4. Osteoarthritis is described as a universal aging process that is usually noninflammatory and involves deterioration and abrasions of the articular cartilage and possibly formation of new bone at the joint surfaces. The examiner must determine whether joint and bone changes are creating symptoms or signs that alter the physical functioning of the client. One author estimates that 15% to 25% of individuals over age 60 years manifest signs or symptoms related to arthritis.*
   a. Risk factors
      (1) Advancing age
      (2) History of excessive use of a given joint (or group of joints)
      (3) Obesity
      (4) Family history of arthritis (especially with involvement of hands and fingers)
      (5) History of injuries to a given joint (or group of joints)
      (6) History of joint abnormalities (e.g., laxness of ligaments)
   b. Joints most frequently involved with symptomatic arthritic changes are weight-bearing areas:
      (1) Knees
         (a) The client frequently notices crepitation.
         (b) Pain, stiffness, and/or joint enlargement may be evident.

---

*Grob, David: Prevalent joint diseases in older persons. In Chinn, Austin B., editor: Clinical aspects of aging, Working with older people, vol. 4, Rockville, Md., 1971, U.S. Department of Health, Education, and Welfare, Public Health Service, p. 163.

(c) The quadriceps may atrophy because of disuse due to pain.

(2) Hips
  (a) Pain may be local or referred to buttock or inner aspect of thigh.
  (b) The hip may be held in partially flexed and adducted position.
  (c) Hip extension and rotation are diminished.

(3) Spine (cervical and lumbar areas most frequently affected)
  (a) Cervical crepitation on movement is noticed by client. Weakness, numbness, or sensory changes may be noticed in upper arm, forearm, and thumb and fingers. "Black-out" spells occasionally occur with neck rotation.
  (b) Spinal changes may result in stiffness, loss of lordotic curve, or exaggerated kyphosis.

(4) Fingers
  (a) May manifest outward changes, especially distal joint enlargement or node formation (Fig. 14-53).
  (b) Range of motion may be limited because of pain.
  (c) Interosseous spaces may be atrophied as a result of decrease in use of fingers and hands.

(5) Shoulders: pain experienced on movement, especially abduction.

(6) Ribs: arthritic changes in the costovertebral joint may produce localized pain on palpation or referred pain to chest wall.

c. Symptoms are often increased by weather changes or prolonged immobility.

d. Temporary relief is often completely or partially provided by rest, heat application, or analgesics. (*Note:* Heat application can be a risk if the client does not check temperature of water or heating device; the client's sensitivity to heat may be impaired. Also, gastrointestinal complaints may result from frequent use of some analgesics.)

5. Osteoporosis is described as a decrease in mass and density of the skeleton, affecting approximately 29% of the aging female population and 18% of aging males.[*] Involvement is more intense in the long bones and vertebral column.

a. Risk factors
  (1) Postmenopausal state
  (2) Immobility
  (3) Cushing syndrome
  (4) Advanced diverticulitis (interferes with calcium absorption)
  (5) Hyperthyroidism (increased bone resorption)
  (6) History of limited calcium dietary intake
  (7) Heparin
  (8) Diabetes mellitus

b. Symptoms are often absent or mild; vague discomfort in back is experienced.

c. The vulnerability to fractures (of the spine, femur, and pelvis) is greatly increased.

d. Loss of height occurs as a result of kyphotic changes and vertebral fractures.

---

[*]Smith, R. W., Jr., Eyler, W. R., and Melinger, R. C.: On the incidence of senile osteoporosis, Ann. Intern. Med. **52**:773, 1960.

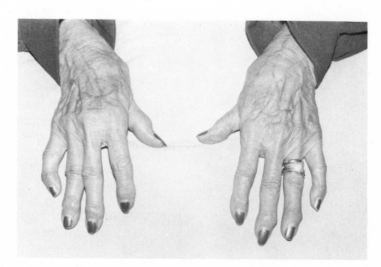

Fig. 14-53. Distal joint deformities associated with osteoarthritis.

e. Point tenderness of the spine is a signal of acute vertebral problems.

6. If the examiner is confronted with a client who is disabled or incapacitated with discomfort or reduced function, the need for safety and performance of activities of daily living should be assessed. Detailed questions regarding activities of daily living are offered on p. 23 in Chapter 1, and inquiries and concerns for safety are described on p. 29 of Chapter 1.

7. Physical assessment. The aging client who is not afflicted with illness or arthritic changes should be able to participate in the musculoskeletal assessment as it is described in the adult section of this chapter. Normal range of motion of joints and muscular strength and tone should be the same as with the younger adult. Even if muscular strength is reduced by 10% to 20%, the client should be able to sustain the opposition of the examiner in the testing for muscular strength. The following general patterns may be noted.

a. The response to examiner commands may be slower.

b. General muscle bulk may be reduced. The arms and legs may appear thinner and flabby.

c. *Note:* Many "normal" clients (including young adults) cannot touch their toes as they bend forward from the waist.

8. Early signs of musculoskeletal deviations. As physical disability and/or advanced aging changes encroach on the elderly client, the response to musculoskeletal physical assessment manifests an increasing number of deviations from normal findings. Some of the early (or more subtle) signs are:

a. Posture (stance) (Fig. 14-54). The appearance is one of general flexion (any or all of these signs may be evident).
   (1) Head and neck thrust forward
   (2) Dorsal kyphosis or kyphoscoliosis
   (3) Flexion at the elbow and wrist
   (4) Hips slightly flexed
   (5) Knees flexed
   (6) Broad stance (feet spread farther apart)

b. Gait should be carefully evaluated in *all* clients. They should be permitted to wear shoes.
   (1) Gait phases
      (a) Heel strike (Fig. 14-55). Dorsiflexors that normally decelerate the foot before striking may be weakened. The flat of the foot strikes the floor. The client may lift the leg farther off the floor with each step.
      (b) Foot at midstance; other foot is pushing off (Fig. 14-56). Weakened quadriceps may not be able to stabilize the knee while the foot is bearing weight. Lateral and anterior-posterior hip stability may not be maintained if gluteus muscles are weakened.
      (c) Foot is pushing off (Fig. 14-57). Weakened gastrocnemius and soleus unable to elevate the body to permit the other foot to swing freely.
      (d) Swing phase (Fig. 14-58). Swing may be shortened, foot may be lifted farther off the ground (marching style), or foot may just fall or slide forward (shuffling pattern).
   (2) Arms may be held out to assist with balance or move in a rowing motion.
   (3) Arm movement may be limited or absent.
   (4) Upper torso may sway from side to side to assist with maintaining balance.
   (5) Feet may be farther apart (broadened base to maintain balance).
   (6) Steps may be uneven or tottering.
   (7) The shortened step and shuffling propulsive gait with limited arm movement are associated with parkinsonism.

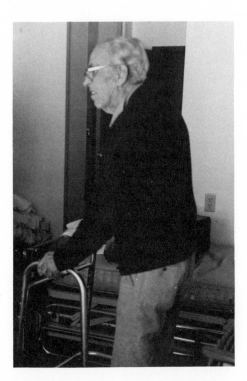

Fig. 14-54. Posture (stance) featuring head and neck thrust forward, dorsal kyphosis, hip flexion, and knees slightly flexed.

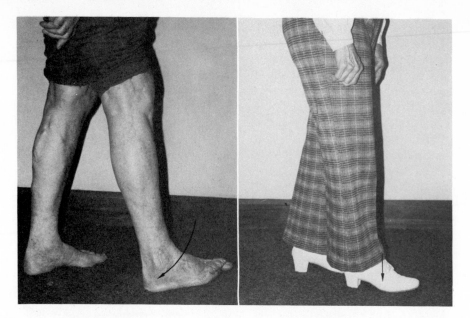

Fig. 14-55. A, Right foot demonstrating normal heel strike; left foot is bearing weight. **B,** Weakened dorsiflexors allow the flat of the right foot rather than heel to strike the floor.

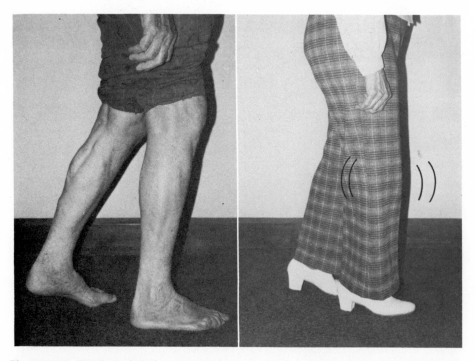

Fig. 14-56. A, Weight is shifted to the right foot, which is in midstance. **B,** Weakened right leg is wobbly while bearing weight (midstance phase). A weakened or painful leg or foot results in a shortened stride, since that weight can be shifted quickly back to the other foot.

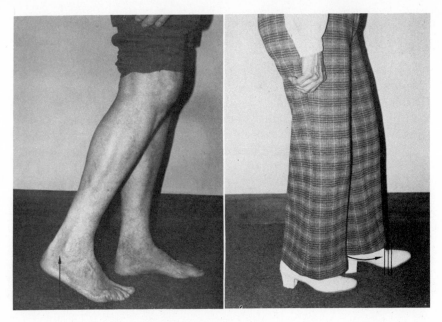

Fig. 14-57. A, Right foot demonstrates normal body lift at the end of push phase; the left leg has swung free to a new step position. **B,** Weakened right leg is unable to lift the body sufficiently to permit the left foot to swing freely.

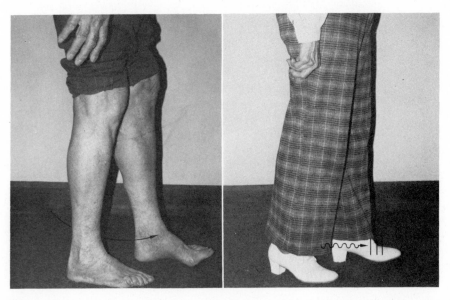

Fig. 14-58. A, Left leg demonstrates normal free swing. **B,** Left leg demonstrates shuffle-forward rather than free swing. Stride is shortened.

(8) Individuals who are weak or unsteady watch their feet as they walk.

c. Range of motion
   (1) Most often limited due to pain (client stops movement abruptly).
   (2) Weight-bearing joints (knees, hips, and lumbar spine) are frequently affected. Joints that are frequently used (cervical spine, shoulder, elbow, and fingers) may have limited range or pain associated with movement.
   (3) Loss of full spinal range of motion, particularly in the lumbar area.

d. Muscle appearance and function
   (1) Muscle wasting may be evident near immobile joints or in extremities that have limited motion (e.g., deep interosseous spaces often appear in severely arthritic hands).
   (2) Mild bilateral muscle weakness (particularly of lower extremities) may not be noticed by the examiner during the opposition testing. Careful evaluation of gait and stair climbing may reveal more subtle weaknesses.

9. Functional testing for activities of daily living. The examiner will be assessing many elderly clients who have permanent muscle or joint function loss or other altered health states that contribute to diminished physical ability. Beyond the assessment of body parts for functional capacity, the examiner needs to assess the client's ability to move about and to perform essential functions at home. The client often compensates for weakened muscle groups by altering posture or assisting movement with other body parts or special devices (e.g., cane, walker). The following assessment tests the ability and combination of major muscle groups to perform vital activities of daily living.

The examiner will observe:	Comments
1. Client rising from a lying to a sitting position (Fig. 14-59)	Often rolls to one side and pushes with arms to raise to elbow position Grabbing siderail or adjacent table may help client to pull up to full sitting position

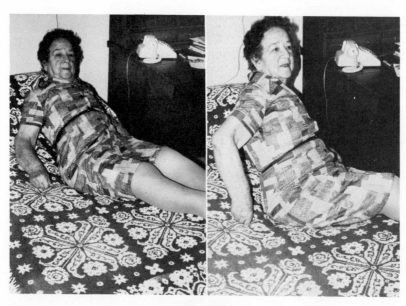

Fig. 14-59.

The examiner will observe:	Comments
2. Client rising from a chair to a standing position (Fig. 14-60)	May supplement weakened leg muscles by pushing with arms Upper torso thrusts forward before body rises; feet spread far apart to provide broad support base

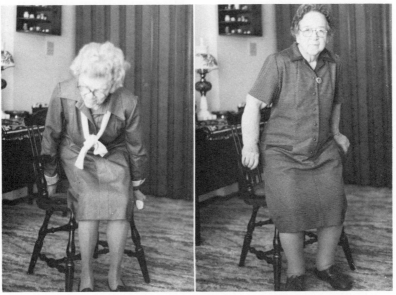

Fig. 14-60.

3. Client walking (Fig. 14-61)	Note heel strike, midstance, push-off, swing phase, arm motion, and upper trunk motion (See comments about gait phases on p. 395.)

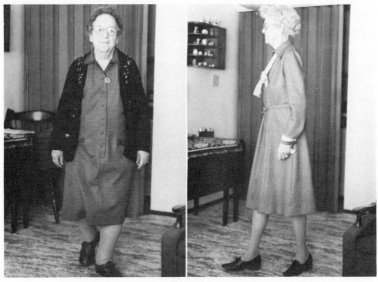

Fig. 14-61.

Continued.

The examiner will observe:	Comments
4. Client climbing a step (Fig. 14-62)	May use favorite leg (stronger one) to climb stair Will usually hold handrail for balance and may pull body up and forward with that arm

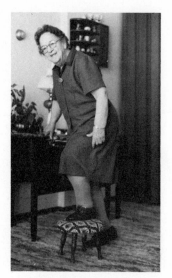

Fig. 14-62.

5. Client descending a step (Fig. 14-63)	Often descends steps sideways, lowering weaker leg first, and holding rail with both hands If unsteady or insecure, client often watches feet while lowering and standing on them

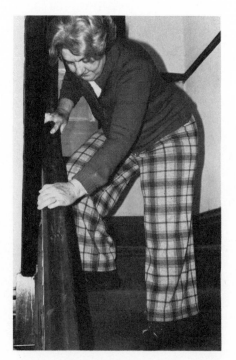

Fig. 14-63.

The examiner will observe:	Comments

6. Client picking up item from the floor (Fig. 14-64) — Grasps or leans on table or handrail for support while lowering body; one hand may be firmly supported on thigh to assist in lowering and in elevating upper torso to standing position; client may avoid bending knees and stoop from waist

Fig. 14-64.

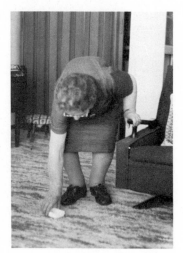

7. Client tying shoes while seated (Fig. 14-65) — Tests for manual dexterity and flexibility of spine
Client may use footstool to reduce need for spinal flexion

Fig. 14-65.

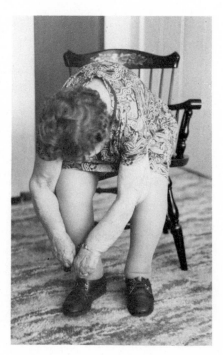

Continued.

The examiner will observe	Comments
8. Client putting on and pulling up trousers (or stockings) (Fig. 14-66)	Clothing often pulled over feet while client seated; final act of pulling up clothing assesses shoulder and upper arm strength

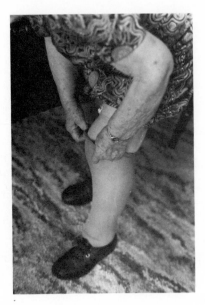

Fig. 14-66.

9. Client putting on sweater or jacket (Fig. 14-67)	Often applies first sleeve to weaker arm or shoulder; may use internal or external shoulder rotation to reach remaining sleeve and to thrust arm into it

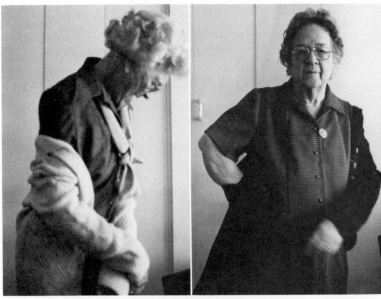

Fig. 14-67.

The examiner will observe:	Comments
10. Client zipping dress in the back (Fig. 14-68) (or fastening brassiere)	Some individuals discard all garments that fasten in back; others find someone else to zip them up This maneuver tests ability to rotate shoulders

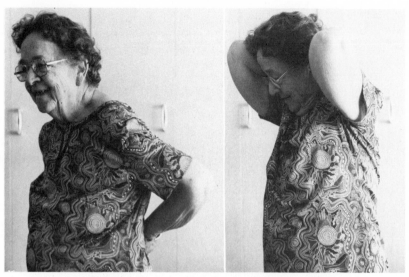

Fig. 14-68.

11. Client combing hair on back and sides (Fig. 14-69)	Assesses ability to grasp and maneuver brush or comb, wrist flexion, and shoulder rotation Some clients will turn back of head toward comb to accommodate diminished external shoulder rotation

Fig. 14-69.

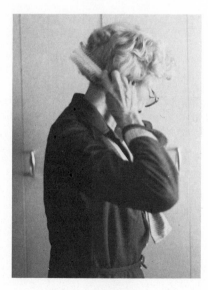

Continued.

The examiner will observe:	Comments

12. Client pushing chair away from table (while seated in chair) (Fig. 14-70)

Assesses upper arm, shoulder, lower arm strength, and wrist motion; some clients will rise to standing position and ease chair out with torso

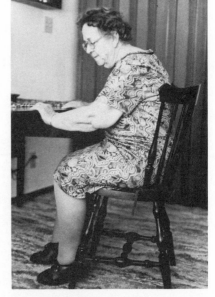

Fig. 14-70.

13. Client buttoning button, writing name, picking up paper from table (Fig. 14-71)

Assesses manual dexterity and finger-thumb opposition

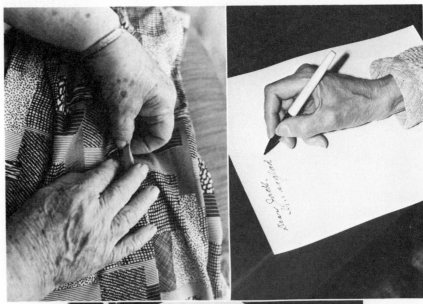

Fig. 14-71.

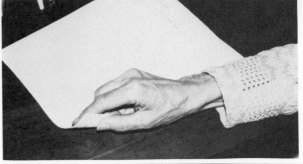

Vocabulary

1. Abduction

2. Adduction

3. Ankylosis

4. Bogginess

5. Bunion

6. Bursa

7. Bursitis

8. Carpal tunnel syndrome

9. Circumduction

10. Clonus

11. Cogwheel motion

12. Crepitus

13. Dorsiflexion

14. Effusion

15. Extension

16. External rotation

17. Fasciculation

18. Flexion

19. Gait: stance

20. Gait: swing

21. Gout

22. Heberden's nodules

23. Internal rotation

24. Kyphosis

↑ convexity of thoracic spine
hunchback

25. Lordosis

↑ concavity in lumbar spine
swayback

26. Myalgia

muscle pain

27. Osteoarthritis

hypertrophic joint degeneration

28. Plantar flexion

29. Pronate

palm down

30. Rheumatoid arthritis

31. Scoliosis

lateral spine curve

32. Spondylitis

inflammation of vertebrae

33. Sprain

partial rupture of ligaments

34. Strain

muscle overstretching

35. Subluxation

partial dislocation

36 Supinate

palm up

37. Tendonitis

38. Tennis elbow

39. Valgus

bent outward

40. Varus

bent inward

Cognitive self-assessment

Mark each statement "T" or "F."

1. ___T___ The two articulating surfaces of a joint are cartilage.

2. __T__ It is important to examine muscles both during relaxation and during contraction.

3. __T__ Varus is a term used to describe an angular deviation of an extremity.

4. __F__ Another name for kyphosis is swayback.

5. __T__ When there is muscle disease, the tendon stretch reflex is greatly altered.

6. __T__ As the client ages, decreased muscle strength is due to an increased amount of collagen in the muscle tissue, followed by fibrosis of the connective tissue.

7. __F__ The kind of arthritis that occurs many times with the aging process is called rheumatoid arthritis.

8. __F__ The normal lumbar curve is convex.

9. __T__ The straight leg raise test is generally a good test to use in evaluation of a disc problem.

10. __T__ The curvature seen in scoliosis is considered to be a varus deformity.

Match the definitions in column B with the terms in column A.

Column A	*Column B*
11. __d__ Supination	a. Potential space, often filled with fluid between two layers that move on each other to decrease friction
12. __i__ Pronation	
13. __f__ Eversion	
14. __e__ Inversion	b. To move toward the medial line
15. __j__ Abduction	c. The rounded protuberance at the end of a bone
16. __b__ Adduction	
17. __c__ Condyle	d. The position of the hand in which the palmar surface faces upward
18. __a__ Bursa	
19. __g__ Varus	e. Turning inward toward the median
20. __h__ Valgus	f. Turning out and away from the median
	g. Bowlegs
	h. Knock-knees
	i. The position of the hand in which the palmar surface faces downward
	j. Movement of the part away from the midline

21. Which of the following musculoskeletal problems does *not* involve the joint?
 ☐ a. Sprain
 ☐ b. Rheumatoid arthritis
 ☐ c. Bursitis
 ☒ d. Tendonitis
 ☐ e. Gout

22. Having the client bend forward to touch his toes is done:
 ☒ a. to check spinal range of motion
 ☐ b. with the examiner standing in front of the client
 ☒ c. to make spinal deformities easier to detect
 ☒ d. with the examiner standing behind the client
 ☐ e. to evaluate balance
 ☐ f. a, c, and e
 ☐ g. a, b, and c
 ☒ h. a, c, and d
 ☐ i. b, c, and e
 ☐ j. all the above

23. The muscle wasting and decreasing muscle strength in an older adult is due to:
    - ☐ a. the muscle tissues collecting increased amounts of collagen
    - ☐ b. stenosis of the muscle fibers
    - ☐ c. fibrosis of connective tissue
    - ☐ d. decompensation of muscle mass due to arteriosclerosis
    - ☐ e. a, b, and d
    - ☐ f. b and d
    - ☑ g. a and c
    - ☐ h. all the above

24. Susan Mulligan, a 24-year-old pregnant client, comes to you because of a repeated "charley horse" in her right leg. Which of the following techniques would you recommend to her to stop the muscle cramp? (Select the *best* answer.)
    - ☐ a. Massage the leg until it stops.
    - ☐ b. Plantar flex the right foot to stop the cramp.
    - ☑ c. Dorsiflex the right foot to stop the cramp.
    - ☐ d. Elevation of the leg from the hip will stop the cramp.

25. Which of the following is not part of a joint?
    - ☐ a. Synovial membrane
    - ☑ b. Bone
    - ☐ c. Ligament
    - ☐ d. Capsule
    - ☐ e. Muscle

26. For which *one* of the following clients would a measurement of muscle mass be most important?
    - ☐ a. Routine physical of a 46-year-old with a 20-year history of polio and resulting crippling of the right side
    - ☐ b. An 18-year-old football player who "sprained" his ankle 2 hours ago
    - ☐ c. A 30-year-old man who just had a cast removed from his right leg following a motorcycle accident 6 weeks ago
    - ☑ d. A 58-year-old man who had a right-sided stroke 2 weeks ago
    - ☐ e. A 24-year-old pregnant woman with a 4-day history of fluid retention

27. Gait evaluation is an important part of muscular skeletal assessment. Which of the following should be included in the client's gait evaluation?
    - ☐ a. Phase
    - ☐ b. Cadence
    - ☐ c. Stride length
    - ☐ d. Trunk posture
    - ☐ e. Pelvic posture
    - ☐ f. Arm swing
    - ☐ g. All except e
    - ☐ h. All except b
    - ☐ i. All except a
    - ☐ j. All except f
    - ☑ k. All the above

28. Painless nodules commonly found around the tendon sheaths of the wrist are:
    - ☑ a. ganglia
    - ☐ b. fovea
    - ☐ c. tophi
    - ☐ d. tenalgia
    - ☐ e. rheumatoid nodules

29. The best instruction you can offer to a client who wants to know what to do in case of a muscle cramp is:
    - ☑ a. tell him to stretch the muscle fibers of the cramping muscle by placing the limb in a position that will stretch the affected muscle
    - ☐ b. rub the area vigorously until the cramp goes away
    - ☐ c. apply ice to the cramping muscle
    - ☐ d. apply heat to the cramping muscle
    - ☐ e. none of the above
30. Basic evaluation of the musculoskeletal system of a nonsymptomatic adult should at minimum include:
    - ☐ a. assessment of activities of daily living
    - ☐ b. gait
    - ☐ c. spine curvature
    - ☐ d. joint evaluation
    - ☐ e. tissue evaluation around joints
    - ☐ f. muscle mass evaluation
    - ☐ g. muscle strength evaluation (make/break)
    - ☐ h. all the above
    - ☐ i. all except e
    - ☑ j. all except f
    - ☐ k. all except g
    - ☐ l. all except c

PEDIATRIC QUESTIONS

31. The normal spinal curvature of the child is different from that of the adult. Identify the *correct* curvature from the following descriptions.
    - ☑ a. The thoracic convexity is decreased and the lumbar concavity is increased.
    - ☐ b. The thoracic concavity is decreased and the lumbar convexity is increased.
    - ☐ c. The thoracic convexity is increased and the lumbar concavity is decreased.
    - ☐ d. The thoracic concavity is increased and the lumbar convexity is decreased.
32. Much of the skeletal makeup of the small child is cartilaginous tissue. Ossification of most bones occurs by _____ of age.
    - ☐ a. 8 months
    - ☐ b. 2 years
    - ☐ c. 5 years
    - ☐ d. 8 years
    - ☑ e. 12 years
33. A parent brings an 18-month-old child for evaluation because the child has "flat feet." All the following statements are true except one. Identify the *false* statement.
    - ☐ a. When a child begins to stand, his feet normally pronate inward.
    - ☐ b. The flap of skin that makes the child's feet appear flat is actually adipose tissue and will disappear as the child grows older.
    - ☑ c. There is no such thing as flat feet in children.
    - ☐ d. Before the weight-bearing period there really is no medial arch of the foot.
    - ☐ e. When the child assumes a wide-base stance, the weight line normally falls on the medial aspect of the foot, giving the appearance that the child has flat feet.

34. Which of the following children should be referred because of a lag in motor development?
    - ☐ a. Four-month-old Kara, who is unable to sit by herself
    - ☑ b. Eight-month-old William, who is unable to roll from prone to supine position and back to prone position
    - ☐ c. Nine-month-old Ryan, who is unable to pull himself into a standing position
    - ☐ d. Two-year-old Lynn, who is unable to build a four-block tower
    - ☐ e. Jason, 3½, who is unable to skip

35. Behaviors for evaluating the gross motor development of 3-year-old Stephen are:
    - ☐ a. able to jump in place
    - ☐ b. able to walk up stairs, alternating feet on steps
    - ☐ c. able to walk down stairs, two feet on each step
    - ☐ d. pedals a tricycle
    - ☐ e. able to walk a straight line, one foot in front of other
    - ☐ f. all the above
    - ☐ g. all except c
    - ☑ h. all except e
    - ☐ i. a, b, and e
    - ☐ j. c, d, and e

36. Certain orthopedic conditions are typically associated with pubertal growth. When developing a routine for evaluating the musculoskeletal system of both teenage boys and girls, thorough emphasis should be placed on:
    - ☐ a. evaluation of the hands
    - ☑ b. evaluation of the knees
    - ☐ c. evaluation of the ankles
    - ☐ d. evaluation of the spine
    - ☑ e. evaluation of the hips
    - ☐ f. none of the above
    - ☐ g. all except a
    - ☐ h. b, c, and e
    - ☑ i. b, d, and e
    - ☐ j. all the above

GERIATRIC QUESTIONS

37. By the time an individual is 70 years old:
    - ☐ a. he usually manifests a 50% loss of muscle strength
    - ☐ b. arthritis of the hip and knee joints are symptomatic
    - ☐ c. he often manifests a longer edurance rate with isometric contractions
    - ☑ d. none of the above

38. Some of the risk factors associated with diminished physical functioning in elderly individuals are:
    - ☐ a. sedentary life style
    - ☐ b. altered mental state
    - ☐ c. obesity
    - ☐ d. pain
    - ☐ e. diminished circulatory supply to body parts
    - ☐ f. a, d, and e
    - ☐ g. a, b, and c
    - ☑ h. all the above
    - ☐ i. a, c, and d

39. Early or mild weakness of lower extremities:
  - ☐ a. is usually easily validated with make/break assessment procedures
  - ☐ b. is always unilateral
  - ☑ c. may be identified by asking client to climb a step
  - ☐ d. none of the above
40. The joints most commonly involved with symptomatic arthritis are:
  - ☐ a. wrists
  - ☑ b. knees
  - ☑ c. hips
  - ☐ d. ankles
  - ☑ e. lumbar spine
  - ☑ f. b, c, and e
  - ☐ g. b, c, and d
  - ☐ h. a, d, and e
  - ☐ i. all the above
41. In a normally functioning gait:
  - ☑ a. the gluteus maximus helps to stabilize the hip while one foot is in stance position
  - ☑ b. the tibial dorsiflexors decelerate the foot as it approaches heel strike
  - ☐ c. the upper torso often sways from side to side to maintain balance
  - ☐ d. none of the above
  - ☑ e. a and b

SUGGESTED READINGS
General

Bates, Barbara: A guide to physical examination, ed. 2, Philadelphia, 1979, J. B. Lippincott Co., pp. 272-310.

DeGowin, Elmer, and DeGowin, Richard: Bedside diagnostic examination, ed. 3, New York, 1976, Macmillan Publishing Co., Inc.

Judge, Richard D., and Zuidema, George, editors: Methods of clinical examination: a physiologic approach, Boston, 1974, Little, Brown & Co., pp. 285-305.

Malasanos, Lois, Barkauskas, Violet, Moss, Muriel, and Stoltenberg-Allen, Kathryn: Health assessment, St. Louis, 1977, The C. V. Mosby Co., pp. 305-366.

Nordmark, Madelyn T., and Rohweder, Anne W.: Scientific foundations of nursing, ed. 2, Philadelphia, 1967, J. B. Lippincott Co., p. 145.

Piercey, Maureen L.: Assessment of low back pain, Nurse Pract. **1**(4):18-21, Mar.-Apr., 1976.

Prior, John A., and Silberstein, Jack S.: Physical diagnosis: the history and examination of the patient, ed. 5, St. Louis, 1977, The C. V. Mosby Co., pp. 424-444.

Pediatric

Alexander, Mary, and Brown, Marie Scott: Pediatric physical diagnosis for nurses, New York, 1974, McGraw-Hill Book Co., pp. 189-208.

Barness, Lewis: Manual of pediatric physical diagnosis, ed. 4, Chicago, 1972, Year Book Medical Publishers, Inc., pp. 144-164.

Coley, Ida Lou: Pediatric assessment of self care activities, St. Louis, 1978, The C. V. Mosby Co.

Daniel, William A., Jr.: Adolescents in health and disease, St. Louis, 1977, The C. V. Mosby Co., pp. 363-377.

DeAngelis, Catherine: Basic pediatrics for primary health care providers, Boston, 1975, Little, Brown & Co., pp. 57-60, 86-93, 231-237.

Erickson, Marcene: Assessment and management of developmental changes in children, St. Louis, 1976, The C. V. Mosby Co.

McMillan, Julia, Nieburg, Phillip, and Oski, Frank: The whole pediatrician catalog, Philadelphia, 1977, W. B. Saunders Co., pp. 38-42.

Pillitteri, Adele: Nursing care of the growing family: a child health text, Boston, 1977, Little, Brown & Co., pp. 128-139, 166-168, 191-193, 219-223.

Geriatric

Andriola, Michael J.: When an elderly patient complains of weakness . . ., Geriatrics **33**(6):79-84, 1978.

Caird, F. I., and Judge, T. G.: Assessment of the elderly patient, London, 1977, Pitman Medical Publishing Co. Ltd., pp. 65-86.

Chinn, Austin B., editor: Clinical aspects of aging, Working with older people: a guide to practice, vol. 4, Rockville, Md., 1971, U.S. Department of Health, Education, and Welfare, Public Health Service, pp. 156-179.

Eliopoulos, Charlotte: Gerontological nursing, New York, 1979, Harper & Row, Publishers, pp. 196-206.

Steinberg, Franz U., editor: Cowdry's the care of the geriatric patient, St. Louis, 1976, The C. V. Mosby Co., pp. 119-132, 403-432.

Woodruff, Diana S., and Birren, James; Aging: scientific perspectives and social issues, New York, 1975, D. Van Nostrand Co., pp. 257-276.

CHAPTER 15

Assessment of the neurological system

Overview

Although the techniques of the neurological examination are fairly easy to implement, the interpretation of findings is complex. The examiner is challenged to understand the physiological interpretations of the elicited responses during neurological testing. References for response interpretations are listed under the suggested readings for this chapter.

Assessment of the neurological system may range from a basic screening of function to a highly detailed and lengthy process. This chapter details the process for performing a *screening* neurological examination for asymptomatic clients. The examination evaluates six major areas:

1. Mental assessment and speech patterns
2. Cranial nerves
3. Proprioception and cerebellar function
4. Muscular function
5. Sensory function
6. Reflex function

If the examiner identifies abnormalities in any of the findings, a more detailed evaluation and referral are warranted.

Cognitive objectives

At the end of this unit the learner will demonstrate knowledge of assessment of the neurological system by the ability to do the following.

1. Define the terms in the vocabulary list.
2. List each of the twelve cranial nerves and define the tests used to assess their integrity and the normal and abnormal responses.
3. List the functions of the cerebellum and define the tests used to assess its integrity and the normal and abnormal responses.
4. Describe the differences between the upper and lower motor neurons.
5. Describe the differences between the pyramidal and extrapyramidal tracts and define the tests used to assess their integrity and the normal and abnormal responses.
6. List the sensory modalities usually tested during a screening neurological examination and discuss the normal and abnormal responses.
7. List the deep tendon reflexes examined during a neurological examination, the site of stimulus, and normal and abnormal responses.
8. Describe the evaluation techniques and the significance of the Babinski reflex and clonus.
9. Explain the relationship of a reflex arc and a deep tendon reflex.
10. Identify selected characteristics of the pediatric neurological examination.
11. Identify selected characteristics of the geriatric neurological examination.

Clinical objectives

At the end of this unit the learner will perform a systematic assessment of the neurological system, demonstrating the ability to do the following:

1. Obtain a health history appropriate to the screening evaluation of the neurological system.
2. Demonstrate testing of the cranial nerves.
3. Demonstrate testing methods to evaluate the intactness of the proprioception and cerebellar systems.
   a. Use two techniques to evaluate general intactness.
   b. Use two techniques to evaluate upper extremity intactness.
   c. Use one method to evaluate lower extremity intactness.
4. Demonstrate testing methods to evaluate the intactness of sensation, including:
   a. Light touch sensation
   b. Painful sensation

c. Vibratory sensation

5. Demonstrate one method by which to evaluate cortical and discriminatory forms of sensation.
6. Demonstrate testing of the deep tendon reflexes, including biceps, triceps, brachioradialis, patellar, and Achilles reflexes.
7. Demonstrate testing of pathological reflexes, including Babinski response, and the test for ankle clonus.
8. Summarize results of the assessment with a written description of findings.

Health history related to neurological assessment additional to data base

1. Any positive finding collected during the screening history should be further explored to describe its characteristics as well as its relation to the client's ability to function. For example, if a client complains of shooting pains in the right leg, the examiner should describe (a) the characteristics of the leg pain (symptom analysis) and (b) how that leg pain interferes with activities of daily living.
2. Complaints such as weakness, nervousness, tremors, or tics should be fully investigated regarding symptom analysis as well as how they interfere with the client's ability to maintain activities of daily living.
3. Clients with complaints of balance problems need further questioning to determine how that problem is precipitated (i.e., position, time of day, activity related, etc.).

4. The term *convulsions* has many meanings. If the client gives this complaint, in-depth data must be collected to document what this term means to the client. Note the following:
   a. What happens to the client's eyes during a convulsion?
   b. Parts of the body involved?
   c. Muscles flaccid vs. stiff, tense vs. twitching?
   d. How long does this last?
   e. How many times during past day, week, month, year, years?
   f. Current medications?
   g. Cause?
   h. Interference with activities of daily living, driving, occupation?
5. Head injury and headache history profiles are discussed under health history in Chapter 4.
6. For the client complaining of pain associated with the neurological system, symptom analysis should be performed. The following may be helpful in evaluating the characteristics of that pain:
   a. Quality of pain: dull ache, throbbing, sharp or stabbing, burning, pressing, stinging, cramping, gnawing, pricking, shooting
   b. Associated manifestation: crying, decreased activities, sweating, muscle rigidity or tremor, impaired mental processes or concentration
7. Objective data can be collected during the history session by noting evidence of factors such as abnormalities in speech, language function, memory, emotional status, and judgment.

Clinical guidelines

The student will:	To identify:	
	Normal	**Deviations from normal**
1. Gather equipment necessary to perform the screening neurological examination: **a.** Penlight **b.** Tongue blade **c.** Safety pin **d.** Tuning fork (200 to 400 cps) **e.** Cotton wisp **f.** Percussion hammer **g.** Odorous materials		
Mental and speech pattern (mental health status has been previously discussed) **1.** Speech pattern **a.** Assess during data base collection	Client gives information requested Speech smooth and flowing Logical thought process Able to relate past events	Error in choice of words or syllables Difficulty in articulation: may involve thought process, tongue, or lips Slurred speech (tone sounds slurred) Poorly coordinated or irregular speech

Continued.

Clinical guidelines–cont'd

The student will:	To identify:	
	Normal	**Deviations from normal**
	Voice tone has inflections Strong voice able to increase volume Clear voice	Monotone voice Weak voice Nasal tone, rasping or hoarse, whisper voice Stuttering

Cranial nerves

1. CN I: olfactory nerve
   a. Obtain information through history or instruct client to close eyes and properly identify aromatic substance held under the nose (Fig. 15-1): coffee, toothpaste, orange, oil of clove; test one nostril at a time

Client correctly identifies item and odor

Unable to smell anything; incorrect identifica-

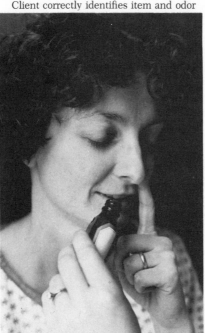

Fig. 15-1. Evaluating CN I (olfactory).

2. CN II: optic nerve(Fig. 15-2) (described in Chapter 7)
   a. Testing visual acuity
   b. Funduscopy examination
   c. Visual fields by confrontation

As previously discussed in Chapter 7

As previously discussed in Chapter 7

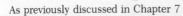
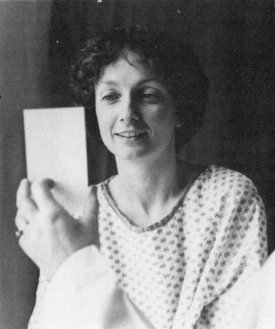

Fig. 15-2. Evaluating CN II (optic).

The student will:	To identify:	
	Normal	Deviations from normal
3. CN III: oculomotor nerve (Fig. 15-3) (described in Chapter 7)	As previously discussed in Chapter 7	As previously described in Chapter 7

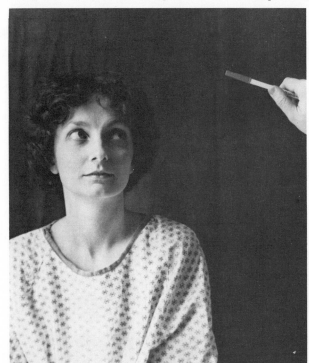

Fig. 15-3. Evaluating CN III (oculomotor).

The student will:	To identify:	
4. CN IV: trochlear nerve (Fig. 15-4) (described in Chapter 7)	As previously described in Chapter 7	As previously described in Chapter 7

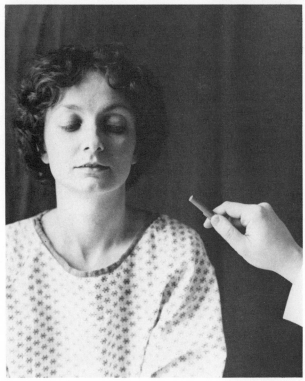

Fig. 15-4. Evaluating CN IV (trochlear).

Continued.

Clinical guidelines–cont'd

The student will:	To identify:	
	Normal	Deviations from normal
5. CN V: trigeminal nerve		
a. Test *motor* function, instructing client to clench the teeth; then palpate temporal and masseter muscles (Fig. 15-5)	Bilaterally strong muscle contractions	Inequality in muscle contractions Pain with muscle contractions Twitching Asymmetry in movement of jaw
b. Test *sensory* function with client's eyes closed		
1. Light sensation: wipe cotton wisp lightly over client's anterior scalp and paranasal sinuses (Fig. 15-6)	Tickle sensation, equally present over palpated areas	Decreased or unequal sensation

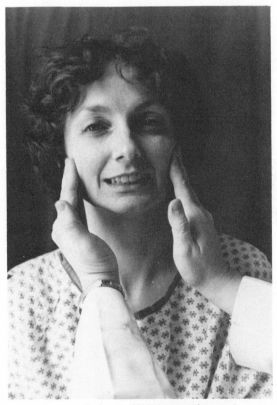

Fig. 15-5. Evaluating CN V (trigeminal—motor).

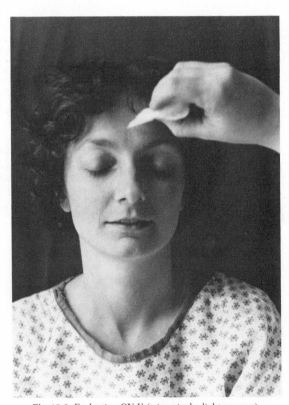

Fig. 15-6. Evaluating CN V (trigeminal—light sensory).

The student will:	To identify:	
	Normal	Deviations from normal
2. Deep sensation: use alternating blunt and sharp ends of safety pin over client's forehead and paranasal sinus areas (Fig. 15-7)	Able to feel pressure and pain equally throughout Able to differentiate between sharp and dull	Decreased or unequal sensation
3. Corneal reflex: use cotton wisp on cornea; instruct client to look up (approach from side) (Fig. 15-8)	Bilateral blink to corneal touch	No blink (make sure abnormal response not due to contact lenses)

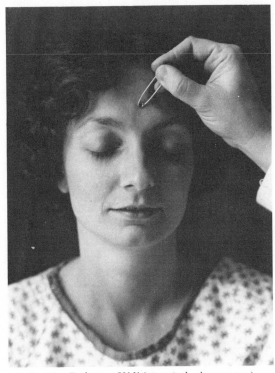

Fig. 15-7. Evaluating CN V (trigeminal—deep sensory).

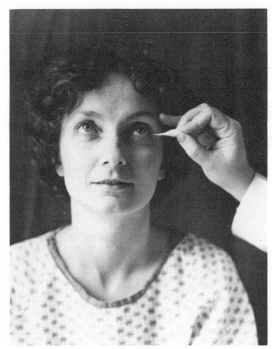

Fig. 15-8. Evaluating CN V (trigeminal—corneal reflex).

Continued.

Clinical guidelines–cont'd

The student will:	To identify:	
	Normal	**Deviations from normal**
6. CN VI: abducens nerve (described in Chapter 7) (Fig. 15-9)	As previously described in Chapter 7	As previously described in Chapter 7

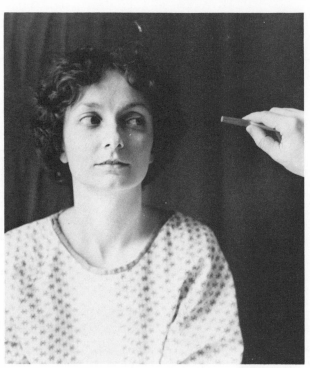

Fig. 15-9. Evaluating CN VI (abducens).

7. CN VII: facial nerve		
a. Inspect face both at rest and during conversation	Symmetry of face	Asymmetry, unequal movements, facial weakness
		Drooping on one side of face or mouth

b. Instruct client to:
    1. Raise eyebrows
    2. Frown
    3. Close eyes tight
    4. Show teeth
    5. Smile
    6. Puff out cheeks (Fig. 15-10)
		Unable to maintain position until instructed to relax

c. Evaluate taste over anterior half of tongue (sensory branch of facial nerve) with sugar, salt, lemon juice (sour), or quinine (bitter); use cotton applicator to place small quantity of substance on client's tongue	Able to correctly identify taste	Unable to identify substance Consistently identifies substance incorrectly

Continued.

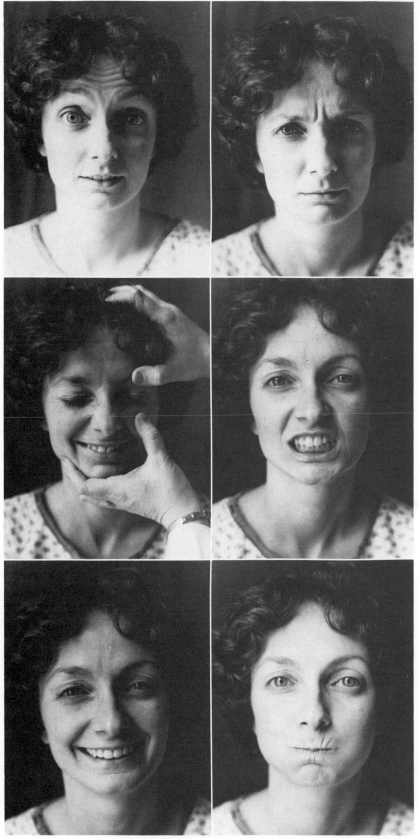

Fig. 15-10. Evaluating CN VII (facial).

Clinical guidelines—cont'd

The student will:	To identify:	
	Normal	Deviations from normal
8. CN VIII: acoustic nerve (Fig. 15-11); hearing assessment described in Chapter 6	As previously described in Chapter 6	As previously described in Chapter 6

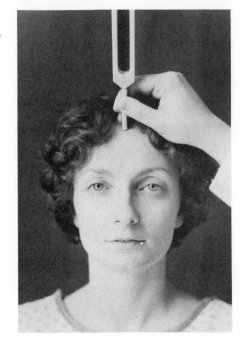

Fig. 15-11. Evaluating CN VIII (acoustic).

9. CN IX: glossopharyngeal nerve CN X: vagus nerve (tested together)		
a. Instruct client to say "ah" (Fig. 15-12)	Bilaterally equal upward movement of soft palate and uvula Speech smooth	Asymmetry of soft palate movement or tonsillar pillar movement; lateral deviation of uvula

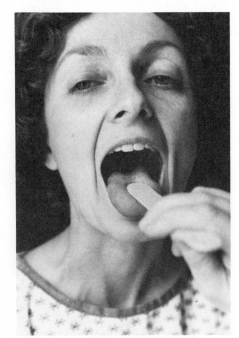

Fig. 15-12. Evaluating CN IX (glossopharyngeal) and CN X (vagus).

The student will:	To identify:	
	Normal	**Deviations from normal**
b. If posterior portion of tongue or pharynx is stimulated:	Gag will occur	Gag reflex absent
1. Taste: posterior third of tongue (by history)	Able to taste sweet, salt, sour	Unable to differentiate tastes
10. CN XI: spinal accessory nerve		
a. Instruct client to shrug shoulders upward against examiner's hand (Fig. 5-13, *A*)	Strength and symmetry of contraction of trapezius muscles	Muscle weakness: unilateral, bilateral Pain or discomfort

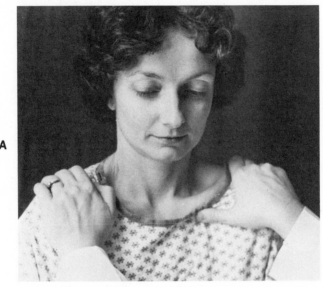

Fig. 15-13. A, Evaluating CN XI (spinal accessory).

b. Have patient turn head to side against examiner's hand; repeat with other side (Fig. 15-13, *B*)	Observe contraction of opposite sternocleidomastoid muscle; note force of movement against examiner's hand	Unable to maintain contracted muscle position Asymmetry, difficulty of movement

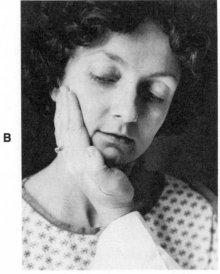

Fig. 15-3, cont'd. B, Evaluating CN XI (spinal accessory).

Continued.

Clinical guidelines–cont'd

	To identify:	
The student will:	**Normal**	**Deviations from normal**

11. CN XII: hypoglossal nerve
   a. Motor development of tongue
      1. Instruct client to stick tongue out and move from side to side (Fig. 15-14)
	As previously described in Chapter 5	As previously described in Chapter 5

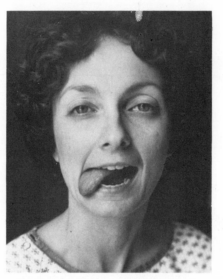

Fig. 15-14. Evaluating CN XII (hypoglossal).

Proprioception, cerebellar, and motor function

Three areas of coordination and motor function will be evaluated:

1. General function
2. Upper extremity function
3. Lower extremity function

Following are examination techniques for the evaluation of proprioception, cerebellar, and motor functions. For the nonsymptomatic client the examiner is encouraged to use at least *two* techniques for each area to be assessed. Which two the examiner chooses may depend on the age and overall physical ability of the client. For example, it is not necessary for every client to perform deep knee bends.

Motor function depends on the intactness of three areas:

1. Intact muscles
2. Functioning of the neuromuscular junction
3. Intact cranial and spinal nerves

More specifically, proprioception and cerebellar function depend on the intactness of the upper and lower neurons and the cerebellar system.

The *upper motor neurons* originate in the cerebral cortex and project downward. These neurons make up the corticobulbar tract, which ends in the brain stem, and the corticospinal tract (or pyramidal tract), which ends in the anterior horn of the spinal cord. This tract is responsible for particularly fine and discrete conscious movement.

Malfunctioning within the corticospinal tract will cause a paralysis or spasticity response. Deep tendon reflexes will increase, and the client will experience decreased voluntary functioning of fine motor ability.

The *lower motor neurons* originate in the anterior horn cells of the spinal cord, leave the spinal cord, and travel to and innervate the muscle fibers. Injury or disease affecting the lower motor neurons will result in decreased or absent muscle tone, reflexes, or strength. The examiner will observe local or general muscle wasting and atrophy as well as fasciculations of affected areas.

The *extrapyramidal motor neurons* originate in the cerebral cortex but lie outside the pyramidal or corticospinal tracts. Their function is to help maintain muscle tone and gross body movements such as walking. Clients may have disease of the pyramidal tract and still maintain gross body functioning because of the intactness of the extrapyramidal and lower motor neurons.

If the client is functioning by using the extrapyramidal system, the examiner would expect to find slow or sluggish voluntary movement, slowed coordination, and decrease in fine motor functioning. The reflexes would be normal.

The *proprioception and cerebellar systems* function to maintain posture and balance. Any malfunctioning of this area would impair muscle coordination or the ability to perform movements smoothly. Muscle tone may be decreased, and the examiner may find that following the deep tendon reflex examination the limb tends to "swing."

The student will:	To identify:	
	Normal	Deviations from normal
1. General (use two for screening of gross motor and balance testing) **a.** Assess client's gait function by asking client to walk across room, turn, and walk back	Maintains upright posture, walks unaided maintaining balance, opposing arm swing	Poor posturing, ataxia, unsteady gait, rigid or no arm movements, wide-base gait, trunk and head held tight, legs bend from hips only, client lurches or reels, scissors gait, steppage gait, staggering gait, parkinsonian gait (stooped posture, flexion at hips, elbows, knees)
b. Perform the Romberg test by asking client to stand with feet together, arms resting at sides, first with eyes open, then with eyes closed (Fig. 15-15)	Slight swaying, but upright posture and foot stance maintained	Unable to maintain foot stance; moves to wider foot base to maintain posture

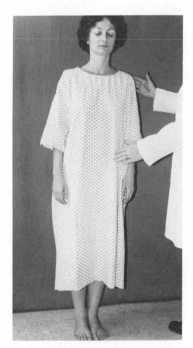

Fig. 15-15. Balance testing using Romberg test.

Continued.

Clinical guidelines–cont'd

The student will:	To identify:	
	Normal	Deviations from normal
c. Instruct client to walk a straight line, placing the heel of one foot directly against the toes of the other foot (Fig. 15-16)	Able to maintain heel-toe walking pattern along straight line	Unable to maintain heel-toe walking pattern Steps to wider-based gait to maintain upright posture

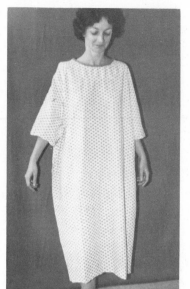

Fig. 15-16. Evaluating balance by having client walk a straight line.

The student will:	Normal	Deviations from normal
d. Instruct client to close eyes and stand on one foot and then the other (Fig. 15-17)	Able to maintain position for at least 5 seconds	Unable to maintain single-foot balancing for 5 seconds

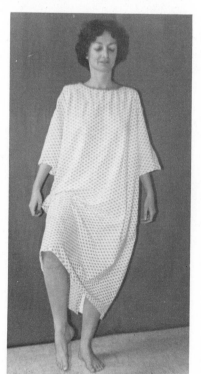

Fig. 15-17. One-foot balance testing with eyes closed.

The student will:	To identify:	
	Normal	**Deviations from normal**
e. Hopping in place: instruct client to first hop on one foot and then the other (Fig. 15-18)	Able to follow directions sucessfully Muscle strength adequate to follow through	Unable to hop or to maintain single-leg balance

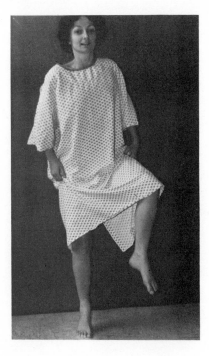

Fig. 15-18. Evaluating balance by having client hop in place.

f. Knee bends: instruct client to hold hands outward and perform several shallow or deep knee bends (Fig. 15-19)	Able to follow directions successfully Muscle strength adequate to follow through	Unable to perform activity due to balance difficulty or muscle strength

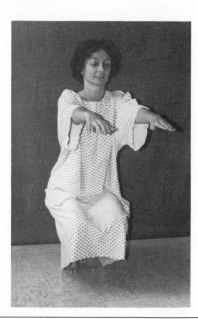

Fig. 15-19. Balance testing by having client perform deep knee bends.

Continued.

Clinical guidelines–cont'd

	To identify:	
The student will:	**Normal**	**Deviations from normal**
g. Walk on toes, then heels	Able to follow directions by walking several steps on toes and then heels May need to use hands to maintain balance	Unable to maintain balance Poor muscle strength Unable to complete activity
2. Upper extremity testing (use two for screening of upper extremity and fine motor testing) **a.** Using pronation and supination of hands, instruct client to alternately tap knees (do both hands together); use rapid movement (see Fig. 14-16)	Bilaterally equal timing Purposeful movement Able to maintain rapid pace	Unequal movement Sloppy or increasingly sloppy movement Unable to maintain rapid pace
b. With arm stretched outward, instruct client to use index fingers to alternately touch nose (eyes closed) rapidly (Fig. 15-20)	Able to repeatedly touch nose Rhythmic response	Sloppy response Misses nose many times Arms unable to maintain testing position, drift downward

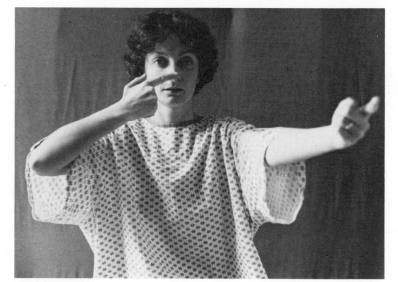

Fig. 15-20. Evaluating fine motor function by having client touch nose with alternating hands.

c. Evaluate client's ability to perform rapid rhythmic alternating movement of fingers (test each hand separately); ask client to touch each finger to the thumb, in rapid sequence (Fig. 15-21)	Can rapidly and purposefully touch each finger to thumb	Unable to coordinate fine, discrete, rapid movement

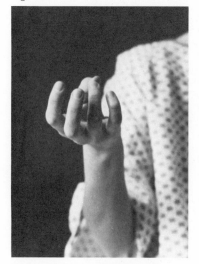

Fig. 15-21. Evaluating fine motor function by rapid rhythmic alternating movement of fingers.

The student will:	To identify:	
	Normal	Deviations from normal
d. Instruct client to rapidly move index finger back and forth between client's nose and examiner's finger (approximately 46 cm [18 inches] apart); test one hand at a time (Fig. 15-22)	Able to maintain activity with conscious coordinated effort	Unable to maintain continuous touch with both own nose and examiner's finger Unable to maintain rapid movement Coordination difficulty obvious

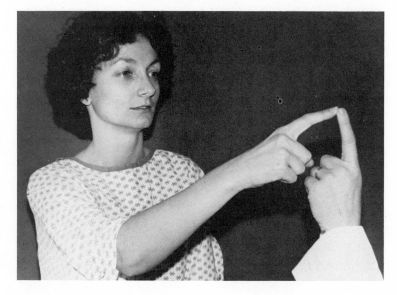

Fig. 15-22. Evaluating fine motor function by rapid movement of client's finger between own nose and examiner's finger.

3. Lower extremity testing for fine motor function		
a. Instruct seated client to place the heel of one foot just below opposite knee on the tibia; then instruct client to run heel down the shin to the foot; repeat with other foot (Fig. 15-23)	Able to purposefully run heel down opposite shin Bilaterally equal coordination	Unable to coordinate activity Heel keeps moving off shin Unequal responses Tremors or awkwardness

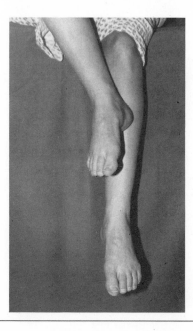

Fig. 15-23. Evaluating fine motor function by having client run heel of one foot down tibia of other leg.

Continued.

Clinical guidelines–cont'd

	To identify:	
The student will:	**Normal**	**Deviations from normal**

Muscular function

Muscle function and strength testing are discussed in Chapter 14.

Sensory function

This component of the examination evaluates the intactness of the dermatomes and major peripheral nerves. The examiner must have knowledge of normal dermatome areas and the spinal nerves represented as well as the major peripheral nerves and areas of sensation.

The examiner should test the peripheral extremities in several areas for sensation. If sensation is intact, no further extremity evaluation is necessary. If the peripheral sensation is impaired, the examiner should move up the extremities, testing periodically until a level or area of sensation is identified. Beyond the extremities the examiner should also evaluate the forehead, the cheeks, and the abdomen.

If a deviation is identified, try to map out the area involved.

The examiner must compare bilateral responses in each of the following sensation testing categories.

1. Primary sensory screening
   a. Light touch sensation: use cotton wisp to lightly touch each designated area (client's eyes closed) (Fig. 15-24)

Client perceives light sensation
Client able to correctly point to spot where touched

Unable to perceive touch
Incorrectly identifies touched location
Asymmetrical response

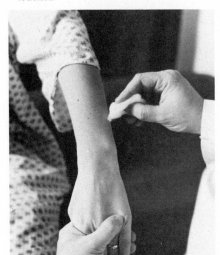
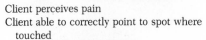

Fig. 15-24. Evaluating light sensory function of forearm (eyes closed).

   b. Painful sensation: using the pointed tip of a pin, lightly prick each designated area (client's eyes closed) (Fig. 15-25); (it may be helpful to alternate light and pain sensations to more accurately evaluate the client's response)

Client perceives pain
Client able to correctly point to spot where touched

Unable to perceive pain sensation
Incorrectly identifies touched location
Asymmetrical response

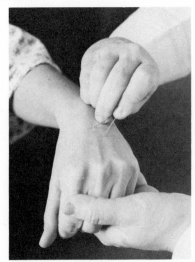

Fig. 15-25. Evaluating pain sensation (eyes closed).

	To identify:	
The student will:	**Normal**	**Deviations from normal**
c. Vibration sensation: have the client verbalize what is felt when a vibrating tuning fork is placed on a bony area of wrist, ankle, and sternum (Fig. 15-26)	Client feels sense of vibration (decreased sensation may be normal response in older adults)	Unequal or decreased vibratory sensations

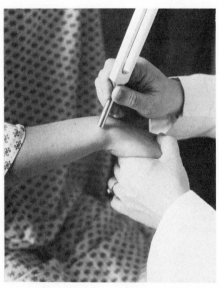

Fig. 15-26. Evaluating vibratory sensation over bony prominence.

2. Cortical and discriminatory forms of sensation (use one for screening)		
a. Stereognosis: place a small familiar object in the client's hand and ask client to identify it (Fig. 15-27)	Appropriate identification	Unable to correctly identify object

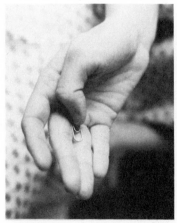

Fig. 15-27. Evaluating stereognosis by client's ability to properly identify a familiar object placed in the hand (eyes closed).

Continued.

Clinical guidelines—cont'd

	To identify:	
The student will:	**Normal**	**Deviations from normal**
b. Two-point discrimination: touch selected parts of the body simultaneously with two sharp objects (client's eyes closed); ask client if one or two objects are used (Fig. 15-28)	Can distinguish two-point discrimination Fingertips: 2.8 mm Palms: 8 to 12 mm Chest-forearm: 40 mm Back: 40 to 70 mm Upper arms-thigh: 75 mm	Unable to tell two-point discrimination within normal limits

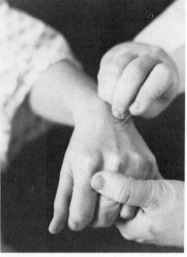

Fig. 15-28. Evaluating two-point discrimination of dorsal surface of hand (eyes closed).

c. Graphesthesia: use a blunt instrument to draw a number or letter on the client's hand, back, or other area (client's eyes closed) (Fig. 15-29)	Client able to recognize drawn number or letter	Client unable to distinguish number or letter

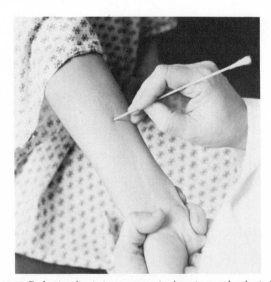

Fig. 15-29. Evaluating discriminatory sensation by using graphesthesia (eyes closed).

	To identify:	
The student will:	**Normal**	**Deviations from normal**
d. Kinesthetic sensation: with client's eyes closed, grasp client's finger and move its position (Fig. 15-30)	Client able to describe how finger position has changed	Unable to distinguish position change

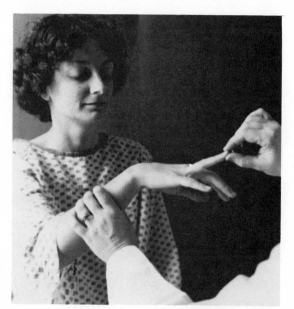

Fig. 15-30. Evaluating discriminatory sensation by using kinesthesia (eyes closed).

Reflex status

The reflex arc consists of five steps:
1. The receptor cells of the tendon are stimulated.
2. The nerve impulse travels along an afferent or sensory neuron from the receptor cells by means of the dorsal root until it synapses with an anterior horn cell.
3. After the synapse the impulse is transmitted directly or indirectly to an efferent neuron.
4. The impulse travels along the efferent or motor neuron by means of the ventral root until it innervates a skeletal muscle.
5. The skeletal muscle contracts.

When evaluating the client's reflexes, irritation or disruption to any portion of the reflex arc will result in disruption of the reflex response. This includes the areas previously discussed regarding corticospinal, sensory, or lower motor neuron disturbances. (See the clinical strategies for description of percussion technique and use of reinforcement.)

Deep tendon reflex responses are commonly scored as follows:
1. 4+ or + + + +: brisk, hyperactive, clonus
2. 3+ or + + +: more brisk than normal but not necessarily indicating disease
3. 2+ or + +: normal
4. 1+ or +: low normal; sluggish response
5. 0: no response

It will take a beginning examiner much practice and working with a preceptor to determine the actual clinical criteria for this scoring. In attempting to elicit an accurate response, the examiner must be confident that the technique being used is correct.

Continued.

Clinical guidelines–cont'd

The student will:	To identify:	
	Normal	**Deviations from normal**
1. Deep tendon reflexes (all are to be tested; client to be seated)		
a. Biceps reflex (tests C_5 and C_6): client's arm should be partially flexed at elbow, with palms down; examiner places thumb on biceps tendon and strikes reflex hammer on thumb toward tendon (Fig. 15-31)	Bilaterally equal response; responds rapidly Contraction of biceps	Hyperactive or diminished response Unequal response bilaterally

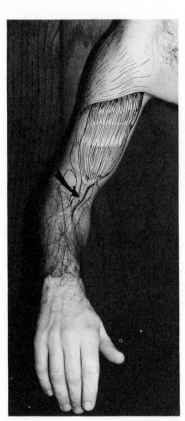

Fig. 15-31. Tendon of biceps brachialis muscle. (Percuss at arrow.)

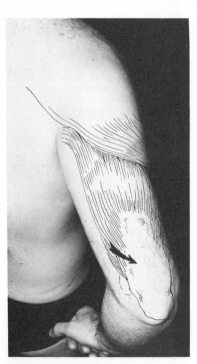

Fig. 15-32. Tendon of triceps muscle. (Percuss at arrow.)

b. Triceps tendon (tests C_6, C_7, and C_8): flex client's arm at elbow, palm relaxed at side of body; abduct elbow; strike triceps tendon above elbow (Fig. 15-32)	Extension of elbow and contraction of triceps muscle Bilaterally equal response	Hyperactive or diminished response Unequal response bilaterally

The student will:	To identify:	
	Normal	**Deviations from normal**
c. Brachioradialis tendon (tests C_5 and C_6: with client's forearm resting on abdomen or lap (palm down), strike radius 2.5 to 5 cm (1 to 2 inches) above wrist over tendon (Fig. 15-33)	Flexion of elbow and pronation of forearm Bilaterally equal response	Hyperactive or diminished response Unequal response bilaterally

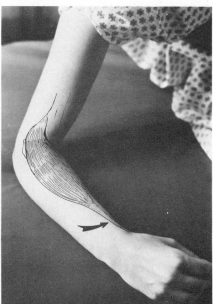

Fig. 15-33. Tendon of brachioradialis muscle. (Percuss at arrow.)

d. Abdominal reflexes (tests T_8, T_9, T_{10}, T_{11}, and T_{12}): with client lying, lightly stroke with sharp instrument both above and below umbilicus in directions as indicated (Fig. 15-34)	Abdominal muscles contract slightly Umbilicus moves slightly toward area of stimulus Bilaterally equal response	Absent or unilateral response

Fig. 15-34. Assessment of abdominal reflexes.

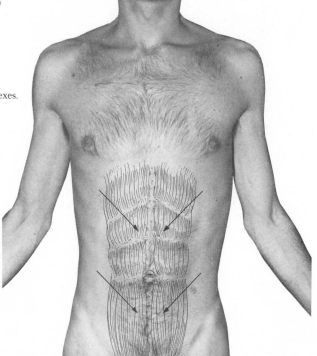

Continued.

Clinical guidelines–cont'd

The student will:	To identify:	
	Normal	Deviations from normal
e. Knee (patellar) reflex (tests L_2, L_3, and L_4): with client sitting or lying and knee flexed and relaxed, tap patellar tendon just below patella (Fig. 15-35)	Contraction of quadriceps with extension of lower leg from knee Bilaterally equal response	Hyperactive or diminished response Unequal response bilaterally
f. Ankle (Achilles) reflex (tests S_1 and S_2): with leg somewhat flexed at knee, dorsiflex ankle; strike Achilles tendon (Fig. 15-36)	Plantar flexion of foot at ankle Bilaterally equal response	Hyperactive or diminished response Unequal response bilaterally

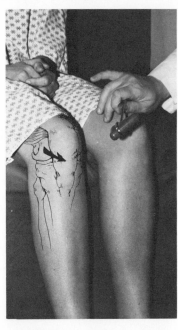

Fig. 15-35. Assessment of patellar tendon. (Percuss at arrow.)

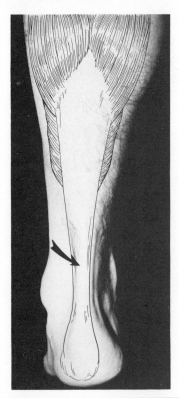

Fig. 15-36. Achilles tendon. (Percuss at arrow.)

The student will:	To identify:	
	Normal	**Deviations from normal**

2. Pathological reflexes
  a. Plantar (Babinski) response: using moderately sharp object, stroke lateral aspect of sole from heel to ball of foot, curving medially across ball (Fig. 15-37)

Flexion of great toe, with fanning of other toes

Extrusion of great toe, with fanning of other toes
Indicates pyramidal tract disease

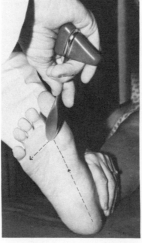

Fig. 15-37. Evaluating for plantar (Babinski) reflex.

  b. Test for ankle clonus (if reflexes are hyperactive): support knee in partly flexed position; with other hand, sharply dorsiflex foot and maintain in flexion (Fig. 15-38)

No movement of foot

Rhythmic oscillations between dorsiflexion and plantar flexion

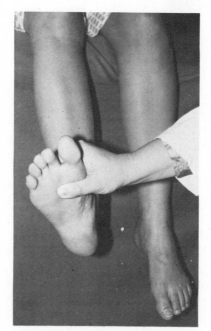

Fig. 15-38. Evaluating for ankle clonus.

Sample recording

Alert, oriented ×3, CN intact I to XII, coordinated movements and gait, negative Romberg. Cerebellar, sensory, and motor testing intact and bilaterally equal for both upper and lower extremities.
DTR intact, bilaterally equal, neither diminished nor hyperactive.

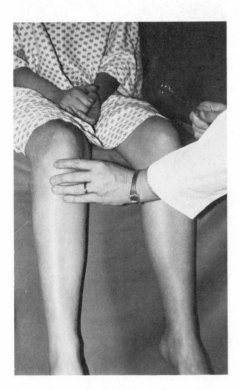

Fig 15-39. Percussing tendon.

Clinical strategies

1. Symmetry is the key!
2. There are numerous tests to screen the various neurological systems. Which specific set the examiner chooses is up to the individual. There should be consideration of the client's functional ability to understand and follow through. For example, deep knee bends or rapid alternating hand movement would not be appropriate for an older adult with osteoarthritis.
3. The important issue is to provide selected screening exercises in each of the designated areas. To skip a total area of assessment is inappropriate.
4. Develop a *method* to examine the neurological system and stick to that general method every time. This will prevent missing any aspect.

5. The percussion hammer, like all other assessment tools, must be correctly used to obtain the desired response. Following are several strategies:
   a. The client must be relaxed and the extremities loose.
   b. The limb should be positioned so that there is slight tension on the tendon to be evaluated. For example, flex the knee to approximately 90° prior to testing the patellar tendon.
   c. The examiner should hold the percussion hammer between the thumb and index finger loosely so that, as the examiner taps the desired tendon, the hammer is able to move in a smooth and rapid yet controlled direction.
   d. The action of percussion with a hammer should be just like the percussion used on the thorax or abdomen. The examiner should use a rapid wrist-flick motion to percuss the desired tendon.
      The tap should be quick, firm, and well directed. As soon as the tendon is tapped, the examiner should flick the wrist back so that the hammer doesn't remain on the tendon.
   e. Prior to the actual percussion, the examiner should palpate the desired tendon so that the precise location will be percussed (Fig. 15-39).
6. If the client is heavy, deep tendon reflexes may be very difficult to elicit. The examiner should spend time trying to specifically locate the tendon prior to striking it with the hammer.
7. If the examiner has difficulty eliciting the deep tendon reflex in a client who shows no signs of neurological dysfunction, several techniques may be tried.
   a. Change the client's position. If the client was sitting, try the technique with the client lying down. Any position may be used, as long as there is slight tension of the muscle or tendon being tested.
   b. If the examiner has difficulty eliciting the deep tendon reflex response of the lower extremity, it may be helpful to use Jendrassik's maneuver of reinforcement. The client locks the fingers together and pulls one hand against the other while the examiner attempts to elicit the lower leg reflexes.
   c. Reinforcement for the upper extremities may include instructing the client to tightly clench the teeth or tighten the muscles in the legs.
   d. If the examiner continues to have difficulty, the percussion technique should be reexamined.
8. Because of the vast complexity of the neurological examination, it must be reemphasized that the clinical guidelines presented in this chapter are

meant to be used for well adult screening. If the examiner is expected to examine a client with neurological dysfunction, there will be a need to gain additional skills.

History and clincial strategies associated with the pediatric client

1. The neurological assessment of children is unlike that of the adult because the central nervous system of babies and very young children is incompletely developed and in fact operates at a subcortical level. The newborn neurological examination reflects brain stem and spinal cord activity. As the child develops, and with increased myelinization and maturation of the neurological system, the examination becomes more like that for the adult client. The clinical guidelines for assessment of the pediatric client have four components: (a) assessment of infants under 1 year of age, (b) assessment of children 1 to 3 years of age, (c) assessment of children over age 3 years, and (d) screening assessment of neurological "soft" signs.

2. The data base history provided evaluative characteristics to accurately assess the maturational and neurological status of the child. In addition to this, the examiner should inquire about the mother's pregnancy when assessing a newborn or infant. Specifically, the mother should be queried regarding history of drug usage, infections, trauma, intoxication, and metabolic disturbances. A careful family history should be gathered regarding seizure disorders or systemic diseases such as muscular dystrophy or cerebral palsy.

3. The parents should be asked if the child has continued to grow and mature normally. Ask how this child's development compares to that of siblings.

4. Has the parent noted any clumsiness, unsteady gait, progressive muscular weakness, or unexplained falling? Describe.

5. Has the child experienced learning or school difficulties associated with attention, interest, activity level, or ability to concentrate?

6. Has the child had a head injury or neurological problems such as seizure, tremor, or weakness in the past? Describe in detail.

7. Have the parents noticed or has the child complained of any problems when going up and down stairs? Is there muscular weakness or weakness when getting up from a lying position on the floor? These are screening questions for muscular dystrophy and should be asked during an examination.

8. The neurological examination, like the musculoskeletal examination, begins as the examiner first meets the child. The examiner should note overall alertness, coordination, and body muscle tone. Observe the child undressing or the parent undressing the child. The examiner should observe for gross floppiness, incoordination, or weakness.

9. In older children, the examiner should evaluate language, as well as adaptive and motor behavior.

10. In younger children, the examiner should watch the child at play. Observe the infant lying on the examination table or sitting in the parent's lap. Observe the toddler moving around the room, taking off shoes, and using a pincer grip. Observations should include purposefulness of movements, symmetry, and motor tone.

11. The examiner must get a general impression of the child's abilities and responsiveness.

12. Even for young children, there must be some structure to neurological assessment. Although the examiner must be alert to neurological function and maturational development throughout the examination, there must be a designated time for actual reflex testing, motor tone evaluation, and cerebellar functioning. When the examiner incorporates these techniques does not matter. We recommend placing them in the middle of the examination. Although they are not considered intrusive procedures, such as the ear and throat examination, their successful evaluation is dependent on the full cooperation and enthusiasm of the child.

13. The Denver Developmental Screening Test (DDST) should be used to evaluate the personal-social, fine motor adaptive, language, and gross motor functioning of all children from ages 1 month through 6 years. This screening evaluation, described in numerous pediatric assessment texts, is meant to uncover "red flags" indicating lag in the child's development. The DDST evaluates neurological, musculoskeletal, and behavioral development. Every examiner should become familiar with this screening test and other similar tests, such as the Goodenough Draw-a-Man test, and incorporate them into practice on a regular screening basis.

14. Table 14 lists the milestones associated with normal neurological development. Note that the fine and gross motor criteria are the same as listed in Chapter 14, on assessment of the musculoskeletal system. These reflect items tested by the Denver Developmental Screening Test.

Table 14. Normal developmental milestones*†

Age	Fine motor	Gross motor	Social-adaptive	Language
1 month	Follows with eyes to midline	Turns head to side Keeps knees tucked under abdomen When pulled to sitting position has gross head lag and rounded swayed back	Regards face	Responds to bell
2 months	Follows objects well; may not follow past midline (major developmental milestone	Holds head in same plane as rest of body Can raise head and maintain position; looks downward	Smiles responsively	Vocalizes (not crying)
3 months	Follows past midline When in supine position puts hands together; will hold hands in front of face	Raises head to 45° angle Maintains posture Looks around with head May turn from prone to side position When pulled into sitting position shows only slight head lag		Laughs
4 months	Grasps rattle Plays with hands together	Actively lifts head up and looks around Will roll from prone to supine position When pulled to sitting position no longer has head lag When held in standing position attempts to maintain some weight support		Squeals
5 months	Can reach and pick up object May play with toes	Able to push up from prone position and maintain weight on forearms Rolls from prone to supine and back to prone Maintains straight back when in sitting position	Smiles spontaneously	
6 months	Will hold spoon or rattle Will drop object and reach for second offered object	Begins to raise abdomen off table Sits, but posture still shaky May sit with legs apart; holds arms straight as prop between legs Supports almost full weight when pulled to standing position		
7 months	Can transfer object, one hand to another Grasps objects in each hand	Sits alone; still uses hands for support When held in standing position bounces Puts feet to mouth		
8 months	Beginning thumb-finger grasping	Sits securely without support (major developmental milestone)	Feeds self crackers	Turns to voice
9 months	Continued development of finger-thumb grasp May bang objects together	Steady sitting; can lean forward and still maintain position		

*For more specific data see clinical guidelines.
†Data from Frankenburg, W. K., and Dodds, J. B.: The Denver Developmental Screening Test, J. Pediatr. **71:**181, 1967.

Age	Fine motor	Gross motor	Social-adaptive	Language
		Begins creeping (abdomen off floor)		
		Can stand holding onto stabilizing object when placed in that position; still may not be able to pull self into standing position		
10 months	Practices picking up small objects Points with one finger Will offer toys to people but unable to let go of objects	Can pull self into standing position; unable to let self down again	Plays peek-a-boo	
11 months		Moves about room holding onto objects Preparing to walk independently, widebase stance Stands securely, holding on with one hand		Imitates speech sound
12 months (1 year)	May hold cup and spoon and feed self fairly well with practice Can offer toys and release them	Able to twist and turn and maintain posture Able to sit from standing position May stand alone at least momentarily		"Dada" or "mama" specific
14 months			Plays pat-a-cake	
15 months	Can put raisins into bottle Will take off shoes and pull toys	Walks alone well Able to seat self in chair		
16 months			Plays ball with examiner	
18 months	Holds crayon Scribbles spontaneously (major developmental milestone)	May walk up and down stairs holding hand May show running ability		
20 months			Imitates housework	Three words other than "mama" or "dada"
24 months (2 years)	Able to turn doorknob Able to take off shoes and socks Able to build two-block tower Dumps raisins from bottle following demonstration	May walk up stairs by self, two feet on each step Able to walk backward Able to kick ball	Uses spoon	
28 months				Combines two words
30 months (2½ years)	Able to build four-block tower Scribbling techniques continue Feeding self with increased neatness Dumps raisins from bottle spontaneously	Able to jump from object Walking becomes more stable, wide-base gait decreases Throws ball overhanded		
36 months (3 years)	Can unbutton front buttons Copies vertical lines within 30° Copies 0 Able to build eight cube tower	Walks upstairs, alternating feet on steps Walks down stairs, two feet on each step Pedals tricycle Jumps in place Able to perform broad jump	Pulls on shoes	Follows two or three simple directions

Continued.

Table 14. Normal developmental milestones—cont'd

Age	Fine motor	Gross motor	Social-adaptive	Language
48 months (4 years)	Able to copy + Picks longer line three out of three times	Walks down stairs, alternating feet on steps Able to button large front buttons Able to balance on one foot for approximately 5 seconds	Dresses with supervision	Gives first and last name
60 months (5 years)	Able to dress self with minimal assistance Able to draw three-part human figure Draws □ following demonstration Colors within lines	Hops on one foot Catches ball bounced to child two out of three times Able to demonstrate heel-toe walking	Dresses without supervision	Recognizes three colors

15. Table 15 lists "red flags," or warning signs, to determine whether the child's neurological development is lagging. Although every expert would agree that children mature at different rates, norms for lag limits must be developed. If the examiner encounters a child who seems to have difficulty, special attention should be given to a thorough neurological examination, implementation of the Denver Developmental Screening Test or similar tool, and, finally, referral to a physician.

16. As with the adult examination, the following clinical guidelines reflect screening procedures for the healthy child. If the child shows significant signs of neurological difficulty, referral and in-depth evaluation are warranted.

Table 15. Developmental lag warning signs*†

Age	General	Hearing and speech	Vision	Arms	Legs
6 weeks	Tremors, asymmetry, or jerky spastic movements	Does not respond to loud noise by startle reflex High-pitched cry	Failure to follow or fix at 22 to 30.5 cm (9-inch to 12-inch) distance	Excessive head lag on pulling to sitting position	Immobility Continued limb extension
6 months	No smiling Jerky or spastic movements Does not seem to recognize parent	Failure to turn toward sound Does not laugh or squeal	Failure to fix or follow both near and distant objects	Failure to keep head steady when pulled to sitting position Persistent fisting Preference, one hand Fails to push up or roll over	Increased adductor tone Increased reflexes Clonus
10 months	Lack of imitation Does not reach for toy Not attempting to feed self or put things in own mouth	Does not babble Does not imitate speech sounds	Displays squint or nystagmus	Abnormal hand posture Fails to pass cube from one hand to other	Absence of weight bearing while held Failure to sit without support
18 months	Absence of constructive play Persistence of drooling Indicates wants only by crying	Lack of words specifically "mama" or "dada"	Any apparent visual defect	No finger-thumb (pincer) grip Does not bang blocks together	Unable to stand bearing weight without support

*See also Table 16.

†Modified from Wood, B., editor: A pediatric vade-mecum, London, England, 1974, Lloyd-Luke (Medical Books) Ltd.

Age	General	Hearing and speech	Vision	Arms	Legs
2 years	Does not play peek-a-boo Not drinking from cup Failure to concentrate	Absence of words other than "mama' and "dada"	Failure to match toys	Does not attempt building with blocks Tremor or ataxia	Unable to walk without aid

Clinical variations associated with the pediatric client

THE INFANT (NEWBORN TO 12 MONTHS)

The examiner assessing the infant is primarily concerned with three factors:
1. Reflex pattern and development
2. Motor skills development
3. Behavioral and socialization development

The infant develops greatly during the first year of life. In fact, there is more neurological maturation during the first year than in any other. The examiner must closely evaluate this development month by month. The infant should be assessed by the DDST as well as according to the following clinical guidelines.

Characteristic or area examined	Normal	Deviations from normal
1. Mental assessment	Appears quiet, content Eyes open Recognizes face of significant other Smiles responsively (after 2 months)	Fretful, tense Tremors or spastic movements
2. Speech	Cry loud and possibly angry Cooing after 3 months Babbles after 4 months One or two words (mama, dada) after 9 months	High pitched, shrill Penetrating cry
3. Cranial nerves: unable to directly test; observe child's functioning, involving at least partial intactness of following cranial nerves:		
a. CN III, IV, VI	Follows movement with eyes Matures from 1 month onward	Response not shown at time appropriate for age
b. CN V	Rooting reflex, sucking reflex	Asymmetry of response Asymmetry of face during response
c. CN VII	Wrinkles forehead, smiles after 2 months	Spastic or movement with tremor
d. CN VIII	Moro reflex to loud noise Turns head toward sound	
e. CN IX, X	Swallowing, gag reflex	
f. CN XII	Evaluated as infant sucks and swallows	
4. Proprioception, cerebellar, and motor function	Observe infant for spontaneous activity, symmetry, and smoothness of movement Ease and passiveness during swallowing Fine and gross motor development as detailed in Chapter 14 (see also Table 14) Gradual purposeful movement after age 2 months	Spasticity, tremors, jerky movements Frequent choking or difficulty with sucking Unable to achieve developmental milestones Any child in question should be evaluated by DDST
5. Sensory function		
a. Light touch	Not normally tested	
b. Pain	Responds by withdrawal of all limbs and crying After 8 months may withdraw only limb tested	Withdrawal of limited limbs, asymmetrical withdrawal, no withdrawal
c. Vibratory	Not normally tested	
d. Discriminatory	Not normally tested	
6. Muscular function (muscle tone)		
a. General observation	Symmetry; limbs semiflexed and slightly abducted (see Fig. 14-37)	Frog position: hips in abduction (almost flat to table) with hips externally rotated

Continued.

THE INFANT (NEWBORN TO 12 MONTHS)–cont'd

Characteristic or area examined	Normal	Deviations from normal
		Opisthotonos: infant prone, maintains back positions with neck hyperextended Hand-over-head position Any asymmetry or spasticity of movement Persistence of fisted hand beyond 3 months
b. Evalution by pulling infant to sitting position using wrists (pull-to-sit maneuver)	Meaningful grasping after age 3 months Newborn will hold head at 45° angle or less until at upright sitting position; then head will flop forward By 4 months head should remain in line with body and should no longer flop forward	Head flop beyond 4 months
c. Range of motion	Able to easily perform range of motion techniques as described in Chapter 14	Spastic muscular response Marked resistance to range of motion attempt Quick spastic response when limbs released
7. Reflex testing: deep tendon reflexes not normally tested; more important to evaluate infant responses, some of the most common of which are detailed in Table 16	Patellar reflex present at birth, followed by Achilles and brachial triceps reflex present by 6 months	If reflexes continue beyond expected disappearance age, examiner should become suspicious

Table 16. Infantile reflexes

Reflex	Technique for evaluation	Appearance age	Disappearance age	Normal response
Reflexes to evaluate position and movement				
Moro	Startle infant by making loud noise, jarring examination surface, or slightly raising infant off examination surface and letting him fall quickly back onto examining table	Birth	1 to 4 months	Infant abducts and extends arms and legs; index finger and thumb assume C position; then infant pulls both arms and legs up against trunk as if trying to protect self

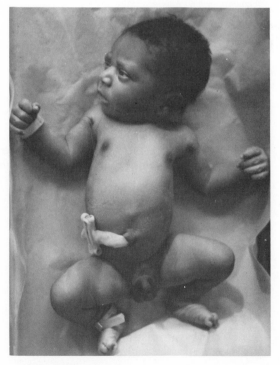

Reflex	Technique for evaluation	Appearance age	Disappearance age	Normal response
Tonic neck	Infant supine; rotate head to side so that chin is over shoulder	Birth to 6 weeks	4 to 6 months	Arm and leg on side to which head turns extends; opposite arm and leg flex; infant assumes fencing position (some normal infants may never show this reflex)

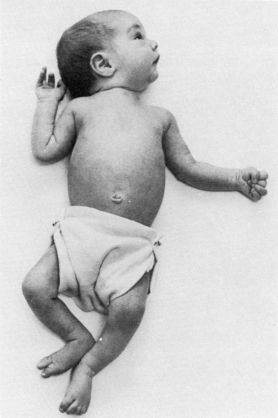

From Jensen, M., Benson, R., and Bobak, I.: Maternity care: the nurse and the family, St. Louis, 1977, The C. V. Mosby Co.

Plantar grasp	Touch object to sole of infant's foot	Birth	8 to 10 months	Toes will flex tightly downward in attempt to grasp

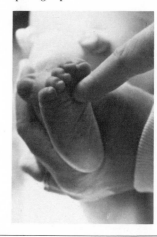

Continued.

Table 16. Infantile reflexes–cont'd

Reflex	Technique for evaluation	Appearance age	Disappearance age	Normal response
Palmar grasp	Touch object against ulnar side of infant's hand; then place finger in palm of hand	Birth	3 to 4 months	Infant will grasp finger with his finger; grasp should be tight, and examiner may be able to pull infant into sitting position by infant's grasp
				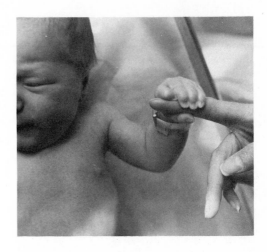
Babinski	Stroke lateral surface of infant's sole, using inverted J curve from sole to great toe	Birth	18 months	Infant response: positive response showing fanning of toes
				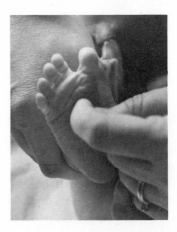
			Starting 18 months	Adult response: occurs after child has been walking for some time; flexion of great toe with slight fanning of other toes

Reflex	Technique for evaluation	Appearance age	Disappearance age	Normal response
Step in place	Infant in upright position, feet flat on surface	Birth	3 months	Will pace forward using alternating steps

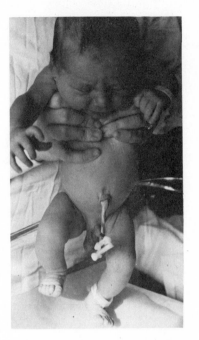

Reflex	Technique for evaluation	Appearance age	Disappearance age	Normal response
Clonus	Dorsiflex foot; pinch sole of foot just under toes	Birth	4 months	May get clonus movement of foot (not always present)

Feeding reflexes

Reflex	Technique for evaluation	Appearance age	Disappearance age	Normal response
Rooting response (awake)	Brush infant's cheek near corner of mouth	Birth	3 to 4 months	Infant will turn head in direction of stimulus and will open mouth slightly
Rooting response (asleep)		Birth	7 to 8 months	

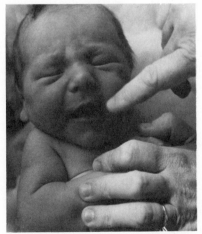

Reflex	Technique for evaluation	Appearance age	Disappearance age	Normal response
Sucking	Touch infant's lips	Birth	10 to 12 months	Sucking motion follows with lips and tongue

THE CHILD FROM 1 TO 3 YEARS

As with the musculoskeletal examination, cleverness will determine the successfulness of data collection. The child has outgrown much of the reflex assessment from the first year but is not yet able to cooperate as an adult. Children 2 years of age and older are said to have mature neurological systems, in that much of the neurological response elicited by the examination will be similar to that of the adult. The problem is that the child's cognitive abilities are not mature enough to allow cooperation. For example, in testing sharp and dull sensory function, the child may not as yet have developed the concepts of sharp and dull. Likewise, the child may have already formed the concept of hurt and will not allow the examiner near with the percussion hammer. Therefore the examiner must still evaluate much of neurological function on the evidence of motor functioning and response. If the child grossly demonstrates motor, social, and language development appropriate for age by climbing, walking, reaching, babbling, smiling, and undressing techniques, a detailed neurological assessment is not always necessary.

Characteristic or area examined	Normal	Deviations from normal
1. Mental assessment	Happy, playful child	Fretful, tense, frightened child
	Shows warm caring relationship with parent; may demonstrate separation anxiety	Demonstrates no concern of relationship with parent
	Recognizes and responds to name	
2. Speech	12 months: 1 to 3 words (nouns)	
	18 months: 10 to 20 words (nouns)	No words by 18 months
	24 months: 200 to 300 words (adds verbs); two- to three-word sentences	
	3 years: 900 words (all types); three- to four-word sentences	Very limited word usage by age 3 years
3. Cranial nerves: may be tested to a limited degree, depending on cooperation		
a. CN III, IV, VI	Follows toy with eyes (not valid if child turns head)	Asymmetry of response
		Asymmetry of face during response
	May have parent immobilize head	Spastic or movement with tremor
b. CN V	Give child cookie or cracker to eat; note bilaterally strong chewing response	Absence of response may be due to lack of cooperation and not actual defect; refer child if in doubt
	Tickle child's forehead with cotton top; child responds by batting with hand	
c. CN VII	Note smile quality and bilaterally equal response	Inability to elicit desired response may be due to lack of cooperation
	Child may imitate frown or show teeth	
	Taste may be evaluated, but examiner may lose child's cooperation; response to salt, sour, or bitter should be negative, batting away	
d. CN VIII	Gross hearing evaluation to bell and whisper	No response
e. CN IX, X	Gag reflex tested during mouth examination	
f. CN XI, XII	Not easily evaluated	
4. Proprioception, cerebellar, and motor function: observe the child at play, bending over, reaching, grasping, returning to standing position	Strong coordinated movements	Continued coordination difficulties beyond normal periods
	One-year-old will show wide-base stance (Fig. 15-40); older child will demonstrate maturity of development (Fig. 15-41) (see clinical strategies for developmental normals)	Unable to achieve developmental milestones
		Any children in question should be evaluated by DDST
5. Sensory function	Not routinely evaluated because almost impossible to separate actual sensory reaction from carefully watching and ready-to-reach toddler	
6. Muscular function	See Chapter 14 for assessment of muscular development of toddler; also see clinical strategies associated with the pediatric client for normal developmental milestones	
7. Reflexes: not normally tested in the healthy child during this time, due to lack of cooperation	Response would be same as for adult	Response would be the same as for adult

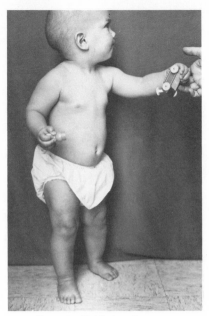

Fig. 15-40. Toddler's wide stance.

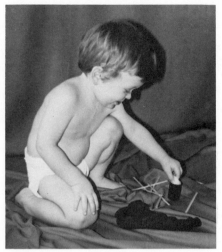

Fig. 15-41. Observing preschooler's coordinated movement.

THE CHILD BEYOND 3 YEARS

Children beyond 3 years of age are normally assessed through the techniques of the adult neurological examination. As the child matures, the actual techniques of evaluation should become easier. The examiner may still need to "play games" with the preschool child to invite cooperation.

Because the actual techniques of the neurological examination are the same as for the adult, the following section was developed to discuss (1) areas to be evaluated, (2) assessment strategies, and (3) developmental variations.

Area to evaluate	Assessment strategies	Normal developmental variations
1. Mental	Questioning about happiness, school success, preferences during play periods	
	Will participate in immediate recall of numbers	4-year-old repeats three-digit number 5-year-old repeats four-digit number 6-year-old repeats five-digit number
2. Speech	Converse with child; personally evaluate type of words used; speech patterns, or problems	4 years old: vocabulary 1500 words; uses plurals; four- to five-word sentences 5 years old: vocabulary approximately 2200 words; uses compound sentences, five to six words in length 6 years old: vocabulary approximately 3000 words; mature sentences over six words in length
3. Cranial nerves	Play games to test CN III to XII CN II not routinely tested until 6 or 7 years; then test as for adult CN III, IV, VI: instruct child to "freeze" the neck, or have parent help immobilize CN V, VII: use imaginary bubble gum; have child chew and blow big beautiful bubbles; then bubble bursts; encourage child to play; may evaluate chewing, muscle function, blowing, frowning, eyes closed tight, smile, frown	

Continued.

THE CHILD BEYOND 3 YEARS–cont'd

Area to evaluate	Assessment strategies	Normal developmental variations
	CN VIII: use whisper game CN IX, X: test during head and neck assessment CN XI: play game; have child show strength by pushing away examiner's hand with face and shoulders CN XII: the famous "tongue dance" will usually aid evaluation of this cranial nerve; instruct child to stick out tongue and wiggle it back and forth	

4. Proprioception, cerebellar, and motor function
  a. General screening
  b. Upper extremity testing
  c. Lower extremity testing
  (Also see following section, testing for neurological soft signs.)
	Use variety of techniques from adult profile
	Even smaller children should be able to do variety of these techniques (Fig. 15-42)
	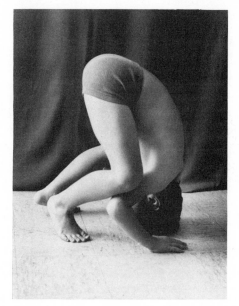
	Fig. 15-42. Observing preschooler's coordinated movements of lower extremities.
		Fine motor coordination not fully developed until child reaches 4 to 6 years of age
		Child should attempt techniques and show continued improvement with maturation; for example, during finger-nose touching, if child brings finger within 2.5 to 5 cm (1 or 2 inches) of end of nose, it is considered normal; *consistent* past pointing should arouse suspicion

5. Sensory function	After age 5 years child usually has enough trust to participate in sensory screening; helpful to show child cotton wisp, blunt end of paper clip, and tip of pin before starting; with child's eyes open, test each and discuss concepts of sharp, dull, and tickle; some authors suggest likening open pin to mosquito bite If child does not understand sharp, dull, and tickle, assessment will fail Two-point discrimination, graphesthesia, stereognosis, and kinesthetic evaluation should first be done with child's eyes open and in educational practice session prior to testing situation For graphesthesia, easy numbers to recognize: 0, 7, 3, 8, 1; for younger children, examiner may use 0, X, + To further vary test, examiner may make mark such as X twice and ask child if it is same or different; child must understand what same and different mean	Developmental progression for one-foot standing: 4 years—5 seconds 6 years—5 seconds with arms folded across chest 7 years—5 seconds with eyes closed

Area to evaluate	Assessment strategies	Normal developmental variations
6. Muscular function	See musculoskeletal examination, Chapter 14	Observe closely for any signs of muscular weakness as child matures Signs associated with muscular dystrophy: 1. Muscle atrophy or hypertrophy 2. Return to wide-base gait 3. Weakness when going up and down stairs 4. Difficulty arising from lying position; necessary to use arms to climb up and legs to push trunk into upright position
7. Reflexes	May be helpful to use reinforcement; if child shows all other healthy neurological signs, not always necessary to evaluate status of reflexes	

SCREENING ASSESSMENT OF "SOFT" NEUROLOGICAL SIGNS IN THE SCHOOL-AGE CHILD

The term "soft" signs, although controversial, is used to describe vague and minimal dysfunctional signs such as clumsiness, language disturbances, inconsistencies, motor overload, mirroring movements of extremities, or perceptual development difficulties.

Following is a series of evaluation techniques recommended by McMillan, Nieburg, and Oski.* If the examiner elicits responses demonstrating difficulty in performing the task, the responses should be clustered and the child referred.

Instructional technique	Important observations	Variables and considerations
1. Evaluation of fine motor coordination: observe child during:		
a. Undressing, unbuttoning	Note child's general coordination	
b. Tying shoe		
c. Rapidly touching alternate fingers with thumb	Note if similar movement on opposite side	For items c to e and h and i, movement of other side noted as associated motor movements, adventitious overflow movements, or synkinesis
d. Rattling imaginary doorknob	Note if similar movement on other side	
e. Unscrewing imaginary light bulb	Note if similar movement on other side	
f. Grasping pencil and writing	Note excessive pressure on penpoint; fingers placed directly over point, or placed greater than 2.5 cm (1 inch) up shaft	May indicate difficulty with fine motor coordination
g. Moving tongue rapidly		
h. Demonstrating hand grip	Note if similar movement on opposite side	
i. Inverting feet	Note similar movement on opposite side	
j. Repeating several times "pa, ta, ka" or "kitty, kitty, kitty"	Accurate reproduction of these sounds indicates auditory coordination	
2. Evaluation of special sensory skills		
a. Dual simultaneous sensory tests (face-hand testing): first demonstrate technique, then instruct child to close eyes; the examiner performs simultaneously:		
1. Touch both cheeks 2. Touch both hands 3. Touch right cheek and right hand 4. Touch left cheek and right hand	Failure to perceive hand stimulus when face simultaneously touched referred to as rostral dominance	About 80% of normal children able to perform this test by age 8 years without rostral dominance

*Data from McMillan, J., Nieburg, P., and Oski, F.: The whole pediatrician catalog, Philadelphia, 1977, W. B. Saunders Co.

Continued.

SCREENING ASSESSMENT OF "SOFT" NEUROLOGICAL SIGNS IN THE SCHOOL-AGE CHILD–cont'd

Instructional technique	Important observations	Variables and considerations
5. Touch left cheek and left hand 6. Touch right cheek and left hand		
b. Finger localization test (finger agnosia test): touch two spots on one finger or two fingers simultaneously; child has eyes closed; ask "How many fingers am I touching, one or two?"	Evaluate number of correct responses with four trials for each hand Six out of eight possible correct responses passes	About 50% of all children pass test by age 6 years About 90% of all children pass by age 9 years This test reflects child's orientation in space, concept of body image, sensation of touch, and position sense
3. Evaluation of child's laterality and orientation in space a. Imitation of gestures: instruct child to use same hand as examiner and to imitate the following movements ("Do as I do."): 1. Extend little finger 2. Extend little and index fingers 3. Extend index and middle fingers 4. Touch two thumbs and two index fingers together simultaneously 5. Form two interlocking rings—thumb and index finger of one hand, with thumb and index finger of other hand 6. Point index finger of one hand down toward the cupped fingers of the opposite hand held below	Note difficulty with fine finger movements, manipulation, or reproduction of correct gesture Note any marked right-left confusion regarding examiner's right and left hands	This test helps to evaluate child's finger discrimination and awareness of body image, right, left, front, back, and up and down orientation Especially important after age 8 years, if there continues to be marked right-left confusion
b. Following directions: ask child to: 1. Show me your left hand 2. Show me your right ear 3. Show me your right eye 4. Show me your left elbow 5. Touch your left knee with your left hand 6. Touch your right ear with your left hand 7. Touch your left elbow with your right hand 8. Touch your right cheek with your right hand 9. Point to my left ear 10. Point to my right eye 11. Point to my right hand 12. Point to my left knee	Note any incorrect responses Note any difficulty with following sequence of directions Items 9 through 12 mastered by age 8	Items 1 through 8 mastered by approximately age 6 years

History and clinical strategies associated with the geriatric client

1. Following are significant symptoms that need careful attention (additional questions for symptom analysis).
   a. "Dizziness," "faintness," "spells," or "attacks"

(1) Describe the sensation: Is the room spinning around? Do you feel as though you are spinning around?
(2) Have you ever fallen down with a dizzy spell or lost consciousness?

(3) If you have lost consciousness, did anyone witness the episode and did they describe your behavior?

(4) Does the dizziness occur when you first sit up or stand up?

(5) Does it occur when you move your head from side to side or up and down?

(6) Does exertion cause you to feel faint? If so, describe the intensity and duration of the exertion.

(7) Are there any associated mood or mental changes?

(8) Are there any associated symptoms (e.g., numbness or tingling of extremities—bilateral or unilateral, weakness or temporary loss of use of extremities, vision changes, facial expression changes such as drooping of side of mouth, difficulty swallowing, difficulty speaking, or chest pain)?

(9) Do your legs ever just "give way" so that you fall to the floor?

(10) Have you (or any observers) noticed your skin color during the episode or during the recovery period (e.g., pallor, flushing)?

(11) Describe the onset of the episode (sudden, slow, any warnings that the episode is going to occur).

(12) Review all new and old prescribed and over-the-counter medications that the client is taking. (*Note:* Some hypotensives, phenothiazines, and antidepressants can cause dizziness). Review alcoholic intake.

b. Weakness

(1) Isolated to a specific body part or generalized (e.g., difficulty swallowing, lid drooping, unilateral or bilateral weakness in feet, ankles, hands, arms)?

(2) Describe specific activities that alerted you to your weakness (e.g., lifting, stair climbing—how many stairs, rising from chair, walking on level ground, holding utensil in hand or manipulating it, such as a toothbrush).

(3) Does weakness occur at onset of activity or after activity has been sustained (how long or how much)?

(4) What are associated symptoms (e.g., dizziness, "black-outs," numbness or tingling, pain, tics [fasciculations], tremors, shortness of breath)?

(5) Associated stiffness of joints, spasms, or muscle tension (do these symptoms occur at night)?

(6) Associated weight gain or loss?

(7) Associated mood or mental changes?

(8) Review all medications and alcoholic beverages being taken.

c. Headaches

(1) Is this a problem that has occurred over a period of years, or is the pattern of headaches new to you?

(2) Do you ever feel localized tenderness over your scalp, forehead, or face?

d. History of injuries, falls (inquire specifically about all recent accidents, minor "spills," or injuries). The client may not be aware that a pattern of increased stumbling, falls, or diminishing agility is emerging if injuries are not obvious or incapacitating.

e. Mental status changes (e.g., mood, thinking process, cognitive functions). (*Note:* A detailed history and observation assessment are covered in Chapter 2.)

f. Speech alterations (content or delivery) details for assessment are covered in Chapter 2.

g. General considerations

(1) Any history of weakness, falling, dizziness, pain, or disability should be explored in terms of loss of ability to carry out activities of daily living and concerns for safety. (The original geriatric data base offers detailed questions in these areas in Chapter 1.)

(2) All symptomatic clients should be asked if they live with someone or have access to someone (relative, neighbor, friend) who can be with them if they need immediate help (day and night).

(3) The symptomatic client should be urged to discuss personal feelings about the symptoms (e.g., what is causing them, how serious it is, and any concerns related to living alone or lack of personal or immediate resources).

(4) Careful exploration of the client's efforts to relieve symptoms or alleviate stress is important. Self medication, self-imposed immobility, use of alcohol, social withdrawal, and denial are examples of new behaviors that might be uncovered with a careful history.

2. The neurological screening examination described in the adult section of this chapter can be used with the majority of elderly clients. The major variations in the aging client's responses to the examination follow:

a. Responses to the examiner's commands may be carried out more slowly.

b. The senses of smell and taste may be diminished.

c. Deep tendon reflexes may be slightly diminished (especially the ankle jerk); however, absence or exaggeration of any of the deep tendon reflexes should be reported as a problem.

d. The vibratory sensation in both feet and ankles may be diminished; however, full sensation should be reported at midcalf. (*Note:* This finding should be reported as a problem by beginning practitioners.)

3. Neurological assessment of the elderly individual becomes complicated when the client is disabled by other problems. Diminished vision or hearing, arthritis, confusion or disorientation, or cardiorespiratory problems may be accompanied by fatigue, weakness, inattentiveness, or other symptoms that mask neurological deficits. Symptoms related to other illnesses may prevent the client from going through the motions of an examination. It might be helpful to conduct the examination over two or three sessions to avoid client fatigue. The beginning practitioner will have to seek advice from a preceptor regarding decisions about which functions are important for the client to complete if the client is greatly disabled.

4. Following are some major physical signs for which the examiner should be alert:

a. Facial asymmetry, drooping of the side of the mouth (flat nasolabial fold), asymmetrical wrinkling on forehead, drooling at side of mouth, or tongue fasciculation (while at rest in the mouth). If any are apparent, ask the client to swallow a sip of water. The observer should be alert for coughing, sputtering, dribbling, or fluid remaining in the mouth after the swallow.

b. Weakness of extremities (unilateral or symmetrical response); note the following:
   (1) Extent of range of motion and strength to opposition
   (2) Accompanying muscle atrophy
   (3) Sensory responses to pain, touch, vibration, and temperature
   (4) Reflexes (normal, present, absent, hyperactive, or diminished)
   (5) Comparison of weakened side to other side in all areas of assessment

c. Gait disturbances (see geriatric section in Chapter 14 for details to observe)

d. Tremors. Some authors state that mild head tremors are normal for elderly individuals; however, the examiner should report all tremors for consultation.
   (1) Anxiety or hyperthyroidism tremors are often fine, rapid, and irregular. Facial tics or twitching may be present. Tremors usually increase with action and decrease with relaxation. Excessive perspiration may be apparent.
   (2) Parkinsonian tremors are slower and occur at rest. The "pill-rolling" pattern of thumb and opposing fingers may be evident. All body movements are slowed or diminished.
   (3) Cerebellar tremors vary in rate and are usually intention tremors.
   (4) Essential tremors (or those associated with aging) occur at a moderate rate and frequently involve the jaw, tongue, or entire head. The head may move up and down or laterally. The tremors disappear on relaxation and are usually not disabling; there is no accompanying rigidity. There may be a familial history of such tremors. The tremors may begin in middle age and continue at same level of severity through the remainder of life.
   (5) Metabolic tremors involve a flapping motion of the wrist, which suddenly drops and then returns to the original position. The client is usually very ill and manifests numerous other signs.

e. Mental acuity alteration (see Chapter 2 for specific behaviors to assess).

f. Labile emotional responses (specific behaviors listed in Chapter 2).

5. Stroke. This is a word commonly used by professional and lay people to describe a sudden neurological deficit that results in a variety of signs, including paralysis or weakness of body parts. The cause of the problem is usually vascular, but the effects are neurological and are therefore described in this chapter. Strokes are often classified in terms of stages of appearance or severity:

a. Transient ischemial attacks are neurological deficits with acute onset and limited duration (5 to 20 minutes). A variety of symptoms or signs might be manifested. Dizziness, confusion, unilateral weakness or numbness, and aphasia are some of the complaints. These episodes often leave few or no aftereffects and sometimes precede a stroke. The frequency and severity of these "spells" or "attacks" vary greatly among individuals.

b. Reversible ischemic neurological deficit is similar to the transient attacks, except that the signs and symptoms linger for several days before disappearing.

c. Stroke-in-evolution is a slowly progressive focal deficit occurring and accumulating in a step-by-step or stuttering fashion over a period of days or weeks. Signs and symptoms become more apparent over this period of time.

d. The onset of signs and symptoms of a completed stroke are abrupt and become stabilized (over a period of days or weeks or years).

6. Risk factors associated with strokes

a. Family history of strokes or vascular disease
b. Client history of hypertension
c. Cardiac enlargement
d. History of myocardial infarction or angina pectoris
e. Congestive heart failure
f. Diabetes mellitus
g. History of peripheral vascular disease
h. History of transient ischemial attacks

Vocabulary

1. Ageusia

2. Anesthesia

3. Anosmia

4. Aphasia

5. Ataxia

6. Athetosis

7. Cerebellar

8. Clonus

9. Decomposition of movement

10. Dysdiadochokinesia

11. Dysmetria

12. Dyssynergia

13. Extrapyramidal tract

14. Fasciculation

15. Graphesthesia

16. Hyperesthesia

17. Hyperkinesis

18. Hypoesthesia

19. Hyposmia

20. Kinesthetic sensation

21. Lower motor neuron

22. Myoclonus

23. Paresthesia

24. Proprioception

25. Rigidity

26. Romberg test

27. Sensory "level"

28. Sensory neuron

29. Spasticity

20. Stereognosis

31. Tics

32. Tremor

33. Two-point discrimination

34. Upper motor neuron

35. Vertigo

Cognitive self-assessment

1. The cranial nerves are outside of the brain and spinal cord. Therefore the cranial nerves are part of the:
   - ☐ a. central nervous system
   - ☑ b. peripheral nervous system
2. Every reflex arc pathway includes:
   - ☐ a. a receptor
   - ☐ b. an efferent fiber
   - ☐ c. an afferent fiber
   - ☐ d. a muscle or gland
   - ☐ e. a brainstem
   - ☐ f. all except c
   - ☐ g. all except a
   - ☑ h. all except e
   - ☐ i. all the above
3. While examining a client's patellar reflexes you get no response. One method you can use to aid you in getting a response is to:
   - ☐ a. have client cross legs, and test the patellar reflexes one at a time
   - ☐ b. have client dorsiflex feet
   - ☑ c. have client lock fingers together and pull one hand against the other
   - ☐ d. have client place both hands under the knees to add more tension on the patellar ligaments
4. A deep tendon reflex _____ dependent on an intact motor nerve fiber.
   - ☑ a. is
   - ☐ b. is not
5. Extension of the elbow is the normal response of the _____ reflex.
   - ☑ a. triceps
   - ☐ b. biceps
6. _____ of the great toe is a normal response to the plantar reflex.
   - ☑ a. Flexion
   - ☐ b. Extension
7. Which of the following is *not* part of a screening neurological assessment?
   - ☐ a. Mental status
   - ☐ b. Proprioception and cerebellar function
   - ☐ c. Cranial nerve evaluation
   - ☐ d. Sensory evaluation
   - ☐ e. Deep tendon reflexes
   - ☐ f. b and e
   - ☑ g. None of the above
8. A function of the cerebellum is the integration of muscle contractions for the maintenance of posture. Characteristics of a client with a "cerebellar gait" are:
   - ☑ a. walking with a wide gait
   - ☑ b. trunk and head held rigidly
   - ☑ c. the legs bent at the hip
   - ☐ d. the arms held outward to maintain balance
   - ☐ e. most walking takes place on the balls and toes of the feet, with no heel strike
   - ☐ f. none of the above
   - ☐ g. a, c, d, and e
   - ☐ h. b, d, and e
   - ☑ i. a, b, and c
   - ☐ j. all the above

9. In assessing the client's proprioceptive or cerebellar function, which of the following tests *are* appropriate?
   □ a. Instruct client to pat his leg as fast as he can with his hand.
   □ b. Instruct client to spread fingers as far as possible and to resist the examiner's attempt to squeeze them together.
   □ c. Instruct client to do a deep knee bend.
   □ d. Instruct client to take the heel of one foot and run it down the opposite shin.
   □ e. Instruct client to close his eyes. The examiner grasps the index finger of the client's hand and changes its position (e.g., up or down). The client then describes how the position was changed.
   □ f. None of the above
   □ g. b, d, and e
   □ h. b, c, and e
   ☑ i. a, c, and d
   □ j. a, b, and c

10. When performing a screening evaluation of sensory function, it is only necessary to evaluate the following areas:
    □ a. lateral aspect of upper thighs
    □ b. inner aspect of upper arms
    ☑ c. dorsal or palmar surface of hands
    □ d. bottom or dorsal surface of feet
    □ e. upper middle aspect of back
    □ f. all the above
    □ g. a, b, and e
    □ h. a and b
    □ i. c, d, and e
    ☑ j. c and d

11. Sensory function testing techniques include:
    □ a. pain sensation
    □ b. light touch sensation
    □ c. temperature identification
    □ d. vibration evaluation
    □ e. position sense
    □ f. stereognosis
    ☑ g. all the above
    □ h. all except a
    □ i. all except c
    □ j. all except e
    □ k. all except f

Mark each statement "T" or "F."

12. __T__ The Romberg test involves asking the patient to stand with feet together and arms outstretched, with eyes open and then closed.

13. __T__ The cerebellum receives both sensory and motor input, coordinates muscular activity, and maintains equilibrium.

14. __T__ The examiner should compare sensitivity in the proximal and distal portions of the extremities.

Match the definitions in column A with the terms in column B.

	Column A	*Column B*
15. __d__	Continuous rapid twitching of a muscle without movement of the limb	a. tic
		b. myoclonus
16. __c__	An involuntary rhythmic rapid back-and-forth movement of a limb	c. chorea
		d. fasciculation

<table>
<tr><td colspan="2">Column A–cont'd</td><td>Column B–cont'd</td></tr>
</table>

Column A–cont'd   *Column B–cont'd*

17. __a__ An occasional twitch of a shoulder or a group of   e. tremor
     facial muscles
18. __c__ Strong involuntary jerks of the body that occur at
     irregular intervals
19. __b__ A hiccup is an example

Match the cranial nerves in column A with the anticipated motor action of that nerve in column B.

Column A   *Column B*

20. __c__ CN V   a. Muscles of the face, including those around eyes and
21. __e__ CN VIII   mouth VII – facial
22. __d__ CN X   b. Movement of the tongue hypoglossal XII
23. __b__ CN XII   c. Temporal and masseter muscles and lateral jaw
                           movement Trigeminal V
                        d. Ability to swallow vagus x
                        e. Hearing and balance acoustic

The testing of the deep tendon reflexes is a rather simple mechanical process. The significance of testing, however, reflects intactness of the neurological system from the tendon to the motor nerve in the spinal cord. Match each reflex in column A with the motor nerve it evaluates in column B.

Column A   *Column B*

24. __d__ Biceps reflex   a. C_7, C_8
25. __a__ Triceps reflex   b. L_4, L_5, S_1, S_2
26. __c__ Knee reflex   c. L_2, L_3, L_4
27. __e__ Ankle reflex   d. C_5, C_6
28. __b__ Plantar response   e. S_1, S_2

PEDIATRIC QUESTIONS

29. It is possible to partially evaluate cranial nerve function by which of the following ages?
    ☑ a. 2 months
    ☐ b. 8 months
    ☐ c. 3 years
    ☐ d. 6 years
    ☐ e. 8 years
30. The correct response to the Moro reflex is which of the following?
    ☐ a. The arm and leg on the side to which the head turns extend; the opposite arm and leg flex.
    ☐ b. The infant grasps the examiner's hand, and the toes flex downward.
    ☐ c. The infant paces in place, alternately lifting each leg.
    ☑ d. The infant responds with rapid abduction of both arms and legs; the index finger and thumb assume a **C** position.
    ☐ e. The infant grasps the examiner's hands, the infant's legs abduct and the toes fan outward.
31. The sucking reflex disappears by approximately which of the following ages?
    ☐ a. 8 months
    ☑ b. 12 months
    ☐ c. 16 months
    ☐ d. 24 months
    ☐ e. 30 months

32. The examiner should expect a child to feed himself crackers or cookies by which of the following ages?
    - ☐ a. 4 months
    - ☐ b. 6 months
    - ☑ c. 8 months
    - ☐ d. 10 months
    - ☐ e. 12 months

33. Which of the following definitions best defines neurological "soft signs"?
    - ☐ a. Objective signs that are present due to an open portion of the spinal column
    - ☐ b. Objective findings of babies prior to mature development of their neurological systems
    - ☐ c. Objective signs found in hyperactive children
    - ☑ d. Objective signs associated with vague complaints such as clumsiness, motor overload, or mirroring of extremity movements
    - ☐ e. There is no such term

GERIATRIC QUESTIONS

34. Neurological signs associated with the normal aging process might include:
    - ☐ a. diminution or absence of ankle jerk response
    - ☐ b. ptosis
    - ☐ c. fasciculations of the tongue
    - ☐ d. all the above
    - ☐ e. none of the above

35. Transient ischemial attacks:
    - ☐ a. may occur in the form of black-out spells
    - ☐ b. may affect speech ability
    - ☐ c. may cause temporary visual changes
    - ☑ d. all the above
    - ☐ e. none of the above

36. Risk factors associated with strokes might include:
    - ☐ a. a history of nervousness
    - ☑ b. a history of transient ischemial attacks
    - ☐ c. a history of hypothyroidism
    - ☐ d. all the above
    - ☐ e. none of the above

SUGGESTED READINGS
General

American Journal of Nursing: Programmed Instruction: Patient assessment: neurological examination. Part I, **75:**9, Sept., 1975.

American Journal of Nursing: Programmed Instruction: Patient assessment: neurological examination. Part II, **75:**11, Nov., 1975.

American Journal of Nursing: Programmed Instruction: Patient assessment: neurological examination. Part III, **76:**4, Apr., 1976.

Bates, Barbara: A guide to physical examination, ed. 2, Philadelphia, 1979, J. B. Lippincott Co., pp. 311-358.

DeMyer, W.: Technique of the neurological examination: a programmed text, ed. 2, New York, 1974, McGraw-Hill Book Co.

Judge, Richard D., and Zuidema, George, editors: Methods of clinical examination: a physiologic approach, Boston, 1974, Little, Brown & Co., pp. 341-366.

Malasanos, Lois, Barkauskas, Violet, Moss, Muriel, and Stoltenberg-Allen, Karthryn: Health assessment, St. Louis, 1977, The C. V. Mosby Co., pp. 379-418.

Prior, John A., and Silberstein, Jack S.: Physical diagnosis: the history and examination of the patient, ed. 5, St. Louis, 1977, The C. V. Mosby Co., pp. 375-423.

SmithKline Corporation: Essentials of the neurological examination, Philadelphia, 1974.

Pediatric

Alexander, Mary, and Brown, Marie Scott: Pediatric physical diagnosis for nurses, New York, 1974, McGraw-Hill Book Co., pp. 212-259.

Barness, Lewis: Manual of pediatric physical diagnosis, ed. 4, Chicago, 1972, Year Book Medical Publishers, Inc., pp. 165-178.

Bates, Barbara: A guide to physical examination, ed. 2, Philadelphia, 1979, J. B. Lippincott Co., pp. 416-426.

Hughes, James: Synopsis of pediatrics, ed. 5, St. Louis, 1980, The C. V. Mosby Co., pp. 718-720.

Johnson, Thomas: Children are different. In Johnson, T. R., Moore, W. M., and Jeffries, J. E., editors: Developmental philosophy, ed. 2, Columbus, Ohio, 1978, Ross Laboratories, p. 34.

Malasanos, Lois, Barkauskas, Violet, Moss, Muriel, and Stoltenberg-Allen, Kathryn: Health assessment, St. Louis, 1977, The C. V. Mosby Co., p. 435.

McMillan, Julia, Nieburg, Phillip, and Oski, Frank: The whole pediatrician catalog, Philadelphia, 1977, W. B. Saunders Co., pp. 74-75, 319-322.

Pillitteri, Adele: Nursing care of the growing family: a child health text, Boston, 1977, Little, Brown & Co., pp. 37-41.

Prior, John A., and Silberstein, Jack S.: Physical diagnosis: the history and examination of the patient, ed. 5, St. Louis, 1977, The C. V. Mosby Co., pp. 471-473.

Van Allen, M. W.: Pictorial manual of neurologic tests, Chicago, 1969, Year Book Medical Publications, Inc.

Geriatric

Caird, F. I., and Judge, T. G.: Assessment of the elderly patient, London, 1977, Pitman Publishing Ltd., pp. 48-52, 65-86.

Chinn, Austin B., editor: Clinical aspects of aging, Working with older people: a guide to practice, vol. 4, Rockville, Md., 1971, U.S. Department of Health, Education, and Welfare, Public Health Service, pp. 45-59.

Ross, Gilbert S., and Klassen, Arthur: The stroke syndrome. Part I. Pathogenesis, Hosp. Med. **9**(3):7-37, March, 1973.

Ross, Gilbert S., and Klassen, Arthur: The stroke syndrome. Part II. Clinical and diagnostic aspects, Hosp. Med. **9**(4):58-81, Apr., 1973.

Steinberg, Franz U., editor: Cowdry's the care of the geriatric patient, St. Louis, 1976, The C. V. Mosby Co., pp. 364-379.

CHAPTER 16

Physical examination integration format

The purpose of this chapter is to discuss the integration of the total physical examination. Throughout, the description of the assessment techniques has been abbreviated. The examiner is referred to the individual chapters for a detailed description. The clinical information has been divided to show the following:

1. The examination format
2. The assessment techniques
3. The systems involved in the assessment procedure
4. Important strategies

At the end of this detailed description is a summary of the pediatric variations and suggested approaches for the pediatric client.

Equipment for physical examination

Eye examination charts
Ophthalmoscope
Otoscope with pneumatic bulb
Stethoscope
Tongue blades
Penlight
4 × 4-inch gauze pads
Examination gloves
Cotton applicator sticks
Lubricant
Drape sheet
Gooseneck light
Examination table with stirrups
Writing surface for examiner
Patient examination gown
Vaginal speculum (for female clients)
Pap smear materials
Percussion hammer
Tuning fork
Odorous material
Cotton balls
Sharp and dull testing instruments
Ruler

Data base history

This should be a time for the examiner to get to know and develop a profile about the client. This profile should be synthesized and provide the examiner with a framework by which to approach the client during the physical assessment.

1. Major concern of client. The examiner must decide whether to examine that area first or whether to wait and examine it during the normal sequence.
2. General approach to the client. The examiner will get to know the client during preparation of the rather lengthy data base. Although the examiner may decide to maintain a systematic and progressive physical examination approach, the client's personality and individual preferences should be incorporated. For example, if the client states that he becomes short of breath when he lies flat, the examiner may decide to keep the head of the examination table up a little and to keep the recumbent period to a minimum.
3. Major areas needing special attention. Many times the examination simply confirms what the examiner already knows. Therefore the examiner should bring to the physical assessment session a "problem list" of areas needing special in-depth evaluation.

Integrated physical assessment

1. The physical examination of each client should begin as the examiner first meets the client. Assessment of objective data should continue throughout the subjective data base collection period.

   During the initial introductory period, collect data by watching the client walk down the hall, come into the examination room, take off and hang up his coat, shake hands with the examiner, sit down on a chair in the office or examination room, and carry on all introductory conversation.

   The examiner may identify areas with obvious difficulties or deviations. Areas requiring primary assessment follow:

   a. Gait: difficulty walking, use of assisting devices

b. Stiffness, weakness
c. Difficulty standing, sitting, rising from sitting position
d. Difficulty taking off coat or hanging it up
e. Obvious musculoskeletal deformities
f. General affect
g. Appearance of interest and involvement
h. Eye contact with examiner
i. Speech pattern or difficulties
j. Dress and posture
k. Overview of mental alertness, orientation, and thought process integrity
l. Tremors or motor difficulties
m. Obvious eye problem or blindness
n. Corrective lenses
o. Difficulty hearing
p. Use of assisting devices
q. Obvious shortness of breath; posture that would facilitate breathing
r. Cyanosis, pale or flushed appearance
s. Language problem or foreign language speaker

t. Cultural orientation
u. Significant others accompanying client
v. Obesity or emaciation
w. Malnourishment

2. Following the initial assessment and data base collection the client should be prepared for the physical assessment.
   a. Instruct client to empty bladder (collect specimen if desired).
   b. Instruct client to remove all clothing (including shoes, socks, bra, and underpants) put on gown, and sit on chair in examination room.

To perform the examination, the approach to body systems must be fragmented for two purposes: (a) to accommodate a regional physical assessment approach and (b) to coordinate client and examiner positions during the assessment process.

Following the assessment the examiner must reunite the body systems for the actual physical assessment write-up. The examiner should not feel compelled to follow the stated outline; the goal should be to develop an individualized routine.

Clinical guidelines for physical examination integration

Procedure or format	Assessment to include	Body part or system involved	Clinical strategies for adults and geriatric clients
1. Assess vital functions and other baseline measurements: client should be in gown and seated on end of examination table or in chair	Temperature Blood pressure (both arms) Radial pulse Respirations Height Weight	Cardiovascular Thorax and lungs	If deviation from normal discovered, reevaluate when associated system assessed

	Vision testing
	  Snellen chart
	  External eye function
		Visual
		Neurological—CN II
		  (optic nerve)	

The client is seated
2. Examine client's hands
	Skin surface
	  characteristics
	Temperature and moisture
	  of hands
		Integumentary	Both examiner and client will be at ease if examiner starts with client's hands

	Characteristics of nails Clubbing	Cardiovascular Respiratory	

	Skeletal characteristics
	  and/or deformities of
	  fingers and hands
	Range of motion and
	  motor strength of fingers
	  and hands
	Muscle wasting
	Asymmetry
		Musculoskeletal	Fine motor neurological assessment may be included at this point; others find it more convenient to perform the neurological assessment as a clustered procedure toward end of the evaluation period

3. Examine client's arms from hands to shoulders	Skin surface characteristics Muscle wasting Asymmetry	Integumentary Musculoskeletal	Examine each arm separately

Continued.

Clinical guidelines for physical examination integration–cont'd

Procedure or format	Assessment to include	Body part or system involved	Clinical strategies for adults and geriatric clients
	Radial pulses: compare one arm to other	Cardiovascular	May have already been done during vital sign evaluation
	Range of motion and motor strength of wrists, elbows, forearms, upper arm, shoulders	Musculoskeletal Neurological	Note that, again, neurological assessment has been delayed Use make/break techniques
	Palpation of epitrochlear lymph nodes	Lymphatic	
4. Examine the client's head and neck	Facial characteristics and symmetry	Head and neck Neurological	Observe head and neck, taking in as much information as possible
	Skin surface characteristics	Integumentary	Do not be tempted to touch until after thorough observation
	Symmetry and external characteristics of eyes and ears		
	Hair characteristics: texture, distribution, quantity		
	Palpation of hair and scalp		Palpate thoroughly; do not be intimidated by hair spray or dirty hair (may need to wash hands before progressing)
	Palpation of facial bones	Musculoskeletal	
	Client opens and closes mouth for evaluation of temporomandibular joint	Neurological—CN V (trigeminal nerve)	
	Clenching teeth		
	Palpation of sinus regions		
	Client clenches eyes tight, wrinkles forehead, smiles, sticks out tongue, and puffs out cheeks	Neurological—CN VII, XII (facial, hypoglossal nerves)	Very straightforward Provide client with step-by-step instructions
	Eye and near vision assessment	Visual	
	External eye examination: eyebrows, eyelids, eyelashes, surface characteristics, lacrimal apparatus, corneal surface, anterior chamber, iris		
	Near vision screening and eye function: pupilary response, accommodation, cover-uncover test	Neurological—CN II, III (optic, oculomotor nerves)	
	Extraocular eye movements; vision field testing	Neurological—CN III, IV, VI (oculomotor, trochlear, abducens nerves)	
	Internal eye examination: red reflex, disc, cup margins, vessels, retinal surface, vitreous		Room must be darkened; should have small amount of secondary light Remember to instruct client to focus on single object at distance
	Ear and hearing assessment	Ear and auditory	
	External ear examination: alignment, surface		

Procedure or format	Assessment to include	Body part or system involved	Clinical strategies for adults and geriatric clients
	characteristics, external canal		
	Use ticking watch to evaluate hearing	Neurological—CN VIII (acoustic nerve)	Room must be quiet
	Otoscope examination: characteristics of external canal, cerumen, eardrum (landmarks, deformities, inflammation)		Use largest speculum that will fit into canal; if necessary, review technique guidelines for using otoscope
	Rinne and Weber tests	Auditory and neurological—CN VIII (acoustic nerve)	
	Nasal examination: note structure, septum position; use nasal speculum to evaluate patency, turbinates, meatuses	Nose, mouth, and oropharynx	Even though uncomfortable, should be part of every thorough assessment
	Evaluation of sense of smell	Neurological—CN I (olfactory nerve)	
	Mouth examination: inspect gingivobuccal fornices, buccal mucosa, and gums	Nose, mouth, and oropharynx	
	Teeth inspection: number, color, surface characteristics		If client has dentures, they should be removed
	Inspection and palpation of tongue: symmetry, movement, color, surface characteristics		
	Inspection of floor of mouth: color, surface characteristics		
	Inspection of hard and soft palates: color, surface characteristics		
	Inspection of oropharynx: note mouth odor, anterior-posterior pillars, uvula, tonsils, posterior pharynx		
	Evaluation of gag reflex	Neurological—CN IX, X (glosso-pharyngeal, vagus nerves)	
	Evaluation of range of motion of the head and neck: instruct client to swing shoulders upward against examiner's resistance; head movement positions, neck flexion, extension, ear to shoulder flexion, chin to shoulder rotation	Musculoskeletal Neurological—CN XI (accessory nerve)	
	Observation of symmetry and smoothness of neck and thyroid		Client's gown should be lowered slightly so that examiner may fully inspect neck

Continued.

Clinical guidelines for physical examination integration–cont'd

Procedure or format	Assessment to include	Body part or system involved	Clinical strategies for adults and geriatric clients
	Palpation of carotid pulses Observation for jugular venous distention	Cardiovascular	
	Palpation of trachea, thyroid (isthmus and lobes), lymph nodes (preauricular, postauricular, occipital, tonsillar, submaxillary, submental, superficial cervical chain, posterior cervical, deep cervical, chain, and supraclav-icular)	Lymphatic	Client may need drink of water to facilitate swallowing during thyroid evaluation
	Completion of assessment of cranial nerves: use cotton swab to evaluate light sensation to forehead, cheeks, chin (trigeminal nerve sensory tract)	Neurological—CN V (trigeminal nerve)	Client should be instructed to close eyes and identify where and when light touch felt
5. Assess posterior chest: examiner moves behind client; client seated; gown to waist for men; gown removed but pulled up to cover breasts for women	Observation of posterior chest: symmetry of shoulders, muscular development, scapular placement, spine straightness, posture	Musculoskeletal	
	Observation of skin: intactness, color, lesions	Integumentary	
	Observation of respiratory movement: excursion, quality, depth, and rhythm of respirations	Thorax and lungs	
	Palpation of posterior chest: evaluate muscles and bone structure, palpate excursion of chest expansion; palpate down vertebral column; note straightness	Musculoskeletal Thorax and lungs	
	Palpation of posterior chest for fremitus		Palpate with base of fingers while client says "how now brown cow" or "ninety-nine"
	Percussion of posterior chest for resonance, respiratory excursion	Thorax and lungs	During excursion evaluation, demonstrate to client how to take deep breath and hold it Measure amount of excursion with ruler
	Percussion with fist along costovertebral angle for kidney tenderness	Genitourinary	
	Inspection, bilateral palpation, and percussion along lateral axillary chest walls	Thorax and lungs	
	Auscultation of posterior and axillary chest walls for breath sounds; note quality of sounds heard	Thorax and lungs	Instruct client to breathe deeply by mouth

Procedure or format	Assessment to include	Body part or system involved	Clinical strategies for adults and geriatric clients
	and presence of adventitious sounds		
6. Assess anterior chest: move around to the front of the client; the client should lower the gown to the waist	Inspection of: skin color, intactness, presence of lesions, muscular symmetry, bilaterally similar bone structure	Integumentary Musculoskeletal	
	Observation of chest wall for pulsations or heaving	Cardiovascular	
	Observation of movement during respirations	Thorax and lungs	
	Observation of client's ease with respirations, posture, pursing lips		
	Female breasts: note size, symmetry, contour, moles or nevi, breast or nipple deviation, dimpling, or lesions; evaluate range of motion of shoulders and regularity of breast tissue during various movements: 1. Client's arms extended over head 2. Client's arm behind head 3. Client's hands behind small of back 4. Client's hands pushed tightly against each other at shoulder level 5. Client leans over slightly so that the breasts hang away from chest wall; note symmetry and pull on suspensory ligaments	Musculoskeletal Breast	It would be helpful to explain to client basically what she will be expected to do and why, prior to actual examination; may help to alleviate client anxiety as well as facilitate active participation During examination, may be helpful to provide discussion as to what is being observed; breast self-examination instruction should follow at some point to reiterate these and other aspects of breast examination
	Male breasts: note size, symmetry, breast enlargement, nipple discharge, or lesions		
	All clients: Palpation of anterior chest wall for stability, crepitations, muscular or skeletal tenderness	Musculoskeletal	
	Palpation of precordium for thrills, heaves, pulsations	Cardiovascular	Be sure to evaluate chest while client is sitting upright and then leaning forward
	Palpation of left chest wall to locate point of maximum impulse (PMI)		
	Palpation of chest wall for fremitus, as with posterior chest	Thorax and lungs	

Continued.

Clinical guidelines for physical examination integration–cont'd

Procedure or format	Assessment to include	Body part or system involved	Clinical strategies for adults and geriatric clients
	Percussion of anterior chest for resonance	Thorax and lungs	If examiner has difficulty percussing woman's anterior chest because of large breasts, percuss downward until breast tissue reached; then postpone continued percussion until client lies down
	For female clients: Palpation of breasts, including all four quadrants, tail of breast, and areolar area; note firmness, tissue qualities, lumps, areas of thickness, or tenderness Palpation of nipples; note elasticity, tissue characteristics, discharge	Breast	Client should be comfortably seated with arms resting comfortably at side As before, discuss what is being done so that client can incorporate similar techniques into breast self-examination
	All clients: Palpation of lymph nodes associated with lymphatic drainage of breast, including supra-clavicular and infraclavicular, central, lateral, axillary, pectoral, subscapular, scapular, brachial, intermediate, and internal mammary areas **For male clients:** Palpation of breast; note swelling or presence of excessive tissue or lumps, nipple discharge, or lesions	Lymphatic	
	All clients: Auscultation of breath sounds of anterior chest from apex to base; note quality, rate, type, presence of adventitious sounds	Thorax and lungs	Instruct client to breathe deeply through mouth
	Auscultation of the heart: aortic area, pulmonary area, Erb's point, tricuspid area, apical area; note rate, rhythm, location, intensity, frequency, timing, and splitting of S_1, S_2, S_3, S_4 murmurs	Cardiovascular	Examiner must decide whether to start at apical area and work upward or start at aortic area and work downward. Examiner should develop routine method of procedure If examining large-breasted woman, part of auscultatory evaluation may be deferred until client lying down
The client is assisted to lying or low Fowler's position 7. Assess anterior chest in recumbent position	Inspection of jugular venous pressure for height seen above sternal angle	Cardiovascular	Be sure to extend footrest for client's legs See clinical strategies for cardiovascular examination techniques to measure jugular venous pressure
	Female breast inspection: symmetry, contour, venous pattern, skin color, areolar area (note size, shape, surface characteristics), nipples (note direction, size, shape,	Breasts	Provide drape for legs and abdomen Place towel under back of side to be evaluated Instruct client to abduct arm overhead Explain procedures to client as performed Following breast palpation, may take time to teach client to palpate her own breasts

Procedure or format	Assessment to include	Body part or system involved	Clinical strategies for adults and geriatric clients
	color, surface characteristics, possible crusting) **Female breast palpation:** note firmness, tissue qualities, lumps, areas of thickness, or tenderness; areolar and nipple area (note elasticity, tissue characteristics, discharge)		
	All clients: Palpation of anterior chest wall for cardiac movement or thrills, heaves, pulsations	Cardiovascular	
	Auscultation of heart: aortic area, pulmonary area, Erb's point, tricuspid area, apical area; note S_1, S_2, S_3, S_4 murmurs (location, rate, rhythm, intensity, frequency, timing, splitting); turn client slightly to left side; repeat assessment of these areas	Cardiovascular	May not need to be done for all clients
8. Assess abdomen: provide chest drape for females; expose abdomen from pubis to epigastric region	Observation of skin characteristics from pubis to midchest region; note scars, lesions, vascularity, bulges, navel	Integumentary	Client should be comfortably positioned with pillow under head and knees slightly flexed to relax abdominal muscles
	Observation of abdominal contour	Abdominal	
	Observation of movement of abdomen, peristalsis, pulsations	Gastrointestinal Cardiovascular	
	Auscultation of abdomen (all quadrants); note bowel sounds, bruits, venous hums	Gastrointestinal Cardiovascular	
	Percussion of abdomen (all quadrants) and epigastric region for tone	Gastrointestinal	
	Percussion of upper and lower liver borders and estimation of liver span		Liver percussion should occur at midclavicular line
	Percussion of left midaxillary line for splenic dullness		
	Light palpation of all four quadrants; note tenderness, guarding, masses		Allow client to become accustomed to examiner's hands
	Deep palpation of all four quadrants; note tenderness, guarding, masses		Gently but firmly move palpation deeper and deeper until examiner convinced that abdomen sufficiently assessed
	Deep palpation of right costal margin for liver border		Examiner must decide whether to use one-hand or two-hand approach
	Deep palpation of left costal margin for splenic border		

Continued.

Clinical guidelines for physical examination integration–cont'd

Procedure or format	Assessment to include	Body part or system involved	Clinical strategies for adults and geriatric clients
	Deep palpation of abdomen for right and left kidneys		
	Deep palpation of midline epigastric area for aortic pulsation	Cardiovascular	Tenderness in epigastric area normal
	Testing abdominal reflexes with pointed instrument	Neurological	
	Client raises head for evaluation of flexion and strength of abdominal muscles	Musculoskeletal	Note use of arms or hands to assist; older client may have difficulty with this technique
	Light palpation of inguinal region for lymph nodes, femoral pulses, and bulges that may be associated with hernia	Lymphatic Cardiovascular Abdominal	
9. Assess lower limbs and hips: client is lying; abdomen and chest should be draped	Inspection of client's feet and legs for skin characteristics, vascular sufficiency, pulses; note deformities of toes, feet, nails, ankles, legs	Integumentary Cardiovascular, peripheral vascular Musculoskeletal	
	Palpation of feet and lower legs; note temperature, pulses, tenderness, deformities	Cardiovascular Musculoskeletal	
	Range of motion and motor strength of toes, feet, ankles, and knees	Musculoskeletal Neurological	Motor strength testing may be postponed until patient seated
	Range of motion and motor strength of hips		
	Palpation of hips for stability		
10. Assess genitalia, pelvic region, and rectum: client is lying and adequately draped	**For males:** inspection and palpation of external genitalia, including pubic hair, penis and scrotum, testes, epididymides, and vas deferens; inspect sacrococcygeal and perianal areas and anus for surface characteristics (with client lying on left side with right hip and knee flexed)	Genitourinary	If mass in scrotal sac suspected, transilluminate
	Palpation of anus, rectum, and prostate gland with gloved finger		Lubricate finger and slowly insert; wait for sphincter to relax before advancing finger
	Note characteristics of stool when gloved finger removed	Gastrointestinal	
	For females (client should be lying in lithotomy position): inspection and palpation of external genitalia, including pubic hair, labia, clitoris, urethral and vaginal orifices, perineal and peri-	Genitourinary	

Procedure or format	Assessment to include	Body part or system involved	Clinical strategies for adults and geriatric clients
	anal area and anus for surface characteristics		
	Insertion of vaginal speculum and inspection of surface characteristics of vagina and cervix		
	Collection of Pap smear and culture specimen		
	Bimanual palpation to assess form, size, and characteristics of vagina, cervix, uterus, adnexa		Lubricate first two fingers of gloved hand to be inserted internally; other hand should be positioned on abdomen directly above internal hand
	Vaginal-rectal examination to assess rectovaginal septum and pouch, surface characteristics, broad ligament tenderness		When examination completed, client should be offered tissue for drying of genital area
	Rectal examination to assess anal sphincter tone, surface characteristics (anal culture may be obtained)		
	Note characteristics of stool when gloved finger removed	Gastrointestinal	
The client is seated			
11. Assess neurological system: assist client to sitting position; should have gown on and be draped across lap	Observation of client moving from lying to sitting position; note use of muscles, ease of movement, and coordination	Neurological Musculoskeletal	
	Testing sensory function of neurological system by using light and deep (dull and sharp) sensation of forehead, paranasal sinus area, hands, lower arms, feet, lower legs	Neurological (sensory function): CN V (trigeminal nerve)	Client's eyes should be closed; instruct client to either point to or verbally report area that has been touched
	Bilateral testing and comparison of vibratory sensations of ankle, wrist, sternum		Alternate light, dull, and pinprick sensations Test bilaterally
	Testing two-point discrimination of palms, thigh, back	Cortical, discriminatory sensory of neurological system	
	Testing stereognosis or graphesthesia		
	Testing fine motor functioning and coordination of upper extremities by instructing client to perform at least two of following: 1. Alternating pronation and supination of forearm	Proprioception and cerebellar function of neurological system	Perform technique bilaterally and compare responses

Continued.

Clinical guidelines for physical examination integration–cont'd

Procedure or format	Assessment to include	Body part or system involved	Clinical strategies for adults and geriatric clients
	2. Touching nose with alternating index fingers 3. Rapidly alternating finger movements to thumb 4. Rapid movement of index finger between nose and examiner's finger Testing and bilaterally comparing fine motor functioning and coordination of lower extremities by instructing client to run heel down tibia of opposite leg Alternately crossing legs over knee	Musculoskeletal	
	Testing and bilaterally comparing deep tendon reflexes, including: 1. Biceps tendon 2. Triceps tendon 3. Brachioradialis tendon 4. Patellar tendon 5. Achilles tendon	Reflex status of neurological system	If client shows any neurological problems, evaluate by Babinski and ankle clonus tests
The client is standing **12.** Palpate scrotum and inguinal region (male)	Palpation of scrotum and inguinal regions for characteristics and hernias	Genitourinary	Instruct client to bear down or cough during hernia evaluation
13. Assess neurological and musculoskeletal system	Assessment of client's gait: observe and palpate straightness of client's spine as client stands and bends forward to touch toes	Musculoskeletal Neurological	Elderly clients may not be able to do this
	With client's waist stabilized, evaluation of hyperextension, lateral bending, rotation of upper trunk		
	Assessment of proprioception and cerebellar and motor function by using at least two of following: 1. Romberg test (eyes closed) 2. Walking straight heel to toe formation 3. Standing on one foot and then other (eyes closed) 4. Hopping in place on one foot and then other 5. Knee bends		Client's age and general ability may help define which technique to use Protect client from falling by remaining close and ready to catch him if necessary Elderly clients may not be able to do this

Integration of the pediatric examination

The procedure for integrating the pediatric examination will depend entirely on the age and cooperation of the child. By the time the child reaches school age, he should be able to participate fully in a cooperative manner. It is the younger child who will present the challenge. The following format changes should facilitate a thorough assessment.

Age and preparation	Procedures	Systems involved
1. Newborn to 6 months: undressed, lying on examination table	1. Obtain history, highlighting developmental or problem areas	
	2. Check vital signs: temperature, pulse, respiration	
	3. Record weight, length, chest and head circumference	
	4. Observe child lying on examination table; note color, general health, body symmetry, gross motor movement, alertness, gross and fine motor development, language development, social adaptive development, skin characteristics, and response to sound and vision stimulation	Cardiovascular, neurological, musculoskeletal, integumentary, visual, auditory
	5. Examine and manipulate hands, arms, shoulders, feet, legs; note range of motion and tone	Musculoskeletal, neurological
	6. Examine skin over extremities, chest, abdomen, and back	Integumentary, cardiovascular
	7. Auscultate thorax, lungs, heart, abdomen	Thorax, lungs, cardiovascular, gastrointestinal
	8. Palpate and examine external characteristics of head, neck, face, axillary region	Lymphatic, head, neck, visual, auditory, oral, nasal
	9. Palpate thorax, abdomen, and umbilical area	Thorax, abdomen
	10. Observe and palpate external genitalia, inguinal area, and hip stability	Genital, musculoskeletal
	11. Examine eyes with ophthalmoscope	Visual
	12. Examine mouth, teeth development, tongue, posterior pharynx, nose	Oral, nasal
	13. Examine ears with otoscope	Auditory
2. Six months to 2 years: child in diaper, sitting on parent's lap; examiner's chair should be in front of parent's chair and examiner's knees should touch parent's; during supine examination, child may lie on parent's and examiner's lap	1. Obtain history highlighting developmental or problem areas	
	2. Perform developmental, social, vision, speech, hearing, and fine and gross motor assessment during play and initial "get acquainted" period	Neurological, visual, speech, auditory, musculoskeletal
	3. Record weight, length, and chest and head circumference (until 18 months)	
	4. Check vital signs, including blood pressure in children over 18 months of age; may be postponed until later if child becomes agitated	
	5. Auscultate lungs and heart	Thorax, cardiovascular
	6. Examine skin over extremities, chest, abdomen, and back	Integumentary, cardiovascular
	7. Examine and manipulate hands, arms, shoulders, feet, legs; note range of motion and tone	Neurological, musculoskeletal
	8. Palpate and examine external characteristics of head, neck, face, axillary region	Lymphatic, head, neck, visual, auditory, oral, nasal
	9. Auscultate abdomen with child in supine position on parent's and examiner's lap	Gastrointestinal
	10. Palpate thorax, abdomen, and umbilical area	Thorax and abdomen
	11. Observe and palpate external genitalia, inguinal area, and hip stability	Genital, musculoskeletal

Continued.

Integration of the pediatric examination–cont'd

Age and preparation	Procedures	Systems involved
	12. Examine eyes with ophthalmoscope	Visual
	13. Examine mouth, teeth development, tongue, posterior pharynx, nose	Oral, nasal
	14. Examine ears with otoscope	Auditory
3. Two to 4 years: undressed to underpants; may be examined either on parent's lap or examination table; much of assessment may be informal as examiner observes and plays with child	Same as for child from 6 months to 2 years; refer to individual chapter details for discussion of strategies	
4. Four to 6 years: undressed to underpants, sitting on examination table; assessment should move toward adult format; the child's developmental immaturity may necessitate that the examiner alter various examination techniques to facilitate the child's participation and a correct response	Same as for child from 6 months to 2 years	
5. Over 6 years old: in gown on examination table	Same as for adult client	

Physical examination write-up

The data base and the information collected during the physical assessment must be organized and documented. The components of the documentation are (1) subjective data base, (2) physical assessment, (3) risk profile, and (4) problem list. Prior to the actual documentation, the examiner must decide whether to record the data on plain paper or on a predesigned form. Each has advantages and disadvantages. We prefer plain paper.

Pro	Con
Plain paper	
Documentation space is not a problem.	The examiner must be organized; if not, rambling and insignificant data may be a problem.
Specific data for individual client may be emphasized as necessary.	All examiners in the agency might not use the same format.
Predeveloped form	
Departmental continuity is maintained.	Individual situations might be difficult to emphasize.
Data will be easy to locate by other examiners.	Examiner may not have adequate space for documentation.
It is a reminder for completeness.	If form was developed prior to examiner's input, it may not include all data the examiner wants to collect.
	Separate forms necessary for pediatric and geriatric clients.

Once the style of documentation is determined, the examiner must synthesize the client's historical and physical data and record information in the following areas. The examiner is urged to record *what* is observed, heard, percussed, or palpated and to avoid vague and nondescriptive terms such as "normal," "negative," "good," or "poor."

Documentation format

1. Subjective data base
   a. Biographical data
   b. Reason for visit
   c. Present health state
   d. Current health statistics: immunizations, allergies, last examination
   e. Past health status: childhood illnesses, serious or chronic illnesses, serious accidents or injuries, hospitalizations, operations, emotional health, obstetrical health
   f. Family history
   g. Review of physiological systems: general, nutritional, integumentary, head, eyes, ears, nose, mouth, neck, breast, cardiovascular, respiratory, hematolymphatic, gastrointestinal, urinary, genital, musculoskeletal, central nervous system, endocrine, and allergic and immunological
   h. Psychological history: general status, response to illness

i. Social history: significant others, occupational history, educational level, activities of daily living, habits, financial status

j. Health maintenance efforts: maintenance of self health, health care patterns

k. Environmental health: general assessment, employment, home, neighborhood, community

2. Physical assessment

a. Vital statistics: height, weight, temperature, pulse, blood pressure (both arms, lying, sitting, standing)

b. General statement of appearance

c. Mental health

d. Integumentary: skin, nails, body hair

e. Head and neck: scalp, hair, face, neck, lymph nodes, thyroid, trachea, sinuses

f. Nose: patency, surface characteristics

g. Mouth, pharynx: oral cavity characteristics, teeth, tongue, voice, tonsillar area and posterior pharynx

h. Ear and auditory: External ear, canal, TM characteristics, hearing, Rinne and Weber tests

i. Eye and visual: external eye characteristics, vision, eye movement, funduscopy

j. Thorax and lungs: thorax characteristics, breathing pattern and rate, percussion tone, auscultatory characteristics

k. Cardiovascular: all pulses, blood pressure, extremity circulation, precordium characteristics, heart sounds

l. Breast: surface characteristics, areolae and nipples, palpation characteristics, lymphatic assessment, breast self-examination assessment

m. Abdominal, rectal: contour, surface characteristics, bowel sounds, percussion tones, palpation characteristics, liver and spleen, bladder, kidney characteristics, CVA tenderness, hernias, rectal examination findings

n. Genital

  (1) Female: external genitalia characteristics, internal-cervical, vagina, uterus, adnexa characteristics

  (2) Male: external genitalia characteristics, palpation characteristics of penis and scrotum, inguinal hernia evaluation

o. Musculoskeletal: muscular development and strength, skeletal and joint characteristics and symmetry, range of motion

p. Neurological: orientation, intactness of CN I to XII, coordination of fine and gross motor movements and gait, sensory evaluation, reflexes

3. Risk profile: those items from the client's history and physical assessment which might indicate risk to the overall health state. These are potential problems. *Examples* that may be considered risk for some clients are detailed in the data base in Chapter 1.

4. Problem list. The problem list should be a synthesis of those items which are currently identified as stresses for the client. The stresses may be physiological, sociological, psychological, or a combination of these. The problems are those items which reduce the client's overall level of health. Once the problems are listed and assigned a priority, it can then be decided which are within the examiner's scope of practice to handle and which must be referred.

It is important for the examiner to cluster subjective and objective data to describe problems. The following unrelated examples demonstrate a holistic approach to problem identification.

a. Weight gain: 18 pounds in past year; exercise limited to game of tennis twice a month; expresses desire to diet but needs direction

b. Short of breath when walking up more than one flight of stairs; moderate edema below midcalf bilaterally; fine rales in lower bases bilaterally

c. Limited range of motion in right shoulder interferes with activities of daily living: dressing, preparing meals

d. Cataracts bilaterally; interfere with reading and driving at night

e. BP 180/120 (right arm) lying, 172/112 (right arm) sitting; retinal A-V ratio appears to be 2/4; arteriolar narrowing

f. Periodic slight urinary incontinence since birth of child 3 years ago; cystocele noted on vaginal examination

g. Complaints of LLQ discomfort for 6 months; cyclic with menses; ↑ discomfort at ovulation time and just prior to menses; thickening in left adnexa area; ↑ tenderness with palpation of left adnexa area; menses regular; pinpoint tenderness on deep palpation in LLQ

h. Smokes one pack of cigarettes a day for past 15 years; deep nonproductive cough for past 5 years, becoming worse; ↑ breathing difficulty when climbing more than one flight of stairs; ↓ breath sounds on right; bilateral rales or rhonchi in base of lungs; slight clearing with cough

i. Death of spouse 2 months ago; since then ↑ periods of depression, 10-pound weight loss, ↓ desire to maintain own health state

Answers

Chapter 2

1. i
2. Any of the following are correct:
   a. Client's initial response to examiner
   b. Body appearance
   c. Body movements
   d. Gait
   e. Facial expression
   f. Vocal tones
   g. Speech
   h. Apparel
   i. Grooming
   j. Odors
   k. General mannerisms

3. c	7. b
4. d	8. f
5. e	9. h
6 b	

Chapter 3

1. T	14. c	27. d
2. T	15. d	28. k
3. T	16. a	29. b
4. F	17. d	30. h
5. T	18. g	31. e
6. T	19. h	32. d
7. T	20. c	33. i
8. T	21. f	34. T
9. T	22. g	35. F
10. T	23. j	36. F
11. e	24. a	37. d
12. b	25. i	38. c
13. a	26. l	39. e

Chapter 4

1. d	8. e	15. b
2. c	9. j	16. i
3. a	10. c	17. f
4. e	11. d	18. i
5. c	12. h	19. d
6. b	13. a	20. g
7. b	14. g	21. e

Chapter 5

1. i	10. b	18. c
2. h	11. f	19. c
3. b	12. i	20. i
4. b	13. f	21. c
5. a	14. h	22. d
6. i	15. i	23. f
7. d	16. h	24. c
8. b	17. b	25. f
9. c		

Chapter 6

1. c	9. j	16. f
2. a	10. h	17. b
3. c	11. h	18. d
4. c	12. f	19. t
5. i	13. t	20. f
6. c	14. f	21. t
7. i	15. t	22. f
8. j		

Chapter 7

1. h	12. b	22. e
2. b	13. j	23. e
3. h	14. i	24. d
4. g	15. e	25. i
5. j	16. h	26. c
6. c	17. i	27. i
7. b	18. b	28. e
8. g	19. a	29. c
9. f	20. j	30. b
10. f	21. a	31. a
11. g		

Chapter 8

1. F	7. >, peripheral lung
2. T	=, first and
3. T	second
4. F	intercostals
5. F	at sternal
6. F	border
	<, over trachea

8. d	13. c	18. a
9. j	14. a	19. e
10. e	15. d	20. i
11. b	16. g	21. f
12. b	17. d	22. c

Chapter 9

1. h	25. aortic; pulmonary;
2. i	diastole
3. g	26. CAI
4. e	27. CAI
5. f	28. CVI
6. i	29. CAI
7. g	30. CVI
8. f	31. CAI
9. f	32. CAI
10. i	33. a
11. g	34. b
12. j	35. b
13. d	36. a
14. f	37. a
15. h	38. a
16. g	39. b
17. b	40. a
18. a	41. b
19. Amplitude	42. b
20. Contour	43. a
21. Amplitude pattern	44. a
22. Symmetry	45. a
23. a. Superior vena cava	46. d
b. Inferior vena cava	47. c
c. Right atrium	48. b
d. Tricuspid valve	49. e
e. Right ventricle	50. a
f. Pulmonary valve	51. e
g. Pulmonary artery	52. d
h. Pulmonary vein	53. a
i. Aorta	54. e
j. Left atrium	55. h
k. Aortic valve	56. a
l. Mitral valve	57. b
m. Left ventricle	
24. mitral; tricuspid;	
systole	

Chapter 10

1. f	7. T	13. T
2. b	8. F	14. T
3. c	9. F	15. T
4. j	10. F	16. F
5. j	11. F	17. c
6. F	12. F	18. j

Chapter 11

1. Student can compare own drawing of major abdominal organs with textbook illustration.
2. Any five of the following are correct:
   a. Client supine with arms on chest or at sides
   b. Small pillow under head
   c. Knees slightly flexed
   d. Warm room
   e. Client draped over breasts and pubis
   f. Examiner's hands warm
   g. Short fingernails
   h. Warm stethoscope
   i. Client breathing slowly through mouth
   j. Examiner explaining procedure

3. c	11. g	19. f
4. b	12. g	20. i
5. b	13. c	21. f
6. d	14. i	22. d
7. c	15. h	23. e
8. a	16. h	24. f
9. a	17. f	25. g
10. d	18. h	26. e

Chapter 12

1. N	14. A	27. d
2. G	15. a	28. f
3. O	16. b	29. e
4. B	17. b	30. a
5. H	18. a	31. c
6. F	19. a	32. b
7. C	20. c	33. d
8. L	21. a	34. c
9. K	22. f	35. i
10. D	23. b	36. c
11. J	24. i	37. a
12. I	25. b	38. i
13. M	26. g	

Chapter 13

1. L	16. D	31. f
2. F	17. G	32. b
3. C	18. B	33. g
4. K	19. H	34. a
5. H	20. K	35. i
6. A	21. C	36. h
7. E	22. M	37. g
8. I	23. F	38. T
9. B	24. A	39. F
10. G	25. L	40. F
11. D	26. I	41. F
12. J	27. E	42. T
13. h	28. J	43. T
14. g	29. j	44. T
15. h	30. f	45. F

Chapter 13—cont'd

46. T	49. F	51. c
47. T	50. g	52. h
48. T		

Chapter 14

1. T	15. j	29. a
2. T	16. b	30. j
3. T	17. c	31. a
4. F	18. a	32. e
5. T	19. g	33. c
6. T	20. h	34. b
7. F	21. d	35. h
8. F	22. h	36. i
9. T	23. g	37. d
10. T	24. c	38. h
11. d	25. b	39. c
12. i	26. d	40. f
13. f	27. k	41. e
14. e	28. a	

Chapter 15

1. b	13. T	25. a
2. h	14. T	26. c
3. c	15. d	27. e
4. a	16. e	28. b
5. a	17. a	29. a
6. a	18. c	30. d
7. g	19. b	31. b
8. i	20. c	32. c
9. i	21. e	33. d
10. j	22. d	34. a
11. g	23. b	35. d
12. T	24. d	36. b